☀HARRISON'S
Manual *of* Oncology

Bruce A. Chabner, M.D.
Thomas J. Lynch, Jr., M.D.
Dan L. Longo, A.B., M.D., F.A.C.P.

FOLLOW THESE INSTRUCTIONS TO DOWNLOAD YOUR FREE PDA SOFTWARE

1) Use your Web browser to go to:
http://www.mhprofessional.com/hmoPDA/

2) Register now

3) Fill in the required fields

4) Enter your unique registration code below

5) Download the free software and sync into your handheld device

Code Listed Here

0945021

Use this code to register and receive your free PDA software.
See above for complete directions.

If you have any problems accessing your download,
please visit: www.books.mcgraw-hill.com/techsupport

For Internal use only:

Card P/N:
ISBN 978-0-07-150812-4
MHID 0-07-150812-0
part of Set
ISBN 978-0-07-141189-9
MHID 0-07-141189-5

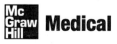

Mc Graw Hill **Medical**

mcgraw-hillmedical.com

HARRISON'S
Manual of
Oncology

NOTICE

Medicine is an ever-changing science. As new research and clinical experience broaden our knowledge, changes in treatment and drug therapy are required. The editors and the publisher of this work have checked with sources believed to be reliable in their efforts to provide information that is complete and generally in accord with the standards accepted at the time of publication. However, in view of the possibility of human error or changes in medical sciences, neither the editors nor the publisher nor any other party who has been involved in the preparation or publication of this work warrants that the information contained herein is in every respect accurate or complete, and they disclaim all responsibility for any errors or omissions or for the results obtained from use of the information contained in this work. Readers are encouraged to confirm the information contained herein with other sources. For example and in particular, readers are advised to check the product information sheet included in the package of each drug they plan to administer to be certain that the information contained in this work is accurate and that changes have not been made in the recommended dose or in the contraindications for administration. This recommendation is of particular importance in connection with new or infrequently used drugs.

HARRISON'S
Manual of
Oncology

Bruce A. Chabner, M.D.

Clinical Director
Massachusetts General Hospital Cancer Center
Associate Director of Clinical Sciences
Dana-Farber/Harvard Cancer Center
Professor of Medicine
Harvard Medical School
Boston, Massachusetts

Thomas J. Lynch, Jr., M.D.

Chief, Hematology-Oncology
Massachusetts General Hospital Cancer Center
Associate Professor of Medicine
Harvard Medical School
Boston, Massachusetts

Dan L. Longo, A.B., M.D., F.A.C.P.

Scientific Director
National Institute on Aging
National Institutes of Health
Bethesda and Baltimore, Maryland

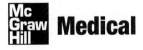

New York   Chicago   San Francisco   Lisbon   London
Madrid   Mexico City   Milan   New Delhi   San Juan
Seoul   Singapore   Sydney   Toronto

Note: Dr. Longo's work as an editor and author was performed outside the scope of his employment as a U.S. Government employee. His work represents his personal and professional views and not necessarily those of the U.S. Government.

Harrison's
Manual of Oncology

1 2 4 3 5 6 7 8 9 0   DOC/DOC   0 9 8 7

Set ISBN 978-0-07-141189-9, Set MHID 0-07-141189-5
Book ISBN 978-0-07-150811-7, Book MHID 0-07-150811-2
PDA Card ISBN 978-0-07-150812-4, PDA Card MHID 0-07-150812-0

This book was set in Times Roman by Aptara.
The editors were James Shanahan and Kim J. Davis.
Project management was provided by Aptara.
The production supervisor was Catherine Saggese.
The cover designer was Janice Bielawa.
The index was prepared by Aptara.
RR Donnelley was printer and binder.

This book is printed on acid-free paper.

Library of Congress Cataloging-in-Publication Data
Harrison's manual of oncology / [edited by] Bruce A. Chabner, Thomas J. Lynch, Dan L. Longo.
    p. ; cm.
Derived from Harrison's principles of internal medicine, 16th ed.
Includes bibliographical references and index.
ISBN-13: 978-0-07-141189-9 (pbk. : alk. paper)
ISBN-10: 0-07-141189-5 (pbk. : alk. paper)
    1. Cancer—Chemotherapy. 2. Antineoplastic agents. I. Chabner, Bruce. II. Lynch, Thomas J. (Thomas James), 1960- III. Longo, Dan L. (Dan Louis), 1949- IV. Harrison's principles of internal medicine. V. Title: Manual of oncology.
    [DNLM: 1. Neoplasms—drug therapy. 2. Antineoplastic Agents—therapeutic use. QZ 267 H322 2008]
RC271.C5H38 2008
616.99'4061—dc22

2007020687

CONTENTS

SECTION 1
CLASSES OF DRUGS

SECTION 2
HORMONAL AGENTS

SECTION 3
BIOLOGIC RESPONSE MODIFIERS

CONTRIBUTORS

Brian M. Alexander, MD
Resident, Harvard Radiation Oncology Program,
Harvard Medical School;
Department of Radiation Oncology,
Massachusetts General Hospital,
Boston, Massachusetts

Philip C. Amrein, MD
Assistant Professor of Medicine,
Harvard Medical School;
Physician,
Massachusetts General Hospital,
Boston, Massachusetts

Eyal C. Attar, MD
Instructor in Medicine,
Harvard Medical School;
Assistant Physician, Center for Leukemia,
Massachusetts General Hospital,
Boston, Massachusetts

Karen Ballen, MD
Associate Professor,
Harvard Medical School;
Director, Center for Leukemia,
Massachusetts General Hospital,
Boston, Massachusetts

Tracy T. Batchelor, MD
Associate Professor of Neurology,
Harvard Medical School;
Executive Director,
Pappas Center for Neuro-Oncology,
Massachusetts General Hospital,
Boston, Massachusetts

Johanna Bendell, MD
Assistant Professor,
Division of Oncology and Transplantation,
Department of Medicine,
Duke University Medical Center,
Durham, North Carolina

Lawrence S. Blaszkowsky, MD
Instructor in Medicine,
Harvard Medical School;
Assistant Physician,
Massachusetts General Hospital,
Boston, Massachusetts

James E. Bradner, MD
Instructor in Medicine,
Harvard Medical School;
Division of Hematologic Neoplasia,
Dana-Farber Cancer Institute,
Boston, Massachusetts

Paul M. Busse, MD, PhD
Associate Professor of Radiation Oncology,
Harvard Medical School;
Clinical Director,
Chief, Center for Head & Neck Cancers,
Department of Radiation Oncology,
Massachusetts General Hospital,
Boston, Massachusetts

Bruce A. Chabner, MD
Professor of Medicine,
Harvard Medical School;
Clinical Director,
Massachusetts General Hospital Cancer Center,
Boston, Massachusetts

Yi-Bin Chen, MD
Clinical Fellow in Medicine,
Harvard Medical School;
Fellow in Hematology/Oncology,
Dana-Farber/Partners CancerCare,
Boston, Massachusetts

Andrew S. Chi, MD, PhD
Fellow in Neuro-Oncology,
Department of Neurology,
Harvard Medical School;
Dana-Farber/Partners CancerCare,
Boston, Massachusetts

Tessa Cigler
Assistant Professor of Medicine,
Weill Cornell Medical College;
Assistant Attending Physician,
New York-Presbyterian Hospital,
New York

Jeffrey W. Clark, MD
Associate Professor of Medicine,
Harvard Medical School;
Associate Physician,
Division of Hematology/Oncology,
Massachusetts General Hospital Cancer Center,
Boston, Massachusetts

John R. Clark, MD
Instructor in Medicine,
Harvard Medical School;
Physician,
Division of Hematology/Oncology,
Massachusetts General Hospital,
Boston, Massachusetts

John J. Coen, MD
Assistant Professor of Radiation Oncology,
Harvard Medical School;
Massachusetts General Hospital,
Boston, Massachusetts

Douglas M. Dahl, MD
Assistant Professor of Surgery,
Harvard Medical School;
Assistant in Urology,
Massachusetts General Hospital,
Boston, Massachusetts

Thomas F. DeLaney, MD
Associate Professor of Radiation Oncology,
Department of Radiation Oncology,
Harvard Medical School;
Medical Director, Francis H. Burr Proton Therapy Center,
Department of Radiation Oncology,
Massachusetts General Hospital,
Boston, Massachusetts

Marcela G. del Carmen, MD
Assistant Professor,
Department of Gynecology/Obstetrics,
Harvard Medical School;
Clinical Director,
Gillette Center for Gynecologic Oncology,
Massachusetts General Hospital,
Boston, Massachusetts

Daniel Deschler, MD
Director,
Division of Head and Neck Surgery,
Massachusetts Eye and Ear Infirmary,
Boston, Massachusetts

April F. Eichler, MD
Instructor in Neurology,
Harvard Medical School;
Assistant Neurologist,
Massachusetts General Hospital,
Boston, Massachusetts

Tracey Evans, MD
Assistant Professor of Medicine,
Abramson Cancer Center;
University of Pennsylvania,
Philadelphia, Pennsylvania

Panos Fidias, MD
Assistant Professor,
Harvard Medical School;
Clinical Director, Center for Thoracic Cancers,
Massachusetts General Hospital,
Boston, Massachusetts

Timothy Gilligan, MD
Cleveland Clinic Lerner College of Medicine,
Case Western Reserve University;
Director, Late Effects Clinic,
Co-Director, Hematology-Oncology Fellowship Program,
Taussig Cancer Center,
Cleveland Clinic,
Cleveland, Ohio

Paul E. Goss, MD, PhD FRCPC, FRCP(UK)
Professor of Medicine,
Harvard Medical School;
Director of Breast Cancer Research,
Massachusetts General Hospital,
Co-Director of the Breast Cancer Disease Program,
Dana Farber/Harvard Cancer Center,
Boston, Massachusetts

David C. Harmon, MD
Assistant Professor,
Harvard Medical School;
Physician, Department of Medicine,
Massachusetts General Hospital,
Boston, Massachusetts

Rebecca Suk Heist, MD, MPH
Instructor in Medicine,
Harvard Medical School;
Assistant Physician,
Division of Hematology/Oncology,
Massachusetts General Hospital,
Boston, Massachusetts

Ephraim Paul Hochberg, M.D.
Instructor in Medicine,
Department of Medicine,
Harvard Medical School;
Assistant Physician, Center for Lymphoma,
Massachusetts General Hospital,
Boston, Massachusetts

Fred H. Hochberg, MD
Associate Professor of Neurology,
Harvard Medical School;
Physician,
Department of Neurology,
Massachusetts General Hospital,
Boston, Massachusetts

Theodore S. Hong, MD
Instructor in Radiation Oncology,
Harvard Medical School;
Assistant in Radiation Oncology,
Director, Gastrointestinal Radiation Oncology,
Massachusetts General Hospital,
Boston, Massachusetts

Francis J. Hornicek, MD, PhD
Associate Professor,
Orthopaedic Surgery,
Harvard Medical School;
Chief, Orthopaedic Oncology Service,
Co-Director, Center for Sarcoma and Connective Tissue Oncology,
Massachusetts General Hospital,
Boston, Massachusetts

Steven J. Isakoff, MD, PhD
Instructor in Medicine,
Harvard Medical School;
Assistant in Medicine,
Gillette Center for Breast Cancer, MGH Cancer Center,
Massachusetts General Hospital Cancer Center,
Boston, Massachusetts

Vicki Jackson, MD, MPH
Instructor in Medicine,
Harvard Medical School;
Associate Director and Fellowship Director,
Palliative Care Service,
Massachusetts General Hospital,
Boston, Massachusetts

Juliet Jacobsen, MD, DPH
Instructor in Medicine,
Harvard Medical School;
Assistant in Medicine,
Massachusetts General Hospital,
Boston, Massachusetts

Pasi A. Jänne, MD, PhD
Assistant Professor of Medicine,
Harvard Medical School;
Lowe Center for Thoracic Oncology,
Dana-Farber Cancer Institute;

Department of Medicine,
Brigham and Women's Hospital,
Boston, Massachusetts

Donald S. Kaufman, MD
Clinical Professor of Medicine,
Harvard Medical School;
Director, The Claire and John Bertucci Center for Genitourinary Cancers,
Massachusetts General Hospital,
Boston, Massachusetts

Carolyn Krasner, MD
Instructor in Medicine,
Harvard Medical School;
Assistant in Medicine,
Division of Hematology/Oncology,
Massachusetts General Hospital,
Boston, Massachusetts

Donald P. Lawrence, MD
Assistant Professor,
Harvard Medical School;
Assistant in Medicine,
Division of Hematology/Oncology,
Massachusetts General Hospital,
Boston, Massachusetts

Geoffrey Liu, MD, FRCPC
Assistant Professor,
University of Toronto and Harvard Medical School;
Alan B. Brown Chair in Molecular Genomics,
Princess Margaret Hospital,
Toronto, Ontario, Canada

Dan L. Longo, MD
Scientific Director,
National Institute on Aging,
National Institutes of Health,
Bethesda and Baltimore,
Maryland

M. Dror Michaelson, MD, PhD
Assistant Professor,
Harvard Medical School;
Assistant in Medicine,
Massachusetts General Hospital,
Boston, Massachusetts

Beverly Moy, MD, MPH
Instructor in Medicine,
Assistant Physician,
Massachusetts General Hospital,
Boston, Massachusetts

Hamza Mujagic, MD, MSc, DRSC
Visiting Scholar and Professor,
Harvard Medical School;
Division of Hematology/Oncology,
Massachusetts General Hospital,
Boston, Massachusetts

Janet E. Murphy, MD
Resident,
Department of Medicine,
Massachusetts General Hospital,
Boston, Massachusetts

Richard T Penson MD MRCP,
Assistant Professor,
Harvard Medical School;
Clinical Director, Gillette Center for Gynecologic Oncology,
Massachusetts General Hospital,
Boston, Massachusetts

William F. Pirl, MD
Assistant professor in Psychiatry,
Harvard Medical School;
Attending Psychiatrist,
Department of Psychiatry,
Massachusetts General Hospital,
Boston, Massachusetts

Scott R. Plotkin, MD, PhD
Assistant Professor of Neurology,
Harvard Medical School;
Director, Neurofibromatosis Clinic,
Assistant Neurologist,
Department of Neurology,
Massachusetts General Hospital,
Boston, Massachusetts

Mark C. Poznansky, FRCP(E), PhD
Assistant Professor,
Department of Medicine,
Harvard Medical School;
Department of Medicine,
Massachusetts General Hospital,
Boston, Massachusetts

Noopur Raje, MD
Assistant Professor,
Department of Medicine,
Harvard Medical School;
Director, Center for Multiple Myeloma,
Division of Hematology/Oncology,
Massachusetts General Hospital Cancer Center,
Boston, Massachusetts

Rachel P.G. Rosovsky, MD, MPH
Instructor in Medicine,
Harvard Medical School;
Assistant in Medicine,
Massachusetts General Hospital,
Boston, Massachusetts

Krista M. Rubin, NP
Division of Hematology/Oncology,
Center for Melanoma,
Massachusetts General Hospital,
Boston, Massachusetts

Kathryn J. Ruddy, MD
Clinical Fellow in Medicine,
Harvard Medical School;
Fellow in Hematology/Oncology,
Dan-Farber/Partners CancerCare,
Boston, Massachusetts

David P. Ryan, MD
Assistant Professor of Medicine,
Harvard Medical School;
Clinical Director,
Tucker Gosnell Center for Gastrointestinal Cancers,
Massachusetts General Hospital,
Boston, Massachusetts

Paula D. Ryan, MD, PhD
Assistant Professor of Medicine,
Harvard Medical School;
Medical Director,
Breast and Ovarian Cancer Genetics and Risk Assessment Program,
Massachusetts General Hospital,
Boston, Massachusetts

Abraham B Schwarzberg
Clinical Fellow in Medicine,
Harvard Medical School;
Fellow in Hematology/Oncology,
Dan-Farber/Partners CancerCare,
Boston, Massachusetts

Lecia V. Sequist, MD, MPH
Instructor in Medicine,
Harvard Medical School;
Assistant Physician in Medicine,
Department of Hematology/Oncology,
Massachusetts General Hospital,
Boston, Massachusetts

Matthew R. Smith, M.D., PhD
Associate Professor of Medicine,
Harvard Medical School;

Director of Genitourinary Malignancies,
The Claire and John Bertucci Center for Genitourinary Cancers,
Massachusetts General Hospital,
Boston, Massachusetts

Thomas R. Spitzer, MD
Professor of Medicine,
Harvard Medical School;
Director, Bone Marrow Transplant Program,
Massachusetts General Hospital,
Boston, Massachusetts

Jerry L. Spivak, MD
Professor of Medicine and Oncology,
Department of Medicine,
Johns Hopkins University;
Attending Physician, Johns Hopkins Hospital,
Baltimore, Maryland

Kathrin Strasser-Weippl, MD
Center for Hematology and Medical Oncology,
Wilhelminen Hospital,
Vienna, Austria

Jennifer Temel, MD
Instructor in Medicine,
Harvard Medical School;
Assistant in Medicine,
Massachusetts General Hospital,
Boston, Massachusetts

Elizabeth Trice, MD, PhD
Clinical Fellow in Medicine,
Harvard Medical School;
Fellow in Hematology/Oncology,
Dana-Farber/Partners CancerCare,
Boston, Massachusetts

Fabrizio Vianello, MD
Attending Hematologist,
Padua University School of Medicine;
Second Chair of Medicine,
Padova, Italy

Sam S. Yoon, MD
Assistant Professor of Surgery,
Harvard Medical School;
Assistant Surgeon,
Division of Surgical Oncology,
Massachusetts General Hospital,
Boston, Massachusetts

Andrew X. Zhu, MD, PhD
Associate Professor,
Harvard Medical School;
Assistant Physician,
Division of Hematology/Oncology,
Massachusetts General Hospital,
Boston, Massachusetts

Dan Zuckerman, MD
Clinical Fellow in Medicine,
Harvard Medical School;
Fellow in Hematology/Oncology,
Dana-Farber/Partners CancerCare,
Boston, Massachusetts

PREFACE

Our intent in writing this book is to provide a concise, straightforward, and well-referenced manual about cancer chemotherapy and biotherapy and to place in context the role of such drugs in the treatment of specific malignant diseases. Further, we offer a condensed version in PDA form for rapid reference on the ward and in the clinic. As physicians actively involved in teaching and patient care, we appreciate the challenge of providing a readily digestible resource for young physicians confronted with a patient with a challenging disease and potentially fatal disease. We have conceived and written this text with the help of our colleagues at the Massachusetts General Hospital and elsewhere, and have intended that it should be particularly useful for a resident training in internal medicine, surgery, or radiation therapy, as well as for cancer subspecialty trainees and practicing clinicians. We have attempted to provide relatively complete information on both diseases and drugs, and on the important underlying rationale for the use of specific therapies in subsets of patients. As a companion to *Harrison's Textbook of Internal Medicine*, this manual is intended to provide expanded and more detailed coverage of the management of malignant tumors, with a particular emphasis on their treatment with chemotherapy, targeted drugs, and hormonal therapy.

Because of the rapid advance of research in cancer biology and treatment, it is impossible for a book to keep pace with all current developments; thus a text such as this must be complemented by the most recent literature and even meeting reports, which are usually available on the internet. We also intend to revise and update the book and its PDA instrument at regular intervals. Please let us know of your reaction to the book and its PDA, and offer any suggestions for their improvement by sending an e-mail to medicine@mcgraw-hill.com. Our hope is that the manual and PDA will expedite and improve our ability to care for patients with cancer.

Bruce A. Chabner, M.D.
Thomas J. Lynch, Jr., M.D.
Dan L. Longo, A.B., M.D., F.A.C.P.

ACKNOWLEDGMENTS

This project would have been impossible without the cooperation of multiple collaborators, who produced their chapters on time and on target, for which we owe our great appreciation. Once again, our families have given us a pass to spend evenings and weekends on yet another project, this one being close to our hearts. Our staff members, particularly Renee Johnson, did an outstanding job of compiling, editing, and tracking manuscripts, keeping us on course, and reassuring our publisher that we would make it to the finish line. In addition, we are grateful to Pat Duffey and Phil Carrieri for providing essential technical assistance. But most of all, we thank our students, residents and fellows, who constantly challenge us to teach what is important and true, and test our ability to teach it in an effective and exciting way. If there is joy in oncology, it comes from two sources; helping our patients, and passing the torch of new knowledge to the next generation.

INTRODUCTION TO CANCER PHARMACOLOGY
Bruce A. Chabner

The treatment of cancer is a complex undertaking that involves, in most patients, a co-ordination of efforts from multiple specialties. Virtually all patients require surgery to establish the diagnosis and to remove the primary tumor, but this effort is only the first part of an extended plan that, with increasing frequency, includes chemotherapy or biological therapy and irradiation. In the succeeding chapters we present the basic information needed by an oncologist for understanding the use of drugs. This information is essential for informed decision making by the medical oncologist or pediatric oncologist, but enhances the integration of treatment planning by the other specialists, who need to know what to expect of their medical colleagues.

In these chapters we present essential information on the mechanism of action, and determinants of response for the standard drugs. In addition, and of particular interest for the medical oncologist, we include valuable data on pharmacokinetics, clearance mechanisms, drug interactions, dose modification for organ dysfunction, and pharmacogenetics, all of which may influence the response to treatment and the development of toxicity. For those that require more detailed information or references, we suggest that the reader consult more comprehensive and specialized texts (1–3).

While individualization of treatment is necessary in certain therapeutic settings, in general readers are urged to administer drugs according to standard and well-tested protocols, and to recognize that intervention with new drugs, with irradiation, or with biological agents in previously unexplored ways may lead to unanticipated toxicity. New interventions or treatment regimens that carry potential risk and uncertain benefit must first be tested in clinical trials to prove their safety and efficacy, with appropriate oversight and approval by an Investigational Review Board.

Finally, it is important for the clinical oncologist to remember that all drugs pose risks and that their use constitutes a balance of risk and benefit. We provide here the latest information available as we go to press. However, because cancer is a potentially fatal disease, drugs are approved after relatively limited clinical testing, and carry incompletely defined potential for toxicity at the time of their first marketing. Cancer drug toxicity affects not only the bone marrow, but extends across a broad spectrum that includes coagulopathy, changes in mental status, immune modulation, cardiovascular effects, pulmonary, hepatic, and renal damage, and second malignancy. With increasing use, these side effects, as well as new indications for the agent, are appreciated and become the subject of FDA alerts published in major cancer journals. It is encumbent upon the oncologist to keep abreast of this new information for both the benefit and the safety of our patients.

REFERENCES

1. Chabner BA, Amrein PC, Druker BJ, et al. Antineoplastic Agents. In JG Hardman and LE Limbird(eds.) "Goodman and Gilmans the Pharmacological Basis of Therapeutics", 11th edition. McGraw-Hill, New York, NY: 2005.
2. Chabner BA. In BA Chabner and DL Longo(eds.), "Cancer Chemotherapy and Biotherapy Principles and Practice", 4th edition, Lippincott Williams & Wilkins Philadelphia, PA, 2006.
3. Kufe DW, Bast Jr, RC, Hait WN, Hong WK, Pollock RE, Weichselbaum RR, Holland JF, Frei III E(eds.), Cancer Medicine, 7th edition. BC Decker Inc, Hamiltion, Unt., 2006.

Bruce A. Chabner

ANTIMETABOLITES: FLUOROPYRIMIDINES AND OTHER AGENTS

FLUOROPYRIMIDINES

5-fluoro-uracil (5-FU) and its prodrug, capecitabine (4-pentoxycarbonyl-5'-deoxy-5-fluorocytidine), are central agents in the treatment of epithelial cancers, particularly cancers of the breast, head and neck, and gastrointestinal tract. They have synergistic interaction with other cytotoxic agents, such as cisplatin or oxaliplatin, with antiangiogenic drugs, and with radiation therapy. As a component of adjuvant and metastatic therapy, fluoropyrimidines have improved survival in patients with colorectal cancer (1).

Mechanism of Action and Resistance

The first agent of this class, 5-FU (Figure 1-1), was synthesized in 1956 by Heidelberger, based on experiments that demonstrated the ability of tumor cells to salvage uracil for DNA synthesis. Later work showed that 5-FU is converted to an active deoxynucleotide, FdUMP, a potent inhibitor of DNA synthesis. Its activation occurs by one of several pathways, as shown in Figure 1-1.

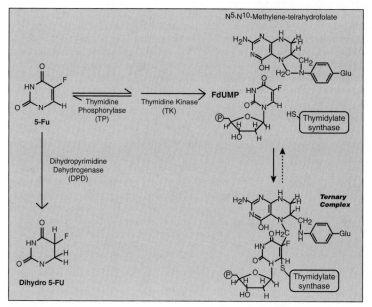

FIGURE 1-1 Routes of activation (via TP and TK) and inactivation (via DPD) of 5-fluorouracil (5-FU).

1

The active product, FdUMP, forms a tight tripartite complex with its target enzyme, thymidylate synthase (TS), and the enzyme's cofactor, 5-10 methylenetetrahydrofolic acid, and thereby blocks the conversion of dUMP to dTMP, a necessary precursor of dTTP (2). dTTP is one of four deoxynucleotide substrates required for synthesis of DNA. Subsequently, it has been shown both in the laboratory and in clinical trials that the addition of an exogenous folic acid source such as leucovorin (5-formyl-tetrahydrofolate) enhances formation of the TS-F-dUMP-folate complex and increases the response rate in patients with colon cancer (3).

5-FU also forms 5-FUTP, and thereby may become incorporated into RNA, where it blocks RNA processing and function. The role of RNA incorporation in determining 5-FU toxicity is incompletely understood. Evidence from studies of 5-FU resistance indicates that inhibition of TS predominates as the mechanism of antitumor action.

Resistance to fluoropyrimidines arises through several different changes in tumor biochemistry (4). Increased expression of TS, or amplification of the TS gene, occurs both experimentally and in a patient's tumors after exposure to FU, and probably represents the primary mechanism. Experimentally, some resistant cells fail to convert 5-FU to its active nucleotide form through decreased expression of one of several activating enzymes, or through increased expression of degradative enzymes. The parent compound is subject to inactivation by dihydropyrimidine dehydrogenase (DPD) (Figure 1-1) and increased expression of DPD has been found in resistant cells. Increased expression of thymidine phosphorylase (TP) reduces the cellular pool of an intermediate in the activation pathway, fluorodeoxyuridine, and increases resistance. Finally, antiapoptotic changes, such as increased expression of bcl-2 or mutation of the cell cycle checkpoint, p53, are associated with resistance in experimental systems.

Capecitabine, an orally active prodrug of 5-FU, has demonstrated antitumor efficacy equal to 5-FU in breast and colon cancer (5). Capecitabine is activated by sequential metabolic steps: carboxylesterase cleavage of the aminoester at carbon 4; deamination of the resulting fluoro-5′ deoxy-cytidine; and lastly cleavage of the 5′-deoxy sugar by TP, releasing 5-FU (Figure 1-2). Steps 1 and 2 are believed to occur in the liver and plasma, while step 3 takes place in tumor cells. Tumor cells with high TP are believed to be particularly sensitive to capecitabine.

Clinical Pharmacology

5-FU is administered intravenously in doses up to 450 mg/m^2/day $\times$ 5 days with 25–500 mg leucovorin orally each day. 5-FU given once weekly causes less neutropenia and diarrhea, and is probably equally effective. More recent regimens employ a bolus of FU on day 1, followed by 48 h infusion of up to 1,000 mg/m^2/day for 2 days, and these infusion regimens appear to be more active than bolus administration. Actual doses vary according to other drugs in the combination regimen and the use of radiation therapy concomitantly. The drug is not readily bioavailable by the oral route due to rapid first pass metabolism in the liver. Following intravenous administration, plasma concentrations of 5-FU decline rapidly, with a $t_{1/2}$ of 10 min, due to the rapid conversion to dihydro-5-FU. Intracellular concentrations of 5-FdUMP and other nucleotides build rapidly, and decay with a half-time of approximately 4 h. Little intact 5-FU appears in the urine. Drug doses do not have to be altered for abnormal hepatic or renal function.

Capecitabine, given in total doses of 2,500 mg/m^2/day for 14 days, is readily absorbed, converted to 5-fluoro-5′-deoxycytidine and 5-fluoro-5′-deoxyuridine (5-F-5′dU) by the liver, and peak levels of these metabolites appear in plasma about 2 h after a dose. Food taken with capecitabine protects the drug from

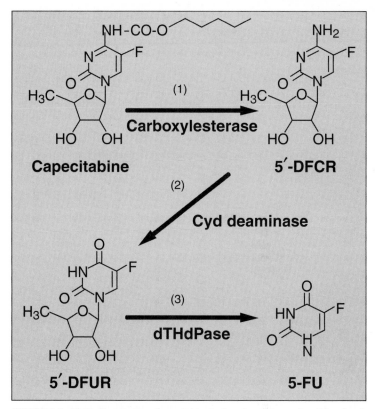

FIGURE 1-2 Metabolic activation of capecitabine by 1, carboxylesterase; 2, cytidine deaminase; 3, thymidine phosphorylase. 5-FU: 5-fluorouracil. 5′-DFCR = 5′-deoxy fluoro-cytosine riboside; 5′-DFUR = 5′-deoxy-fluorouracil riboside.

degradation and leads to higher active metabolite concentrations in plasma. 5-F-5′dU, the primary active precursor of 5-FU, exits plasma with a $t_{1/2}$ of 1 h. There is no evidence that leucovorin enhances the activity of capecitabine. The clearance of 5-F-5′-dU is delayed in patients with renal dysfunction, leading to recommendations that capecitabine should not be used in patients with severe renal failure (6). Patients with moderately impaired renal function (CCr of 30–50 ml/min) should receive 75% of a full dose.

In fluoropyrimidine therapy, the clinician must be prepared to make dose adjustment according to white blood count, gastrointestinal symptoms, and cutaneous toxicity, given the variability in drug clearance rates among patients.

Toxicity

Fluoropyrimidines cause significant acute toxicity to the gastrointestinal tract and bone marrow. Of primary concern are mucositis and diarrhea, which may lead to dehydration, sepsis, and death in the presence of myelosuppression. Persistent watery diarrhea should alert the patient to receive immediate medical attention. Women are more often affected than men, and elderly patients (above 70) are particularly vulnerable to 5-FU toxicity. Myelosuppression follows a typical pattern of an acute fall in white cell and platelet count over a 5–7 day period, followed by recovery by day 14. Occasional patients deficient in DPD due to inherited polymorphisms may display overwhelming toxicity to first doses of the drug (7). A test for DPD in white blood cells is now available, and can confirm this deficiency, which, if present, should preclude further attempts to use fluoropyrimidines. Other toxicities encountered with 5-FU include cardiac vasospasm with angina and rarely myocardial infarction and cerebellar dysfunction, predominantly after high-dose infusion or intracarotid infusion.

Capecitabine has the additional significant toxicity of palmar–plantar dysesthesias, with redness, extreme tenderness, and defoliation over the palms and plantar regions.

A third fluoropyrimidine, 5-F-deoxyuridine (5-F-dU), is used almost exclusively in regimens of hepatic artery infusion (0.3 mg/kg/day for 14 days) for metastases from colon cancer, in which setting it has a greater than 50% response rate (8). Given in this manner it has the advantage of achieving higher intratumoral concentrations, but is cleared by hepatic parenchyma and produces modest systemic toxicity. Intrahepatic arterial infusion may lead to serious hepatobiliary toxicity, including cholestasis, hepatic enzyme elevations, and ultimately biliary sclerosis. Corticosteroids given with 5-F-dU decrease the incidence of biliary toxicity. Thrombosis, hemorrhage or infection at the catheter site, and ulceration of the stomach or duodenum may further complicate this treatment approach.

NUCLEOSIDE ANALOGS OF DEOXYCYTIDINE AND CYTIDINE: GENERAL CONSIDERATIONS

The base, cytosine, is one of four primary building blocks of DNA and RNA, the other bases being the purines, guanine and adenine, and a second pyrimidine, either uracil for RNA or thymine for DNA. In order for these bases to function as substrates for DNA synthesis, ribose (for RNA) or deoxyribose (for RNA) must be attached to the base, forming a (deoxy)nucleoside, and three phosphate molecules must then be attached to the 5′ position of the nucleoside's sugar, forming a (deoxy)nucleotide. These synthetic reactions, which lead to formation of the four kinds of triphosphates required for making RNA and DNA, occur within the cancer cell, as well as within normal tissues.

Where do these bases come from? They can be made by tumor cells de novo, in a complex, multistep system of reactions. Alternatively, the bases can be salvaged from the breakdown of RNA and DNA and the release of their component bases or nucleosides into the bloodstream. Some bases, such as uracil and guanine, can be salvaged from the bloodstream as simple bases, while other bases, including cytosine, are salvaged from the circulation only if they are still attached to the appropriate sugar (as ribose or deoxyribose nucleosides).

Many of the earliest effective anticancer agents were designed as analogs of these bases or nucleosides. The specific form of these antitumor analogs was determined by the ability of cells to take up and activate either the base itself, or a ribose or deoxyribose derivative. Thus 5-FU proved to be an effective analog of uracil, and 6-mercaptopurine an analog of hypoxanthine, a precursor of both adenine and guanine. In the case of cytosine, cells could not utilize nonribosylated analogs of the base, but effective (deoxy)ribosylated analogs of cytosine have become valuable anticancer drugs.

CYTOSINE ARABINOSIDE

Effective analogs of deoxycytidine triphosphate have become critical components of the therapy of both leukemia and solid tumors. The first of these, cytosine arabinoside (araC) (Figure 1-3), was isolated from a fungal broth and proved to be the single most effective drug for inducing remission in acute

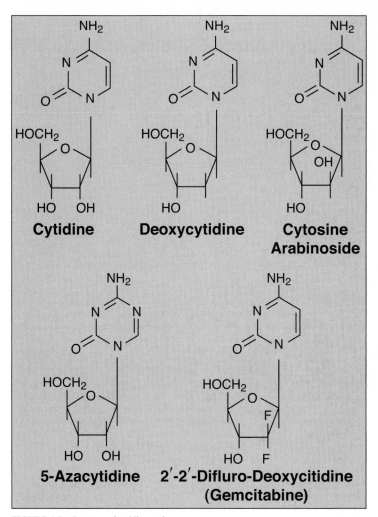

FIGURE 1-3 Structure of cytidine analogs.

myelogenous leukemia (AML) (9). It differs from deoxycytidine in having an arabinose sugar rather than a deoxyribose, with a 2'OH group in the beta configuration, rather than the H group found on deoxyribose. The presence of the beta-2'OH does not inhibit entry into cells or its further metabolism to an active triphosphate, or even its subsequent incorporation into the growing DNA strand. However, once incorporated, araC blocks further elongation of the DNA strand by DNA polymerase, and initiates apoptosis (programmed cell death). The incorporation of ara CMP into DNA in the ratio of 5 molecules per 10^4 bases is sufficient to initiate the cell death pathway (10).

The steps leading from polymerase inhibition to cell death are not clearly understood. Exposure of cells to araC induces a complex set of reactive signals, including induction of the transcription factor AP-1, and the damage response

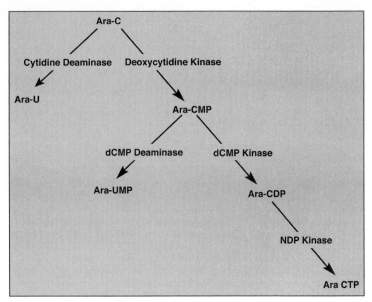

FIGURE 1-4 Metabolic pathway for conversion of deoxycytidine and its anticancer analog, cytosine arabinoside, to a triphosphate. ara-CMP: ara-C monophosphate; ara-CDP: ara-C diphosphonate; ara-CTP: ara-C triphosphate; ara-U: ara-uracil; dCMP: deoxycytidine monophosphate; NDP: nucleoside diphosphate.

factor, NF-κB. At low concentrations of araC, some leukemic cell lines in culture may differentiate, while others activate the apoptosis pathways. Levels of proapoptotic and antiapoptotic factors within the leukemic cells appear to influence susceptibility to cell death (11). Exposure to araC leads to stalling of the replication fork for cells undergoing DNA synthesis, and this event activates checkpoint kinases, ATR and Chk 1, which block further cell cycle progression, activate DNA repair, and stabilize the replication fork. Loss of ATR or Chk 1 function sensitizes cells to araC.

The specific steps in araC uptake and activation to a triphosphate within the cancer cell are important (12) (Figure 1-4). It is taken into cells by an equilibrative cell membrane transporter, hENT1, which also transports physiologic nucleosides. AraC is then converted to its monophosphate by deoxycytidine kinase, a key rate-limiting step in its activation and antitumor action. Ara CMP requires further conversion to its triphosphate, but the enzymes involved are found in abundance and do not limit its activity.

The drug and its monophosphate, ara-CMP, are both subject to degradation by deaminase enzymes. The resultant ara-U or ara UMP is inactive as a substrate for either RNA or DNA synthesis. Cytidine deaminase is found in most human tissues, including epithelial cells of the intestine, the liver, and even in plasma. Elevated concentrations of cytidine deaminase have been implicated as the cause of araC resistance in AML, but the evidence is as yet not convincing. The most important cause of resistance appears to be a deletion of deoxycytidine kinase activity in a few well-studied cases (13). Other evidence suggests that the formation and duration of persistence of ara-CTP in leukemic cells determine the therapeutic outcome. The intracellular half-life of ara-CTP is only approximately 4 h.

For unexplained reasons, certain forms of AML (those with mutations involving the core binding factors (CBPs) found on chromosomes 8 and 16 seem particularly sensitive to araC and derive benefit in terms of a longer duration of remission and improved survival, when treated with high-dose araC (14). High-dose araC has become the standard for consolidation of remission in AML, following remission induction. Cure rates for patients under 60 years of age now approach 30–40%, but vary with patient age and with cytogenetics, the poorest results coming in older patients who have leukemia with complex karyotypes, leukemia secondary to cytotoxic therapy, or leukemia following a period of myelodysplasia.

Clinical Pharmacology

AraC, in doses of 100–200 mg/m^2/day × 7 days, is commonly used with daunomycin or idarubicin for remission induction in AML. The drug may be given by bolus injection or continuous infusion. Once remission has been induced, high-dose araC is given in doses of 3 g/m^2 as a 3 h infusion for consolidation therapy (15). Doses are repeated every 12 h twice daily on days 1, 3, and 5. Continuous infusion regimens are designed to maintain cytotoxic levels (above 0.1 μM) of drug throughout a several-day period, in order to expose dividing cells during the DNA synthetic phase of the cell cycle.

AraC disappears rapidly from plasma, with a half-time of 10 min, due primarily to its rapid deamination by cytidine deaminase (see above). High-dose araC follows similar kinetics in plasma, although a slow terminal phase of disappearance becomes apparent, and may contribute to toxicity. The primary metabolite, ara-U, has no known toxicity, but, in patients with renal dysfunction, through feedback inhibition of deamination ara-U may contribute to the slower elimination of high-dose araC from plasma, resulting in greater risk of toxicity. High-dose regimens provide cytotoxic drug concentrations in the cerebrospinal fluid, but direct intrathecal injection of 50 mg, either as a standard formulation of drug, or in a depot form of araC immersed in a gel suspension for slow release (DepoCyt), is the preferred treatment for lymphomatous or carcinomatous meningeal disease. AraC has comparable intrathecal activity to methotrexate in these settings. DepoCyt produces sustained CSF concentrations of araC above 0.4 μM for 12–14 days, thus avoiding the need for more frequent lumbar punctures (16).

Toxicity

AraC primarily affects dividing tissues such as the intestinal epithelium and bone marrow progenitors, leading to stomatitis, diarrhea, and myelosuppression, all of which peak at 7–14 days after treatment. In addition, araC may cause pulmonary vascular/epithelial injury, leading to a syndrome of noncardiogenic pulmonary edema. It is associated with an increased incidence of streptococcal viridans pneumonitis in children. Liver function abnormalities and rarely jaundice may occur as well, and are reversible with discontinuation of therapy.

High-dose araC may cause cerebellar dysfunction, seizures, dementia, and coma; this neurotoxicity is most common in patients with renal dysfunction and those over 60, thus leading to recommendations that high-dose consolidation not be used in such patients. The same neurotoxicities, as well as arachnoiditis, may follow intrathecal drug injection.

GEMCITABINE

A second deoxycytidine analog, Gemcitabine (2′, 2′difluorodeoxycytidine, dFdC), has become an important component of treatment regimens for pancreatic cancer, nonsmall cell lung cancer, ovarian and breast cancer, and bladder cancer, and its range of activity is constantly expanding. Its metabolic pathways are very similar to those of araC (Figure 1-4), although its triphosphate has a much longer intracellar half-life, perhaps accounting for its broader solid tumor activity. In vitro, sensitive tumor cells are killed by exposure to gemcitabine concentration of 0.01 μM for 1 h or longer, levels achieved by usual intravenous doses.

Its pathway of uptake and activation in tumor cells is much the same as araC, requiring the hENT1 transporter, initial phosphorylation to dFdCMP by deoxycytidine kinase, conversion to the triphosphate, and incorporation into DNA, where it allows the addition of one more nucleotide before terminating DNA synthesis. However, it has additional sites of action. Its diphosphate inhibits ribonucleotide reductase (RNR), and therefore lowers intracellular levels of its physiologic competitor, dCTP, allowing greater incorporation of dFdC into DNA. Incorporation into DNA correlates with apoptosis. Exposure of cells to gemcitabine activates the same ATR/Chk 1 kinases that block further cell cycle progression after araC treatment, but, in addition, it activates an alternative, p53-dependent pathway, which includes the checkpoint monitor, ATM. Activation of ATM implies a response to double-strand breaks, and thus differs from the single break pathway activation by araC (17).

Resistance in experimental tumors arises by several mechanisms, including deletion of the hENT1 transporter, deletion of deoxycytidine kinase, increased phosphatase activity, or by increased expression or amplification of either the large, catalytic subunit of RNR, or its smaller tyrosyl containing subunit (17). Inhibition of RNR expression by small interfering RNA potentiates gemcitabine activity. These findings regarding RNR imply that the cytotoxic action of the drug requires inhibition of this enzyme. In addition, src kinase activity may potentiate gemcitabine resistance in pancreatic tumor cells, possibly through src kinase activation of expression of RNR.

Clinical Pharmacology

The standard regimen of administration is 1,000 mg/m^2 given as a 30 min infusion on days 1, 8, and 15 of a 28 day cycle. More prolonged periods of infusion, up to 150 min, may produce higher intracellular levels of dFdCTP, but also greater toxicity, and perhaps greater antitumor effects. Comparative trials of short- and long-infusion strategies are ongoing.

Doses may be modified for myelosuppression. Gemcitabine markedly sensitizes both normal and tumor tissues to concurrent radiation therapy, thus requiring drug dose reductions of 70–80%. The mechanism of radiosensitization appears to be related to inhibition of repair of double-strand breaks and to inhibition of cell cycle progression (18). The drug is cleared rapidly from plasma by deamination, with a half-life of 15–20 min. Women and elderly patients may clear the drug more slowly, and all patients should be watched carefully for extreme myelosuppression.

Toxicity

The primary toxicity of gemcitabine is myelosuppression, which peaks in the third week of a four-week schedule, blood counts usually recovering rapidly thereafter. Mild liver enzyme abnormalities may appear with longer term use. Pulmonary toxicity, with dyspnea and interstitial infiltrates, may occur in up to a quarter of patients treated with multiple cycles of the drug (19). In addition, patients on repeated cycles of gemcitabine experience progressive anemia, which appears to have several components, including the direct effects of drug on red cell production, and the induction of hemolysis. After multiple cycles of treatment, a small but significant fraction of patients will experience a hemolytic-uremic syndrome (HUS), including anemia, edema and effusions, and a rising BUN (20). The HUS reverses with drug discontinuation, but in patients with pancreatic cancer, there may be no alternative effective therapy, and careful reinstitution of gemcitabine at lower doses may be tried.

Severe toxicity has been reported in a single patient with a polymorphism of the cytidine deaminase gene, in which a homozygous substitution of threonine for alanine at position 208 was found (21). The patient had a fivefold slower clearance of the parent drug, as compared to nontoxic controls.

5-AZACYTIDINE (5AZAC)

5-azacytidine (5azaC) (Figure 1-3) is both a cytotoxic and a differentiating agent, and has become a standard drug for treatment of myelodysplasia (22). In this syndrome, characterized by refractory cytopenias and diverse chromosomal abnormalities, 5azaC reduces blood transfusion requirements and improves thrombocytopenia or leukopenia in one-quarter to one-third of patients. It is unclear whether these effects are mediated by its antiproliferative activity or its ability to demethylate and thereby to reactivate genes that induce maturation of hematopoietic cells.

5azaC is transported into cells by one of several nucleoside transporters, and converted to a nucleoside monophosphate by cytidine kinase. After further conversion to a triphosphate, it becomes incorporated into RNA and DNA and, when incorporated into DNA, acts as a suicide inhibitor of the enzyme responsible for cytidine methylation, inducing expression of silenced genes (23). Thus, in noncytotoxic concentrations in tissue culture, it is able to promote differentiation of both normal and malignant cells. In patients with sickle cell anemia, 5azaC induces synthesis of hemoglobin F and thereby reduces the frequency of sickle cell crisis and acute chest syndrome. However, DNA synthesis inhibitors, such as hydroxyurea, have a similar effect on patients with sickle cell anemia; thus it is unclear whether 5azaC's beneficial effects are mediated by DNA demethylation or by inhibition of DNA synthesis.

The mechanism of 5azaC cytotoxic action is incompletely understood (24). The azacytidine ring is less stable than cytidine, undergoing spontaneous hydrolysis and ring opening. At high-drug concentration, DNA synthesis is blocked and cells undergo apoptosis. The elimination of 5azaC occurs through its rapid deamination in plasma, liver, and other tissues by cytidine deaminase. The primary metabolite, 5-azauridine, undergoes spontaneous hydrolysis and is thought to be inactive.

Clinical Pharmacology

Toxicity is primarily myelosuppression, with recovery 10–14 days after treatment, but the drug does cause significant nausea and vomiting when administered in high doses as antileukemic therapy. In the usual regimen for myelodysplasia, 30 mg/m^2/day subcutaneously, it has minimal side effects aside from leukopenia. A closely related agent, decitabine (5aza deoxycytidine) has similar but more potent cytotoxic and differentiating properties and is also approved for treatment of myelodysplasia (24).

HYDROXYUREA

Hydroxyurea (HU), an inhibitor of RNR, is a useful agent for acutely lowering the white blood cell count in patients with myeloproliferative disease, especially acute or chronic myelogenous leukemia (CML). It also effectively lowers the platelet count in essential thrombocythemia. It has little value as a remission-inducing agent. Prior to Gleevec, HU was a component of the maintenance regimen for CML but is rarely employed for that purpose, currently. Its effects on myelopoiesis are seen within 24 h, and reverse rapidly thereafter. Because of its minimal side effects and predictable and reversible action, it is commonly used to lower extremely high white blood cell counts at the time of initial presentation of leukemia. During the course of its clinical evaluation it was also found to be a potent radiosensitizer, and has been used with radiation therapy in experimental protocols for treatment of cervical cancer and head and neck cancer. It potently induces fetal hemoglobin expression, and has become the standard agent for prevention of sickle cell crisis (25). It has multiple effects on sickling including a reduction of adhesion of red cells to vascular endothelium and a lowering of the white cell count, all of which may contribute to its beneficial action.

$$H_2N - \overset{\overset{\displaystyle O}{\|}}{C} - \overset{\overset{\displaystyle H}{|}}{N} - OH$$

Hydroxyurea

HU inhibits RNR by binding to the iron required for catalytic reduction of nucleoside diphosphates. Through deoxynucleotide depletion, it blocks progression of cells through the DNA synthetic phase of the cell cycle, an inhibition mediated by p53 and other checkpoints (26). P53 deficient cells may exhibit blockage of cell cycle progression in the presence of HU. Through its effects on deoxynucleotide pools, it enhances incorporation of other antimetabolites into DNA, and inhibits repair of alkylation. Despite these multiple potentiating effects, it has not achieved broad usage in solid tumor combination chemotherapy. Resistance arises through outgrowth of cells that amplify or over-express the catalytic subunit of RNR.

In addition to its effects on DNA synthesis, HU stimulates production of nitric oxide by neutrophils; NO in turn may function as an inducer of differentiation and a vasodilator, effects that may contribute to its control of sickle cell crisis (27).

Clinical Pharmacology

HU is well absorbed after oral administration, but is available for intravenous infusion as well for emergent situations. Usual daily oral doses are 15–30 mg/kg, although higher doses are used for acute lowering of the white cell count. It is cleared by renal excretion, and its plasma half-life is approximately 4 h in patients with normal renal function. Doses should be adjusted according to creatine clearance in patients with abnormal renal function.

Its toxicity is manifest primarily as acute myelosuppression, affecting all three lineages of blood cells. It may also cause a mild chronic gastritis, an interstitial pneumonitis, skin hyperpigmentation, ulcerations on the lower extremities, and neurologic dysfunction. It is a potent teratogen and should not be used without contraception in women of childbearing age. It has uncertain potential as a carcinogen, a concern in patients with nonmalignant disease and in chronic myeloproliferative syndromes such as p. vera.

PURINE ANTAGONISTS

At least three general classes of purine antagonists have proven useful for treatment of cancer. The first were the thiopurines, 6-mercaptopurine (6-MP), and 6-thioguanine (6-TG), which were introduced as antileukemic drugs in

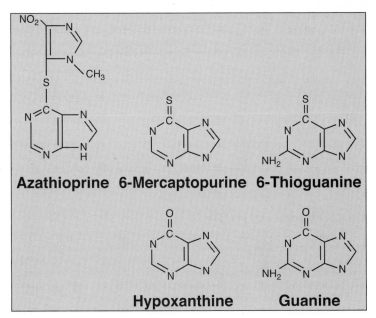

Azathioprine 6-Mercaptopurine 6-Thioguanine

Hypoxanthine **Guanine**

FIGURE 1-5 Structure of the naturally occurring purine, hypoxanthine and guanine, and related antineoplastic agents 6-mercaptopurine, 6-thioguanine, and azathioprine.

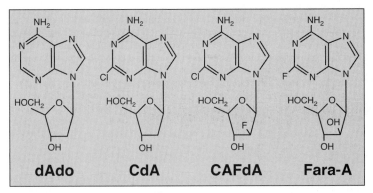

dAdo **CdA** **CAFdA** **Fara-A**

FIGURE 1-6 Structures of deoxyadenosine, Cladribine (CdA), Clofarabine (CAFdA), and Fludarabine (Fara-A). Substitution with a chloro or fluoro atom at the 2-position of the adenine ring makes the compounds resistant to deamination by adenosine deaminase. At the 2′-arabino position, CAFdA has a fluoro atom and Fara-A has a hydroxy group.

the early 1950s (Figure 1-5). 6-MP remains a standard drug for maintenance of remission in childhood acute lymphocytic leukemia, in combination with methotrexate.6-MP, which is also the active metabolite of Imuran, is a potent immunosuppressive and in common use for Crohn's disease. The second group (Figure 1-6) of purine analogs consists of halogenated adenosine derivatives, fludarabine, clofarabine, and cladribine. Unlike adenosine, these drugs are resistant to deamination, and are toxic to both normal and malignant lymphoid cells (28). Cladribine is highly effective, and possibly curative for hairy cell leukemia, while fludarabine has become a first-line agent for chronic lymphocytic leukemia and is frequently used in a broad array of other lymphoid tumors, including follicular lymphomas (29). Fludarabine, a potent immunosuppressant, is often used to suppress graft versus host disease after allogeneic bone marrow transplantation. Finally, nelarabine, a pure arabinosyl guanine analog (araG), is specifically effective against T-cell lymphoid tumors (30). The various structures and their physiologic counterparts are shown in Figure 1-6.

Why are these purine analogs so specific in their inhibitory effects against lymphoid tumors? The purine analogs are readily activated to nucleotides (mono-, di-, and triphosphates) in such tumors, and the active purine nucleotides are long lived ($t_{1/2}$ up to 16 h) and only slowly degraded, as compared to their rapid disappearance in nonlymphoid tissue. All of these compounds, to varying degrees, are both cytotoxic to tumors and to normal lymphocytes. Immunosuppression is a common feature.

Clinical Pharmacology of 6-MP

6-MP is converted to 6-thio-inosine monophosphate (6-IMP) by hypoxanthine-guanine phosphoribosyl transferase (HGPRT'ase). 6-IMP has multiple actions. It inhibits the first step in de novo purine synthesis. It is also converted to a triphosphate, which is incorporated into RNA and DNA, potentially inhibiting RNA and DNA synthesis. Resistance to 6-MP arises through loss of HGPRT'ase, or by increased degradation of the active nucleotides.

6-MP is administered in doses of 50–100 mg/m^2/day, and is titrated according to the degree of leukopenia. Oral absorption is erratic, and may contribute to therapeutic failure, further strengthening the need for titration of dose to leukopenia (31).

6-MP is cleared by two pathways, leading to a half-life in plasma of 90 min. The first pathway requires its oxidation by xanthine oxidase (XO), a ubiquitous enzyme. In the presence of allopurinol, a potent inhibitor of XO used for treating gout, breakdown of orally administered 6-MP is inhibited by 75%, and thus the dose of 6-MP must be reduced by 75% in that circumstance. In the second degradative pathway, the sulfur group undergoes methylation by thiopurine methyltransferase to the less potent 6-methyl MP. Polymorphisms of the methyltransferase responsible for this conversion are found with reasonable frequency (32). Fewer than 1% of the Caucasian population is homozygous for inactive forms of the enzyme, but these affected individuals become severely toxic with standard doses of 6-MP. About 10–15% of Americans are heterozygotes for one allele of a relatively less active form of the methyltransferase, and may require dose reduction, which is titrated according to the white blood cell count. A hyperactive polymorphism of methyl transferase has been identified in rare individuals of African descent; these patients may require increased doses of 6-MP, again titrated to produce modest leukopenia. While direct genetic testing of patients is not routinely available, many larger pediatric cancer centers test the content of red cell methylthiopurine nucleotides after 6-MP in order to detect patients at risk of over or under treatment.

The principal toxicities of 6-MP, as mentioned above, are myelosuppression and immunosuppression. It predisposes patients to opportunistic infection caused by fungal, viral, and parasitic organisms. It causes biliary stasis and hepatocellular necrosis in up to one-third of patients on treatment, although these effects rarely lead to permanent discontinuation of treatment. The drug is teratogenic, and is associated with an increased incidence of squamous cell carcinomas of the skin.

Clinical Pharmacology of Fludarabine and Cladribine

Fludarabine is administered as a water-soluble monophosphate that is rapidly hydrolyzed to a nucleoside in plasma, while cladribine, clofarabine, and nelarabine are administered as the parent nucleoside in solution. The cellular uptake of the fludarabine nucleoside, cladribine, clofarabine, and nelarabine proceeds via nucleoside transporters. Inside the cell, fludarabine, clofarabine, and cladribine are activated to the monophosphate by deoxycytidine kinase, while nelarabine is activated by guanosine kinase. All four are then converted to their active triphosphate, and act as inhibitors of DNA synthesis. In addition, fludarabine diphosphate inhibits RNR, thereby depleting the physiologic triphosphates and enhancing the analog's incorporation into DNA. The triphosphates have long intracellular half-lives of 12–16 h. All four analogs lead to apoptosis, an effect that, in the case of fludarabine, depends on activation of cytochrome c released by the intrinsic apoptosis pathway.

Fludarabine and cladribine share many common features with respect to their clinical pharmacology. Both are cleared by renal excretion of the parent drug, leading to plasma half-lives of 7 h for cladribine and 10 h for fludarabine. Both cause prolonged immunosuppression (low CD4 counts) and moderate and reversible myelosuppression at therapeutic doses. Opportunistic infection is common, particularly in CLL patients who are hypogammaglobulinemic prior to treatment. Fludarabine also causes a host of autoimmune phenomena, including hemolytic anemia, pure red cell aplasia, idiopathic thrombocytopenic purpura, arthritis, and antithyroid antibodies (33). It may also cause peripheral neuropathy, renal dysfunction, and altered mental status. Doses of both fludarabine and cladribine should be reduced in proportion to the reduction in creatinine clearance in patients with abnormal renal function. Recent reports describe anecdotal cases of AML with deletion of the long arm of chromosome 7, suggesting therapy induced disease, in CLL patients treated with fludarabine (34).

The usual dose and schedule of fludarabine is 25 mg/m^2/day intravenously for five days, repeated every four weeks for six cycles of treatment. Lower doses may be given in combination with Cytoxan and with Rituxan in treating CLL. Fludarabine is well absorbed (60% bioavailability) when given orally in doses of 40 mg/m^2/day, and preliminary results indicate equal activity by this route. Cladribine is administered in a single course of 0.09 mg/kg/day for seven days to patients with hairy cell leukemia.

NELARABINE

Nelarabine, a 6-methoxy prodrug of arabinosylguanine (Figure 1-7), has received approval for treatment of relapsed T-cell acute leukemia and for lymphoblastic lymphoma, for which it gives a complete response rates of approximately 20%, but with a few long-term remissions.

The mechanism of action of nelarabine proceeds through its activation by adenosine deaminase, which removes the 6-methoxy group, generating the active ara-G. AraG is resistant to purine nucleoside phosphorylase, an enzyme essential for regulation of T-cell function, and the primary mechanism of protecting T-cells against build up of toxic purine nucleotides. Intracellular araG is converted to its monophosphate by either deoxycytidine kinase or by deoxyguanosine kinase, and then further to its triphosphate. Incorporation of araGTP into DNA terminates DNA synthesis and induces apoptosis in a manner similar to the effects of other Ara nucleotides (35). T-cells, either normal or malignant, accumulate greater concentrations of araGTP, and retain the triphosphate for longer periods, than do B-cells, perhaps explaining its preferential effects on T-cell malignancy. Maximal cellular concentrations of araGTP are reached within 4 h of the end of

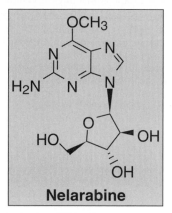

FIGURE 1-7   Molecular structure of Nelarabine.

infusion, decline thereafter with a $t_{1/2}$ of up to 24 h, and $t_{1/2}$ in individual patients closely correlates with complete response (36).

The conversion of nelarabine to araG occurs rapidly in blood and tissues, with a $t_{1/2}$ of 15 min. Ninety-four percent of the parent drug is converted to araG in 1 h. AraG is cleared from plasma with a $t_{1/2}$ of 2–3 h; clearance occurs primarily by metabolism, with a minor renal component (37). No modification of dose is required in patients with renal dysfunction.

Adults receive 1,500 mg/m^2/day infused over 2 h on days 1, 3, and 5, while pediatric patients are given 650 mg/m^2/day for five days. Courses are repeated every 21 days until remission. Almost half of adult patients experience serious neurologic side effects, including somnolence, confusion, lethargy, or peripheral neuropathy. Other significant side effects include neutropenia and transaminase elevations. However, neurologic side effects are in general dose-limiting, and may be irreversible. In isolated cases, patients may develop an ascending neuropathy resembling the Guillain–Barre syndrome.

CLOFARABINE

The most recent addition to the ranks of anticancer purine analogs is clofarabine, which contains a chlorine substitution at position 2 of the adenosine ring, as found in cladribine, and a fluorine in the beta-2′ position of the arabinose sugar (38) (Figure 1-6). It thus has the general properties of cladribine: it becomes incorporated into DNA, thereby inhibiting DNA synthesis; it also inhibits RNR; and it is resistant to adenosine deaminase. The 2′ fluorine in the arabinosyl configuration confers resistance to purine nucleoside phosphorylase, and probably increases the stability of the intracellular triphosphate. It has the additional feature of promoting apoptosis through mitochondrial toxicity. Clofarabine is approved for treatment of relapsed or refractory AML, for which as a single agent it induces complete remission in 30–50% of patients, but other indications are being explored, including combination therapies in AML and other hematologic malignancies.

Clofarabine is administered as a 1 h infusion of 30–40 mg/m^2 daily for five consecutive days in the treatment of AML (39). The drug is eliminated by renal excretion. Its half-life in plasma varies from 4 to 10 h, occuring the shortest half-life in children, and less rapid clearance as body weight increases in adolescents and adults. Intracellular clofarabine triphosphate levels reach a maximum at doses of 40 mg/m^2/day, and at steady state, plasma clofarabine concentrations peak at 2–3 μM. The intracellular triphosphate persists at near peak levels (10 μM or higher) for longer than 24 h and accumulates with each dose. The mechanism of resistance of clofarabine has not been defined in clinical use, but experimental evidence suggests deletion or decreased expression of deoxycytidine kinase, its initial activating enzyme, as the likely event (40).

The primary toxicity encountered at low doses (2 mg/m^2/day for 5 days) in nonleukemic patients is myelosuppression. However, in patients with leukemia, treated with much higher doses, hepatic dysfunction (enzyme elevations and increased bilirubin) develops in 50–75%. Hepatic function tests normalize within 14 days after drug discontinuation.

A skin rash is noted in 50% of leukemia patients receiving clofarabine, and palmoplantar dysesthesia may also develop.

It is not known whether clofarabine treatment is associated with long-term immunosuppression, as occurs after fludarabine and cladribine.

REFERENCES

1. Meyerhardt JA, Mayer RJ. Systematic therapy for colorectal cancer. N Engl J Med. 2006; 352: 476–487.
2. Santi DV, McHenry CS, Sommer H. Mechanism of interaction of thymidylate synthetase with 5-fluorodeoxyuridylate. Biochemistry. 1974; 13: 471–481.
3. Grogan L, Sotos GA, Allegra CJ. Leucovorin modulation of fluorouracil. Oncology. 1993; 7: 63–72.
4. Washtein WL. Thymidylate synthetase levels as a factor in 5-fluorodeoxyuridine and methotrexate cytotoxicity in gastrointestinal tumor cells. Mol Pharmacol. 1982; 21: 723–728.
5. Ishikawa T, Sekiguchi F, Fukase Y, et al. Positive correlation between the efficacy of capecitabine and doxifluridine and the ratio of thymidine phosphorylase to dihydropyrimidine dehydrogenase activities in tumors in human cancer xenografts. Cancer Res. 1998; 58: 685–690.
6. Milano G, Ferrero JM, Francois E. Comparative pharmacology of oral fluoropyrimidines: a focus on pharmacokinetics, pharmacodynamics and pharmacomodulation. Br J Cancer. 2004; 91: 613–617.
7. Milano G, Etienne MC, Pierrefite V, et al. Dihydropyrimidine dehydrogenase deficiency and fluorouracil-related toxicity. Br J Cancer. 1999; 79: 627–630.
8. Kemeny N, Huang Y, Cohen AM, et al. Hepatic arterial infusion of chemotherapy after resection of hepatic metastases from colorectal cancer. N Engl J Med. 1999; 341: 2039–2048.
9. Ellison RR, Holland JF, Weil M, et al. Arabinosyl cytosine: a useful agent in the treatment of acute leukemia in adults. Blood. 1968; 32: 507.
10. Kufe DW, Munroe D, Herrick D, et al. Effects of 1-beta-D-arabinofuranosylcytosine incorporation on eukaryotic DNA template function. Mol Pharmacol. 1984; 26: 128.
11. Campos L, Rouault J, Sabido O, et al. High expression of bcl-2 protein in acute myeloid leukemiacells in association with poor response to chemotherapy. Blood. 1993; 81: 3091.
12. Wiley JS, Taupin J, Jamieson GP, et al. Cytosine arabinoside transport and metabolism in acute leukemias and t-cell lymphoblastic lymphoma. J Clin Invest. 1985; 75: 632–642.
13. Tattersall MNH, Ganeshaguru K, Hoffbrand AV. Mechanisms of resistance of human acute leukemia cells to cytosine arabinoside. Br J Haematol. 1974; 27: 39.
14. Bloomfield CD, Lawrence D, Byrd JC, et al. Frequency of prolonged remission duration after high-dose cytarabine by cytogenetic subtype. Cancer Res. 1998; 58: 4173.

15. Bishop JF, Matthews JP, Young GA, et al. A randomized study of high-dose cytarabine in induction in acute myeloid leukemia. Blood. 1996; 87: 1710.

16. Cole BF, Glantz MJ, Jaeckle KA, et al. Quality-of-life-adjusted survival comparison of sustained-release cytosine arabinoside versus intrathecal methotrexate for treatment of solid tumor neoplastic meningitis. Cancer. 2003; 97: 3053.

17. Rosell R, Danenberg KD, Alberola V, et al. Ribonucleotide reductase messenger RNA expression and survival in Gemcitabine/Cisplatin-treated advanced non-small cell lung cancer patients. Clin Cancer Res. 2004; 10: 1318.

18. Pauwels B, Korst AEC, Lardon F, Vermorken JB. Combined modality therapy of Gemcitabine and radiation. Oncologist. 2005; 10: 34.

19. Dimopoulou I, Efstathiou E, Samakovli A, et al. A prospective study on lung toxicity in patients treated with gemcitabine and carboplatin: clinical, radiological and functional assessment. Ann Oncol. 2004; 15: 1250.

20. Humphreys BD, Sharman JP, Henderson JM, et al. Gemcitabine-associated thrombocitic microangiopathy. Cancer. 2004; 100: 2664.

21. Yonemori K, Ueno H, Okusaka T, et al. Severe drug toxicity associated with a single-nucleotide polymorphism of the cytidine deaminase gene in a Japanese cancer patient treated with gemcitabine plus cisplatin. Clin Cancer Res. 2005; 11: 2620–2624.

22. Kaminskas E, Farrell AT, Wang YC, Sridhara R, Pazdur R. FDA drug approval summary: azacitidine (5-azacytidine, VidazaTM) for injectable suspension. Oncologist. 2005; 10: 176.

23. Lee T, Karon MR. Inhibition of ribosomal precursor RNA maturation by 5-azacytidine and 8-azaguanine in Novakoff hepatoma cells. Arch Biochem Biophys. 1974; 26: 1737.

24. Carr BI, Rahbar S, Asmeron Y, et al. Carcinogenicity and haemoglobin synthesis induction by cytidine analogs. Cancer. 1988; 57: 395.

25. Galanello R, Stamatoyannopolous G, Papayannopoulou T. Mechanism of Hb F stimulation by s-stage compounds: in vitro studies with bone marrow cells exposed to 5-azacytidine, Ara-C or hydroxyurea. J Clin Invest. 1988; 81: 1209.

26. Elford HL. Effect of hydroxyurea on ribonucleotides reductase. Biochem Biophys Res Commun. 1968; 33: 129.

27. Cokic VP, Smith RD, Belesin-Cokic BB, et al. Hydroxyurea induces fetal hemoglobin by the nitric oxide-dependent activation of soluble guanylyl cyclase. J Clin Invest. 2003; 111: 231.

28. Fidias P, Chabner BA, Grossbard ML. Purine analogs for the treatment of low-grade lymphoproliferative disorders. Oncologist. 1996; l(3): 125.

29. Keating MJ, O'Brien S, Albitar M, et al. Early results of a chemoimmunotherapy regimen of fludarabine, cyclophosphamide, and rituximab as initial therapy for chronic lymphocytic leukemia. J Clin Oncol. 2005; 23: 4079.

30. Kisor DF. Nelarabine: a nucleoside analog with efficacy in t-cell and other leukemias. Ann Pharmacother. 2005; 39: 1056.

31. Balis FM, Holcenberg JS, Zimm S, et al. The effect of methotrexate on the bioavailability of oral 6-mercaptopurine. Clin Pharmacol Ther. 1987; 41: 384.

32. Holme SA, Dudley JA, Sanderson J. Erythrocyte thiopurine methyl transferase assessment prior to azathioprine use in the UK. Q J Med. 2002; 95: 439.

33. Fujimaki K, Takasaki H, Koharazawa H, et al. Idiopathic thrombocytopenic purpura and myasthenia gravis after fludarabine treatment for chronic lymphocytic leukemia. Leuk Lymphoma. 2005; 46: 1101.

34. Lam CCK, Ma ESK, Kwong YL. Therapy-related acute myeloid Leukemia after single-agent treatment with fludarabine for chronic lymphocytic leukemia. Am J Hematol. 2005; 79: 288.

35. Rossi JF, Van Hoof A, De Boeck K, et al. Efficacy and safety of oral fludarabine phosphate in previously untreated patients with chronic lymphocytic leukemia. J Clin Oncol. 2004; 22: 1260.

36. Kurtzberg J, Ernst TJ, Keating MJ, et al. Phase I study of 506U78 administered on a consecutive five day schedule in children and adults with refractory hematologic malignancies. J Clin Oncol. 2005; 23: 3396.
37. Kisor D, Plunkett W, Kurtzberg J, et al. Pharmacokinetics of nelarabine and 9-beta-D-arabinofuranosyl guanine in pediatric and adult patients during a phase I study of Nelarabine for the treatment of refractory hematologic malignancies. J Clin Oncol. 2000; 18: 995.
38. Faderl S, Gandhi V, Keating MJ, Jeha S, Plunkett W, Kantarjian HM. The role of clofarabine in hematologic and solid malignancies—development of a next-generation nucleoside analog. Cancer. 2005; 103: 1985–1995.
39. Kantarjian H, Gandhi V, Cortes J, et al. Phase 2 clinical and pharmacologic study of clofarabine in patients with refractory or relapsed acute leukemia. Blood. 2003; 102: 2379–2386.
40. Mansson E, Flordal E, Liliemark J, et al. Down-regulation of deoxycytidine kinase in human leukemic cell lines resistant to cladribine and clofarabine and increased ribonucleotide reductase activity contributes to fludarabine resistance. Biochem Pharmacol. 2003; 65: 237–247.

ANTIFOLATES

The antifolates were first introduced as antileukemic drugs in 1948; in landmark experiments treating children with acute lymphocytic leukemia (ALL), Sidney Farber produced the first evidence that chemotherapy could lead to complete remissions, with normalization of bone marrow morphology (1). These first experiments were conducted with aminopterin, a close congener of methotrexate. Because of its more predictable toxicity, methotrexate subsequently became the standard antifolate in treatment of ALL. It has gained an important role in regimens for lymphomas, and choriocarcinoma, and as an immuno-suppressive. It is used following allogeneic bone marrow transplantation to suppress grant versus host rejections and in the treatment of autoimmune diseases such as rheumatoid arthritis and Weggener's granulomatosis. The structure of methotrexate and related antifolates is shown in Figure 2-1, and closely resembles that of the naturally occurring folates, except for the key substitution of the amino group on the C-4 position of the pteridine ring. This change in structure confers the ability to bind with extreme affinity to dihydrofolate reductase, the enzyme responsible for maintaining an adequate pool of intracellular tetrahydrofolates required for DNA synthesis. Subsequent experiments revealed that methotrexate, like the physiologic folates, is converted intracellularly to a series of highly charged, long-chain polyglutamates. These metabolites are retained preferentially within cells and inhibit with high affinity other folate dependent enzymes, including thymidylate synthase (TS, the same target as fluoro-uracil), and two early enzymes in purine

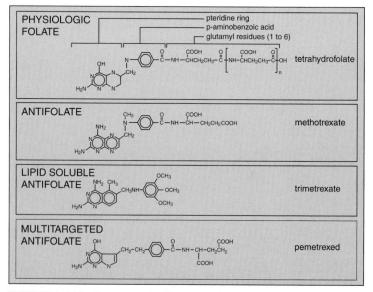

FIGURE 2-1 Molecular structure of methotrexate and related structures.

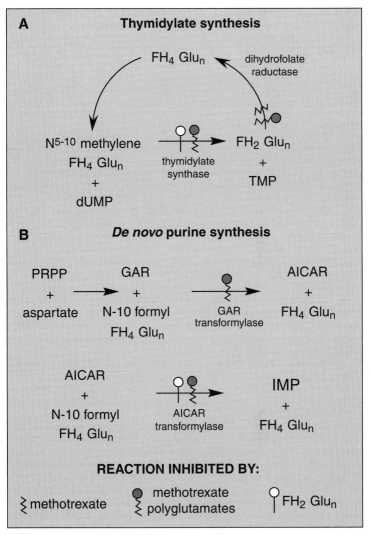

FIGURE 2-2 Multiple sites of inhibitory action of methotrexate, its polyglutamate metabolites, and dihydrofolate polyglutamates the substrate that accumulates when dihydrofolate reductase is inhibited. AICAR: aminoimidazole carboxamide; TMP: thymidine monophosphate; dUMP: deoxyuridine monophosphate; FH_2Glu_n: dihydrofolate polyglutamate; FH_4Glu_n: tetrahydrofolate polyglutamate; GAR: glycinamide ribonucleotide; IMP: inosine monophosphate; PRPP: 5-phosphoribosyl-1-pyrophosphate.

biosynthesis (Figure 2-2). The cumulative effects of inhibition of multiple enzymatic sites lead to depletion of intracellular folates and direct blockage of both purine and pyrimidine biosynthesis (2).

Because of its strong electro-negative charge at physiologic pH, the parent methotrexate crosses cell membranes slowly and, like physiologic folates, requires active transport into cells via the reduced folate carrier (3). In selected cells, such as choriocarcinomas, a second carrier, the folate binding protein, mediates methotrexate transport, and may become the preferred transporter. Polyglutamates, because of their multiple negative charges, are retained preferentially inside normal and tumor cells, and extend the duration of drug action. High-dose methotrexate (1 gm/m^2 or higher), as administered for childhood ALL, achieves a median intracellular antifolate concentration of 500 p moles/10^9 cells, overcoming interpatient variability in transport and polyglutamation (4). The parent compound is subject to efflux by members of the MRP (multidrug resistance protein) transporter family.

PHARMACOLOGIC CONSIDERATIONS

Methotrexate kills cells through its inhibition of DNA synthesis, and is thus most effective against rapidly growing tumors, such as leukemias and lymphomas. Cell kill by methotrexate depends on both drug concentration and duration of exposure. The threshold of drug toxicity for normal cells lies in the range of 10 nM. Classic studies of methotrexate resistance have shown that cells can delete the reduced folate transporter, lose the ability to polyglutamate folates, or amplify the gene coding for dihydrofolate reductase, all of which have been demonstrated in ALL cells in association with relapse (5). In addition, it is likely that alterations in apoptotic pathways can lead to resistance.

Recent studies have established that leukemic cells vary greatly in their ability to transport and polyglutamate methotrexate; thus ALL cells positive for the TEL-AML1 or E2A-PBX1 translocations have high expression of the ABC-G2 efflux transporter and accumulate low concentrations of the drug and its polyglutamates (6). Surprisingly, these subsets of ALL have a favorable prognosis, perhaps due to their sensitivity to other drugs. T-cell ALL cells have a reduced capability of polyglutamation of folates and methotrexate, and have a less favorable therapeutic outcome.

In addition to tumor specific factors that influence response, individual genetic variation modifies folate metabolism. The methylene tetrahydrofolate reductase variant C677T increases the intracellular level of 5–10 methylene tetrahydrofolic acid, the substrate for TS, and is associated with an increased rate of relapse in childhood ALL (7).

An alternative antifolate, Alimta or pemetrexed, has become an important addition to the available antifolates (8). It is more avidly transported and converted to a polyglutamate than is methotrexate. Alimta has notable activity against mesothelioma as a single agent, and enhances the effectiveness of cisplatin in this disease. Because of its mild toxicities, it has become a preferred agent for second line therapy of metastatic nonsmall cell lung cancer, ovarian cancer, and breast cancer. Following its intracellular conversion to polyglutamate forms, its primary target appears to be thymidylate synthesis and the purine synthetic enzymes, as it only modestly reduces the intracellular tetrahydrofolate pool. Unlike methotrexate, Alimta is given with folic acid (0.4–1.0 mg per day, beginning 1 week prior to treatment, and continuing throughout therapy) and with B-12 (1 mg on day 1), as these vitamins ameliorate its unpredictable toxicity to bone marrow (9).

CLINICAL PHARMACOLOGY

Methotrexate is well absorbed orally in doses of 25 mg/m^2 or less, and is used by that route in maintenance therapy of ALL. Otherwise it is given primarily by the intravenous route in doses of 50–500 mg/m^2, or in higher dose regimens with leucovorin rescue. Individual drug regimens vary considerably, and are tailored to specific indications. Careful adherence to proven regimens is critical, with particular attention to the status of the patient's pretreatment renal function, which may drastically alter tolerance to the drug.

Methotrexate is cleared primarily by renal excretion. Small amounts are metabolized to a nontoxic 7-OH derivative. In patients with normal renal function, it has a primary elimination half-life from plasma of 2–4 h, followed by a secondary elimination phase of 8–10 h (10). The terminal phase of disappearance is critical in determining the duration of exposure to cytotoxic concentrations of drug, and becomes much longer in patients with compromised renal function. Doses should be modified in proportion to the reduction in renal function for patients with a creatinine clearance of less than 60 ml/min. NSAIDS reduce renal blood flow and displace methotrexate from plasma protein binding, thereby slowing clearance and increasing unbound drug concentrations in plasma. They should not be used in conjunction with methotrexate administration. Penicillins reduce methotrexate secretion by renal tubules and may also increase the risk of toxicity.

High doses of methotrexate are administered to patients with ALL, osteosarcoma, and non-Hodgkin lymphoma in order to increase intracellular drug concentration and polyglutamate formation. These potentially lethal doses (3–20 g/m^2) are infused over 6–24 h, and are followed several hours later by intravenous leucovorin (5-formyl-tetrahydrofolate), 15–100 mg/m^2, which restores the intracellular pool of tetrahydrofolates and rescues normal tissue from drug toxicity. Various regimens have proven safe and effective, and should be followed strictly to assure lack of toxicity. Because of the tendency of methotrexate to precipitate in the renal tubules at acid pH, patients require alkalinization of the urine prior to drug administration, and profuse hydration and diuresis during methotrexate infusion to prevent renal shut down (10). Drug levels in plasma and renal function should be monitored post infusion. Concentrations of methotrexate above 1 μM at 24 h after the completion of infusion, usually in conjunction with evidence of renal failure, should alert clinicians to impending serious toxicity. The first step should be to increase and extend leucovorin administration (up to 500 mg every 6 h), along with hydration to prevent drug precipitation in the renal tubules. In extreme cases, when drug levels remain above 10 μM and show a very slow decline, leucovorin may be ineffective, and other measures need to be instituted. Continuous flow hemodialysis is able to reduce drug levels at a clearance rate of about 50 ml/min, but very rapid clearance of drug and effective rescue from toxicity can be achieved through the use of a bacterial folate-cleaving enzyme, Carboxypeptidase G-2, which is available from the Cancer Therapy Evaluation Program at the National Cancer Institute (11). Greater than 95% clearance of drug from plasma is achieved within 15 min of administration of 50 units/kg, and life-threatening toxicity will be avoided in most, but not all, patients.

Methotrexate is routinely administered intrathecally in doses of 12 mg for prevention or treatment of meningeal lymphoma, leukemia, or meningeal carcinomatosis. In patients with no evidence of meningeal tumor, the drug clears with a half-life of 2 h from the cerebral spinal fluid. In patients with active meningeal tumor, its clearance may be slowed and it may penetrate poorly into the ventricles, requiring the placement of a reservoir for direct intraventricular therapy. High-dose methotrexate regimens do produce modestly cytotoxic drug concentrations in the spinal fluid. Intrathecal use, particularly in patients with active meningeal disease and slow drug clearance, may lead to arachnoiditis, seizures, coma, and death (12). High-dose systemic methotrexate may rarely cause seizures or status epilepticus. Leucovorin is not an effecter antidote to CWS toxicity.

Alimta pharmacokinetics closely follow those of methotrexate, with a 3 h terminal half-life in plasma, clearance by renal excretion, and dose adjustment for renal dysfunction. The usual dose of Alimta administration is 500 mg/m^2 every 3 weeks, with B-12 and folate supplementation as described previously.

Toxicity

Virtually every organ system may be affected by antifolate toxicity. Acutely, bone marrow suppression, mucositis, and gastrointestinal symptoms are the primary side effects, and usually resolve within 10–14 days of completion of therapy. High-dose methotrexate may be accompanied by very minimal evidence of toxicity, aside from acute and completely reversible elevations in hepatic enzymes in the peripheral blood. Cirrhosis is occasionally reported in psoriasis or rheumatoid arthritis patients on long-term oral methotrexate, and is heralded by elevations in plasma type III procollagen aminopeptide (PIIIAP). Patients with elevated PIIIAP levels in plasma are at 20% risk of drug-related cirrhosis and should undergo a liver biopsy (13). An interstitial pneumonitis, likely related to hypersensitivity to the drug, with eosinophilic infiltrates, is occasionally seen with methotrexate. As stated previously, renal dysfunction, usually completely reversible with hydration, may result from high-dose therapy.

Alimta is toxic to bone marrow and gastrointestinal and oral mucosa. Toxicity tends to be predictably mild in patients receiving concurrent folic acid and B-12. Early trials without vitamin protection witnessed a significant (15–20%) incidence of severe toxicity, primarily in patients with high levels of homocysteine in plasma, an indicator of folate deficiency, prior to treatment. Pulmonary toxicity, manifested as an interstitial pneumonitis, may complicate therapy with Alimta (14). Up to 40% of patients may experience a bothersome erythematous rash, which can be largely prevented by dexamethasone, 4 mg twice daily on days –1,0, and +1 of treatment.

REFERENCES

1. Farber S, Diamond LK, Mercer RD, et al. Temporary remission in acute leukemia in children produced by folic acid antagonist 4-amethopteroylglutamic acid (aminopterin). N Engl J Med. 1948; 238: 787.
2. Allegra CJ, Hoang K, Yeh CG, et al. Evidence for direct inhibition of de novo purine synthesis in human MCF-7 breast cells as a principal mode of metabolic inhibition by methotrexate. J Biol Chem. 1985; 260: 9720–9726.
3. Moscow JA, Gong M, He R, et al. Isolation of a gene encoding a human reduced folate carrier (RFC1) and analysis of its expression in transport deficient, methotrexate-resistant human breast cancer cells. Cancer Res. 1995; 55: 3790–3794.
4. Whitehead VM, Shuster JJ, Vuchich MJ, et al. Accumulation of methotrexate and methotrexate polyglutamates in lymphoblasts and treatment outcome in children with B-progenitor-cell acute lymphoblastic leukemia: a Pediatric Oncology Group study. Leukemia. 2005; 19: 533–536.
5. Longo GS, Gorlick R, Tong W, Lin S, Steinherz P, Bertino JR. Gamma-glutamyl hydrolase and folylpolyglutamate synthetase activities predict polyglutamylation of methotrexate in acute leukemia. Oncol Res. 1997; 9: 259.
6. Kager L, Cheok M, Yang W, et al. Folate pathway gene expression differs in subtypes of acute lymphoblastic leukemia and influences methotrexate pharmacodynamics. J Clin Invest. 2005; 115: 110–117.
7. Aplenc R, Thompson J, Han P, La M, Zhao H, Lange B, Rebbeck T. Methylenetetrahydrofolate reductase polymorphisms and therapy response in pediatric acute lymphoblastic leukemia. Cancer Res. 2005; 65: 2482–2487.
8. Walling J. From methotrexate to pemetrexed and beyond: a review of the pharmacodynamic and clinical properties of antifolates. Invest New Drugs. 2006; 24: 37–77.
9. Scagliotti GV, Shin DM, Kindler HL, et al. Phase II study of pemetrexed with and without folic acid and vitamin B12 as front-line therapy in malignant pleural mesothelioma. J Clin Oncol. 2003; 21(14): 1556–1561.

10. Stoller RG, Hande KR, Jacobs SA, et al. Use of plasma pharmacokinetics to predict and prevent methotrexate toxicity. N Engl J Med. 1977; 297: 630–634.

11. Buchen S, Ngampolo D, Melton RG, Hasan C, Zoubek A, Henze G, Bode U, Fleischhack G. Carboxypeptidase G2 rescue in patients with methotrexate intoxication and renal failure. Br J Cancer. 2005; 92: 480–487.

12. Glantz MJ, Cole BF, Recht L, et al. High-dose intravenous methotrexate for patients with nonleukemic leptomeningeal cancer: is intrathecal chemotherapy necessary? J Clin Oncol. 1998; 16: 1561–1567.

13. Chalmers RJ, Kirby B, Smith A, et al. Replacement of routine liver biopsy by procollagen III aminopeptide for monitoring patients with psoriasis receiving long-term methotrexate: a multicentre audit and health economic analysis. Br J Dermatol. 2005; 152: 444–450.

14. Cohen MH, Johnson JR, Wang YC, Sridhara R, Pazdur R. FDA drug approval summary: pemetrexed for injection (Alimta) for the treatment of non-small cell lung cancer. Oncologist. 2005; 10: 363–368.

THE TAXANES AND THEIR DERIVATIVES

INTRODUCTION

In the past decade, the taxanes have emerged as one of the most powerful group of compounds active against malignant tumors. Two taxanes are approved for clinical use (paclitaxel and docetaxel). An albumin-stabilized paclitaxel (Abraxane) is also available for treatment of breast cancer. Despite their similar structures and a common mechanism of action, the two taxanes differ in their pharmacological profiles and their patterns of clinical activity. Taxanes are predominantly employed in solid tumor chemotherapy in combination with platinum derivatives, with other cytotoxics, or with monoclonal antibodies such as herceptin (traztuzumab). Both taxanes act synergistically with trastuzumab against Her2/neu overexpressed breast cancer cells in vitro and in vivo and lead to an improved response rate and an extension of time to progression in previously untreated metastatic breast cancer patients. Docetaxel appears to be somewhat more active than paclitaxel against breast cancer but is also more myelotoxic. The two taxanes differ in their interaction with doxorubicin, paclitaxel potentiating the anthracycline's cardiac toxicity, while docetaxel and doxorubicin are a well tolerated and highly active combination, both for metastatic disease and adjuvant therapy (3). The taxanes are active in a number of other malignant tumors including ovarian, lung, and bladder cancer.

STRUCTURE

Paclitaxel is a diterpenoid first isolated from the bark of the Pacific yew, Taxus brevifolia, while docetaxel, a semisynthetic analog of paclitaxel, is synthesized from 10-deacetylbaccatin III, a precursor found in the leaves of the European yew Taxus baccata (4). Both molecules are complex esters containing a 15-member taxane ring system linked to a four-member oxetan ring at the C-4 and C-5 positions of the molecule. The structures of paclitaxel and docetaxel differ in substitutions at the C-10 taxane ring position and on the ester side chain attached at the C-13 ring position. Docetaxel is slightly more water-soluble than paclitaxel and a more potent inhibitor of tubulin in cell free systems. The substitutions at C-13 position are essential for antimicrotubule activity. The chemical structures of paclitaxel and docetaxel are shown in Figure 3-1.

MECHANISM OF ACTION

The taxanes are microtubule stabilizers. They bind to the interior surface of the β-microtubule chain and enhance microtubule assembly by promoting the nucleation and elongation phases of the polymerization reaction and by reducing the critical tubulin subunit concentration required for microtubules to assemble. Unlike the vinca alkaloids, which prevent microtubule assembly, the taxanes decrease the lag time and dramatically shift the dynamic equilibrium between tubulin dimers and microtubule polymers toward polymerization (5).

The β-tubulin binding sites are distinct from those of vinca alkaloids, podophyllotoxin, colchicines, and exchangeable GTP. Paclitaxel binds reversibly to amino acid residues at 217–233 positions, and requires a higher

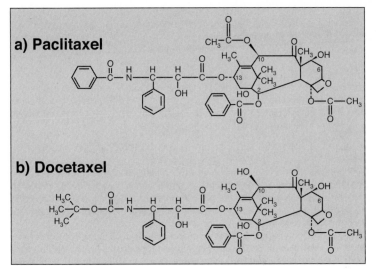

FIGURE 3-1   The chemical structure of taxanes.

concentration of tubulin than does docetaxel in order to stabilize microtubules. The initial slope of the assembly reaction and the amount of polymer formed are also greater for a given concentration of docetaxel, as compared to paclitaxel. These effects are accompanied by an increase in bundles of stabilized microtubules, which can be visualized by special stains for microtubules in treated cells. Disruption of the orderly array of microtubules not only halts progression through mitosis, but also alters signaling pathways and promotes apoptosis. Taxanes block the antiapoptotic effects of the BCL-2 gene family, and induce p53 gene activation with consequent mitotic arrest, formation of multinucleated cells, and cell death. Of additional interest are the biological effects of paclitaxel and docetaxel as inhibitors of angiogenesis, leading to the use of paclitaxel on coated intracoronary stents. It is not known whether the antiangiogenic effects of these drugs contribute to their antitumor activity. Finally, paclitaxel and docetaxel enhance the cytotoxic effects of radiation at clinically achievable concentrations.

DRUG RESISTANCE

Two major mechanisms of acquired taxane resistance in vitro have been characterized (6). Taxanes are one of several drugs affected by multidrug resistance (MDR) as mediated through increased expression of the 170-kilodalton P-glycoprotein efflux pump encoded by the MDR1 gene. The p-glycoprotein promotes rapid efflux of taxanes, anthracyclines, and vinca alkaloids, as well as other natural products. MDR resistance can be reversed in animal test systems by calcium channel blockers, tamoxifen, hormones, cyclosporine A, and even by cremaphor, the principal lipid used to formulate paclitaxel. The precise role of MDR-1 in conferring resistance to the taxanes in the clinical setting is not firmly established. For example, clinical observations to date suggest that in breast cancer, there is incomplete cross-resistance between taxanes and anthracyclines, implying that MDR-1 expression is not responsible for drug resistance in some cases. This finding supports the combined use of taxanes and anthracycline in clinical chemotherapy. A second form of resistance to taxanes is seen in cells that express an altered β-tubulin phenotype. These cells have an impaired ability to polymerize tubulin dimers into microtubules. Amplification of β-tubulin encoding genes, mutation of the β-tubulin binding sites and isotype switching of β-tubulin all have been reported in taxane resistant cell lines.

Two additional mechanisms potentially responsible for taxane resistance have also been reported: (1) upregulation of caveolin-1, a protein that acts as a scaffold for intracellular kinases and participates in the formation of membrane-derived vesicles involved in transmembrane drug transport, and (2) increased expression of genes that inhibit the apoptotic cycle, such as BCL-2.

CLINICAL PHARMACOLOGY AND METABOLISM

The taxanes are active in their parent form. Their metabolites are inactive. The oral bio-availability of either paclitaxel and docetaxel is poor owing in part to the constitutive overexpression of P-glycoprotein and other ABC transporters in intestinal epithelium, and first-pass metabolism of taxanes in the liver or intestines.

The metabolism of taxanes is mediated through hepatic cytochrome P450 mixed-function oxidases. Paclitaxel is metabolized to one primary metabolite, 6α-OH paclitaxel, to a lesser extent to C3′-OH, and to a minor extent to the dihydroxyl metabolite (7). The formation of hydroxylated metabolites results from stepwise catalysis by cytochrome 2C8 producing 6α-OH and CYP3A4 producing 6α-OH-3′OH. Docetaxel is oxidized at C13 by CYP3A4. The involvement of cytochrome enzymes in taxane biotransformation has two important implications: first, comedications capable of inducing or inhibiting cytochromes influence the rate of inactivation and the metabolic fate of taxanes. Second, polymorphisms have been described for both 2C8 and 3A4 of cytochrome isoforms, thereby providing an explanation for the interpatient variability of pharmacokinetics.

The taxanes are commonly administered by intravenous infusion. Pharmacokinetic data for paclitaxel and docetaxel are shown in Table 3-1.

Table 3-1

Comparative Pharmacokinetic Characteristics of Taxanes

Characteristic	Paclitaxel	Docetaxel
Dose and schedule	135–175 mg/m², 3 h infusion every 3 weeks	75–100 mg/m², 1 h infusion every 3 weeks
Pharmacokinetic behavior	Nonlinear	Linear
Volume of distribution	182 l/m²	74 l/m²
Plasma protein binding	>95%	>90%
Peak plasma concentration	5–10 μM (175 mg/m²/3 h)	2–5 μM (100mg/m²/1 h)
Average terminal plasma half-life/h	11.5	12
Tissue distribution	Extensive except CNS and testes	Extensive except CNS
Clearance	~350 ml/min/m²	300 ml/min/m²
Primary route of clearance	Hepatic metabolism and biliary elimination	Hepatic metabolism and biliary elimination
Renal clearance	<10%	<10%

Table 3-2

Pharmacokinetic Parameters For Paclitaxel

Dose range mg/m²	Infusion duration (h)	Peak plasma concentration (μM)	AUC (ng/ml/h)	Terminal half-life (h)	Clearance (l/h/m²)
100–135	1	6.0–19.3	9918–35018	10.6–15.8	8.05–11.64
135–175	3	1.3–4.3	6568–15007	6.3–20.2	12.2–17.2
135–175	24	0.2–0.4	6300–7993	15.7–24.6	21.7–23.8

Paclitaxel

Pharmacokinetic studies have disclosed substantial interpatient variabilities and nonlinearity of the relationship between paclitaxel dose and drug concentration in plasma (Table 3-2).

The pharmacokinetics of this drug have been evaluated in doses ranging from 100 to up to 300 mg/m² infused in time periods of 1, 3, and 24 h. Following intravenous administration, the drug exhibits a biphasic decline in plasma concentration, reaching peak concentrations between 5 and 10 μM on most schedules, and remaining in the inhibitory range for myelopoiesis (above 50 nM) for 12–24 h. Both the terminal half-life of 24 h and the mean clearance of paclitaxel appear to either remain unchanged or may slightly increase as the infusion time is increased. Approximately 80% of paclitaxel is excreted in feces in the form of metabolites, 6α-hydroxy-paclitaxel accounting for 20% of the dose. Renal clearance of paclitaxel and its metabolites is minor, accounting for about 15% of administered dose and only 5% is excreted unchanged. The dose should be reduced by 50% in patients with a bilirubin greater than 1.5 mg/dl, and the drug should be withheld in patients with severe hepatic dysfunction.

Docetaxel

The pharmacokinetic behavior of docetaxel on a 1 h schedule at doses of 75–115 mg/m² or less is linear. The terminal half-life is about 16.7 h and clearance 22.7 l/h/m². As with paclitaxel, docetaxel is widely distributed among tissues except for central nervous system.

DRUG INTERACTIONS

Because of its reliance for clearance upon the P450 system, there are many opportunities for drug interactions of taxanes with other cancer drugs. Clinically significant taxane interactions are shown in Table 3-3. Pharmacokinetic interactions of taxanes with other antineoplastic agents may be sequence dependent, a first shown for the combination of paclitaxel and cisplatin and later confirmed for the combination of docetaxel and cisplatin (8). Cisplatin, when administered prior to paclitaxel, causes a significantly higher incidence of neutropenia as a result of a 25% reduction in paclitaxel clearance. Reversing the sequence eliminates this detrimental effect. The combination of carboplatin and paclitaxel has emerged as safe and well tolerated, causing less thrombocytopenia than the administration of carboplatin alone.

Paclitaxel preceding doxorubicin increases the frequency of mucositis, cardiotoxicity, and neutropenia than would be anticipated from additive effects of the two drugs. Pharmacokinetic studies indicate that paclitaxel decreases doxorubicin clearance. Administration of these drugs 24 h apart may ameliorate this effect.

Alternating sequences of paclitaxel and cyclophosphamide revealed that cytopenias were profound when paclitaxel was infused first. Docetaxel given

Table 3-3

Clinically Significant Taxane–Drug Interaction

Paclitaxel and doceel	Interacting drug	Mechanism	Comment
	Doxorubicin epirubicin	Increased C_{max} and decreased clearance of doxorubicin	Administer doxorubicin before paclitaxel
	Cisplatin	Decreased taxane clearance	Administer taxane 24 h before cisplatinum
	Carboplatin	Increased carboplatin clearance, decrease in thrombocytopenia	
	Anticonvulsants	CYP induction decreases plasma concentration and increases clearance of paclitaxel	Increase dose of taxane
	Warfarin	Taxane displaces coumadin from protein-binding sites	Decrease dose of coumadin
	Gemcitabine	Increased level of gemcitabine triphosphate by unknown mechanism	Decrease dose of gemcitabine

before ifosfamide increases the clearance of the alkylator, and dose-limiting toxicity occurred at lower doses of docetaxel when ifosfamide preceded the taxane (9).

Enzyme-inducing anticonvulsants increase cyp3A4 activity, accelerate taxane clearance, and markedly increase the dose of paclitaxel requires to reach cytotoxicity. Treating patients on taxanes with CYP3A inhibitors, such as ketoconazol profoundly, slows taxane clearance.

TOXICITY

Neutropenia is the principal and dose-limiting toxicity of both taxanes. The severity and frequency of paclitaxel induced neutropenia increases when infusion is prolonged from 3 to 24 h and at doses above 175 mg/m². However, neutropenia is noncumulative, and its duration even in heavily pretreated patients, is usually brief. Weekly treatments with lower doses of 80–100 mg/m² of paclitaxel yield antitumor activity equivalent to higher doses given every three weeks in breast and nonsmall cell lung cancer. Severe thrombocytopenia and anemia are uncommon except in heavily pretreated patients.

Paclitaxel administration causes a high incidence of acute hypersensitivity reactions in the absence of antihistamines and corticosteroids; the cremaphor solvent contributes significantly to this reaction. The incidence and intensity of hypersensitivity to paclitaxel are significantly diminished by preventive treatment with dexamethasone and histamine inhibitors, diphenhydramine, and ranitidine.

Cardiac arrhythmias, especially asymptomatic bradycardias, are seen after paclitaxel. The presence of an implanted pacemaker or a prior history of cardiac conduction disturbances is a relative contraindication to its use. As discussed previously, paclitaxel increases the incidence of anthracycline-induced congestive heart failure (CHF), when the two drugs are used together. There is no conclusive evidence for an increased rate of CHF in patients receiving docetaxel/anthracycline combinations. Neither taxane increases the cardiac toxicity of herceptin. Dose-related myalgia and neuropathy, especially an increase in neurosensory symptoms (numbness in a symmetrical glove and stocking distribution), may become significant complaints with paclitaxel, particularly with higher doses and when used with cisplatin. Neurotoxicity is more frequently associated with shorter (1–3 h) infusion schedules indicating that peak plasma concentrations are a principal determinant. Mild to moderate peripheral neurotoxicity occurs in approximately 40% of patients receiving paclitaxel, especially with those who had received cisplatin, but asthenia and muscular weakness have been a prominent complaint in patients who have been treated with large cumulative doses and on a long-term weekly schedule (10).

The toxicity of docetaxel closely mimics that of paclitaxel with several important exceptions. Docetaxel is more myelosuppressive at clinically useful doses. Stomatitis appears to be a more frequently side effect of docetaxel than paclitaxel. Nausea, vomiting, and diarrhea have been observed with both taxanes, but severe gastrointestinal toxicity is uncommon.

During its early phases of development, docetaxel treatment led to a cumulative fluid retention syndrome in approximately 50% of patients after three to five cycles of therapy. Ankle edema, pleural effusions, and even ascites may become dose limiting. Premedication with dexamethasone, 8 mg twice daily for 3–5 days, beginning 1 day before drug administration, significantly decreases the severity and incidence of the fluid retention syndrome.

FORMULATION AND ADMINISTRATION

Paclitaxel

Taxanes are insoluble in water. Paclitaxel is formulated in 50% alcohol and 50% polyoxyethylated castor oil derivative. An initial dose of 135 mg/m^2 of paclitaxel on a 24 h schedule was approved for patients with refractory or recurrent ovarian cancer, but later regulatory approval was obtained for a dose of 175 mg/m^2 on a 3 h schedule in ovarian cancer as well as for other indications. Data obtained from mostly ovarian and breast cancer patients treated on different schedules of 3, 24, and 96 h every 3 weeks indicated that the various schedules were largely equally effective with regard to disease free and overall survival (11). Later trials limited the infusion duration to 3 h, or even 1 h with the weekly regimen. The recommended dose of paclitaxel as a single agent or in combination now ranges from 135 to 250 mg/m^2, generally as a 3 h infusion repeated every 3 weeks.

In general, children tolerate higher doses of paclitaxel and the recommended phase II dose for a 24 h infusion was 350 mg/m^2 for pediatric studies (12).

Docetaxel

Docetaxel is formulated in polysorbate 80, and it can be administered after dilution in 0.9% saline, or 5% dextrose solution to a confirmed concentration of between 0.3 mg/ml and 0.9 mg/ml. It is administered in doses of 60–100 mg/m^2 over 1 h every 3 weeks in patients with breast and nonsmall cell lung cancers, respectively. Weekly schedules of 30–40 mg/m^2 have been associated with a higher incidence of cumulative muscular weakness and neurotoxicity. This toxicity was especially noticeable with docetaxel doses exceeding 36 mg/m^2.

NOVEL TAXANES OF CLINICAL IMPORTANCE

Attempts at developing more active, less toxic, and orally administered taxanes are summarized in Table 3-4.

Table 3-4

The Characteristics of Novel Taxanes

Analogue	Characteristics	Potential advantage	Preliminary clinical activity in phase I/II studies
Abraxane	Albumin stabilized 100–200 nm paclitaxel particles	Delivers 50% more drug to tumor, improved safety profile	Equal or better against breast cancer, longer time to tumor progression
Tocosol	Vitamin E-based emulsion of paclitaxel	Shorter infusion time (15 min), reduced side effects, better efficacy	Partial regression according to RECIST criteria, or stabilized disease in 61% of breast cancer patients
LEP-EDU	Liposome entrapped paclitaxel	Designed for urothelial cancers, less toxicity	Thus far activity seems to be comparable to that of classic paclitaxel
Xyotax	Paclitaxel-based polymer conjugate	Improved therapeutic index, favorable safety profile, shorter administration time, minimal side effects	Objective response rates varry from 33% in metastatic colorectal to over 45% in platinum resistant ovarian cancers
BMS-784476	7-methylthiomethyl ether derivative of paclitaxel	More soluble in aqueous solvents, markedly reduced concentration of castor oil, shorter administration schedule, no severe allergies	Seems to be more potent than classic taxanes
MST-997	Intralipid-trapped paclitaxel	Improved pharmacokinetic characteristics, favourable toxicity profile	Objective responses in various cancers in early trials
DHA-paclitaxel	Conjugate of docosahexanoic fatty acid and paclitaxel	sixfold increase in drug delivery, increased activity, improved therapeutic ratio	Awaiting clinical data

REFERENCES

1. Eisenhauer EA, Vermorken JB. The taxoids: comparative clinical pharmacology and therapeutic potential. Drugs. 1998; 55(1): 55–30.

2. Gradishar WJ, Tjulandin S, Davidson N, Shaw H, Desai N, Bhar P, Hawkins M, O'Shaughnessy J. Phase III trial of nanoparticle albumin-bound paclitaxel compared with polyethylated castor oil-based paclitaxel in women with breast cancer. J Clin Oncol. 2005; 23: 7794–7803.

3. Crown J, O'Leary M, Wei-Seong O. Docetaxel and paclitaxel in the treatment of breast cancer: a review of clinical experience. Oncologist. 2004; 9(suppl.2): 24–32.

4. Wani MC, Taylor HL, Wall ME, Coggan P, McPhail AT. Plant antitumor agents. VI. The isolation and structure of taxol, a novel antileukemic and antitumor agent from *Taxus brevifolia*. J Am Chem Soc. 1971; 93: 2325–2327.

5. Dumontet C, Sikic BI. Mechanism of action of and resistance to anti-tubulin agents; microtubule dynamics, drug transport and cell death. J Clin Oncol. 1999; 17: 1061–1070.

6. Orr AG, Verdier-Pinnard P, McDaid H, Horwitz BS. Mechanisms of taxol resistance related to microtubules. Oncogene. 2003; 22: 7280–7295.

7. Vaishampayan U, Parchament ER, Jasti RB, Maha H. Taxanes: an overview of pharmacokinetics and pharmacodynamics. Urology. 1999; 54(6): 22–29.

8. Baker AF, Dorr RT. Drug interactions with the taxanes: clinical implications. Cancer Treat Rev. 2001; 27: 221–233.

9. Viganol L, Locatelli A, Granelli G, Gianni L. Drug interactions of paclitaxel and docetaxel and their relevance for the design of combination chemotherapy. Invest. New Drugs. 2001; 19: 179–196.

10. Rowinsky EC. Taxanes: paclitaxel (taxol) and docetaxel (taxotere). In "Cancer Medicine," 6th edition, BC Decker, Hamilton, Canada, 2003.

11. Ghersi D, Wilcken N, Simers RJ. A systematic review of taxane-containing regimens for metastatic breast cancer. Br J Cancer. 2002; 93: 293–301.

12. Hurwitz CA, Relling VM, Weitman SD, Yadanapoudi R, Vietti TJ, Strother DR, Ragab AS, Pratt CB. Phase I trial of paclitaxel in children with refractory solid tumors: a pediatric Oncology group study. J Clin Oncol. 1993; 11: 2324–2329.

VINCA ALKALOIDS

The vinca alkaloids, derived from the vinca rosacea plant, have been a mainstay of the treatment of hematologic malignancies for almost 50 years. They were first discovered in an in vitro antileukemic screen at Eli Lilly and Co. in the early 1950s, and reached prominence in the combination therapy of childhood acute lymphocytic leukemia and Hodgkin Disease a decade later. They continue as part of curative regimens for the lymphomas and testicular cancer, and new derivatives (vinorelbine and vindesine) have proven active in other solid tumors. The vinca alkaloids are similar in structure and share common pharmacologic properties, but differ in their profile of toxicity and specific disease indications (Figure 4-1).

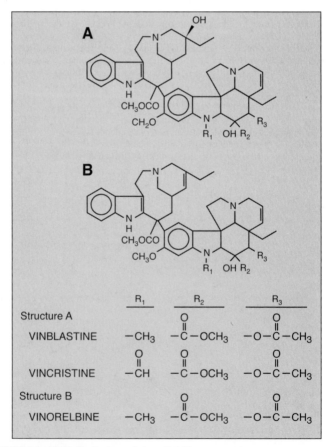

FIGURE 4-1 Metabolic structures of vinca alkaloids.

MECHANISM OF ACTION

The vincas bind to a common site on beta tubulin and prevent dimerization of tubulin alpha and beta subunits to form microtubules (1). They block cells in mitosis due to the absence of a microtubular apparatus required for chromosomal separation. Apoptosis follows. Resistance arises through up-regulation or amplification of one of several drug exporters, including the MDR gene product (p-glycoprotein), or through mutations in the tubulin-binding site (2). The latter mutations appear to stabilize microtubules and slow its rate of disassembly; in contrast mutations that destabilize microtubules confer resistance to taxanes. A variety of changes may affect the apoptosis pathway, such as increased expression of bcl-2 and can lead to vinca resistance as well.

In addition to their effects on microtubules, the vincas, like the taxanes and other antimitotics drugs, have potent antiangiogenic activity, inhibiting proliferation of human endothelial cells in culture at subnanomolar concentrations, below concentrations that inhibit sensitive tumor cells.

Clinical Pharmacology

The drugs share a common pharmacokinetic pattern of inactivation through hepatic metabolism by P-450 isoenzymes, primarily CYP3A4, and have long half-lives in plasma of up to several days. Vincristine has the longest terminal plasma $t_{1/2}$ (23–85 h), while vinorelbine is intermediate (18–49 h) and vinblastine is the most rapidly cleared ($t_{1/2}$ of 24 h), clearance depending on hepatic function. While there is no clear relationship of vinca clearance to any single liver function test, patients with abnormal hepatic function (bilirubin > 1.5 mg/dl) should receive no more than 50% of a full dose for their initial infusion (3). The drugs are given intravenously as bolus infusions every 1–3 weeks, depending on the regimen employed. Usual single doses of the vinca alkaloids are vincristine, 1–2 mg lm; vinorelbine, 15–30 mg lm^2; and vinblastine, 6–8 mg lm^2.

TOXICITY

All vinca alkaloids cause neurotoxicity, primarily a peripheral sensory neuropathy. Vincristine is the most highly neurotoxic, may cause motor dysfunction in severely toxic patients, and should not be given to patients with significant neurologic dysfunction due to other drugs, diabetes, stroke, or inherited neurologic disease. Neurotoxicity due to Vinorelbine occurs with repeated cycles of therapy, but is usually mild and reversible. Vinblastine has minimal neurotoxicity, but like vinorelbine is a potent myelosuppressant, with rapid recovery of blood counts in 10–14 days. Vincristine has little effect on the bone marrow. In high doses (not used in common practice) vincristine causes prolonged abdominal distention and ileus.

Because the vinca alkaloids depend for their clearance on CYP-3A4, the most important drug metabolizing enzyme in the liver, drug interactions are likely if the vincas are given with inducers or inhibitors of CYP-3A4 (4). Thus Dilantin induces vinca clearance, and vincas may accelerate Dilantin metabolism and lead to seizures in patients treated with both drugs. Imidazole antifungal drugs, such as ketoconazole or itraconazole, inhibit CYP-3A4 and slow vinca clearance, leading to severe toxicity if the dose of vinca alkaloid is not reduced.

REFERENCES

1. Jordan MA, Wilson L. Microtubules as a target for anticancer drugs. Nat Rev Cancer. 2004; 4: 253.

2. Grant CE, Valdmarsson G, Hipfner R, et al. Overexpression of multidrug resistance associated protein (MRP) increases resistance to natural product drugs. Cancer Res. 1994; 54: 356.

3. Robieux I, Sorio R, Borsatti E, Cannizzaro R, Vitali V, Aita P, Freschi A, Galligioni E, Monfardini S. Pharmacokinetics of vinorelbine in patients with liver metastases. Clin Pharmacol Ther. 1996; 59: 32–40.

4. Villikka K, Kivisto KT, Maenpaa H, Joensuu H, Neuvonen PJ. Cytochrome P450-inducing antiepileptics increase the clearance of vincristine in patients with brain tumors. Clin Pharmacol Ther. 1999; 66: 589–93.

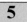
TOPOISOMERASE INHIBITORS: CAMPTOTHECINS, ANTHRACYCLINES, AND ETOPOSIDE

INTRODUCTION

The camptothecins are a class of antineoplastic agents that inhibit the enzyme topoisomerase I and that have activity in several different tumors. Camptothecin was originally isolated from the Chinese tree *Camptotheca acuminata* in 1966 and was demonstrated to have antitumor effects in animal systems. Topotecan (Hycamptin) and irinotecan (Camptosar), two agents in this class, have been subsequently approved for clinical use in the United States by the FDA. Topotecan is currently used as second-line chemotherapy for ovarian cancer and small cell lung cancer (SCLC). Irinotecan is indicated for the treatment of metastatic colon cancer, both as first-line and salvage therapy, and has been incorporated into combination regimens to treat small cell lung, gynecologic, and upper gastrointestinal malignancies and glioblastoma multiforme. This chapter reviews the mechanistic, pharmacokinetic, and clinical properties of the camptothecins and provides some insight into future directions for development of these drugs.

CAMPTOTHECINS: STRUCTURE AND FUNCTION

Structure

The camptothecins are based on a five-ring structure in which a quinolone moiety on one end is joined to an α-hydroxy-δ-lactone ring on the other end (Figure 5-1). The electrophilic center of the lactone subunit is responsible for the camptothecins' biological activity. At the same time, the lactone is also vulnerable to reversible hydrolysis to a less active carboxylate species at neutral and alkaline pH. Substitutions of the C-9 and C-10 positions on the quinolone ring can enhance the potency of topoisomerase inhibition by stabilizing the lactone form over the carboxylate form in human blood (1).

Mechanisms of Action

Camptothecin and its analogs exert their antitumor activity by inhibiting the enzyme DNA topoisomerase I, a nuclear enzyme that relieves torsional strain in supercoiled DNA during replication and transcription (Figure 5-2). It accomplishes this action by forming a transient, intermediate complex with single-stranded DNA that allows either for passage of the intact single strand through the nicked strand and/or for rotation about the intact strand. The camptothecins stabilize this otherwise transient topoisomerase I-DNA complex and prevent the enzyme from dissociating from single-stranded DNA, which eventually leads to double-stranded breaks and apoptosis. Since DNA synthesis is a prerequisite for this interaction, the camptothecins are S-phase specific drugs (1). The clinical implication is that tumor cells must be exposed to a minimum concentration of the drug for a prolonged period of time and, therefore, lower dose, infusional schedules may prove more efficacious and less toxic (2).

Mechanisms of Resistance

Several mechanisms of resistance to the camptothecins have been demonstrated in vitro, including the presence of the multidrug resistance (MDR) efflux pump, P-glycoprotein; cellular redistribution of topoisomerase I away from the nucleoli;

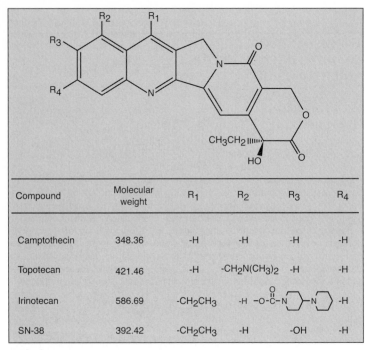

Compound	Molecular weight	R₁	R₂	R₃	R₄
Camptothecin	348.36	-H	-H	-H	-H
Topotecan	421.46	-H	-CH₂N(CH₃)₂	-H	-H
Irinotecan	586.69	-CH₂CH₃	-H	-O-C-N⬡-N⬡ (O)	-H
SN-38	392.42	-CH₂CH₃	-H	-OH	-H

FIGURE 5-1 Structure of the camptothecins.

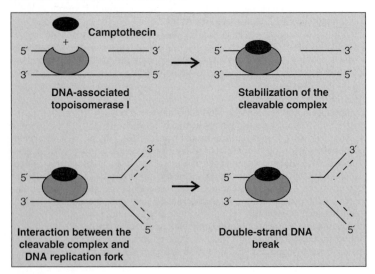

FIGURE 5-2 Mechanism of the camptothecins. (Used with permission from www.scielo.br.)

down-regulation of topoisomerase I expression; mutations in the catalytic or DNA binding sites of topoisomerase I; up-regulation of topoisomerase II; and up-regulation of NFκB and inhibition of chemotherapy-induced apoptosis. The clinical significance of these mechanisms of resistance observed in vitro is unclear. For example, topotecan is the only member of this class of agents that is unequivocally a substrate for the MDR efflux pump, P-glycoprotein, yet tumor models that overexpress MDR are not particularly resistant to topotecan (1).

CAMPTOTHECINS: CLINICAL APPLICATIONS

Topotecan

PHARMACOKINETICS   Topotecan (Hycamptin) is a semisynthetic derivative of camptothecin in which an N,N-dimethylaminomethyl substituent at C-9 allows for greater solubility. A great deal of pharmacokinetic data have been gathered about topotecan in both adult and pediatric cancer patients. Topotecan is usually given as a 30 min intravenous infusion. Plasma concentrations of the inactive carboyxlate species begin to predominate over the active lactone form within 5–10 min after the end of infusion. Topotecan can also be given orally and the bioavailability ranges from 30 to 40%. The degree of absorption is not affected by taking it with food, although there is a slight delay to peak plasma concentration (1).

The plasma half-life of topotecan is 2.4–4.3 h. Topotecan is eliminated primarily by plasma hydrolysis to the inactive carboxylate form followed by renal excretion. Approximately one-third to one-half of unmetabolized drug is seen in the urine. The clearance of plasma total topotecan is reduced by 33% in patients with creatinine clearance between 40 and 59 ml/min and by 75% in patients with creatinine clearance between 20 and 39 m/min. There is no significant change in elimination or toxicity in patients with liver disease, even in patients with total bilirubin levels up to 10 mg/dl. There is evidence to suggest that administration of cisplatin decreases topotecan clearance, presumably through renal tubular damage. Topotecan pharmacokinetics are not altered in the presence other chemotherapies with which it has been combined, including anthracyclines, cyclophosphamide, cytarabine, etoposide, and paclitaxel (1).

DOSING AND SCHEDULE   The standard dosing schedule for topotecan is 1.5 mg/m^2 given as a 30 min intravenous infusion on 5 consecutive days, repeated every 21 days. Continuous infusion regimens ranging from 24 h infusions to 21 day infusions have been used in phase II clinical trials in attempts to take advantage of the in vitro observation that prolonged exposures of low concentrations are more efficacious than intermittent exposures to high concentrations. In experimental trials, topotecan has been given orally as 2.3 mg/m^2 daily for 5 consecutive days every 21 days (3).

TOXICITY   Neutropenia is the most significant dose-limiting toxicity for all schedules of topotecan administration, with grade 4 neutropenia in up to 81% of patients and febrile neutropenia in 26%. Severe neutropenia is observed even with a 33% reduction in dose in patients with moderate to severe renal dysfunction. Therefore, a 50% reduction to 0.75 mg/m^2 per day is recommended for previously untreated or minimally pretreated patients with creatinine clearance between 20 and 40 ml/min. Further reduction to a daily dose of 0.5 mg/m^2 is warranted in heavily pretreated patients with this degree of renal insufficiency. There is no dose modification required for patients with hepatic dysfunction. Nonhematologic toxicities of topotecan include nausea, vomiting, mucositis, elevated transaminases, fatigue, and rash. These side effects are generally minimal and easily managed (1).

CLINICAL INDICATIONS   The two FDA approved indications for topotecan are as a second-line agent in advanced, platinum refractory or resistant ovarian carcinoma and as a treatment for relapsed SCLC. Its use in relapsed ovarian cancer is supported by a phase III trial in which topotecan 1.5 mg/m²/day for 5 days was shown to have an equivalent response rate and improved median time to disease progression when compared to paclitaxel 175 mg/m² (4). There was no difference in overall survival and rates of hematologic toxicity were significantly greater in the topotecan arm.

The role for topotecan in SCLC was confirmed in a randomized study in which single-agent topotecan was compared to cyclophosphamide, doxorubicin (DX), and vincristine in relapsed SCLC (5). Response rates, time to disease progression, and overall survival were the same in both groups, but topotecan provided greater clinical benefit based on control of disease-related symptoms.

Topotecan has also demonstrated activity in some hematologic malignancies and pediatric malignancies, such as rhabdomyosarcoma, neuroblastoma, osteosarcoma, and retinoblastoma.

Irinotecan

PHARMACOKINETICS Irinotecan (Camptosar) is a congener of camptothecin specifically designed to facilitate the administration of its active metabolite, the 7-ethyl-10-hydroxy analog, SN-38, which is a 1000-fold more potent inhibitor of topoisomerase I than the parent, irinotecan. Irinotecan is converted primarily by hepatic carboxylesterases to SN-38. The half-life of the lactone (active) form of SN-38 is 11.5 h (1).

Irinotecan is primarily eliminated through the liver via two clinically relevant mechanisms (Figure 5-3). First, irinotecan is a substrate of the cytochrome P450 system and is metabolized in part by CYP2B6 and CYP3A4. It has been shown that irinotecan clearance is increased when administered to glioblastoma patients on phenobarbital or phenytoin for seizure prophylaxis (1). Second, irinotecan is converted to its active form, SN-38, and SN-38 is then glucuronidated and excreted in the biliary system. SN-38 undergoes glucuronidation by the polymorphic enzyme uridine diphosphoglucuronosyl-transferase (UGT1A1), which is also responsible for bilirubin glucuronidation. The activity of this enzyme is reduced in patients who are homozygous for the allele UGT1A1*28, which is the same defect seen in subjects with Gilbert's syndrome.

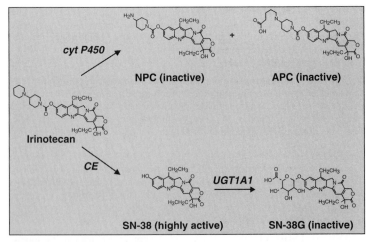

FIGURE 5-3 Metabolic pathway for irinotecan showing the conversion to inactive metabolites NPC and APC via cytochrome P450 enzymes and the conversion by liver carboxyxylesterase (CE) to the active form, SN-38, and its subsequent inactivation to SN-38G by the enzyme UGT1A1.

This deficiency is found in approximately 10% of patients. When treated with standard doses of irinotecan such patients are exposed to higher levels of plasma SN-38 and encounter higher rates of toxicity, particularly diarrhea and neutropenia (6). In patients with a personal or family history of Gilbert's, or with an unexplained elevated indirect bilirubin level, lower staring doses of irinotecan should be used. There is a commercially available test for the UGT1A1*28 polymorphism (Invader UGT1A1*28 Molecular Assay), although it has not been widely accepted in clinical practice. Several studies have suggested that polymorphisms in either UGT1A1 or drug transporter may account for differences in response rates and toxicities between Asian and Caucasian patients (7).

Oral bioavailability of irinotecan is only 8%, but the little irinotecan that is absorbed undergoes rapid first-pass conversion to SN-38 in the intestine and liver. Although actively under study, there is currently no role for oral irinotecan.

DOSING AND SCHEDULE   Irinotecan, as a single agent, can be given at a dose of 125 mg/m2 over a 90 min intravenous infusion every week for 4 of 6 weeks or at a dose 350 mg/m^2 over a 90 min intravenous infusion every 3 weeks. There are data to support equal efficacy in the weekly versus every 3 week administration, although there are lower rates of diarrhea with the every 3 week regimen (8). When given in combination with leucovorin and 5-FU, irinotecan is often given at 180 mg/m^2 as a 90 min infusion every 2 weeks (see Toxicity below). As with topotecan, regimens involving prolonged, lower dose continuous infusions are being explored in phase I trials to take advantage of the drug's S-phase specificity.

TOXICITY   The most common adverse effects of irinotecan are diarrhea, which can be life-threatening in some instances, myelosuppression, and a cholinergic syndrome consisting of nausea, vomiting, mucositis, and flushing. Interstitial pneumonitis has been reported in Japanese patients receiving irinotecan. Grade 3–4 diarrhea was observed in up to 35% of patients in early clinical studies. Irinotecan given at 125 mg/m^2 on a weekly basis for 4 of 6 weeks, when studied in combination with 5-FU and leucovorin in the Saltz regimen (9), led to toxic deaths due to severe diarrhea and neutropenia, leading to the widespread adoption of biweekly irinotecan at 180 mg/m^2, whether as single agent or combined with 5-FU and leucovorin (9). Loperamide starting at 4 mg should be given at the first sign of diarrhea and administered at 2 mg every 2 h until resolution of the diarrhea.

Myelosuppression is common with irinotecan use and grade 3–4 neutropenia occurs in 14–47% of patients, occurring more frequently in the every 3 week regimen than with weekly administration.

Irinotecan can inhibit acetylcholinesterase activity and can lead to a cholinergic syndrome characterized by acute diarrhea, diaphoresis, abdominal cramping, hypersalivation, lacrimation, rhinorrhea, and, occasionally, asymptomatic bradycardia. This constellation of symptoms responds rapidly to atropine.

CLINICAL INDICATIONS   Irinotecan is most commonly used in advanced colorectal cancer. Response rates of 10–35% were consistently noted in phase II trials examining single-agent irinotecan in patients with metastatic colon cancer. It is usually given to metastatic colorectal cancer patients at 180 mg/m^2 every 2 weeks, in combination with 5-FU, leucovorin, and bevacizumab as first-line therapy, or as second-line after failure of an oxaliplatin-based regimen (9, 10). It can also be given as a single agent in the second line or combined with cetuximab in irinotecan-refractory patients (11).

Single-agent activity of irinotecan is also seen in cervical cancer, ovarian cancer, gastric cancer, pancreatic cancer, and malignant gliomas.

CAMPTOTHECINS IN DEVELOPMENT

Several newer camptothecins have entered into early clinical trials, including exatecan (DX-8951f), rubitecan, OSI-211 (liposomal formulation of lurtotecan), and gimatecan, an orally available camptothecin. Gimatecan has demonstrated the greatest promise, with response rates ranging from 10 to 27% in phase II trials in advanced ovarian and breast cancer (12, 13).

TOPOISOMERASE INHIBITORS: ANTHRACYCLINES

Drugs of this class, derived from the fungal culture broths of S. peucetius, have become critical components of many regimens that contribute to the cure of a broad array of tumors, including leukemias, lymphomas, and breast cancer. The two original members of this family, daunorubicin (DN) and doxorubicin (DX), remain in active clinical practice, DN for acute myelogenous leukemia (AML), and DX for lymphomas and solid tumor chemotherapy. Two semisynthetic derivatives, idarubicin (IDA) and epirubicin (EPI), have made inroads as valuable agents for leukemia and breast cancer, respectively. Liposomal formulations of DN and DX have found limited niches. Each of the anthracyclines and the liposomal formulations have distinct pharmacological properties that have led to their continued clinical roles.

Mechanism of Action

The anthracyclines share a rigid planar four-ring structure complemented by a glycosidic substitution on the D ring and variable side groups of the A and D rings (Figure 5-4). The planar configuration allows anthracyclines to intercalate between strands of DNA, and this action was originally thought to be responsible for its inhibition of DNA synthesis. However, the anthracyclines possess other important features. The quinone on ring C readily undergoes oxidation/reduction cycling in the presence of metals such as Fe^{++}, producing free radicals from oxygen and/or lipids (14). These free radicals are believed to be responsible for the cardiac toxicity inherent in this class of agents. Most

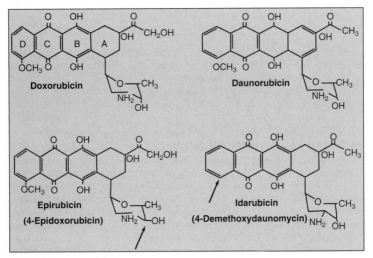

FIGURE 5-4   Anthracyclines in current clinical use. For epirubicin and idarubicin, arrows point to the sites where these new drugs differ from doxorubicin and daunomycin, respectively.

recently, it was shown that these drugs bind to and inhibit topoisomerase II (topo II), an enzyme which promotes DNA strand unwinding essential for DNA synthesis and repair. Topo II binds to DNA and creates a double strand break that allows strand passage. The anthracyclines bind to the covalent DNA–topo II complex, and the tripartite complex is sufficiently stable to prevent resealing of the strand break (15). Accumulation of strand breaks signals the p53 system to halt cell cycle progression, and to initiate DNA repair. If the breaks are sufficiently numerous, the cell undergoes apoptosis. The extrinsic apoptosis pathway, initiated by the fas receptor, may also play a role in anthracycline toxicity.

Levels of topo II expression correlate positively with response to DX in patients with breast cancer (16). Cells become resistant to anthracyclines through diminished expression of topo II activity or through topo II mutations that diminish binding affinity of the enzyme for the drugs of this class. An interesting correlation has been observed between amplification of the isoenzyme topo IIa and the Her 2/neu receptor. The topo IIa gene is located on chromosome 17 adjacent to the gene coding for the Her 2/neu. Her 2/neu is amplified in about one quarter of breast cancers, and is a marker for sensitivity to herceptin. Thirty-five per cent of breast cancers that amplify her 2/neu coamplify topo IIa, and patients with tumors that contain coamplified topo II experience a greater benefit from DX-based adjuvant therapy, as compared to those with low levels of topo II expression.

Drug Resistance

Transporters that export anthracyclines and other natural products influence response to this class of agents. Expression of the MDR gene, which codes for the membrane transporter p-glycoprotein, increases resistance to anthracyclines, and seems to play an important role in anthracycline resistance in patients with AML, multiple myeloma, and lymphomas. Other membrane exporters, including the MRP family, and the breast cancer resistance transporter, have been implicated as causing resistance in cell lines and in preliminary studies in patients with solid tumors, but their clinical role is uncertain. IDA is less affected by the presence of MDR, than is DX, and has greater toxicity toward hematopoietic stem cells in vitro (17).

Other intracellular processes that recognize DNA strand breaks and initiate apoptosis appear to influence sensitivity to anthracyclines. High levels of BCL-2 expression, an antiapoptotic factor, render cells insensitive to anthracyclines, as does a loss of function of the mismatch repair complex that recognizes defective strand pairing. Mutations in p53 and in ATM, a sensor of free radicals and an activator of p53, also confer resistance to DX (18). There is some evidence that defective repair of double strand breaks, as found in patients with BRCA-1 or -2 mutations, increases sensitivity to anthracyclines.

Clinical Pharmacology

To a variable extent, all anthracyclines are converted to an active alcohol (-ol) intermediate by the ubiquitous enzyme, aldoketoreductase, but for DX and EPI, the parent compounds are believed to be more potent and are responsible for their clinical efficacy. Metabolism of IDA to its alcohol metabolite occurs rapidly and the alcohol becomes the predominant species in plasma 1–4 h after drug administration (19). The metabolite is slightly less potent than the parent, and is believed to be at least partially responsible for the drug's antitumor activity in vivo.

The important pharmacokinetic features of the various anthracyclines are shown in Table 5-1. The parent compounds (DX, DN, and EPI), or in the case of idarubicin, the active alcohol metabolite, have a prolonged terminal half-life in plasma of 1 day or longer, thus allowing intermittent dosing once every week to once every 3 weeks. Clearance occurs primarily through hepatic nonmicrosomal conversion to sulfates, aglycones, and other inactive metabolites. Anthracycline semiquinone radicals may also be inactivated by enzymatic or chemically mediated conjugation with sulfhydryls such as glutathione. Because of the importance of hepatic enzymatic clearance of parent compounds and alcohol metabolites, hepatic dysfunction, with bilirubin greater than 1.5 mg/dl, is associated with delayed drug clearance and a probable increased risk of toxicity (20). In this case, most regimens call for a 50% dose reduction, with subsequent escalation if the dose is well tolerated. Renal dysfunction (creatinine clearance less than 60 ml/min) also slows DX and IDA clearance, probably through changes in hepatic blood flow or hepatic clearance of parent drug.

IDA is the only anthracycline that has acceptable (40%) oral bioavailability; the AUC of the alcohol metabolite, as compared to the AUC of parent drug, is increased by this route, the ratio of IDA-OL/ IDA varying from 3 to 18 (19). In the oral regimens, total IDA doses of 30–60 mg/m^2 are given every 3 weeks, either as a single dose or in split doses daily for 3 days. Oral IDA has received preliminary evaluation in non-Hodgkin lymphoma and in AML in elderly patients, and has modest efficacy.

Intravenous IDA in total doses of 40–60 mg/m^2 given over 2–3 days has also been studied as a component of high-dose chemotherapy regimens for patients with AML or multiple myeloma, followed by autologous stem cell transplantation. There was no significant cardiac toxicity, but patients experienced severe mucositis and there was uncertain clinical benefit.

Toxicity

All anthracyclines cause myelosuppression, mucositis, and alopecia. Recovery of peripheral blood counts occurs within 10–14 days. Their most significant late toxicity is cardiac. Initial clinical experience with DX, as documented by sequential endomyocardial biopsy, disclosed myocardial necrosis, both in animals and

Table 5-1

Anthracycline Pharmacokinetics

Drug	Route of elimination	Plasma $t_{1/2}$ (h)	Primary metabolites	Typical dose & schedule
Doxorubicin	Hepatic metabolism, biliary excretion of conjugated metabolites (glucuronides, sulfates)	30	13-alcohol (minor), aglycone, conjugates	45–60 mg/m^2 q.3.w
Daunorubicin	"	20–50	13-alcohol (predominant), conjugates	30–45 mg/m^2 qd.x3
Epirubicin	"	18	13-alcohol, glucuronide of parent and alcohol	90 to 110 mg/m^2 q.3.w
Idarubicin	Hepatic conversion to 13-alcohol, urinary excretion of alcohol	13–18 (parent) 40–60 (–ol)	13-alcohol predominates	10–15 mg/m^2 q.3.w

in patients receiving multiple doses of drug. Subsequent studies in children have revealed elevations of troponin T in the days following drug administration, and an elevated risk of late events in patients demonstrating such elevations. Cardiac function is ordinarily monitored through tests of left ventricular ejection fraction (scintigraphy or echocardiography). Decreases of greater than 10% from baseline values, or a fall below 40% signal a high risk of later congestive failure. These changes should prompt discontinuation of anthracycline treatment (21). Symptomatic cardiac disease, manifested primarily as congestive heart failure in most cases does not occur until total doses of DX exceed 450 mg/m^2, with a marked increase in risk above 550 mg/m^2. However, in DX-treated children receiving a total dose of 300 mg/m^2 or less, a significantly elevated risk of cardiac disease (arrythmias, sudden death, myocardial infarcts, or congestive failure) emerges later in adult life (22).

EPI appears to be less cardiotoxic than DX in studies of breast cancer patients receiving adjuvant chemotherapy. The incidence of congestive failure following adjuvant therapy reaches 1–1.5% of patients treated with EPI, and is slightly higher (approximately 2%) for DX-containing regimens (23). It appears that cardiac toxicity may be less in patients receiving DX by continuous infusion over 4 days, or in small weekly doses, but the convenience of single bolus doses every 2–3 weeks has compelled the use of this schedule in standard adjuvant therapy.

In both children and adults, oncologists usually limit total doses of DX to less than 300 mg/m^2. Dezrozoxane, an iron chelating drug, clearly decreases troponin T elevations and lessens the risk of cardiac toxicity, and is routinely administered with DX to children who are receiving treatment for potentially curable malignancy.

Radiation therapy to the chest delivered with chemotherapy increases the risk of cardiotoxicity. Because of this potentiation of effects of irradiation, anthracyclines are not given simultaneously with irradiation. Other chemotherapy drugs potentiate anthracycline cardiotoxicity. Paclitaxel, administered with DX, decreases the rate of DX clearance and significantly enhances the rate of DX cardiotoxicity, an effect attributed to inhibition of DX metabolism and/or biliary excretion (24). Herceptin, the anti-Her 2/neu antibody, when given with DX, causes a marked increase in cardiotoxicity when the combination is given for four cycles (27% of patients show cardiac toxicity). Sequential administration of DX–cytoxan, followed by four cycles of Herceptin, is associated with a more than twofold increase in cardiac events. EPI given with Herceptin or with docetaxel causes no obvious increase in cardiotoxicity, although less data are available for these regimens (25).

In addition to cardiac toxicity, the anthracyclines as a class increase the risk of myelodysplasia and AML (26). The onset of MDS occurs within 1–3 years of treatment in patients receiving cytoxan/EPI as adjuvant therapy, and the risk increases markedly in patients receiving greater than 720 mg/m^2 EPI or 6300 mg/m^2 cytoxan. With cytoxan/EPI treatment, leukemias displayed either chromosome 5 or 7 deletions, or more commonly balanced translocations involved 11q23 or 21q22, a finding characteristic of leukemia secondary to topo II inhibitors.

LIPOSOME ENCAPSULATED ATHRACYCLINES

In an effort to increase drug uptake selectively in tumor cells, and to decrease cardiac toxicity, both DX and DN have been reformulated in lipid spheres (liposomes). In this form, the drug has a half-life in plasma of greater than 50 h. Liposomal DX (Doxil) has proven useful in platinum-refractory ovarian cancer, while liposomal DN is approved for treatment of Kaposi's sarcoma. These preparations have less cardiotoxicity but uncertain effectiveness in other tumors.

ETOPOSIDE

The enzymatic activity of topo II exists in two discrete forms (alpha and beta) both of which play a critical role in unwinding DNA and allowing strand passage. These functions are required for transcription, replication, and repair of DNA. As discussed previously, topo II inhibitors are found in nature as potent cellular poisons. Among these are etoposide and its close congener teniposide. These drugs are semisynthetic derivatives of podophyllotoxin, a plant product (Figure 5-5). Both derivatives have found useful roles in cancer chemotherapy, etoposide for the treatment of leukemias, lymphomas, and germ cell tumors, and teniposide for the treatment of AML in children.

Mechanism of Action and Resistance

The mechanism of enzymatic activity of topo II isoforms begins with the cleavage of a DNA strand mediated by ATP hydrolysis and attachment of an enzyme tyrosyl group to the 5′ end of the broken strand. Under physiologic conditions, the cleavage of DNA allows passage of an unbound strand of DNA, thus promoting unwinding and relieving torsion. After strand passage, the enzyme reseals the 3′ and 5′ ends, restoring DNA integrity. Etoposide and teniposide bind to the complex of DNA and enzyme, inhibiting the resealing activity of the enzyme and perpetuating strand breaks (Figure 5-6) (27). Most breaks are single stranded, but about 5% are double stranded. These double-stranded breaks require repair and, through p53, signal a halt to cell cycle progression, and, if sufficiently numerous, prompt apoptosis.

The cytotoxic action of these drugs requires the presence of topo II. The alpha isoform of the enzyme is tightly regulated, increasing significantly in concentration during the S-phase of the cell cycle. It may be coamplified with the *her 2* gene on chromosome 17, and its amplification identifies tumors highly sensitive to topo II inhibition (28). As natural products, the epipodophyllotoxin derivatives are subject to transport by the p-glycoprotein, a product of the *MDR* gene. Resistance may also arise through deletion of topo II (via methylation of the gene or loss of promoter activity) or through mutation of its binding site for these drugs (29). Finally, disruptions of apoptotic pathways, and the capacity to repair double strand breaks, may also determine the outcome of therapy.

Clinical Pharmacology

Etoposide is eliminated by both renal excretion and hepatic metabolism, and doses should be adjusted for either kind of organ dysfunction (30). Approximately 40% of a dose of etoposide is excreted unchanged in the urine, and dose should be reduced in proportion to changes in creatinine clearance. The remainder is eliminated by glucuronidation. A smaller fraction of drug undergoes p450 3A4 metabolism through demethylation, producing a cytotoxic catechol metabolite and other quinine derivatives of uncertain significance. The drug has a terminal half-life of 8 h in plasma in patients with normal renal and hepatic function. In patients with elevated serum bilirubin of 1.5–3.0 mg/dL, the dose should be reduced by 50%, while in those with higher bilirubin, alternative therapies should be used until liver function improves.

High-dose etoposide (1.5 g/m^2 or above) is used alone, or in combination with cyclophosphamide, carboplatin, or other drugs (31). It is the only topo II agent that can be significantly escalated in dose without encountering serious non-myeloid toxicity. At these high doses, mucositis and hepatic enzyme elevations become dose limiting. Its pharmacokinetics remain linear at these high doses.

Teniposide is eliminated primarily by the liver, with a variety of p450 and other metabolites appearing in the bile. Its half-life in plasma is 10–21 h. Very

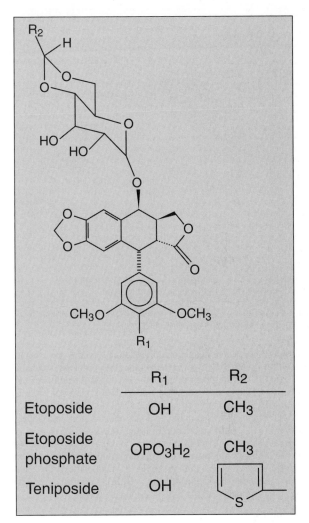

	R₁	R₂
Etoposide	OH	CH₃
Etoposide phosphate	OPO₃H₂	CH₃
Teniposide	OH	

FIGURE 5-5 Molecular structure of etoposide, etoposide phosphate, and Teniposide.

little drug is excreted in the urine, and no dose adjustment for renal dysfunction is indicated.

Toxicity

At usual doses of 100 mg/m^2 per day for 3 days every 3 weeks, bone marrow suppression is the primary toxicity of etoposide, with recovery 10 to 14 days after treatment. Hypotension, fever, and asthmatic episodes may follow drug infusion, probably a hypersensitivity response to the cremophor diluent in which the drug is administered. Liver function abnormalities and mucositis supervene at higher doses, and especially after myelo-ablative doses given with bone marrow transplantation.

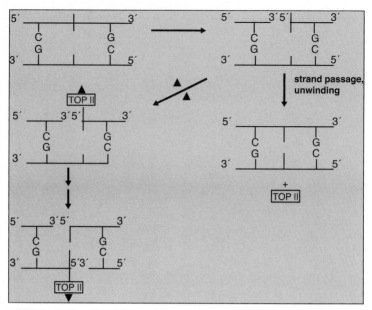

FIGURE 5-6 Formation of single and double strand breaks by topoisomerase II (TOP II), and prevention of break resealing in the presence of etoposide(▲).

Etoposide causes acute myelogenous leukemia as a later toxic event, usually 2–3 years after treatment (32). The leukemia often involves a translocation in the *MLL* gene on the long arm of chromosome 11 at AT-rich sites favored for topo II cleavage. The leukemia may be preceded by a period of myelodysplasia. Acute promyelocytic leukemia has also been reported following etoposide. The risk of AML increases with cumulative doses above 6 g/m² and with schedules of weekly or biweekly administration of drug (33).

Tenoposide side effects follow the same pattern as these of etoposide; acute myelosuppression and mucositis are the most common toxicities. The incidence of acute hypersensitivity reactions is higher for teniposide, probably related to the greater concentration of lipid diluent used in its clinical formulation. Like etoposide, it is associated with a risk of secondary AML.

REFERENCES

1. Garcia-Carbonero R, Supko JG. Current perspectives on the clinical experience, pharmacology, and continued development of the camptothecins. Clin Cancer Res. 2002; 8: 641–661.
2. Fujitani K, Tsujinaka T, Hirao M. Pharmacokinetic study of two infusion schedules of irinotecan combined with cisplatin in patients with advanced gastric cancer. Oncology. 2003; 64: 111–115.
3. Gore M, Oza A, Rustin G, et al. A randomized trial of oral versus intravenous topotecan in patients with relapsed epithelial ovarian cancer. Eur J Cancer. 2002; 38: 57–63.
4. ten Bokkel Huinik W, Gore M, Carmichael J, et al. Topotecan versus paclitaxel for the treatment of recurrent epithelial ovarian cancer. J Clin Oncol. 1997; 15: 2183–2193.

5. von Pawel J, Schiller JH, Shepherd FA, et al. Topotecan versus cyclophosphamide, doxorubicin, and vincristine for the treatment of recurrent small-cell lung cancer. J Clin Oncol. 1999; 17: 658–667.

6. Massacesi C, Terrazzino S, Marcucci F, et al. Uridine diphosphate glucuronsyl transferase 1A1 promoter polymorphism predicts the risk of gastrointestinal toxicity and fatigue induced by irinotecan-based chemotherapy. Cancer. 2006; 106: 1007–1016.

7. Zhou Q, Sparreboom A, Tan E-H, et al. Pharmacogenetic profiling across the irinotecan pathway in Asian patients with cancer. Br J Clin Pharmacol. 2005; 59: 415–424.

8. Fuchs CS, Moore MR, Harker G, et al. Phase III comparison of two irinotecan dosing regimens in second-line therapy of metastatic colorectal cancer. J Clin Oncol. 2003; 21: 807–814.

9. Saltz LB, Cox JV, Blanke C, et al. Irinotecan plus fluorouracil and leucovorin for metastatic colorectal cancer. N Engl J Med. 2000; 343: 905–914.

10. Douillard JY, Cunningham D, Roth AD. Irinotecan combined with fluorouracil compared with fluorouracil alone as first-line treatment for metastatic colorectal cancer: a multicentre randomized trial. Lancet. 2000; 355: 1041–1047.

11. Cunningham D, Humblet Y, Siena S, et al. Cetuximab monotherapy and cetuximab plus irinotecan in irinotecan-refractory metastatic colorectal cancer. N Engl J Med. 2004; 351: 337–345.

12. Pecorelli S, Ray-Coquard I, Colombo N, et al. A phase II study of oral gimatecan (STI481) in women with progressing or recurring advanced epithelial ovarian, fallopian tube and peritoneal cancers. J Clin Oncol. 2006; 24: 5088 (abstract).

13. Mariani P, Moliterni A, Da Prada D, et al. A phase II trial of the novel oral camptothecin gimatecan in women with anthracycline and taxane pre-treated advanced breast cancer. J Clin Oncol. 2006; 24: 662 (abstract).

14. Doroshow JH. Anthracyclines and anthracenediones. In BA Chabner, DL Longo (eds.), "Cancer Chemotherapy and Biotherapy: Principles and Practice" Lippincott, Williams and Wilkins, Philadelphia, PA, 2006, pp. 416.

15. Liu LF. DNA topoisomerase poisons as antitumor drugs. Annu Rev Biochem. 1989; 58: 351.

16. Durbecq V, Paesmans M, Cardoso F, et al. Topoisomerase-II expression as a predictive marker in a population of advanced breast cancer patients randomly treated either with single-agent doxorubicin or single-agent docetaxel. Mol Cancer Ther. 2004; 3: 1207.

17. Kroschinsky F, Schleyer E, Renner U, et al. Increased myelotoxicity of idarubicin: is there a pharmacological basis? Cancer Chemother Pharmacol. 2004; 53: 61.

18. Kurz EU, Douglas P, Lees-Miller SP. Doxorubicin activates ATM-dependent phosphorylation of multiple downstream targets in part through the generation of reactive oxygen species. J Biol Chem. 2004; 279: 53272.

19. Crivellari D, Lombardi D, Spazzapan S, et al. New oral drugs in older patients: a review of idarubicin in elderly patients. Crit. Rev. Oncol./Hematol. 2004; 49: 153.

20. Camaggi CM, Strocchi E, Carisi P, et al. Idarubicin metabolism and pharmacokinetics after intravenous and oral administration in cancer patients: a crossover study. Cancer Chemother Pharmacol. 1992; 30: 307.

21. Lu P. Monitoring cardiac function in patients receiving doxorubicin. Semin Nucl Med. 2005; 35: 197.

22. Nysorn K, Holm K, Lipsitz SR, et al. Relationship between cumulative anthracycline dose and late cardiotoxicity in childhood acute lymphoblastic leukemia. J Clin Oncol. 1998; 16: 545.

23. Bonneterre J, Roche H, Kerbrat P, et al. Epirubicin increases long-term survival in adjuvant chemotherapy of patients with poor-prognosis, node-positive, early

breast cancer: 10-year follow-up results of the French adjuvant study group 05 randomized trial. J Clin Oncol. 2005; 23: 2686.

24. Partridge AH, Burstein HJ, Winer EP. Side effects of chemotherapy and combined chemohormonal therapy in women with early-stage breast cancer. J Natl Cancer Inst Monogr. 2001; 30:135.

25. Buzdar AU, Ibrahim NK, Francis D, et al. Significantly higher pathologic complete remission rate after neoadjuvant therapy with trastuzumab, paclitaxel, and epirubicin chemotherapy: results of a randomized trial in human epidermal growth factor receptor 2-positive operable breast cancer. J Clin Oncol. 2005; 23: 3676.

26. Praga C, Bergh J, Bliss J, et al. Risk of acute myeloid leukemia and myelodysplastic syndrome in trials of adjuvant epirubicin for early breast cancer: correlation with doses of epirubicin and cyclophosphamide. J Clin Oncol. 2005; 23: 4179.

27. Minford J, Pommier Y, Filipski J, Kohn KW, Kerrigan D, Mattern M, Michaels S, Schwartz R, Zwelling LA. Isolation of intercalator-dependent protein-linked DNA strand cleavage activity from cell nuclei and identification as topoisomerase II. Biochemistry. 1986; 25(1): 9–16.

28. Pritchard KI, Shepherd LE, O'Malley FP, Andrulis IL, Tu D, Bramwell VH, Levine MN. National Cancer Institute of Canada Clinical Trials Group. HER2 and responsiveness of breast cancer to adjuvant chemotherapy. N Engl J Med. 2006; 354(20): 2103–2111.

29. Tan KB, Mattern MR, Eng WK, McCabe FL, Johnson RK. Nonproductive rearrangement of DNA topoisomerase I and II genes: correlation with resistance to topoisomerase inhibitors. J Natl Cancer Inst. 1989; 81(22): 1732-1735.

30. D'Incalci M, Rossi C, Zucchetti M, Urso R, Cavalli F, Mangioni C, Willems Y, Sessa C. Pharmacokinetics of etoposide in patients with abnormal renal and hepatic function. Cancer Res. 1986; 46(5): 2566–2571.

31. Beyer J, Kramar A, Mandanas R, et al. High-dose chemotherapy as salvage treatment in germ cell tumors: a multivariate analysis of prognostic variables. J Clin Oncol. 1996; 14(10): 2638–2645.

32. Smith MA, McCaffrey RP, Karp JE. The secondary leukemias: challenges and research directions. J Natl Cancer Inst. 1996; 88(7): 407–418.

33. Le Deley MC, Leblanc T, Shamsaldin A, et al. Societe Francaise d'Oncologie Pediatrique. Risk of secondary leukemia after a solid tumor in childhood according to the dose of epipodophyllotoxins and anthracyclines: a case-control study by the Societe Francaise d'Oncologie Pediatrique. J Clin Oncol. 2003; 21(6): 1074–1081.

ADDUCT-FORMING AGENTS: ALKYLATING
AGENTS AND PLATINUM ANALOGS

Since the first experiments with nitrogen mustards at Yale in the early 1940s, alkylating agents have played a primary role in cancer treatment (1). They have gradually been replaced by platinum-based compounds in most regimens for treating epithelial cancers, but remain primary components in the treatment of childhood solid tumors, lymphomas, and adult sarcomas, and in high-dose chemotherapy. As a class, they have the features of the prototypical cytotoxic drugs, affecting virtually every organ system in addition to tumors. They share common characteristics of a significant improvement in response as doses are escalated above standard doses: acute toxic effects on bone marrow, epithelium of the gastrointestinal tract, and hair follicles; significant toxicity to lung, heart, and central nervous systems at bone marrow ablative doses; and late induction of myelodysplasia and acute leukemia.

MECHANISM OF ACTION

Three general classes of alkylating agents have found clinical application. The first are the chloroethyl nitrogen mustards, exemplified by cyclophosphamide, ifosfamide, and chlorambucil (Figure 6-1). These drugs activate through spontaneous formation of an unstable imonium intermediate and transfer of their ethyl group to nucleophilic (electronegative) sites on DNA and other macromolecules (Figure 6-2). Many of these drugs contain two chloroethyl groups and can therefore crosslink strands of DNA, creating a lesion that is difficult to repair. The second group consists of drugs that transfer single-methyl radicals to DNA. This second class, which includes procarbazine, DTIC, temozolomide, busulfan, and others, tends to require more complex activation, either enzymatic or chemical, and attacks the O-6 position of guanine or the N-7 position of adenine. The resulting methylation is repaired by guanine-O-6 methyltransferase, the activity of which, in cancer cells, determines the response of tumors to this group of drugs (2). The third group of drugs, while not strictly alkylators, include the platinum analogs, which attach activated platinum coordinate complexes to

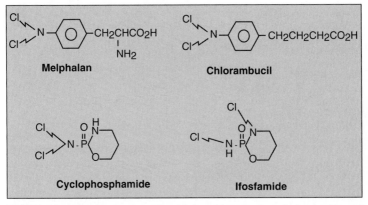

FIGURE 6-1 Molecular structures of melphalan, chlorambucil, cyclophosphamide, and ifosfamide.

nucleophilic sites on DNA, in much the same way as the classical alkylators attach methyl or ethyl groups. The platinum activation pathway begins with the displacement of chloride or other leaving groups by water, with the formation of a reactive −OH intermediates (Figure 6-3). The platinum analogs have two chloride leaving groups and, thus, upon full activation, are capable of crosslinking DNA.

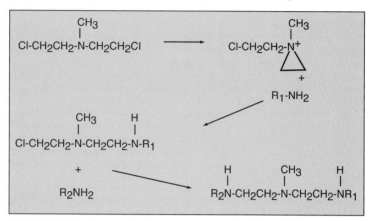

FIGURE 6-2 Nitrogen mustard undergoes spontaneous chemical rearrangement to form an unstable, positively charged, aziridinium ring, which reacts with nucleophilic sites on DNA such as amines. (R_1NH_2 and R_2NH_2).

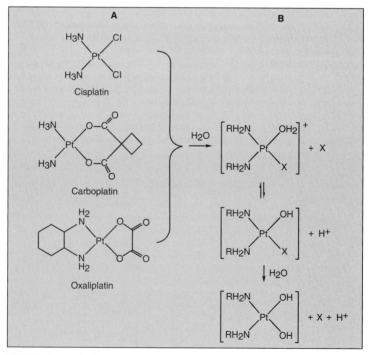

FIGURE 6-3 Activation of platinum analogs.

Cellular Pharmacology of Alkylating Agents

As a class, the alkylating agents are lipid soluble and easily cross cell membranes. However, at least two members of the class, nitrogen mustard and melphalan are actively transported into cells, the former by the choline transporter, and the latter by leucine or neutral amino acid transporters. Resistance may arise experimentally by deletion of these transporters.

Following their uptake, most alkylating agents, and in particular the chloroethyl mustards, spontaneously undergo activation to an unstable, electrophilic intermediate. Some agents, such as dimethyl triazinoimidazolecarboxamide (DTIC), require metabolic activation, but the closely related temodar generates the same unstable methyltriazino derivative spontaneously, and has surpassed DTIC in treatment of gliomas and melanoma (4). Procarbazine, cyclophosphamide, and ifosfamide require prior P450 activation in the liver in order to generate chemically active end products. In the case of cyclophosphamide and the closely related ifosfamide, the active end product is a simple phosphoramide mustard (Figure 6-4).

Once inside cells, alkylating agents or their active intermediates form unstable intermediates such as the aziridinum ion, and seek sites capable of donating electrons and relieving the tension of the unstable aziridinium ring (Figure 6-5). They attack sites such as sulfhydryl groups on proteins, sulfhydryls offered by glutathione (the sulfhydryl found in highest concentration within cells), and various electron rich sites on nucleic acids, including the N-2 and N-7 groups on guanine, the O-6 on guanine, and the N-3 on adenine. Single-base alkylations are recognized by the DNA nucleotide excision repair (NER) complex, while crosslinks must be repaired by a more complex process of excision of the alkylated bases, and accurate repair of the resulting double stand break through homologous recombination. An accumulation of crosslinks, particularly those of the interstrand variety, signals p53 and its downstream partners to initiate apoptosis.

Specific enzymes may be critical to the process of DNA repair and survival. Methylating agents and the nitrosoureas have a particular propensity for alkylation

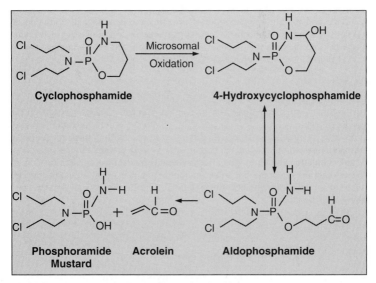

FIGURE 6-4 Microsomal activation of cyclophosphamide.

of the O-6 position of guanine, and this alkylation is removed by a specific O-6 alkyl guanine transferase (AGT). AGT gene methylation and its lack of expression in primary brain tumors are associated with greater sensitivity to procarbazine, temodar, the nitroso-ureas, and other alkylators. The ability to repair alkylating damage varies among tumors and is influenced by inherited polymorphisms. Low levels of expression of repair enzymes, such as various polymorphisms of enzymes in the NER pathway, have been correlated with greater host toxicity in lung cancer patients (5).

Resistance

Any one of the critical steps in the action of alkylating agents may present an opportunity for development of resistance. In experimental systems, tumor cell resistance can arise through increased levels of sulhydrils, increased activity of glutathione transferases, and increased expression of AGT or other repair enzymes. Competence of the double strand break repair sequence, which includes BRCA-1, Rad-51, and other proteins, is required for effective elimination of potentially lethal crosslinks. Finally, changes that interfere with apoptosis, including increased expression of bcl-2, may alter the threshold for cell death. On the clinical level, the understanding of alkylating resistance is incomplete. P53 mutation, a hallmark of advanced, drug-resistant tumors is believed to play a prominent role (6).

Clinical Pharmacology

In general, because of their reactivity in aqueous solution, parent compounds or their reactive metabolites have a brief residence time in plasma. Because their decomposition is primarily through chemical reactivity, doses do not have to be decreased for renal or hepatic dysfunction.

The pharmacokinetics of busulfan, a drug used frequently in bone marrow transplantation, have been carefully studied in both adults and children. In adults, its half-life averages about 2.5 h in plasma, while in children it is cleared much faster, leading to the use of higher doses in the pediatric transplantation setting (see below) (7). Busulfan, the nitrosoureas, temodar, thiotepa, and the active metabolite of procarbazine penetrate into the central nervous system well. Busulfan causes seizures in high-dose regimens and, because it accelerates the metabolism of phenytoin, the latter must be used in higher doses to prevent seizures.

Toxicity

The alkylating agents as a class actively inhibit hematopoiesis. They suppress the immune system and injure intestinal epithelium and gonadal tissue. Multiple cycles of treatment may lead to epithelial pulmonary injury, pneumonitis, and pulmonary fibrosis (especially after treatment with busulfan and the nitrosoureas, and other agents in high doses), as well as renal tubular injury and bladder toxicity. Alkylators as a class are teratogenic and carcinogenic. Most of these toxicities are acute but some, including gonadal injury, accumulate with successive cycles of treatment, and leukemia and solid tumors may appear many years after treatment.

Bone marrow recovers 10–14 days after conventional doses, except in the case of nitrosourea treatment, which produces a nadir in neutrophil and platelet count 5–6 weeks after administration. Busulfan typically causes a prolonged suppression of the white blood count, probably due to its toxicity to marrow stem cells, and is used in high doses to produce host marrow ablation. Cyclophosphamide tends to have modest effects on platelet production in conventional doses.

Male spermatogenesis is typically lost after a complete course of chemotherapy for Hodgkin Disease, lymphomas, or leukemia in adults, and sperm banking prior to treatment may be indicated; female fertility is less affected and the degree of injury correlates with age. Alkylators cause the early induction of menopause, as in premenopausal women who are receiving cyclophosphamide for adjuvant therapy of breast cancer. Younger women (15–35) often remain fertile after such treatment.

Acrolein, an alkylating metabolite of both cyclophosphamide and ifosfamide, causes injury to the bladder mucosa and renal tubules, necessitating the use of a sulfhydryl, MESNA (2-mercaptoethanesulonate), in patients receiving high doses of these drugs. MESNA is an inactive disulfide at neutral pH in plasma or tissues, but becomes a reactive sulfhydryl in the acid pH of urine. Hemorrhagic cystitis may become life threatening in patients receiving low-dose or single high-dose cyclosphosophamide without MESNA. The nitrosoureas also cause interstitial renal fibrosis and renal failure when used in higher doses and for multiple cycles of treatment.

All alkylating agents cause leukemia, which in many cases is preceded by a myelodysplastic phase. Cytogenetic studies of bone marrow cells reveal a deletion of portions of chromosomes 5, 7, or 11. Full-blown leukemia appears on average 3–5 years after chemotherapy administration, and responds poorly to antileukemic treatment (8). There is also an increased risk of solid tumors after alkylating agent chemotherapy, most obvious in the second decade after treatment. Concomitant radiation therapy increases the risk of leukemia, and of solid tumors, which occur 10–20 years after exposure to alkylating agents.

PLATINUM ANALOGS: MECHANISM OF ACTION

The cytotoxic effects of the platinum analogs result from the formation of adducts with purine bases in DNA. Intrastrand and cross-strand crosslinks are formed by the replacement of the dichloride arms of the platinum complex with two $-OH$ groups (Figure 6-4), and subsequent displacement of the $-OH$ leaving groups by nucleophilic sites such as the N-7 position of guanine or adenine. A variety of single adducts, as well as intrastrand and interstrand crosslinks result from reaction of the platinum analogs with DNA. The intrastrand adducts formed between adjacent bases in d(GpG) or d(ApG) sequences appear to be most important in blocking DNA and RNA polymerase activity and promoting apoptosis. Adducts cause a bending of the DNA strand, a distortion recognized by DNA repair complexes. Mismatch repair genes recognize the adducts and are required for full expression of the cytotoxicity of cisplatin and carboplatin; these genes trigger an attempt to excise the adduct-bearing sequence and rebuild the damaged strand by the NER complex. When the number of DNA adducts exceeds repair capacity, p53 initiates the process of apoptosis.

Resistance

Resistance to platinum analogs has been studied experimentally, and has been ascribed to failure of DNA damage recognition due to defective mismatch repair, increased detoxification of reactive platinum species by glutathione, increased efflux of platinum complexes by active transport, increased NER capacity, loss of p53, and overexpression of antiapoptotic genes such as bcl-2. It is unclear which of these responses leads to clinical resistance, although tumors that recur after extensive platinum-based chemotherapy often show crossresistance to alkylating agents, and irradiation, and exhibit loss of p53 function. The greater activity of oxaliplatin than that of the other platinum analogs in combination with 5-fluorouracil in colon cancer is well established, but not understood. DNA polymerase has greater difficulty bypassing the bulky diaminocyclohexyl substitution on oxaliplatin, as compared to the other platinum analogs. Additionally, oxaliplatin seems to down-regulate the expression of thymidylate synthase, perhaps contributing to its synergy with 5-fluorouracil.

Clinical Pharmacology

The three clinically useful analogs differ in their reactivity, pharmacokinetics, and toxicity profiles. Cisplatin is highly reactive at neutral pH and in aqueous solution. It rapidly disappears from plasma, as it forms adducts with protein sulfhydryls in the extracellular space, and reacts with nucleic acids and glutathione intracellularly. Little of the platinum found in plasma hours after its administration is intact, or reactive drug species; most is bound to protein. Carboplatin, by virtue of is more stable dicarboxylate leaving group, persists in plasma as unchanged drug with a $t_{1/2}$ of 2 h, and is eliminated by renal excretion. Doses should be corrected according to creatinine clearance, according to the Calvert formula:

$$\text{Dose (mg)} = \text{target AUC (5–6 mg/ml} \times \text{min)} \times \text{(glomerular filtration rate (ml/min)} + 25)$$

Oxaliplatin is rapidly eliminated through its reaction with nucleophilic targets. No dose adjustment is required for patients with a creatinine clearance of greater than 20 ml/min.

TOXICITY

The toxicity profiles of the three analogs differ significantly. Cisplatin causes severe acute nausea and vomiting, which responds to pretreatment with antiemetics and glucocorticoids. It causes renal tubular damage unless a high-chloride diuresis is maintained, usually with generous saline hydration. It also causes a progressive high-tone hearing loss. It is only mildly myelosuppressive, but with repeated doses, patients develop a progressive anemia that responds to erythropoietin. Renal tubular toxicity of cisplatin may lead to calcium and magnesium wasting, and tetany, but hydration and electrolyte replacement decrease the frequency and severity of this problem.

Carboplatin is less nephrotoxic and otototoxic than cisplatin, but causes greater myelosuppression, particularly thrombocytopenia. Oxaliplatin is minimally nephrotoxic but causes moderate leukopenia and thrombocytopenia. Its most bothersome toxicity is a neuropathic throat pain and a progressive peripheral sensory neuropathy. Carboplatin and cisplatin may also cause a disabling peripheral motor and sensory neuropathy after multiple cycles of therapy. In high-dose regimens, carboplatin may be associated with interstitial pneumonitis and pulmonary fibrosis.

All three platinum derivatives may cause allergic reactions, including rash, wheezing, and diarrhea, in up to 10% of patients, but usually only after multiple cycles of treatment. Pretreatment with glucocorticoids and antihistamines may allow continued treatment in patients displaying mild allergy.

The platinum analogs have been associated with myelodysplasia and acute myelogenous leukemia as a late complication of therapy.

REFERENCES

1. Chabner BA, Roberts TG Jr. Timeline: chemotherapy and the war on cancer. Nat Rev Cancer. 2005; 5: 65.
2. Dolan ME, Pegg AE. O6-Benzylguanine and its role in chemotherapy. Clin Cancer Res. 1997; 8: 837.
3. Lim MC, Martin RB. The nature of *cis* amine Pd(II) and antitumor *cis* amine Pt(II) complexes in aqueous solutions. Inorg Nucl Chem. 1976; 38: 1911.

4. Yung A, Levin VA, Brada M, et al. Randomized, multicenter, open-labeled, phase II, comparative study of temozolomide and procarbazine in the treatment of patients with glioblastoma multiforme at first relapse. Br J Cancer. 2000; 83: 588.

5. Suk R, Gurubhagavatula S, Park S, et al. Polymorphisms in ERCC1 and grade 3 or 4 toxicity in non-small cell lung cancer patients. Clin Cancer Res. 2005; 15: 1534.

6. Kirsch D, Kastan M. Tumor suppressor p53: implications for tumor development and prognosis. J Clin Oncol. 1998; 16: 3158.

7. Grochow LB, Krivit W, Whitely CB, et al. Busulfan disposition in children. Blood. 1990; 75: 1723.

8. Tucker MA, Coleman, CN, Cox RS, et al. Risk of second cancers after treatment for Hodgkin's disease. N Engl J Med. 1988; 318: 76.

THALIDOMIDE AND ITS ANALOGS

Thalidomide was originally developed in Germany in 1954 as an antihistamine, but it produced significant sedation. The drug was therefore further developed and marketed as a nonbarbiturate hypnotic. It had a notable prompt onset of action and lack of hangover, and alleviated symptoms of morning sickness associated with pregnancy. However, in 1963 it was withdrawn from the market when its use was associated with stunted limb growth (dysmelia) in children born of women who used the drug during pregnancy. Thirty years later it was reintroduced as an oral agent for the management of cutaneous leprosy (erythema nodosum leprosum) (1). Based on its ability to suppress certain components of the immune response and angiogenesis, thalidomide became the subject of trials against a spectrum of diseases, including cancer, and most notably against multiple myeloma (2). Thalidomide and its newer analogs have also shown clinical activity in patients with the 5q-subset of myelodysplastic syndrome (3) and in suppressing graft versus host disease. Ongoing clinical studies are addressing its potential role in other neoplasms as well.

STRUCTURE

Thalidomide is piperidinyl isoindole $\{(\pm)$-α-(N-phtalimido)$\}$ glutarimide. It is a neutral racemic compound derived from glutamic acid, and is structurally related to the analeptic drug bemegride (α-ethyl-α-methyl-glutarimide, $C_{18}H_{13}NO_2$), and to a sedative and antiepileptic drug, glutethimide (β-ethyl-β-phenyl-glutarimide, $C_{15}H_{23}NO_4$). It has two ring systems: a left-sided phthalimide, and a right-sided glutarimide with an asymmetric carbon atom at position 3' of the glutarimide ring. The drug consists of equimolar amounts of (+)-R, and (−)-(S) enantiomers. Thalidomide is sparingly soluble in water (< 0.1 g/l) and spontaneously hydrolyses in solution at ph 6.0 or higher to produce at least 12 different products.

MECHANISM OF ACTION

The precise mechanism responsible for thalidomide's clinical activity and the potential contribution of thalidomide versus that of its numerous metabolites have not been elucidated. Thalidomide has immunomodulatory, antiinflammatory and antiangiogenic properties attributed to downregulation of signaling molecules such as IL-6, VEGF, and TNFα (4). The antitumor activity of thalidomide and its derivatives may derive from any, or a combination of, effects:

1. A direct antiproliferative/proapoptotic effect probably mediated by downregulation of nuclear factor kappa B (NF-κB), a transcription factor that promotes a protective response to cell injury, and TNFα, a tumor stimulating and immunomodulatory, cytokinine.
2. An indirect antitumor effect mediated by downregulation of tumor cell adhesion molecules (I-CAM 1) and stimulatory cytokines such as IL-6.
3. Inhibition of secretion of angiogenic cytokines such as basic FGF and VEGF.
4. Suppression of activity of cyclo-oxygenase, an enzyme that stimulates proliferation through the synthesis of prostaglandins and related products.

METABOLISM AND CLINICAL PHARMACOLOGY

Thalidomide absorption from the gastrointestinal tract of human subjects is slow due to its poor aqueous solubility, with peak levels in plasma at 3 to 6 h after ingestion. Absorption at doses at or below 200 mg is variable, but becomes linear as doses increase to 800–1,200 mg. Thalidomide is loosely bound to serum albumin and to α_1-acid glycoprotein and is widely distributed throughout the body. It is mainly broken down through nonenzymatic hydrolytic cleavage, but some 20% of the drug is also metabolized by hepatic cytochrome p450 2C19 to form hydroxylated metabolites (Figure 7-1).

The extent of hydrolysis has been estimated to be 8% at 1 h and 80% at 24 h. Hydrolysis cleaves the two-imide bonds of both enantiomers opening the glutarimide and phthalimide rings, yielding 12 products, 11 of which are chiral (5). These products are further broken down to yield numerous optically active compounds.

Thalidomide disappears from plasma with an apparent half-life of 4.7 h for both the (S)- and (R)-enantiomers, which are rapidly interconvertible in vivo. Thalidomide and its metabolites are excreted in the urine, while the nonabsorbed portion of the drug is excreted unchanged in feces, but clearance of the parent compound is primarily metabolic and nonrenal. Studies of multiple oral doses in healthy subjects showed that thalidomide capsules 200 mg/day over 18–21 days did not produce accumulation and the AUC on days 1 and 21 were equivalent. It is not known if accumulation occurs with higher daily dosages, although pharmacokinetic simulations of 400 and 800 mg once daily suggest that this would not occur (6).

THALIDOMIDE DERIVATIVES

In an effort to improve upon the side effects and the efficacy profile of thalidomide, analogs have entered clinical evaluation. They belong to two main groups. The first class, called immunomodulatory drugs or imids, is represented by revlimid. The imids strongly inhibit production of TNF-α along with IL-1β, IL-6, and IL-12 while augmenting production of IL-10 and costimulation of T-lymphocytes. They also induce FAS and caspase-mediated apoptosis of myeloma cells. The second class, termed selective cytokine inhibitory drugs (SelCids), represented by actimid, are phosphodiesterase-4 inhibitors and potently and selectively inhibit TNF-α, having considerably less effect on other inflammatory cytokines. Experimental and early clinical studies indicate that both new classes of analogs are active in multiple myeloma. Revlimid has won approval for the treatment of patients with 5q-variant of myelodysplastic syndrome (7). In this syndrome, which accounts for 5–10% of patients with MDS, revlimid produces a normalization of blood counts in 55% of patients, when given in doses of 10 mg per day for 21 days with a seven day rest period between cycles.

Revlimid is absorbed rapidly after oral intake, reaches maximum plasma concentration after 1–1.5 h and disappears from plasma with a half-life of 3.1–4.2 h. Approximately two-thirds of the drug is excreted intact in the urine; its renal clearance exceeds glomerular filtration. The remainder of the drug is excreted unchanged in feces, with little evidence for metabolism. In vitro, it displays a broad spectrum of antitumor activities: it induces apoptosis or growth arrest even in chemotherapy resistant myeloma cells, decreases binding of myeloma cells to bone marrow stromal cells (BMSCs), inhibits the production in the bone marrow milieu of cytokines (IL-6, VEGF, and TNF-α), blocks angiogenesis, stimulates host antimyeloma natural killer (NK) cell immunity, and inhibits tumor growth.

Patients with myeloma become refractory to thalidomide after prolonged use, but the changes responsible for resistance are incompletely understood. On the

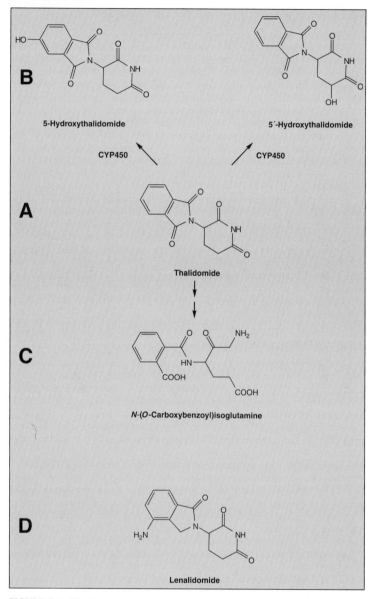

FIGURE 7-1   The Structure of thalidomide, hydroxylated metabolites with their hydrolytic products and analogs revlimid and actimid. (a) Thalidomide, (b) its p450 hydroxylation product, (c) a spontaneous hydrolytic breakdown product, and (d) its analog, revlimid.

other hand, studies in vitro and in mice indicate that thalidomide can increase the efficacy of other chemotherapy in otherwise drug resistant myeloma cells. Like thalidomide, imids also cause growth arrest in myeloma cells that are resistant to dexamethasone, melphalan, and doxorubicin (8).

TOXICITY

Sedation and constipation are the most important side effects of thalidomide and become dose-limiting at daily doses of 400 mg or greater. Other side effects include dizziness, mood changes, headaches, skin rash, and, rarely, neutropenia. Peripheral neurotoxicity, primarily peripheral sensory changes, is reported in up to one-third of patients, usually at doses of 400 mg or greater taken for more than 60 days. Hematologic toxicity, primarily a decrease in the neutrophil and platelet counts, is modest and seen only at doses of 400 mg or greater. As a single agent, thalidomide causes a 5% incidence of deep vein thromboses, but both revlimid and thalidomide in combination with dexamethasone or velcade cause major thrombotic events in up to 15% of patients especially in these receiving 400 mg doses of thalidomide or greater (9).

Revlimid does not cause significant sleepiness, or constipation, and neuropathy is infrequent. However, it causes neutropenia and thrombocytopenia in 20% of patients. Revlimid enhances myelosuppression caused by concomitant chemotherapy. SelCIDs are well tolerated with a safety profile similar to imids.

FORMULATION, DOSAGE, AND ADMINISTRATION

Thalidomide is available as tablets or capsules containing the racemic mixture. Recently a chemically stable formulation of separate enantiomers has been developed, but has not been approved for marketing. The therapeutic dose of racemic thalidomide in myeloma is usually given, either divided into a morning and evening dose or as a single evening dose each day (10). The starting dose is 200 mg/day, increasing to a maximum of 800 mg/day as tolerated. The approved dosing regimen for revlimid in treating MDS is 25 mg daily for 21 days followed by a seven day rest period.

REFERENCES

1. Sheskin J. Thalidomide in the treatment of lepra reaction. Clin Pharm Ther. 1965; 6: 303–306.
2. Barlogie B, Desikan R, Eddlemon P, et al. Extended survival in advanced and refractory multiple myeloma after single-agent thalidomide: identification of prognostic factors in a phase 2 study of 169 patients. Blood. 2001; 98(2): 492–494.
3. Zorat F, Shetty V, Dutt D, et al. The clinical and biological effects of thalidomide in patients with myelodysplastic syndromes. Br J Haematol. 2001; 115(4): 881–94.
4. Richardson P, Hideshima T, Anderson K. Thalidomide: emerging role in cancer medicine. Annu Rev Med. 2002; 53: 629–657.
5. Eriksson T, Bjorkman S, Roth B, Bjork H, Hoglund N. Hydroxylated metabolites of thalidomide:formation in vitro and in vivo in man. J Pharm Pharmacol. 1998; 50: 1409–1416.
6. Teo KS, Colburn WA, Tracewell GW, Kook AG. Clinical pharmacokinetics of thalidomide. Clin Pharmacokinet. 2004; 43(5): 311–327.
7. Dredge K, Dalgleish KA, Mariott BJ. Thalidomide analogs as emerging anticancer drugs. Anticancer Drugs. 2003; 14: 331–335.
8. Hideshima T, Dharminder C, Yoshihito S, et al. Thalidomide and its analogs overcome drug resistance of human multiple myeloma cells to conventional therapy Blood. 2000; 96: 2943–2950.
9. Cavenagh DJ, Oakervee H. On behalf of UK myeloma forum and the BCSH hematology/oncology task forces-Guidelines. Br J Hematol. 2003; 120: 18–26.
10. Mujagic H, Chabner BA, Mujagic Z. The mechanisms of action and potential therapeutic use of thalidomide. Croat Med J. 2002; 43(3): 274–285.

BLEOMYCIN

Traditional fermentation research has been the backbone of efforts to discover anti-infective agents. A few of these products have proven to possess valuable antitumor activity as well, among them bleomycin, a drug important in the curative combination therapy of Hodgkin Disease and testicular germ cell tumors. Among the natural products with antitumor activity, none is more uniquely designed by nature than bleomycin, which was isolated from the broth of the fungus, S. verticillus. The clinical bleomycin preparation consists of a family of peptides that share a common C-terminal metal binding core, attached to a variable DNA binding portion with different substitutions on the animo-terminal end of the molecule (Figure 8-1). The various bleomycin peptides have a molecular weight of about 1,500, and vary in their potency for DNA cleavage, but share a common chemistry. The predominant peptide, bleomycin A2, comprises 70% of the clinical preparation.

MECHANISM OF ACTION

The bleomycin peptides function as carriers for a catalytic metal that undergoes rapid cycles of oxidation/reduction (1). The metal may be copper, iron, cobalt, zinc, or others, bound in a hexagonal co-ordination complex of amine groups contributed by the unusual amino acids of the peptide. All metals but the cobalt species are readily exchangeable; thus 57 Co (II) bleomycin is sufficiently stable to be used as a tumor-imaging agent. The clinical preparation of bleomycin is metal-free, but upon administration rapidly acquires Cu (II) or Fe (II), the latter probably representing the active form of the drug. Bleomycin binds to DNA by intercalation of its C-terminal bithiazole groups between guanine bases in adjacent DNA strands. Intercalation brings the bleomycin metal group into proximity with the deoxyribose backbone of DNA. The radicals released by cycles of oxidation/reduction of the Fe^{++} core oxidize adjacent deoxyribose groups at the 3′-4′ bond, releasing propenal or propenal-thymine as its most frequent products (Figure 8-2). DNA single and double strand breaks (in the ratio of 10:1) result, and must be repaired if the cell is to survive. If double strand breaks are sufficient in number, the cell undergoes apoptosis. Cells deficient in

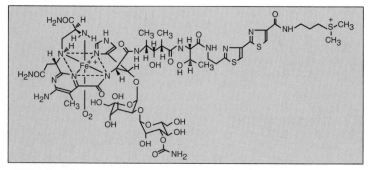

FIGURE 8-1   Bleomycin A₂.

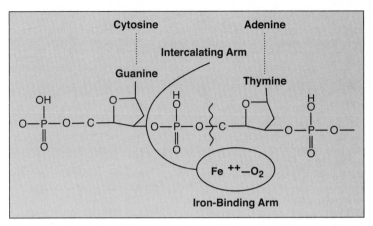

FIGURE 8-2 Intercalation of bithiazole groups between DNA strands in which one strand has the preferred sequence of GpT or GpC. The Fe^{++}-O_2 complex bound to bleomycin comes in opposition to the deoxyribose of DNA, abstracting a proton and cleaving the deoxyribose phosphate bond.

double strand break repair, such as those from tumors with BRCA-1 mutation are highly sensitive to bleomycin (2).

Bleomycin, a large, positively charged molecule, crosses the cell membrane slowly, possibly entering through vesicles. In the cytoplasm it is subject to cleavage by a specific aminohydrolase, which is found in both malignant and normal tissues, and which may play a role in determining both response and toxicity (3). For example, the hydrolase is found in low concentrations in lung tissue and skin, both of which are highly susceptible to bleomycin toxicity. Mice deficient in hydrolase are extremely sensitive to the drug's toxicity. Tumor cells with high levels of hydrolase are resistant to the drug.

A number of factors determine sensitivity to bleomycin in experimental studies. Defects in mismatch repair are often associated with mutations of genes involved in double strand break repair, and lead to hypersensitivity to the drug (3). Inhibition of RAD21, a gene that participates in double strand break repair, also leads to bleomycin sensitization. Resistance arises by several other mechanisms in experimental cells (4). These changes include an increase in hydrolase activity, decreased drug uptake by an as yet unidentified transporter, increased DNA repair capacity, or increased detoxification of free radicals.

CLINICAL PHARMACOLOGY

Bleomycin is administered i.v. or i.m. in doses of 10–20 units/m^2 every 2 weeks. Single doses above 25 mg/m^2 are associated with an increased risk of pulmonary toxicity. The disposition of bleomycin is characterized by its slow uptake in tissues and selective hydrolysis in certain tissues, including liver and kidney. Most of an administered dose is excreted in the urine as an intact molecule. After intramuscular or intravenous administration, it disappears from plasma with a half-life of 2–3 h. Patients with renal dysfunction, such as those treated with cisplatin, may exhibit much delayed clearance and may develop overwhelming systemic toxicity (see below). Doses should be reduced at least 50% in patients with reduced renal function (creatinine clearance below 80 ml/min), and should not be given in any dose to patients in renal failure (creatinine clearance below 30 ml/min) (5).

Bleomycin is also given by intrapleural instillation in doses of 60 mg or greater, dissolved in 50–100 ml of saline, to ablate the pleural space. Given in this manor it has a 75% success rate for ablation of effusions, and has little systemic toxicity (6). It has been used as an experimental therapy by direct injection to cause regression of warts, keloids and hemangiomas, and other vascular abnormalities.

TOXICITY

The primary acute toxicity of bleomycin is cutaneous erythema, tenderness, and ulceration over the joints or the distal extremities, and frank Raynaud's phenomenon in occasional patients. Hyperpigmentation, nail changes, and alopecia may occur after prolonged use.

The most serious long-term toxic effects are those that affect the lung. Pulmonary toxicity is usually dose-related and most frequent (10% or greater) in patients receiving total doses of 450 mg or more, but may appear at lower total doses in selected patients, and particularly in patients above 70 years of age, in those treated with single doses above 20 mg/m^2 and in those who have received or are receiving chest irradiation. Concomitant treatment with gemcitabine and bleomycin leads to unacceptable rates of pulmonary toxicity (7). Acute deterioration in pulmonary function may be seen as a postoperative complication in patients exposed to high concentrations of inspired O$_2$ subsequent to bleomycin treatment, as, for example, in patients undergoing surgical resection of residual tumor after chemotherapy for germ cell tumors of the testis. In combination therapy of Hodgkin Disease, 20% of patients will have a greater than 20% decrease in diffuse capacity after a full course of combination therapy including bleomycin (8).

The pathophysiology of bleomycin pulmonary toxicity is not well understood. Experimental intertracheal injection of small doses of bleomycin or its terminal amine fragment evokes an acute inflammatory response and subsequent pulmonary fibrosis in mice and hamsters. Bleomycin induces macrophage secretion of proinflammatory cytokines such as interleukins 1 and 6, TNF-alpha, and TGF-beta. Mice deficient in metalloproteinases or plasminogen activators are resistant to bleomycin pulmonary fibrosis, suggesting that inhibitors of these enzymes might be useful in preventing fibrosis (9).

Clinically, bleomycin pulmonary toxicity manifests as a dry cough, shortness of breath, and in some patients fever, with pulmonary alveolar infiltrates on chest x-ray. Computerized tomography may reveal extensive changes in patients with minimal evidence on routine chest x-rays. Pleural thickening and even cavitary lesions have been reported. In later stages, there is evidence of extensive pulmonary parenchymal fibrosis. The acute syndrome must be distinguished from opportunistic infection or other causes of pulmonary infiltrates in cancer patients. In such patients, biopsy discloses inflammatory alveolar infiltrates, hyaline membrane formation, and fibrosis. Patients on bleomycin experience a steady decrease in pulmonary diffusion capacity and, in later stages, develop evidence of restrictive disease and desaturation. There is no proven therapy for bleomycin pulmonary toxicity other than discontinuation of the drug. Corticosteroids may produce temporary improvement of symptoms, but there is no evidence that they change the incidence of late pulmonary fibrosis, which is in general irreversible. With discontinuation of the drug, the inflammatory component may resolve and pulmonary function may improve in less severe cases. Approximately a quarter of patients who develop full-blown evidence of bleomycin toxicity, with symptoms and bilateral infiltrates, will have a fatal outcome.

Limitation of total doses to less than 250 units, selection of patients without risk factors (see above), and careful clinical monitoring for evidence of toxicity have reduced the incidence of serious pulmonary injury to less than 5% in patients treated for Hodgkin Disease or testicular cancer. The drug remains a unique and important component of their treatment regimens.

REFERENCES

1. Lazo JS, Chabner BA. Bleomycin. In BA Chabner, DL Longo (eds.), "Cancer Chemotherapy & Biotherapy Principles and Practice," 4th edition, Lippincott Williams & Wilkins, Philadelphia, 2006, pp. 344.
2. Quinn JE, Kennedy RD, Mullan PB, et al. BRCA1 Functions as a differential modulator of chemotherapy-induced apoptosis. Cancer Res. 2003; 63: 6221.
3. Li HR, Shagisultanova EI, Yamashita K, Piao Z, Perucho M, Malkhosyan SR. Hypersensitivity of tumor cell lines with microsatellite instability to DNA double strand break producing chemotherapeutic agent bleomycin. Cancer Res. 2004; 64: 4760.
4. Atienza JM, Roth RB, Rosette C, et al. Suppression of RAD21 gene expression decreases cell growth and enhances cytotoxicity of etoposide and bleomycin in human breast cancer cells. Mol Cancer Ther. 2005; 4: 361.
5. O'Sullivan JM, Huddart RA, Norman AR, et al. Predicting the risk of bleomycin lung toxicity in patients with germ-cell tumors. Ann Oncol. 2003; 14: 91.
6. Sartori S, Tassinari D, Ceccotti P, et al. Prospective randomized trial of intrapleural bleomycin versus interferon alfa-2b via ultrasound-guided small-bore chest tube in the palliative treatment of malignant pleural effusions. J Clin Oncol. 2004; 22: 1228.
7. Bredenfield H, Franklin J, Nogova L, et al. Severe pulmonary toxicity in patients with advanced-stage Hodgkin's disease treated with a modified bleomycin, doxorubicin, cyclophosphamide, vincristine, procarbazine and gemcitabine (BEACOPP) regimin is probably related to the combination of gemcitabine and bleomycin: a report of the German Hodgkin's Lymphoma Study Group. J Clin Oncol. 2004; 22: 2424.
8. Martin WG, Ristow KM, Habermann TM, Colgan JP, Witzig TE, Ansell SM. Bleomycin pulmonary toxicity has a negative impact on the outcome of patients with Hodgkin's lymphoma. J Clin Oncol. 2005; 23: 7614.
9. Zuo F, Kaminski N, Fugui E, et al. Gene expression analysis reveals matrilysin as a key regulator of pulmonary fibrosis in mice and humans. Proc Natl Acad Sci. 2002; 99: 6292.

L-ASPARAGINASE

Most anticancer drugs are small molecular weight molecules designed to inhibit enzymes or to interact with DNA. Newer drugs may be proteins, such as monoclonal antibodies or biologicals that interact with cell surface receptors. L-asparaginase (L-ASP) is unique as a bacterial protein that hydrolyzes an essential amino acid, L-asparagine, which some tumors are unable to synthesize, and must derive from the blood stream. Initial experiments by Broome described the antitumor effects of this enzyme against lymphoid tumors, leading to the purification and commercial use of enzyme from *E. coli* (1). L-ASP is now an essential component of the remission induction and consolidation regimen for childhood acute lymphocytic leukemia (ALL). Its enzymatic activity is highly specific for asparagine hydrolysis. A broad range of toxicities result from asparagine depletion, including inhibition of the synthesis of various clotting factors, insulin, and other essential proteins.

L-ASP is a 144,000 tetrameric protein that catalyzes the deamination of the circulating blood pool of L-asparagine. Enzyme from *E. coli*, and an alternative protein from Erwinia Chrysanthemi, are highly specific for L-asparagine, but retain minor cleaving activity against glutamine. The two enzymes lack immunologic cross-reactivity; therefore the Erwinia enzyme may be used with relative assurance of safety in patients hypersensitive to *E. coli* enzyme. The Erwinia enzyme must be used in higher doses, as it has a shorter plasma $t_{1/2}$ (16 h versus 30 h for *E. coli*). A third form of L-ASP, the *E. coli* enzyme conjugated to polyethylene glycol (pegaspargase), has a much longer $t_{1/2}$ of 6 days and is less immunogenic than either unconjugated enzyme, and is often used in patients demonstrating hypersensitivity to the unconjugated enzymes, 70% of whom will not react to the pegylated enzyme (2). It is unclear whether either Erwinia or pegaspargase is as effective as *E. coli* in depleting L-asparagine.

CLINICAL PHARMACOLOGY

A comparison of the primary features of the three drugs is shown in Table 9-1. No single dosing schedule of the various L-ASP preparations has been established. While in theory intravenous dosing may be less immunogenic, evidence is lacking, and the drug is given by intramuscular injection in the United States. Higher doses are associated with more complete and prolonged asparagine depletion, but cause a higher incidence of side effects, particularly thrombotic events, and more frequent hypersensitivity responses. In general, most regimens strive to maintain enzyme activity in plasma of 0.05–0.1 units/ml for the duration of therapy (for 7–21 days), a level associated with total asparagine depletion in plasma, but not in the cerebrospinal fluid.

Clinical effectiveness of L-ASP appears to be a function of the duration of therapy (less or more than 25 weeks), the development of neutralizing antibodies, and the tolerance to treatment, which is less in older children and adults. Cellular resistance to L-ASP arises by induction of asparagine synthetase in tumor cells. In the TEL-AML1 negative subset of ALL, higher levels of this enzyme correlate with clinical resistance. However, in the 25% of ALL patients with translocations involving the TEL gene, ALL cells are highly sensitive

Table 9-1

Comparison of the Primary Features of Three Drugs

Preparation	Typical dose/schedule IU/m^2 / dose	Elimination from plasma (half-life)	Antibody positive patients (%)*
E. coli	5–10,000 IU/m^2 3 d/wk × 2–4wks 25,000 IU/m^2 q.wk	30 h	45–75
Erwina	10,000 IU/m^2 qd × 7	16 h	30–50
Pegaspargase	2,500 IU/m^2 q 1–4 wks	6 days	5–18

*Following completion of a course of therapy, with no prior asparaginase exposure, and with no concurrent corticosteroids.

despite high levels of the synthetase, perhaps indicating a defect in aspartate uptake or transamination (3).

TOXICITY

In ALL patients, antibodies are detected in up to 50% of patients receiving single agent L-ASP, but in only 20% of patients receiving L-ASP with immunosuppressive drugs, such as methotrexate 6-mercaptopurine or corticosteroids. About half of patients with neutralizing antibodies will have clinical evidence of hypersensitivity, but some asymptomatic patients will have "silent inactivation" and undetectable L-ASP levels in plasma and will be at increased risk of leukemic relapse (4). Monitoring of L-ASP levels during therapy is recommended. Patients hypersensitive to *E. coli* enzyme should be switched to Erwinia L-ASP or to pegaspargase.

Other toxicities of L-ASP include its effects on coagulation and protein synthesis. It depletes both antithrombotic (protein C and protein S, antithrombin III) and procoagulant factors (prothrombin), and is associated with a significant risk of stroke related to cortical sinus thrombosis. The risk of thrombosis seems highest in patients with underlying inherited defects in anticoagulant factors, such as homocystinemia, factor V Leiden deficiency, or prothrombin mutations (5). Protein synthesis inhibition may cause extreme hypertriglyceridemia and pancreatitis (lipoprotein lipase deficiency), hyperglycemia (insulin deficiency), and, infrequently, hemorrhage (prothrombin, factor IX, and factor X deficiency). The same spectrum of side effects occurs in patients receiving pegaspargase, although the frequency of hypersensitivity reactions is significantly reduced.

The only significant drug interaction is the ability of L-ASP to terminate methotrexate action through its inhibition of cell cycle progression. Sequential therapy with L-ASP followed in 10 days by methotrexate may yield synergistic antileukemic effects.

Considerable uncertainty remains regarding the best regimen, including dose and schedule (Table 9-1), for treating ALL, and the best use of the various L-ASP preparations. Alternative regimens employing higher doses, more extended periods of treatments, and various drug combinations are undergoing clinical evaluation (2).

REFERENCES

1. Cooney DA, Handschumacher RE. L-asparaginase and L-asparaginase metabolism. Annu Rev Pharmacol. 1970; 10: 421–440.
2. Boos J. The best way to use asparaginase in childhood acute lymphatic leukemia—still to be defined? Br J Haematol. 2004; 125: 117–127.

3. Stams WAG, den Boer ML, Holleman A, et al. Asparaginase synthetase expression is linked with L-asparaginase resistance in TEL-AML1-negative but not TEL-AML1-positive pediatric acute lymphoblastic leukemia. Blood. 2005; 105: 4223–4225.

4. Muller HJ, Boos J. Use of L-asparaginase in childhood ALL. Crit Rev Oncol Hematol. 1998; 28: 97–113.

5. Nowak-Gottl U, Wermes C, Junker R, et al. Prospective evaluation of the thrombotic risk in children with acute lymphoblastic leukemia carrying the MTHFR TT 677 genotype, the prothrombocin G20210A variant, and further prothrombotic risk factors. Blood. 1999; 93: 1595–1599.

MOLECULAR TARGETED DRUGS

INTRODUCTION

Discoveries important for survival, proliferation, and metastasis of different cancer cells combined with technological advances have produced agents that target proteins or genes critical in the neoplastic process (Figure 10-1). These agents include monoclonal antibodies (mAbs), designed small molecules, peptidomimetics, small interfering RNAs (siRNAs), antisense oligonucleotides, vaccines, and other targeted therapies. A number of these have sufficient clinical activity to be important components of standard therapy for malignancies, including (1–11):

Monoclonal antibodies

- *Trastuzumab:* breast cancer
- *Rituximab, ibritumomab tuixetan, and tositumomab + I131*: follicular B-cell non-Hodgkin's lymphomas (NHLs)
- *Alemtuzumab*: B-cell chronic lymphocytic leukemia (B-CLL)
- *Gemtuzimab ozogomicin*: AML
- *Bevacizumab*: combined with chemotherapy: colorectal cancer, non-small cell lung cancer (NSCLC)
- *Cetuximab*: colorectal cancer (with or without chemotherapy and squamous cell head and neck cancer (with radiation therapy)
- *Panitumumab*: colorectal cancer

Peptide immunotoxins

- *Denileukin diftitox* (diphtheria toxin-interleukin 2 (IL-2) fusion protein): cutaneous T-cell lymphoma (CTCL)

Targeted small molecule kinase inhibitors

- *Imatinib*: chronic myelogenous leukemia (CML) and gastrointestinal stromal tumors (GIST)
- *Sunitinib*: renal cell cancer (RCC) and GIST
- *Sorafenib*: RCC
- *Dasatinib*: imatinib resistant CML or PH+ ALL
- *Gefitinib and erlotinib*: (NSCLC)
- *Erlotinib* (with gemcitabine): pancreatic cancer
- *Lapatanib* (breast cancer)
- *Temsirolimus* (RRC)

Proteosome inhibitor

- *Bortezomib*: multiple myeloma (MM)

A large number of agents are in clinical trials, and this list continues to grow.

MOLECULAR TARGETS IN CANCER

Increased understanding of cancer biology has led to a more rational approach to therapeutic discovery through targeting pathways and proteins essential for cancer cell survival, growth or metastasis and, either quantitatively or qualitatively, unique to cancer (Figure10-1). Some of the mechanisms that have been

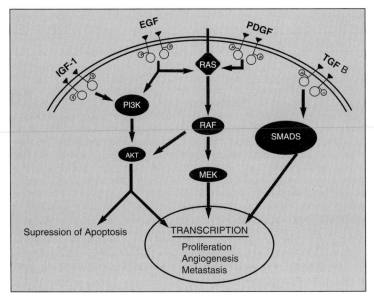

FIGURE 10-1   Schematic of growth factor receptor signaling in tumor cells.

discovered include: mutant genes that alter a critical cellular function leading to uncontrolled growth, inhibition of apoptosis, or inappropriate spread to another organ; overexpression of growth factors or their receptors, such as the epidermal growth factor receptor (EGFR) family, including *HER-2-neu;* angiogenic pathways (e.g., vascular endothelial growth factors (VEGFs) and their receptors); antiapoptotic mechanisms that antagonize cell death, such as overexpression of Bcl-2 or decreased BAX expression; inappropriate telomerase expression leading to antiapoptotic effects; and enhanced activity of intracellular signaling pathways that promote growth, inhibit apoptosis, or lead to invasion/metastasis.

1. *Mutant genes in cancer cells provide unique targets.*
   Examples include BCR-ABL in CML, c-KIT in GIST and EGFR in certain cases of NSCLC all of which have proven to be clinically useful targets for small molecular inhibitors of their tyrosine kinase activity (2, 3, 10). Mutations of genes in signal transduction pathways, such as activation of one of the Ras families of proteins (found frequently in pancreatic adenocarcinoma, thyroid cancer, and several other malignancies), can lead to unrestrained growth. Sorafenib may mediate part of its antitumor effect by inhibiting the Raf kinase, which is one of the proteins immediately downstream of Ras (9). Activating mutations of Raf are found in malignant melanoma and other solid tumors. Mutations in tumor suppressor genes such as p53, retinoblastoma (RB), or the phosphate and tensin homolog (PTEN) that regulates the PI3-kinase pathway can produce loss of important brakes on proliferation leading to unrestrained growth. These have been harder to target because it is more difficult to return normal function than to inhibit aberrant function. However, extensive research is ongoing in attempts to accomplish this.
2. *Growth factor receptors or their ligands.*
   These are overexpressed in a number of malignancies, mutated in several, and in both cases have increased activity making them good targets for

inhibition (1–4). Growth factors and their receptors are important in a number of cellular processes essential for proliferation, survival, and metastasis of neoplastic cells. Their expression on the cell surface makes them accessible to monoclonal antibodies. Examples of growth factors and receptors currently being targeted include:

- *EGFR family, including HER-1 (EGFR)* and *HER-2* (EGFRs are present on epithelial cells which give rise to the majority of cancers; overexpressed in many cancers; mutated in a subset of NSCLC with adenocarcinoma or adenocarcinoma with bronchoalveolar cancer histologies (Some tumors with mutated receptors appear to be more sensitive to anti-EGFR therapy). HER-2 is a major target for a subset of breast cancers).
- *c-KIT* (mutations are frequently found in GIST tumors).
- *VEGF/VEGFR* (play important role in angiogenesis).
- *PDGFR's* (e.g., overexpressed in brain tumors or mutated in a subset of GIST).
- *MET* (overexpressed in a number of malignancies).
- mTOR (an anti-apoptotic signaling element in the PI-3 kinase pathway)

Responses in patients treated with mAbs to HER-2 (e.g., trastuzumab) or the EGFR (e.g., cetuximab), and small molecular weight inhibitors (e.g., erlotinib) demonstrate that interruption of growth factor signaling can be a useful strategy for cancer therapy (1, 2). Bevacizimab's success (combined with chemotherapy) in treating colorectal cancer has established the benefit of inhibiting VEGF (critical in tumor angiogenesis). Anti-angiogenesis is likely mechanism by which the small molecules sorafenib and sunitinib mediate their antitumor activity (4, 9).

3. *Signal transduction.* A number of signaling pathways downstream of GFRs have been identified and shown to play important roles in malignancies. These include Ras, Src, and PI3 kinase. Approaches targeting these and multiple other signal transduction proteins are currently being investigated.

4. *Cell cycle control.* This has been the nonspecific target of many of the currently available chemotherapeutic agents. Now, more specific approaches (e.g., targeting specific overexpressed cyclin dependent kinases or proteins that inactivate pRB) are being evaluated based on increased understanding of the critical proteins involved in this process.

5. *Apoptosis.* As the complex protein interactions involved in controlling the apoptotic process continue to be elucidated, a number of agents aimed at enhancing apoptosis in cancer cells are in clinical trials, including inhibitors of the PI-3 kinase pathway.

6. *Tumor suppressor proteins.* Extensive research is ongoing to try to overcome the difficulty in restoring normal protein function to cancer cells.

7. *Telomerase.* Although much has been learned about the role of telomerase in maintaining telomeres in neoplastic cells and thus allowing continued proliferation, significant preclinical work is needed to translate this into a useful anticancer approach.

8. *Targeted molecules for imaging.* Although this is in its relative infancy clinically, preclinical studies suggest that this holds great promise for earlier diagnosis or the ability to detect smaller lesions that might be more treatable.

9. *Multiple targets.* Most cancers represent the evolution of multiple mutations, and targeting multiple different genes may be necessary to kill individual clones of cells. In addition, targeting the environment within which cells are growing might also be important (4, 6, 8, 9). Lenalomide which affects multiple targets (e.g., modulation of growth factor pathways including VEGF, inhibiting proinflammatory proteins (e.g., TNF-alpha)

and immunostimulation) is active against 5q- MDS. Bortezomib (a proteosome inhibitor) that inhibits destruction of a number of ubiquinated proteins including ones involved in controlling cell cycle, cell survival, and tumor growth is active against MM. Either combinations of agents specifically targeting several processes or individual agents that target a number of processes may be required for control of many types of cancer. Both of these approaches are actively being pursued.

CURRENTLY APPROVED TARGETED AGENTS IN CANCER THERAPY (USA)

Monoclonal Antibodies

The ability to generate highly specific antibodies against the antigen of choice makes mABs excellent targeting agents (1, 4). They can be used alone or to deliver radionuclides, toxins, or chemotherapy to malignant cells or specific tissues. mAbs directed against GFRs and other cell surface antigens have undergone extensive testing in treatment of a number of cancers. Approved mAB agents for treating cancer include trastuzumab against HER-2 (breast cancer); bevicizumab against VEGF (colorectal, NSCLC); anti-EGFR antibodies cetuximab (for colorectal and head and neck cancer) and panitumumab (colorectal); three antibodies directed against the CD20 antigen: rituximab, ibritumomab (coupled to yttrium 90 to deliver radiation therapy) (zevelin), and tositumomab (coupled to I131 to deliver radiation therapy) (Bexxar) (for B-cell NHL); alemtuzumab which binds to CD52 (for B-CLL); and gemtuzamab ozogomicin (Mylotarg) which binds to CD33 and contains a cytotoxic agent (for AML). The most serious toxicities for each of these are shown in Table 10-1. A number of other mABs are currently undergoing clinical evaluation. Continued improvements utilizing antibodies to target agents, such as radioactive compounds or chemotherapeutic agents, in an attempt to slectively kill tumor cells, continue to be explored. Combinations of antibodies with radiation therapy or chemotherapeutic agents are also being investigated. (See Chapter 16 for additional details on monoclonal antibodies.)

Small Molecules

Because they can be subjected to high throughput screening and can be readily modified to incorporate favorable pharmacologic properties, small molecules have become the most attractive agents to utilize for targeted therapy (2–4, 6–10). High-throughput screening against recombinant proteins allows identification of molecules with high affinity for the specific target site of interest. Subsequent preclinical evaluation allows development of compounds that retain the biological effect of interest while having properties (e.g., oral bioavailability, extended plasma half-life, decreased toxicity) that aid clinical development.

IMATINIB   *Mechanism of action*: The 9:22 translocation in CML places the Abl tyrosine kinase on chromosome 9 in juxtaposition to the breakpoint cluster region (BCR) of chromosome 22 with a resultant protein that has a complex variety of functions including constitutively active tyrosine kinase activity that affects a number of signaling pathways. Like most other kinase inhibitors that have been developed, imatinib blocks the ATP binding site leading to potent inhibition of the tyrosine kinase activity of BCR-Abl (7). Imatinib also potently inhibits c-KIT, which is frequently mutated in GIST, and PDGFR-alpha, which is mutated in a smaller percentage of GIST tumors, but is also over expressed on a other types of malignant cells (10).

Toxicity: Neutropenia, thrombocytopenia, anemia; hepatotoxicity (usually manifested by elevated liver enzymes but rarely severe); fluid retention/edema;

musculoskelatal pains/cramps; rash; diarrhea; GI irritation; bleeding (gi or intratumoral); hypophosphatemia; congestive heart failure. Imatinib is metabolized by cyp3A4. It is therefore important to monitor the dose when given with cyp3A4 inhibitors (e.g., itraconazole, erythromycin) and decrease as necessary. Similarly, serum imatinib levels may be decreased by inducers of cyp3A4 (e.g., phenytoin) and the dose may need to be increased.

Clinical effectiveness (CML): Imatinib produces clinical hematologic responses in the majority of CML patients in chronic phase and cytogenetic complete remission in approximately half of previously untreated patients (3, 7). At higher dose it also has activity against CML in accelerated phase. Although less active for patients with blast crisis, it still produces a small percentage of complete hematological responses. It has had less clinical activity against acute lymphoblastic leukemia with the 9:22 translocation.

GIST: GISTs are the most common mesenchymal tumors arising from the GI tract (10). They can arise from any site in the gastrointestinal tract or even the omentum, mesentery, or retroperitoneum, but they most commonly occur in the stomach. Surgical resection is the primary treatment. However, there is a fairly high rate of recurrence or metastatic disease. GISTS have been unresponsive to standard chemotherapeutic agents. Imatinib inhibits the c-KIT receptor and the PDGF receptor (PDGFR). KIT is mutated in a high proportion (approximately 85%) of patients with GIST. Evidence strongly indicates that clinical antitumor activity of imatinib against GIST correlates with specific mutations in KIT. The PDGFR-alpha is mutated in approximately 35% of tumors with wild-type GIST and these tumors are also often responsive to imatinib. Imatinib has also recently been approved for dermatofibrosarcoma protuberans, myelodysplastic/myeloproliferative diseases associated with PDGFR rearrangements, hypereosinophilic syndrome/chronic eosinophilia, and aggressive systemic mastocytosis.

DASATINIB   *Mechanism of action*: Similar to imatinib, dasatinib is a potent inhibitor of the tyrosine kinase activity of BCR-Abl (7). It also inhibits a number of other tyrosine kinases including src family members, c-kit, EPHA 2, and PDGFR.

Toxicity: Similar to imatinib, including neutropenia, thrombocytopenia, anemia; hepatotoxicity (usually manifested by elevated liver); fluid retention/edema; musculoskelatal pains/cramps; headaches; fatigue; rash; diarrhea; GI irritation; bleeding; hypophosphatemia; congestive heart failure; cardiac dysrhythmias. It also can cause prolongation of the QT interval. Similar to imatinib, it is metabolized by cyp3A4. It is therefore important to monitor the dose when given with cyp3A4 inhibitors.

Clinical effectiveness (CML): Imatinib produces clinical hematologic responses in the CML or PH+ ALL patients who have become resistant to imatinib therapy (7) through mutation that affect Imatinib binding to the ATP-Catalytic site on the enzyme.

GEFITINIB (ATP POCKET-BINDING INHIBITOR OF EGFR)
Mechanism of action: Gefitinib (Iressa) is a specific inhibitor of the EGFR tyrosine kinase by targeting the ATP binding site (2). Since EGFR signaling is involved in survival and proliferation of certain neoplastic cells, inhibition of the tyrosine kinase activity can lead to inhibition of cell proliferation and/or apoptosis.

Toxicity: Diarrhea and skin rash (often acneiform) are the most common toxicities. Nausea, pruritis, elevated liver function tests, fatigue, and asthenia can be seen. Uncommon but potentially serious toxicities include corneal erosion or ulcer and interstitial pneumonitis that can be life-threatening or fatal.

Clinical effectiveness: It has activity against approximately 10–12% of NSCLC that have progressed after two lines of chemotherapy. The activity of gefitinib appears to correlate with activating somatic mutations in the EGFR(2). Mutations are found primarily in adenocarcinomas (including those with bronchoalveolar features) and are more frequent in nonsmokers, women, and oriental subjects.

ERLOTINIB (ATP POCKET-BINDING INHIBITOR OF EGFR)
Mechanism of action: Erlotinib (Tarceva) is a potent specific inhibitor of the EGFR tyrosine kinase (2). Similar to gefitinib, it targets the ATP binding site of the protein.

Toxicity: Rash, dermatitis, and pruritis in the majority of patients, diarrhea (although uncommonly severe), nausea, fatigue, uncommon bleeding or clotting, and rare cases of interstitial pneumonitis.

Clinical effectiveness: Erlotinib has a similar level of activity to gefitinib against NSCLC (approximately 12% response rate in unselected patients, and a several fold higher rate in patients whose tumors have activating mutations). However, erlotinib was associated with a statistically significant (approximately 2 month) prolongation of median survival as compared with placebo in patients who had failed previous chemotherapy for metastatic NSCLC. A phase III trial has also shown a survival advantage (albeit small) for pancreatic adenocarcinoma patients receiving gemcitabine plus erlotinib as compared to those receiving gemcitabine alone and it has also been approved for this indication.

LAPATANIB *Mechanism of action*: An oral inhibition of EGFR and HER2, the Latter is thought to primary target in traztuzumab resistant breast cancer (12).
Toxicity: Diarrhea, rash.
Clinical effectiveness: Approved for patients who have received prior traztuzumab; used in combination with capecitabine.

SORAFENIB *Mechanism of action*: Sorafenib is an orally available multigarted kinase inhibitor including inhibition of Raf, VEGFR2, VEGFR3, PDGFR-beta, Flt3, and c-KIT (9). Raf is one of the immediate downstream targets of Ras in signal transduction and thus inhibiting Raf potentially inhibits proliferative signaling from GFRs. However, given its activity against a number of other kinases, it also has antiangiogenic and other effects that may be important for its antitumor activity.
Toxicity: Rash, hand–foot syndrome, hypertension, diarrhea, elevated amylase/lipase (usually without clinical pancreatitis), alopecia, myalgias/arthralgias, mild bone marrow suppression, and uncommonly bleeding or clotting.
Clinical effectiveness: Approved for treatment of RCC based on a phase III study showing a doubling of progression free survival (PFS). Being evaluated in other diseases, especially hepatocellular cancer.

SUNITINIB *Mechanism of action*: Sunitinib is an orally available small molecular inhibitor of the tyrosine kinase activity of the VEGFR-2, PDGFR, and c-KIT receptors (9, 10).
Toxity: Cytopenias, bleeding, skin discoloration, diarrhea, mucocutaneous inflammation, altered taste, asthenia, left ventricular dysfunction (uncommon), GI perforation (rare), and pancreatitis (rare).
Clinical effectiveness: It has shown sufficient activity against GIST (either intolerant of imatinib or after progression on imatinib) and RCC to be approved for these indications. It is being evaluated in other diseases.

TEMSIROLIMUS *Mechanism of action*: An intravenous inhibitor of mTOR, a critical enzyme in the PI-3 kinase-AKT pathway, important in the regulation of a number of processes within cells including cell survival and proliferation (13).

Toxicity: Rash, edema, anorexia, nousea, asthemia, mucositis, hyperglycemia, hyperlipoemia, elevated liver function tests, bone marrow suppression, and increased creatinine.

Clinical effectiveness: It has activity against advanced RRC.

BORTEZOMIB (VELCADE) (PROTEOSOME INHIBITOR) *Mechanism of action*: Bortezomib is a reversible inhibitor of the proteosome, which is involved in degrading ubiquitinated proteins and thus maintaining cellular homeostasis (8). Since many of these proteins play essential roles in cell signaling and survival, disruption can lead to cell death. It is not yet certain which proteins are critical for bortezomib's antitumor activity.

Toxicity: Fever, infection, diarrhea, nausea/vomiting, fatigue, hypotension, and peripheral neuropathy.

Clinical effectiveness: Bortezomib is approved for treatment of patients with multiple myeloma who have received at least two prior chemotherapy regimens and have progressive disease based.

Targeting Cytotoxic Agents via Modified Peptides

DENILEUKIN DIFTITOX (IL-2–DIPHTHERIA HYBRID TOXIN)
Mechanism of action: The fusion protein delivers a potent cellular toxin (diphtheria) to CD25 expressing malignant cells inhibiting cellular protein synthesis and leading to cell death (5).

Toxicity: Hypersensitivity reactions (although most are controllable/preventable by slowing the rate or temporarily interrupting the infusion and treating with antihistamines, acetaminophen, and possibly steroids, they can be severe or life-threatening); respiratory (dyspnea); gastrointestinal; constitutional (flu-like); vascular leak syndrome; rash; elevations of hepatic enzymes (not usually accompanied by other liver abnormalities); renal insufficiency; anemia; thrombocytopenia; hemolysis; proteinuria; increased risk of infections. Most patients develop antibodies against the toxin/IL-2 and these may impact on clearance rates which tend to be two to three times more rapid by the third course.

Clinical effectiveness: Approved for treatment of persistent or recurrent cutaneous T-cell lymphomas (CTCL) expressing the CD25 antigen.

FUTURE OF TARGETED THERAPY FOR TREATING CANCER

A large number of other agents targeting a wide variety of proteins (primarily kinases) are currently undergoing clinical investigation. Some of these have been chosen to have greater specificity for one protein whereas others have activity against a number of protein targets. It is not known whether having agents with specific activity (and potentially combining different agents each with specific activity) or having broader activity within one agent will be more clinically effective. This will likely vary depending on disease indications, targets and agents. Strategies for combining different classes of targeted agents (e.g., mAbs and small molecules) are also being pursued, including combining inhibitors targeting different sites on the same molecule. Approaches targeting multiple steps in a given pathway (such as a signal transduction pathway) or multiple receptors or pathways in parallel are also being evaluated. Similar to the situation with chemotherapy, efforts are ongoing to understand and prevent or overcome resistance to targeted agents.

In addition to development of agents targeted against cell surface receptors, much (13) current interest is to test inhibitors of steps in signal transduction pathways from cell surface to nucleus. For example, identification of the mammalian target for rapamycin (mTOR which is a downstream effector in the PI-3 kinase/Akt pathway) has led to the development of a number of analogues that are currently in clinical evaluation (13). Clearly, there are many other potential targets within cells, including proteins involved in other signaling pathways, enzymes, or important protein–protein interactions.

To date, clinically useful targeted compounds have come from one of three classes of agents (mABs, small molecules, or modified peptides). However, there continues to be significant research evaluating other classes of compounds for potential utility as anticancer agents. An example is the discovery of RNA interference with small inhibitory oligonucleotide (siRNA). The ability of siRNAs to bind to complementary RNA molecules leading to their cleavage and thus produce post-transcriptional gene silencing (PTSG) has provided a very powerful tool for studying the effects of silencing a specific gene. In addition to the power this approach has brought to elucidating biological processes, it is also being actively pursued as a potential treatment approach (14).

CONCLUSION

Increased understanding of the biology of cellular processes combined with tools that allow manipulation of molecular systems for therapeutic benefit has led to rational design of molecules directed at specific proteins or genes important for survival, growth, or spread of malignant cells. A number of molecularly targeted agents have been developed over the past decade, which are now part of standard anticancer therapy. Targets include mutant proteins, proteins expressed in malignant cells that can be utilized to differentially target those cells as opposed to normal cells, and angiogenic factors. These include GFRs and their ligands as well as proteins involved in downstream signaling processes from GFRs. Most targeted therapies have been designed to inhibit the target directly although several are used to deliver cytotoxic compounds to malignant cells. Continued improvement in understanding critical processes in cancer development, growth, and metastasis is providing new targets and agents for attacking these.

REFERENCES

1. O'Mahony D, Bishop MR. Monoclonal antibody therapy. Front Biosci. 2006; 11: 1620–1635.
2. Sequist LV, Bell DW, Lynch TJ, et al. Molecular predictors of response to epidermal growth factor receptor antagonists in non-small-cell lung cancer. J clin oncol 2007; 25: 587–595.
3. Kuriakose P. Targeted therapy for hematologic malignancies. Cancer Control. 2005; 12: 82–90.
4. Cardones AR, Banez LL. VEGF inhibitors in cancer therapy. Curr Pharm Des. 2006; 12: 387–394.
5. Foss F. Clinical experience With Denileukin diftitox (ONTAK). Semin Oncol. 2006; 33: 11–16.
6. Larson RA. Myelodysplasia: When to treat and how. Best Pract Res Clin Haematol. 2006; 19: 293–300.
7. O'Hare T, Corbin AS, Druker BJ. Targeted CML therapy: controlling drug resistance, seeking cure. Curr Opin Genet Dev. 2006; 16: 92–99.
8. Richardson PG, Schlossman R, Hideshima T, et al. New treatments for multiple myeloma. Oncology. 2005; 19: 1781–1792; discussion 1792, 1795–1787.
9. Schoffski P, Dumez H, Clement P, et al. Emerging role of tyrosine kinase inhibitors in the treatment of advanced renal cell cancer: a review. Ann Oncol. 2006; 17: 1185–96.
10. Rubin BP. Gastrointestinal stromal tumours: an update. Histopathology. 2006; 48: 83–96.
11. Bendell J, Goldberg RM. Targeted agents in the treatment of pancreatic cancer: history and lesson learned. Curr Opin Oncol 2007; 19: 390–5.

12. Mayer EL, Lin NU, Burstein HJ. Novel approaches to advanced breast cancer: bevacizumab and Lapatinib. J Natt Compr Canc Netur 2007; 5: 314–323.

13 Easton JB, Houghton PJ, mTOR and cancer therapy. Oncogene 2006; 25: 6436–6446.

14. Aagaard L, Rossi JJ. RNAi therapeutics: Principles, prospects and challenges. Adv Drug Deliv Rev 2007; 59: 75–86.

DIFFERENTIATING AGENTS

One of the most obvious features of malignant cells is their failure to differentiate, this is, their failure to acquire the histologic, biochemical, and functional features of the mature cells of the tissue from which they arise. Thus, leukemia cells resemble the more primitive normal progenitors of the myeloid or lymphoid series, and some may be indistinguishable from "stem cells." Growing evidence suggests that malignant cells arise through a series of mutations that progressively impair their ability to differentiate. Malignant cells in general display patterns of gene expression and cell surface markers, and the histologic appearance of a progressively more primitive cell. Indeed it has been possible to isolate a small fraction of continuously self-renewing cells from frankly malignant tissues that have the capacity for infinite self-renewal, but which are able to reproduce multiple differentiated cell lineages when appropriately stimulated by "differentiating" agents. The progression from mature cell phenotype to malignancy is recapitulated in serial observations of premalignant human cancer. One of the earliest signs of the premalignant state is the presence of a highly proliferative cell population blocked in a state of intermediate differentiation, as seen in chronic myelogenous leukemia or in adenomatous polyps of the intestinal tract. With further mutation and evolution, these intermediate states become frankly malignant.

These observations have led to research efforts that have defined pathways responsible for a block in differentiation in malignant cells, with the hope of pharmacologic intervention. Vitamin A and its derivatives and analogs were the first compounds to show differentiating effects in cell culture, and all-trans retinoic acid (ATRA) (Figure 11-1) was subsequently found to be highly effective

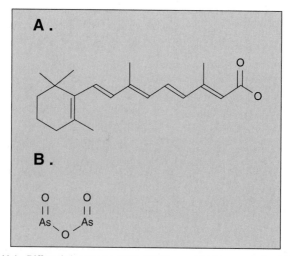

FIGURE 11-1 Differentiating agents useful in APL therapy. (a) All-trans retinoic acid (ATRA) and (b) arsenic trioxide.

in inducing remission in promyelocytic leukemia, a disease characterized by a translocation involving the retinoic acid receptor, RAR-alpha (1). Subsequently, other pathways have been exploited as targets for development of differentiating agents, including histone deacetylase (HDAC), DNA cytidine methyl transferase (CMT), and vitamin D signaling. Of these, CMT is targeted by both 5-azacytidine and decitabine, as discussed in the section on antimetabolites, while HDAC inhibitors and vitamin D analogs are currently in clinical trial. Here we will present a description of three clinically useful agents that promote differentiation, ATRA and arsenic trioxide (ATO), both of which are effective in APL, and vorinostat for cutaneous T-cell lymphoma.

ATRA

Retinoids (vitamin A and its derivatives) were one of the first classes of small molecules shown to induce differentiation of malignant cells in cell culture systems. Early work showed that retinoids caused promyelocytic leukemia (APL) (HL-60) cells to undergo maturation into granulocytes at micromolar drug concentrations easily achievable in humans. The mechanism of ATRA action has been elucidated by in vitro studies of its effects on differentiation of normal myeloid cells and APL cells. In normal cells, RAR-alpha exists in a multiprotein complex with the PML transcription factor and the retinoid X receptor (RXR). This complex, when bound to ATRA, then activates transcription of a series of genes that induce differentiation (2). In APL cells, the normal pathway for vitamin A action is disrupted. APL is characterized by a translocation involving the retinoic acid receptor—alpha gene (RAR-alpha) on chromosome 15 and the PML gene on chromosome 17. When not bound to ATRA, the fusion protein acts as a repressor of differentiation and, through the FOS gene, promotes proliferation. The RAR-alpha/PML fusion protein has low affinity for ATRA and requires pharmacologic concentrations of retinoid to activate the normal differentiation pathway in APL cells. ATRA activation of the pathway frees HDAC, a gene expression modifier, from a repressor complex with PML. It also upregulates transcription factors (CEBP beta, OCT-1, and most importantly, PU. 1) required for myeloid differentiation (2). Resistance to ATRA arises through mutation of the fusion protein to decrease its binding affinity, and possibly by induction of the ATRA metabolizing P450 isoenzyme (CYP26A1) in the liver or in APL cells after prolonged exposure to the drug (3).

CLINICAL PHARMACOLOGY

ATRA induces complete remission in more than 90% of patients with APL, alone or in combination with an anthracycline (1). The initial clinical experience in patients relapsing after intensive cytotoxic chemotherapy revealed clear evidence of leukemic cell maturation in bone marrow and peripheral blood, culminating in complete remission in the majority of such patients. Remission duration for single agent ATRA tends to be brief, and the recurrent tumor is usually refractory to a second cycle of treatment due to further mutation in the RAR-alpha gene. However, when ATRA is used in combination with anthracyclines, the regimen is curative for 70% or more of patients with this disease. It is effective in all PML patients with the PML/RARa translocation, including those with a masked translocation, only detectable by PCR. The "long" form of the translocation is more sensitive to APL and has a greater disease free survival after remission than does the "short" form (4).

ATRA is given in daily intravenous doses of 45 mg per m^2 per day with an anthracycline until remission is achieved. It is now used as the initial therapy in APL, as it quickly aborts the life-threatening coagulopathy associated with this disease. In patients with significant comorbidities or in elderly patients, it efficiently induces remission when used with ATO, without a cytotoxic agent. It may also be effective in maintenance therapy, but continuous use leads to cutaneous toxicity and abnormal lipids. Therefore intermittent schedules of maintenance ATRA may be better tolerated and equally efficacious, when given with methotrexate and mercaptopurine. ATRA concentrations in plasma reach 400 ng/ml, and ATRA is rapidly eliminated by p450-mediated metabolism. The rate of clearance increases markedly with repeated doses.

TOXICITY

ATRA's primary side effects are cutaneous and pulmonary. Retinoids cause a redness, dryness, and sensitivity of the skin and cracking of the lips (cheilosis). Through its differentiating effects on APL cells, it causes an accumulation of leukemic neutrophil precursors in pulmonary vessels, leading to hypoxia, pleural and pericardial effusions, and, in extreme cases, to death. Concurrent corticosteroids and cytotoxic chemotherapy, given with ATRA, control the increase in leukemic granulocytes in the peripheral blood, decease their adhesion to endothelium, and greatly lessen the risk of the "retinoic acid syndrome." Prophylactic dexamethasone should be given to patients with a presenting white blood cell count of 5×10^9 per l or higher (5).

Other ATRA toxicities include pseudotumor cerebri, with headaches, change in mental status, and papilledema; liver function test abnormalities; bone tenderness; and elevated plasma triglycerides, all of which are reversible with cessation of therapy.

ARSENIC TRIOXIDE (ATO)

A second unique therapy, ATO (Figure 11-1) has been identified for APL, with differentiating effects that mimic those of ATRA. ATO induces a high rate of complete response in patients refractory to ATRA and chemotherapy, and has become a component of first line regimens (6). Its mechanism of action is less well understood than that of ATRA. It promotes differentiation and apoptosis of cultured APL cells. It alters the phosphorylation and promotes the degradation of RAR-α/PML, and promotes degradation of NF-κB, an antiapoptotic transcription factor (7). It also generates potentially cytotoxic free radicals. The relative contribution of each of these properties to the antileukemic action of APL is not clear.

CLINICAL PHARMACOLOGY

The standard regimen for ATO administration as a single agent is a 2 h infusion of 0.15 mg/kg/day for up to 60 days, or until achievement of a complete response. Further treatment is given after a three week break. Alternative schedules of a five day loading dose, followed by twice weekly drug infusions until remission, are being explored. Its use in combination with ATRA and cytotoxic chemotherapy for primary therapy of APL is evolving. Early trials indicate that it is highly effective in inducing remission when used with ATRA, both in low-risk and high-risk patients (WBC count $>5 \times 10^9$/l) (8).

Peak concentrations of total arsenic achieved during the 2 h infusion reach 5 μM. The parent compound is eliminated through interaction with sulfhydrils and through enzymatic methylation. The concentration of parent drug, the active principle, is probably significantly lower (less than 1 μM) (9).

TOXICITY

ATO causes a long list of side effects, the most important of which is a leukemic cell maturation syndrome similar to that caused by ATRA, with pulmonary distress, pleural and pericardial effusions, and alteration in mental status. It may cause hyperglycemia, hepatic enzyme abnormalities, and acute, fatal hepatic failure. Myositis manifested as muscle tenderness and swelling, accompanied at times by fever, has also been reported. ATO inhibits ion channels in the cardiac conduction system, causing a prolongation of the QT interval and predisposing to atrial and ventricular arrhythmias. During ATO therapy, a weekly EKG should be monitored for signs of QT changes and arrhythmias, and serum K^+ and Mg^{2+} should be monitored weekly and replenished as necessary to maintain their concentrations above 4 and 2 meq/l, respectively. An absolute QT interval of >500 ms should lead to drug discontinuation and repletion of electrolytes.[*]

VORINOSTAT (ZOLINZA), AN HDAC INHIBITOR

The most recent addition to the list of differentiating agents approved for clinical use is vorinostat, an HDAC inhibitor also known as SAHA based on its chemical structure, suberoylanalide hydroxamic acid (11). It is one of a series of planar-polar compounds that inhibit the ezymatic activity of HDACs, which remove acetyl groups from amino groups of the lysines found in chromatin. Deacetylation of histones promotes the compacting of chromatin and DNA and prevents gene expression; inhibitors of HDACs reverse this process, promoting the transcription of DNA and leading to terminal differentiation and apoptosis.

Vorinostat was approved based on its ability to cause partial or complete responses in 22 of 74 patients (30%) with cutaneous T-cell lymphoma (CTCL) after failure of at least two prior regimens (12). Responses were achieved after a median of 55 days of treatment on a schedule of 400 mg per day, and lasted a median of 5.5 months. The primary toxicities were mild to moderate fatigue, diarrhea, thrombocytopenia, and anemia, but serious side effects were uncommon, the most frequent being thrombocytopenia in 6 %. While the hydroxamic acids as a class cause lengthening of the Q-T interval, no cardiac arrhythmias were reported in this trial.

Other HDAC inhibitors, including depsipeptide, a complex natural product, have shown significant activity in CTCL and peripheral T-cell lymphoma, and are in later stages of clinical evaluation.

REFERENCES

1. Sanz MA, Tallman MS, Lo-Coco F. Practice points, consensus, and controversial issues in the management of patients with newly diagnosed acute promyelocytic leukemia. Oncologist. 2005; 10: 806–814.

2. Mueller B, Pabst T, Fos J, et al. ATRA resolves the differentiation block in t(15; 17) acute myeloid leukemia by restoring PU 1 expression. Blood. 2006; 107(8): 3330–3338.

3. Idres N, Marill J, Chabot G. Regulation of CYP26A1 expression by selective RAR and RXR agonists in human NB4 promyelocytic leukemia cells. Biochem Pharmacol. 2005; 10: 1595–1601.

4. Tussie-Luna MI, Rozo L, Roy AL. Pro-proliferative function of the long Isoform of PML-RARα involved in acute promyelocytic. Oncogene. 2006; 25(24): 3375–3386.

5. Wiley JS, Firkin FC. Reduction of pulmonary toxicity by prednisolone prophylaxis during all-trans-retinoic acid treatment of acute promyelocytic leukemia. Australian Leukaemia Study Group. Leukemia. 1995; 9: 774–778.

6. Dover D, Tallman MS. Arsenic trioxide: new clinical experience with an old medication in hematologic malignancies. J Clin Oncol. 2005; 23(10): 2396–2410.

7. Mathieu J, Besancon F. Clinically tolerable concentrations of arsenic trioxide induce p53-independent cell death and repress NF-κB activation in Ewing sarcoma cells. Int J Cancer. 2006; 10: 1–6.

8. Estey E, Carcia-Manero G, Ferrajoli A, et al. Use of all-trans retinoic acid plus arsenic trioxide as an alternative to chemo in untreated acute promyelocytic leukemia. Blood. 2006; 107(9): 3469–3473.

9. Fukai Y, Hirata M, Ueno M. Clinical pharmacokinetic study of arsenic trioxide in an acute promyelocytic leukemia patient: speciation of arsenic metabolites in serum and urine. Bio Farm Bull. 2006; 29(5): 1022–1027.

10. Mari F, Bertol E, Fineschi V, Karch S. Channelling the Emperor: what really killed Napoleon? J R Soc Med. 2004; 97: 397–399.

11. Minucci S, Pelicci PG. Histone deacetylase inhibitors and the promise of epi-genetic (and more) treatments for cancer. Nat. Rev Cancer 2006; 6: 38–51.

12. Mann BS, Johnson JR, Cohen, MH, et. al. FDA approval summary: Vorinostat for treatment of advanced primary cutaneous T-cell lymphoma. The Oncologist 2007 (in press).

---

* On a historical note, Napoleon appears to have been the victim of arsenic cardiac toxicity. An analysis of Napoleon's hair has demonstrated high levels of arsenic, indicating chronic arsenic poisoning; it is believed his acute fatal episode was a ventricular arrhythmia (torsades de pointes) induced hypokalemia that resulted from treatment with emetics and cathartics (10) given for his chronic gastrointestinal symptoms. At autopsy he was discovered to have a gastric carcinoma.

12	Kathrin Strasser-Weippl, Paul E. Goss

HORMONAL AGENTS: ANTIESTROGENS

ANTIESTROGENS

Antiestrogen treatment options for the therapy of hormone-receptor positive breast cancer currently include the use of selective estrogen-receptor modulators (SERMs), selective estrogen-receptor down-regulators (SERDs), and aromatase inhibitors (AIs).

Selective Estrogen-Receptor Modulators

Tamoxifen citrate, which is the most widely used antiestrogenic therapy, is the lead compound of a class of agents referred to as selective estrogen-receptor modulators (SERMs) (Figure 12-1). These agents bind to the estrogen receptor (ER) and exert either estrogenic or antiestrogenic effects depending on the specific organ.

TAMOXIFEN   *Mechanism of action*   Tamoxifen is a competitive inhibitor of estradiol binding to the ER. In addition to its estrogen antagonist effects on breast cancer, tamoxifen exerts estrogenic effects in nonbreast tissues which influence its overall therapeutic index. Organs other than the breast that are affected by the administration of tamoxifen include:

- the uterine endometrium: endometrial hypertrophy, vaginal bleeding, and endometrial cancer
- the coagulation system: increased incidence of thromboembolism
- bone metabolism: bone mineral density preserved in postmenopausal women
- liver function: favorable influence on blood lipid profile (reduction of total and LDL cholesterol levels).

The variable response to tamoxifen in hormone-receptor positive breast cancer is accounted for by many factors that may modulate the effects of estrogen or the SERMs on the target cells. These include different levels of ER expression in the tumors and of coregulator proteins and transcriptional activating factors, of which over 50 have been described.

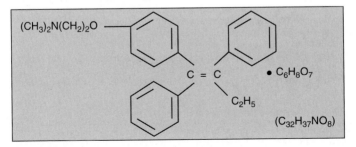

FIGURE 12-1   Structure of tamoxifen.

Absorption, fate, and excretion   Tamoxifen is readily absorbed following oral administration, with peak concentrations measurable after 3–7 h and steady-state levels being reached at 4–6 weeks. The drug is metabolized predominantly to N-desmethyltamoxifen and to 4-hydroxytamoxifen, a more potent metabolite. Both of these metabolites can be further converted to 4-hydroxy-N-desmethyltamoxifen, which retains high affinity for the ER. The parent drug has a terminal half-life of 7 days, while the half-lives of N-desmethyltamoxifen and 4-hydroxytamoxifen are significantly longer at about 14 days (1). After enterohepatic circulation, glucuronides and other metabolites are excreted in the stool; excretion in the urine is minimal.

Therapeutic uses   Tamoxifen citrate (Nolvadex®) is marketed for oral administration. The usual dose prescribed is 20 mg daily.

Tamoxifen is used for:

- treatment of ER positive metastatic breast cancer until disease progression
- adjuvant endocrine treatment of ER positive premenopausal breast cancer alone or in combination with ovarian ablation for 5 years
- adjuvant endocrine treatment of ER positive postmenopausal breast cancer for 2–3 or for 5 years prior to administration of an AI
- prevention of breast cancer in women at increased risk for the disease.

Tamoxifen only affects ER positive tumors leaving ER negative tumors, which contribute disproportionately to breast cancer mortality, unaffected.

Clinical toxicity   The clinical adverse reactions to tamoxifen compared to placebo include (2):

- vasomotor symptoms (hot flashes)
- atrophy of the lining of the vagina
- hair loss
- nausea
- vomiting
- menstrual irregularities
- vaginal bleeding and discharge
- pruritus vulvae
- dermatitis.

These clinical symptoms may occur in as many as 25% of patients and are rarely sufficiently severe to require discontinuation of therapy as overall quality of life (QoL) appears not to be impaired.

Other side effects of tamoxifen are:

- increased risk of endometrial cancer by two- threefold, particularly in postmenopausal women over 60 years taking tamoxifen for 2 years or longer; it is recommended to monitor abnormal vaginal bleeding with prompt gynecological evaluation in women with an intact uterus
- increased risk of thromboembolic events; it is recommended to discontinue tamoxifen before elective surgery
- increased risk of cataracts, retinal deposits, and decreased visual acuity
- slowing of the development of osteoporosis in postmenopausal women
- lowering of total serum cholesterol, LDL cholesterol, and lipoproteins and elevation of apolipoprotein AI levels.

Selective Estrogen-Receptor Down-Regulators

SERDs, also termed "pure anti-estrogens," include compounds such as fulvestrant (ICI 182780), RU 58668, SR 16234, ZD 164384, and ZK 191703. SERDs, unlike SERMs, are devoid of any estrogen agonist activity. The lead compound of this class currently approved for the treatment of advanced breast cancer is fulvestrant (Figure 12-2).

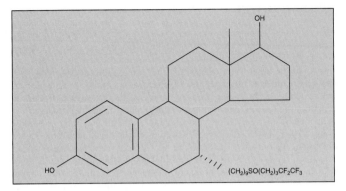

FIGURE 12-2 Structure of fulvestrant.

FULVESTRANT *Mechanism of action* Fulvestrant is a steroidal antiestrogen that binds to the ER with an affinity over 100 times that of tamoxifen, inhibits its dimerization, and increases its degradation. In contrast to tamoxifen, which increases the level of ER expression, fulvestrant is associated with a reduction in the number of detectable ER molecules in cells. It was hypothesized that fulvestrant and other SERDs, through their pure ER antagonist activity, were to have an improved safety profile, faster onset, and longer duration of action than the SERMs (3).

Absorption, fate, and excretion Fulvestrant is administered intramuscularly (i.m.) once monthly. Maximum plasma concentrations are reached at about 7 days after i.m. administration and are maintained over a period of 1 month. The plasma half-life is approximately 40 days. Steady-state concentrations are reached after 3–6 i.m. monthly injections. There is extensive and rapid distribution predominantly to the extravascular compartment.

Various pathways similar to those of steroid metabolism extensively metabolize fulvestrant. The putative metabolites possess no estrogenic activity and only the 17-keto compound demonstrates a level of antiestrogenic activity about 4.5-fold less than that of fulvestrant. The major route of excretion is via the feces, with less than 1% being excreted in the urine (3).

Therapeutic uses Fulvestrant (Faslodex®) is available as a long-acting 50 mg/ml solution that is typically administered as a 250 mg i.m. injection at monthly intervals. Fulvestrant is used for:

- treatment of postmenopausal women with hormone-receptor positive metastatic breast cancer after progression on first-line antiestrogen therapy such as tamoxifen or an aromatase inhibitor

Clinical toxicity Clinical side effects of fulvestrant include:

- nausea
- asthenia
- pain
- vasodilatation (hot flushes)
- headache
- injection site reactions.

Fulvestrant is generally well tolerated and QoL outcome measures are maintained over time (4).

Aromatase Inhibitors

Aromatase (estrogen synthetase) is responsible for the conversion of the androgens androstenedione and testosterone to the estrogens estrone (E1) and estradiol (E2), respectively. In postmenopausal women, this conversion occurs primarily in peripheral tissues while the production of estrogen in premenopausal women is primarily from the ovary. AIs inhibit the function of the aromatase enzyme. In postmenopausal women, AIs can suppress most of the peripheral aromatase activity leading to profound estrogen deprivation.

AIs have been classified as first-, second-, or third-generation. In addition, they are further classified as type 1 (steroidal aromatase inactivator) or type 2 (nonsteroidal AI) inhibitors according to their structure and mechanism of action (Figure 12-3). Type 1 inhibitors are steroidal analogues of androstenedione and bind to the same site on the aromatase molecule, but unlike androstenedione bind irreversibly because of their conversion to reactive intermediates by aromatase. Thus they are commonly known as aromatase inactivators. Type 2 inhibitors are nonsteroidal and bind reversibly to the heme group of the enzyme by way of a basic nitrogen atom (5).

Third-Generation Aromatase Inhibitors

The third-generation inhibitors, developed in the 1990s, include the type 1 steroidal agent, exemestane, and the type 2 nonsteroidal imidazoles anastrozole and letrozole.

ANASTROZOLE   *Mechanism of action*   Anastrozole, like letrozole, binds competitively and specifically to the heme of the cytochrome P450 subunit of the aromatase enzyme. Anastrozole 1 mg administered once daily for 28 days

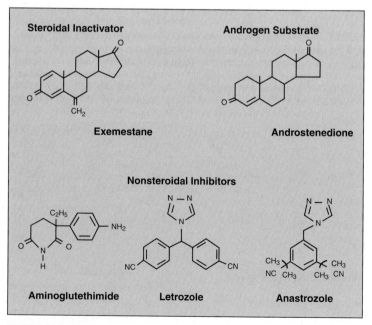

FIGURE 12-3   Structures of aromatase inhibitors.

reduces total body aromatization by 96.7%. In addition, anastrozole reduces in situ aromatization in large, ER+ breast tumors.

Anastrozole has no clinically significant effect on adrenal corticoid synthesis in postmenopausal women, or on plasma concentrations of luteinising hormone or follicle stimulating hormone and thyroid hormone.

Absorption, fate, and excretion Anastrozole is absorbed rapidly after oral administration with maximal plasma concentrations occurring after 2 h. Repeated dosing increases plasma concentrations of anastrozole and steady state is attained after 7 days. Anastrozole is metabolized by N-dealkylation, hydroxylation, and glucuronidation. The main metabolite is a triazole. Less than 10% of the drug is excreted as the unmetabolized parent compound. The principal excretory pathway is via the liver. The pharmacokinetics of anastrozole can be affected by drug interactions via cytochrome P450 (6).

Therapeutic uses Anastrozole (Arimidex®) 1 mg is administered once daily orally. Anastrozole is used for:

- treatment of postmenopausal women with advanced, hormone-receptor positive breast cancer until disease progression
- adjuvant treatment of postmenopausal breast cancer for 5 years or for 2–3 years following 2–3 years of tamoxifen.

Clinical toxicity Anastrozole has not been compared to placebo in a randomized, double-blind fashion.

Compared to tamoxifen, anastrozole causes

- less vaginal bleeding and vaginal discharge
- less hot flushes
- less endometrial cancer
- less ischemic cerebrovascular events and venous thromboembolic events
- more musculoskeletal disorders and fractures (7).

LETROZOLE   ***Mechanism of action***   In postmenopausal women, letrozole inhibits whole body aromatization and reduces in situ aromatization within breast cancers. The drug has no significant effect on the synthesis of adrenal corticoids, aldosterone, or thyroid hormone, and does not alter levels of a range of other hormones. Letrozole also reduces cellular markers of proliferation to a significantly greater extent than tamoxifen in human estrogen-dependent tumors that overexpress human epidermal growth factor receptors (HER)1 and/or HER2.

Absorption, fate, and excretion   Letrozole is rapidly absorbed after oral administration and the maximum plasma levels are reached about 1 h after ingestion. Steady-state plasma concentrations of letrozole are reached after 2–6 weeks on treatment. Following metabolism by cytochrome P450, CYP2A6, and CYP3A4, letrozole is eliminated as an inactive carbinol metabolite mainly via the kidneys. The elimination half-life is about 40–42 h (8).

Therapeutic uses   Letrozole (Femara®) 2.5 mg is administered orally once daily. Letrozole is used for:

- treatment of postmenopausal women with advanced, hormone-receptor positive breast cancer until disease progression
- adjuvant treatment of postmenopausal breast cancer for 5 years or for 2–3 years following 2–3 years of tamoxifen
- adjuvant treatment of postmenopausal breast cancer for 5 years following 4.5–6 years of tamoxifen

Clinical toxicity   The side effects of letrozole compared to placebo include (9):

- hot flushes
- arthralgia, myalgia, arthritis
- osteoporosis, fractures
- nausea
- hair thinning.

Generally, letrozole is well tolerated.

EXEMESTANE   *Mechanism of action*   Exemestane is a potent, orally administered analog of the natural substrate androstenedione. In contrast to the reversible competitive inhibitors, anastrozole and letrozole, exemestane irreversibly inactivates the enzyme; therefore it is referred to as a "suicide substrate." Doses of 25 mg per day inhibit aromatase activity by 98% and lower estrone and estradiol levels in plasma by about 90%.

Absorption, fate, and excretion   Exemestane is rapidly absorbed from the gastrointestinal tract reaching maximum plasma levels after 2 h. Its absorption is increased by 40% after a high fat meal. Exemestane has a terminal half-life of approximately 24 h. It is extensively metabolized in the liver to metabolites that are inactive against aromatase. A key metabolite, 17-hydroxyexemestane, has weak androgenic activity, which might contribute to antitumor activity and androgenic end-organ effects. Excretion is distributed almost equally between the urine and feces. Since significant quantities of active metabolites are excreted in the urine, doses of exemestane should be adjusted in patients with renal dysfunction (10).

Therapeutic uses   Exemestane 25 mg is administered orally once daily. Exemestane is used for:

- treatment of postmenopausal women with advanced, hormone-receptor positive breast cancer until disease progression
- treatment of postmenopausal women with advanced, hormone-receptor positive breast cancer after failure of a nonsteroidal inhibitor until disease progression
- adjuvant treatment of postmenopausal breast cancer for 2–3 years after 2–3 years of tamoxifen.

Clinical toxicity   Exemestane has not been compared to placebo in a randomized double-blind fashion.

Compared to tamoxifen, exemestane causes

- arthralgia more frequently
- more diarrhea
- less gynecological symptoms including vaginal bleeding
- less muscle cramps
- more clinical fractures
- more visual disturbances.

REFERENCES

1. Ellis M, Swain SM. Steroid hormone therapies for cancer. In BA Chabner, DA Longo (eds.), "Cancer Chemotherapy and Biotherapy: Principles and Practice," 3rd edition, Wilkinson & Wilkins, Phildelphia, 2001, pp. 85–138.
2. Fisher B, Costantino JP, Wickerham DL, et al. Tamoxifen for prevention of breast cancer: Report of The National Surgical Adjuvant Breast and Bowel Project P-1 Study. J Natl Cancer Inst. 1998; 90(18): 1371–1388.
3. Robertson JF, Harrison M. Fulvestrant: pharmacokinetics and pharmacology. Br J Cancer. 2004; 90(suppl)1: S7–10.

4. Vergote I, Robertson JF. Fulvestrant is an effective and well-tolerated endocrine therapy for postmenopausal women with advanced breast cancer: results from clinical trials. Br J Cancer. 2004; 90(suppl)1: S11–S14.

5. Strasser-Weippl K, Goss PE. Advances in adjuvant hormonal therapy for postmenopausal women. J Clin Oncol. 2005; 23(8): 1751–1759.

6. Koberle D, Thurlimann B. Anastrozole: pharmacological and clinical profile in postmenopausal women with breast cancer. Expert Rev Anticancer Ther. 2001; 1(2): 169–176.

7. Baum M, Buzdar AU, Cuzick J, et al. ATAC Trialists' Group. Anastrozole alone or in combination with tamoxifen versus tamoxifen alone for adjuvant treatment of postmenopausal women with early breast cancer: first results of the ATAC randomised trial. Lancet. 2002; 359(9324): 2131–2139.

8. Lonning PE, Geisler J, Bhatnager A. Development of aromatase inhibitors and their pharmacologic profile. Am J Clin Oncol. 2003; 26(4): S3–S8.

9. Goss PE, Ingle JN, Martino S, et al. Randomized trial of letrozole following tamoxifen as extended adjuvant therapy in receptor-positive breast cancer: updated findings from NCIC CTG MA.17. J Natl Cancer Inst. 2005; 97(17): 1262–1271.

10. Lonning PE. Pharmacology and clinical experience with exemestane. Expert Opin Invest Drugs. 2000; 9(8): 1897–1905.

Bruce A. Chabner

ANTIANDROGEN THERAPY

The initial attempt at treating cancer with hormone ablation was implemented by Charles Huggins at the University of Chicago in 1941, when he hypothesized that the prostate depended on testosterone (and, ultimately, its metabolite dihydrotestosterone) for its growth (1). Orchiectomy of patients with advanced prostate cancer reduced serum testosterone to barely detectable levels (less than 50 ng/dl) and produced dramatic relief of bone pain in 90% of such patients. The median duration of response was about 1 year, and hormone-independent tumor emerged in most cases. Huggins was awarded a Nobel Prize for his work.

Since that time, androgen ablation has not changed in concept, but drugs have largely taken the place of orchiectomy. Two basic classes of drugs are used: (1) gonadotrophin releasing hormone (GnRH) agonists, a family of small peptides that promote release, and exhaustion of GnRH from the hypothalamus, thus lowering Gn levels in plasma and blocking androgen release from the testes (medical castration); and (2) small molecular weight androgen analogs that inhibit androgen interaction with its receptor in normal and tumor cells.

GnRH AGONISTS

Two GnRH Agonists approved for clinical use in the United States are leuprolide and goserelin. These drugs are given by intermittent, monthly to 4-monthly subcutaneous injection, and produce a flair response of testosterone release for several days to weeks, followed by a rapid decline in serum testosterone levels. The flair may induce an increase in bone pain and, in the presence of significant vertebral metastases, symptoms of spinal cord compression may result. In such patients a GnRH antagonist, abarelix, is available to ablate the flair response and offers protection from the short-term progression of disease (3), but is only occasionally used. A more important consideration in the use of GnRH agonists is their lack of effect on adrenal androgen, which makes a small contribution to serum androgen activity and theoretically could be sufficient to maintain or promote tumor growth in the absence of testicular androgen. However, clinical trials of complete androgen blockade with a GnRH agonist and an inhibitor of androgen receptor binding have not yielded conclusively positive results (4), as compared to GnRH agonists alone.

Side effects of GnRH agonists are those of acute androgen deprivation, including vasomotor instability (flushing and sweating), loss of libido, gynecomastia, acute and dramatic bone and muscle loss with an increase in hip fracture rates, truncal obesity, diabetes, and an increased risk of myocardial infarction and sudden cardiac death (5). A "metabolic syndrome" of insulin resistance, increased body fat mass, and changes in plasma lipids can be detected within weeks of initiation of GnRH therapy (6). Bone preservation with bisphosphonates is recommended for patients on long-term GnRH agonist therapy (7).

The GnRH analogs are cleared by both renal excretion and by hepatic metabolism, with an elimination half-life of 3–7 h. Depending on their formulation and dose, plasma concentrations of analog are sufficient to suppress testosterone levels for 1–4 months.

Table 13-1

Clinical Pharmacology of Antiandrogens

Compound	Elimination half-life (h)	Daily dose (mg)
Bicalutamide	140	50
Flutamide (active metabolite)	8	250 every 8 h
Nilutamide	50	300 for 30 days, 150 thereafter

ANDROGEN RECEPTOR INHIBITORS

Three such compounds (Table 13-1), all nonsteroidal in structure, have been approved for treatment of prostate cancer (8). They are most commonly used with GnRH agonists to block the temporary surge in adrenogens released in response to GnRH agonists and to inhibit the residual effects of adrenal androgens, but may be used without GnRH agonists in selected cases. As single agents, they have not been proven to be equally effective as the GnRH agonists but their side effect profile is somewhat advantageous. They elevate testosterone levels as a result of inhibition of androgen receptors in the hypothalamus and increased GnRH secretion; thus as single agents they cause less loss of libido and gynecomastia, and have little effect on bone and muscle mass. However, all three drugs cause rare cases of severe hepatic injury, flutamide causes diarrhea, and nilutamide causes interstitial pneumonitis and visual disturbances (dark adaptation). All are eliminated by hepatic metabolism, and may inhibit the clearance of Coumadin, phenytoin, and other agents cleared by hepatic cytochrome-dependent enzymes. Flutamide is rapidly converted to its active alpha-hydroxy-metabolite after oral administration. The doses and pharmacokinetics of the antiandrogens are given in Table 13-1.

The mechanism of resistance to GnRH agonists and to receptor inhibitors is not clearly delineated. In a few cases, resistant cells may develop androgen receptor mutations that allow the small molecule inhibitors to act as agonists (9). In other instances, changes in intracellular signaling may allow very small concentrations of androgen/receptor complex to activate proliferation. Still other tumors lose androgen receptor and may depend on other signaling pathways, such as the IGF-1 pathway, for proliferation (10).

REFERENCES

1. Huggins C, Hodges CV. Studies on prostate cancer. I. The effects of castration, of estrogen, and of androgen injection on serum phosphatases in metastatic carcinoma of the prostate. Cancer Res. 1941; 1: 293–297.
2. Sharifi N, Gulley JL, Dahut WL. Androgen deprivation therapy for prostate cancer. J Am Med Assoc. 2005; 294: 238–244.
3. Weckermann D, Harzmann R. Hormone therapy in prostate cancer LHRH antagonists versus LHRH analogues. Eur Urol. 2004; 46: 279–284.
4. Prostate Cancer Trialists' Collaborative Group. Maximum androgen blockade in advanced prostate cancer: an overview of randomized trials. Lancet. 2000; 355: 1491–1498.
5. Keating NL, O'Malley AJ, Smith MR. Diabetes and cardiovascular disease during androgen deprivation therapy for prostate cancer. J Clin Oncol. 2006; in press.
6. Smith MR, Finkelstein JS, McGovern FJ, et al. Changes in body composition during androgen deprivation therapy for prostate cancer. J Clin Endocrinol Metab. 2002; 87: 599–603.

7. Shahinian VB, Kuo YF, Freeman JL, Goodwin JS. Risk of fracture after andro-
    gen deprivation for prostate cancer. N Engl J Med. 2005; 352: 154–164.
8. Reid P, Kantoff P, Oh W. Antiandrogens in prostate cancer. Invest New Drugs.
    1999; 17: 271–284.
9. Taplin ME, Balk SP. Androgen receptor: a key molecule in the progression of
    prostate cancer to hormone independence. J Cell Biochem. 2004; 91(3): 483–490.
10. Majumder PK, Sellers WR. Akt-regulated pathways in prostate cancer.
    Oncogene. 2005; 24(50): 7465–7474.

| 14 | Dan L. Longo |

INTERFERONS

The interferons are a family of proteins that are grouped into three classes, α, β, and γ. They were discovered based on their ability to "interfere" with viral infection of cells. Subsequent study has revealed a panoply of biological actions including immunomodulatory, antiproliferative, and antiangiogenic effects (1). Nearly all the oncologic applications of the interferons have been uses of the α class.

The α and β interferons are encoded by a series of genes on chromosome 9p. At least 12 varieties of α interferon exist. A product composed of several species of α interferon produced by stimulated lymphoblasts exists (Wellferon, Burroughs Wellcome), but the predominant forms of interferon in clinical use are recombinant molecules of a single species of α, specifically α2. Interferon-α2 is 165 amino acids in length with a molecular weight of about 23 kD. Interferon-α2a (Hoffmann–LaRoche) differs from interferon-α2b (Schering Plough) by a single amino acid; -α2a has a lysine at position 23, -α2b has an arginine. Interferon-β has no established role in cancer treatment but is widely used to suppress relapses in multiple sclerosis.

Interferon-γ maps to chromosome 12, is 143 amino acids in length, and has minimal sequence homology with interferons α and β. Its cellular receptor is distinct from the receptor for interferons α and β, but both types of receptors are widely expressed on all nucleated cells and tissues. Each cell expresses 100 to 2,000 receptors and the binding constants (K_d) are between 10^{-11} and 10^{-9} M. The α receptor has two chains, one of which is associated with Tyk2 tyrosine kinase and one with JAK1 kinase (2). The genes for the α receptor map to chromosome 21q22.1. The γ receptor also has two chains one of which is associated with JAK1 kinase and one with JAK2 kinase. The γ receptor genes are on chromosome 6q. Figure 14-1 shows the two forms of receptor for the three classes of interferons.

Interferons have been approved for use in seven types of cancer, several viral diseases, an autoimmune disease (multiple sclerosis; interferon-β) and an immune deficiency disease (chronic granulomatous disease; interferon-γ) (Table 14-1). In addition to the tumors listed in Table 14-1, interferon-α also has antitumor activity in cutaneous T-cell lymphoma. However, for most of these cancers, interferon is a second- or third-line alternative.

MECHANISM OF ACTION

The wide range of biologic effects of the interferons has made it difficult to determine a single central mechanism of action. The fact that responses appear to correlate roughly with dose suggests that direct antitumor mechanisms predominate. Interferon-α and -β may exert direct antitumor effects and are capable of boosting mainly innate host defenses. Interferon-γ appears to have minimal direct effects on tumor cells but is a potent mediator of effects on immune cells. As a cytokine produced by CD4+ Th1 cells, interferon-γ promotes cytolytic activity from CD8+ cytotoxic T cells. Cells exposed to interferons are induced to express literally hundreds of new gene products (see http://www.lerner.ccf.org/labs/williams/der.html).

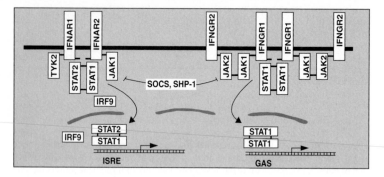

FIGURE 14-1 Components of the interferon (IFN) signaling pathways. The major components responsible for relaying IFN-mediated signals from the cell surface to the regulatory elements of IFN-stimulated genes are represented. GAS, IFN-γ activated site; IFNAR, IFN-α receptor; IFNGR, IFN-γ receptor; ISRE, IFN-stimulated response element; JAK, Janus Kinase; SHP, src-homology 2 domain-containing protein tyrosine phosphatase; SOCS, suppressor of cytokine signaling; STAT, signal transducer and activator of transcription; Tyk, JAK family kinase. Small black bars represent tyrosine residues that become phosphorylated and induce complex formation.

Table 14-1

Uses for Interferon

Cancers
        Hairy cell leukemia
        Follicular lymphoma
        Myeloma
        Chronic myeloid leukemia
        Kaposi's sarcoma
        Renal cell carcinoma
        Melanoma
Viruses
        Hepatitis C
        Hepatitis B
        Herpes keratitis
        Papillomavirus infections
          Genital warts
          Laryngeal warts
Myeloproliferative syndromes
        Essential thrombocytosis

They induce cyclin-dependent kinase inhibitors to cause cell cycle arrest and induce FAS and caspases, components of apoptosis pathways (3). Interferons also induce alterations in host defenses. They increase CD8+ cytotoxic T-cell activity, increase NK activity, and stimulate macrophages and dendritic cells. They induce an upregulation of class I MHC molecules in tumors, which could result in more effective recognition of target cells by cytotoxic T cells. In addition, interferons induce the expression of some known tumor-associated antigens. Many cell effects of interferons are mediated through the action of a family of proteins called interferon regulatory factors or IRFs (4). Interferons also inhibit the expression of basic fibroblast growth factor and vascular endothelial growth factor, cytokines involved in tumor angiogenesis.

The in vivo mechanisms of action have not been defined. When biological effects of interferon are measured in man, the assays usually test levels of neopterin (produced by IFN-stimulated monocytes) or β2-microglobulin (shed by IFN-stimulated cells) in the serum or measure the induction of the IFN-inducible 2–5 oligo A synthetase in mononuclear cells.

PHARMACOLOGY

IFN-α is generally administered intramuscularly or subcutaneously. About 80% of an injected dose is absorbed. It is absorbed with a $t_{1/2}$ of 2–2-1/2 h and eliminated with a $t_{1/2}$ of 3–8 h. An intramuscular dose of 72 million units usually produces peak serum levels of 300–500 U/ml (5). The intravenous administration of 20 million units/m^2 produces peak serum levels of about 2,500 U/mL. The maximum tolerated dose of IFN-α depends on the route of administration, the frequency of dosing, the duration of treatment, and the patient's willingness to accept toxicities (see below). Most people can tolerate 3–5 million units three times a week on a continuous basis.

Efforts to alter the pharmacokinetics of the molecule have been made by attaching polymers of polyethylene glycol (PEG) to the parent molecule (6). Hoffmann–LaRoche attached a 40 kD branched chain molecule of PEG to its interferon-α2a and Schering Plough attached a 25 kD linear chain of PEG to its interferon-α2b. PEG-IFN-α2a has an absorption half-life of 50 h, an elimination half-life of 65 h, and time to maximum serum concentration of 48–80 h. The maximum tolerated dose for PEG-IFN-α2a is 450 micrograms per week. PEG-IFN-α2b has an absorption half-life of 4–5 h, an elimination half-life of about 40 h, and a time to maximum serum concentration of 15–44 h. The maximum tolerated dose for PEG-IFN-α2b is around 6 μg/kg per week. These pegylated forms sustain measurable blood levels of interferon over a longer period of time. Pegylation may improve the antiviral efficacy of interferon in hepatitis C treatment, but comparisons of efficacy between native and pegylated IFN preparations have been limited in cancer indications. Unpegylated and pegylated IFN appear to be comparably active in chronic myeloid leukemia (7).

TOXICITIES

Interferon induces severe flu-like symptoms including fever, chills, rigors, myalgias, arthralgias, malaise, and somnolence in the initial stages of treatment (Table 14-2). If treatment continues, over time these symptoms abate as a reflection of tachyphylaxis. If the course of therapy is interrupted for even short periods, the flu-like symptoms may return upon restarting IFN treatment. With chronic administration, patients often develop severe fatigue, depression, anorexia, and weight loss. These are the major symptoms that may cause an interruption in the course of therapy. Aside from the systemic and nervous system toxicities, myelosuppression and hepatic toxicity are the major organ toxicities. Hypertriglyceridemia is common. Rare patients, particularly those with T-cell tumors, can develop nephrotic syndrome and acute renal failure. Some patients develop autoimmune disorders such as thyroiditis and some with preexisting autoimmune disease experience an exacerbation of symptoms on interferon.

Myelotoxicity and hepatic toxicity are generally addressed by lowering the dose. Mood changes may be affected by addition of paroxetine. Hypertriglyceridemia can be managed with gemfibrosil. Mechanisms of the toxicity are actively being investigated (8). A surprising level of tolerance for the fatigue and weakness develops among patients chronically receiving interferon. Many patients report not realizing how tired they were until they stopped the drug. For this reason, patient self-evaluation of toxicity often underestimates the level of functional decline associated with IFN administration.

Table 14-2

Toxicities Associated with Interferon

Acute
    Fever
    Chills and rigors
    Malaise
    Somnolence
    Myalgias
    Arthralgias
    Neutropenia
    Thrombocytopenia
    Anemia
Chronic
    Fatigue
    Depression
    Exhaustion
    Anorexia
    Weight loss
    Sleep disturbances
    Transaminase elevations
    Hypertriglyceridemia
    Nephrotic syndrome
    Development of or exacerbation of preexisting autoimmune disease

INTERFERON RESISTANCE

Resistance to interferon has not been extensively studied. Cellular resistance can be mediated by a defects in STAT1 signaling, down-regulation of interferon receptors, increased expression of SOCS or SHP1 proteins (these alter interferon signaling), and increased expression of antiapoptotic proteins such as BCL-2. Viruses have adopted a number of mechanisms to resist IFN effects. For example, EBNA-2 of the Epstein–Barr virus and E1A of adenovirus can both inhibit the cellular response to interferon. However, the mechanisms that make most human cancers interferon resistant are not defined.

The development of resistance to interferon in a patient who was responding to it can signal the development of neutralizing antiinterferon antibodies (9). In one study, 16 of 51 patients chronically receiving interferon developed neutralizing antibodies and 6 of the 16 with antibodies acquired interferon resistance. Every patient who had initially responded to interferon and then stopped responding had neutralizing antibodies.

Aggregated forms of interferon are believed to be responsible for the development of antibodies.

REFERENCES

1. Pestka S, Krause CD, Walter MR. Interferons, interferon-like cytokines, and their receptors. Immunol Rev. 2004; 202: 8–32.
2. Darnell JE, Jr, Kerr IM, Stark GR. Jak-STAT pathways and transcriptional activation in response to IFNs and other extracellular signaling proteins. Science. 1994; 264: 1415–1421.
3. Stark GR, Kerr IM, Williams BR, et al. How cells respond to interferons. Annu Rev Biochem. 1998; 67: 227–264.
4. Taniguchi T, Ogasawara K, Takaoka A, Tanaka N. IRF family of transcription factors as regulators of host defense. Annu Rev Immunol. 2001; 19: 623–655.

5. Lindner DJ, Taylor KL, Reu FJ, Masci PA, Borden EC. Interferons. In BA Chabner, DL Longo (eds.), "Cancer Chemotherapy and Biotherapy: Principles and Practice," 4th edition, Lippincott Williams and Wilkins, Philadelphia, 2006, pp. 699–717.

6. Zeuzem S, Welsch C, Herrmann E. Pharmacokinetics of peginterferons. Semin Liver Dis. 2003; 23(suppl1): 23–28.

7. Michallet M, Maloisel F, Delain M, et al. Pegylated recombinant interferon alpha-2b vs recombinant interferon alpha-2b for the initial treatment of chronic-phase chronic myelogenous leukemia: a phase III study. Leukemia. 2004; 18: 309–315.

8. Kirkwood JM, Bender C, Agarwala S, et al. Mechanisms and management of toxicities associated with high-dose interferon alfa-2b therapy. J Clin Oncol. 2002; 20: 3703–3718.

9. Steis RG, Smith JW II, Urba WJ, et al. Resistance to recombinant interferon alfa-2a in hairy-cell leukemia associated with neutralizing antiinterferon antibodies. N Engl J Med. 1988; 318: 1409–1413.

CYTOKINES, GROWTH FACTORS, AND IMMUNE-BASED INTERVENTIONS

Cytokines are soluble proteins or glycoproteins that exert trophic effects on a variety of targets based on the expression of particular ligand-specific receptors on the target. All of the cytokines have not yet been identified; but at this time, more than 80 different molecules have been defined. The same cytokine can exert different effects on different cells and tissues. However, the biochemical consequences of ligand binding to its cellular receptor are similar among all the targets. A number of cytokines have been evaluated for their antitumor effects including the interferons, interleukin-1 (IL1), tumor necrosis factor, IL4, IL12, and others. The rationale for testing these agents as antitumor agents is twofold. First, many of these agents stimulate cells of the immune system, an effect that could promote the immunological killing of the tumor cells. Second, many neoplastic cells retain the cytokine receptors of their normal counterparts; thus, direct biological and potentially antitumor effects are theoretically possible.

Currently, only interferon-α (Chapter 14) and IL2 are approved for use as anticancer agents. Most other tested cytokines have either had little or no antitumor effect or were too toxic when administered systemically as a pharmacologic agent. In general, cytokines work physiologically as paracrine signals coordinating cellular responses in a localized area of release. It has been estimated that in the course of trying to develop IL2 as a therapeutic agent, we administered more of the agent to a few hundred patients than had been produced physiologically in the courses of their entire lives by every man and woman who ever lived.

INTERLEUKIN-2

Interleukin-2 (IL2) is a glycoprotein composed of 133 amino acids and has a molecular weight of 15 kD. It is structurally related to IL4, IL15, and granulocyte-macrophage colony-stimulating factor (GM-CSF). It is normally produced by stimulated T cells and NK cells and acts to promote the proliferation of activated T cells. Resting T cells do not express IL2 receptors and do not respond to the cytokine.

The IL2 receptor has three components: an α-chain, a 55 kD component, also known as CD25, that has only 13 amino acids located intracellularly and functions mainly in binding to IL2; a β-chain, a 75 kD component with a large intracellular component involved in signaling; and the common γ-chain, a 64 kD component called "common" because it is also a shared signaling component of receptors for IL4, IL7, IL9, IL15, and IL21. IL2 binds to the three-component high-affinity receptor with a Kd of 10 pmol/l; in the absence of the α-chain, IL2 binding is termed intermediate and is about 100-fold reduced. High-affinity receptors are mainly expressed on activated T cells; intermediate affinity receptors are expressed on monocytes and NK cells.

Biologic activity. IL2 stimulates the proliferation of activated T cells and promotes the secretion of cytokines from monocytes and NK cells. The main biologic consequence of IL2 stimulation is an increase in cytotoxicity in both T cells and NK cells. IL2 also has a negative regulatory effect on T cells to prevent them from overexpanding or attacking self as IL2 knockout mice have lymphadenopathy and autoimmunity.

Pharmacology. The serum half-life of IL2 after intravenous administration has an α-phase of about 13 min and a more prolonged β-phase of about 90 min. Peak serum levels vary with the dose; 6×10^6 IU/m² by IV bolus produces serum levels near 2,000 IU/ml. IL2 has been conjugated to polyethylene glycol to prolong its half-life (α 3 h; β 12-1/2 h), but this form is not FDA approved. It is mainly excreted as an inactive metabolite in the urine. When 6×10^6 IU/m² IL2 is administered by continuous infusion, it reaches steady state levels within 2 h at 123 IU/ml and levels fall rapidly after the infusion is stopped. When 6×10^6 IU/m² IL2 is administered subcutaneously, peak serum levels of 32–42 IU/ml are reached within 2–6 h.

Method of administration. Chiron IL2 (aldesleukin) is the only form of IL2 currently FDA approved. It is administered in one of three ways. High-dose IL2 is 600,000 or 720,000 IU/kg administered by IV bolus every 8 h until dose-limiting toxicity is reached or a maximum of 15 doses. Low-dose IL2 is 60,000 or 72,000 IU/kg administered by IV bolus every 8 h for 15 doses. A third regimen is for more chronic administration: 250,000 IU/kg subcutaneously daily for 5 days then 125,000 IU/kg daily for 6 weeks. Considerable data exist on high-dose and low-dose schedules. Much less information is available on the activity of the subcutaneous regimen. Treatment is generally repeated at least once in responding patients.

Because of its life-threatening toxicities (see below), patients must be carefully screened before embarking on a course of IL2 treatment. Patients should undergo cardiac stress testing, pulmonary function tests, brain MRI, and a thorough physical examination and laboratory testing before treatment. They should have a good performance status (0.1 on ECOG scale), no active infections, and normal renal, hepatic, and thyroid function.

Clinical effects. IL2 was approved for use in metastatic renal cell cancer in 1992 and in metastatic melanoma in 1998 (1, 2). High-dose IL2 produces an overall response rate of about 19% in patients with renal cell cancer; however, 8% of patients get complete responses. Both complete and partial responses appear to be quite durable with median response durations of 8–9 years. Thus, median survival is not affected appreciably but a subset of patients receives substantial benefit from the therapy. Unfortunately, it is not possible to distinguish in advance patients more likely to respond.

High-dose IL2 produces an overall response rate of 16% in metastatic melanoma and 6% of patients achieve complete responses, many of which are long lasting. Median response duration is about 5 years.

The role of high-dose therapy versus low-dose therapy is controversial. Many argue that response rates are the same with the two regimens. However, response durations do not seem to be as durable when low-dose IL2 is used, at least in some studies. Other groups have not seen dramatic differences in efficacy between high- and low-dose regimens, but all groups have noted dramatic differences in toxicities. The mechanism of action of IL2 against these cancers is undefined.

Toxicities. The toxicities from IL2 are life threatening and are dominated by the capillary leak syndrome (3). Intravascular fluid leaks into the extravascular space, tissues, and alveoli of the lungs. As a consequence, patients develop hypotension, edema, respiratory difficulties, confusion, tachycardia, oliguric renal failure, and electrolyte abnormalities including hypokalemia, hypomagnesemia, hypocalcemia, and hypophosphatemia. Patients may also experience nausea and vomiting, fever, chills, malaise, and thrombocytopenia. Diarrhea, abnormal liver functions, and neutropenia may occur. Patients often develop a pruritic skin rash over most of the body. Hypothyroidism may also occur. Arrhythmias are a rare complication.

Despite the severity and widespread distribution of the toxic effects of IL2, nearly all the toxicities are reversible within 24–48 h of stopping the drug.

COLONY-STIMULATING FACTORS

The relatively disappointing antitumor efficacy of cytokines has been counterbalanced by the more effective use of a group of cytokines in supportive care of the cancer patient. The lesson learned from these development efforts is that cytokines are more effectively applied to people when they are used to influence their known physiologic targets. Thus, colony-stimulating factors are capable of increasing the production of the cells they normally regulate. However, here, too, we have learned the physiologic limitations of the hematopoietic system. Generally, when we make a patient anemic or granulocytopenic or thrombocytopenic with chemotherapy or radiation therapy, the problem is not that the physiologic response to the cytopenia is limited by poor production of the relevant colony-stimulating factor. Instead the limitation is the number of surviving marrow precursors and the obligate time period for their differentiation into end-stage cells. Thus, even when a cytokine is used to perform its physiologically relevant task, it does not act as a cure-all that erases the prior damage of disease and therapy. Nevertheless, colony-stimulating factors have made a modest contribution to more rapid recovery of blood counts after treatment.

Unfortunately, the magnitude of the effect of colony-stimulating factors has not been sufficient to influence the maximally tolerated doses of myelotoxic agents, a result that was hoped for when these agents were first introduced. However, clinical experience has defined settings in which their use can be beneficial, and guidelines for clinical use have been developed.

Granulocyte-Colony-Stimulating Factor

Granulocyte-colony-stimulating factor (G-CSF) is a 174 amino acid glycoprotein (MW 19,600) encoded by a gene on chromosome 17q11-12 that acts late in myeloid cell differentiation to promote the development of granulocytes. Not only is granulocyte production increased by G-CSF, but the generation of reactive oxygen species by granulocytes is also augmented. Over time additional functions have been uncovered and its use is now being evaluated in cardiac disease and stroke. It may have a role in suppressing immune reactions.

G-CSF production is usually induced by inflammatory cytokines and it is produced by fibroblasts, macrophages, and endothelial cells. The receptor for G-CSF is in the cytokine type I receptor family and signals through Janus-like kinase (JAK)/signal transducer and activator of transcription (STAT) pathways.

Biologic activity. When added to bone marrow cell cultures, G-CSF mainly stimulates the development of neutrophils, in contrast to GM-CSF, which induces neutrophil, eosinophil, basophil, monocyte, and dendritic cell development. In addition to increasing neutrophils in the marrow, G-CSF promotes the early release of these cells into the peripheral blood and promotes their ability to phagocytose and kill bacteria. Through the release of metalloproteinases, they also promote the mobilization of hematopoietic stem cells into the peripheral blood.

Pharmacology. Intravenous administration of G-CSF (filgrastim) shows an α-phase half-life of about 8 min and a β-phase half-life of about 2 h. When given subcutaneously, the half-life is 2.5–5.8 h. To prolong the half-life, a 20 kD polyethylene glycol molecule was covalently attached to the N-terminal methionine of filgrastim to produce pegfilgrastim. The half-life of subcutaneously administered pegfilgrastim is 27–47 h.

Method of administration. Filgrastim is generally administered at a dose of 5 μg/kg subcutaneously daily. When given to promote granulocyte recovery, the daily dose is continued until the neutrophil count has increased above 10,000/μl. Pegfilgrastim is usually administered only once at a dose of 100 μg/kg or a total dose of 6 mg subcutaneously. A single dose of pegfilgrastim appears comparable in efficacy to a 10–14 day course of filgrastim. For mobilization of stem cells, the usual dose of filgrastim is 10 μg/kg/day or 5–8 μg/kg twice daily.

Clinical effect. Based on expert opinion and analysis of the world's literature on G-CSF use (4, 5), guidelines have been developed to aid in decision-making on who should and who should not receive G-CSF during chemotherapy (Table 15-1). In general, G-CSF is overused in clinical practice. The guidelines suggest that it be used with regimens that have a greater than 20% likelihood of inducing febrile neutropenia. Only a small fraction of frequently used regimens are in this category. Risk of developing febrile neutropenia is reduced by about 50%. In the setting of febrile neutropenia, G-CSF may speed neutrophil recovery by 2 or 3 days. However, its use has not permitted dose escalation of chemotherapy. G-CSF is extremely effective in mobilizing hematopoietic stem cells into the peripheral blood. It is so effective that bone marrow harvest has become unnecessary in the vast majority of stem cell donors. Not only are peripheral blood stem cells easier to collect from the donor, but G-CSF-mobilized cells are also more efficient at reestablishing normal hematopoiesis than bone marrow erived cells and are associated with shorter periods of neutropenia and thrombocytopenia.

Table 15-1

Clinical Indications for Neutrophil Growth Factors

Medically necessary

The use of colony-stimulating factors (CSFs) is considered *medically necessary* for patients with cancer with *any* of the following indications:

1. *Primary prophylaxis.* For the prevention of febrile neutropenia (FN) in patients who have a risk of FN of 20% or greater when there are no equally effective regimens not requiring CSFs available. Patients are at high risk based on:
   - Age
   - Medical history
   - Disease characteristics
   - Myelotoxicity of the chemotherapy regimen.
2. *For the prevention of FN even when the risk of developing FN is less than 20%* in patients who have other risk factors for FN including any of the following:
   a. Patient age greater than 65 years; or
   b. Poor performance status; or
   c. Previous episodes of FN; or
   d. Extensive prior treatment including large radiation ports; or
   e. After completion of combined chemoradiotherapy; or
   f. Bone marrow involvement by tumor producing cytopenias; or
   g. Poor nutritional status; or
   h. The presence of open wounds or active infections; or
   i. More advanced cancer; or
   j. Other serious comorbidities.
3. *Secondary prophylaxis* with CSFs is recommended for patients who experienced a neutropenic complication from a prior cycle of chemotherapy (for which primary prophylaxis was not received), in which a reduced dose may compromise disease-free or overall survival or treatment outcome. In many clinical situations, dose reduction or delay may be a reasonable alternative.

Table 15-1 (*Continued*)

4. *Use in febrile neutropenic patients.* Adjunctive use with antibiotics in *high-risk, febrile, neutropenic* patients who are at high risk for infection-associated complications or have *any of the following* prognostic factors predictive of clinical deterioration:
   a. Expected prolonged (greater than 10 day) and profound (less than $0.1 \times 10^9/l$) neutropenia; or
   b. Age greater than 65 years; or
   c. Uncontrolled primary disease; or
   d. Pneumonia; or
   e. Hypotension and multi organ dysfunction (sepsis syndrome); or
   f. Invasive fungal infection; or
   g. Hospitalized at the time of the development of fever.
5. *Use for dose-dense therapy.* Dose-dense regimens (treatment given more frequently, such as every 2 weeks instead of every 3 weeks) should only be used within an appropriately designed clinical trial or if supported by convincing efficacy data. (For "dose-dense" regimens CSFs are required and recommended by American Society of Clinical Oncology (ASCO) specifically in the treatment of node positive breast cancer, small cell lung cancer, and diffuse aggressive non-Hodgkin's lymphoma.)
6. *Use as adjunct to progenitor cell transplantation.* Administration of CSFs to mobilize peripheral blood progenitor cells (PBPC) often in conjunction with chemotherapy and their administration after autologous, but *not* allo-geneic, PBPC transplant.
7. *Use for patients with leukemia or myelodysplastic syndromes*
   A. *Initial or repeat induction chemotherapy (acute myeloid leukemia (AML) and consolidation chemotherapy (AML).* For administration shortly after the completion of induction chemotherapy of *AML with patients over* 55 years of age most likely to benefit *or* for patients of any age, after the completion of consolidation chemotherapy for AML. Use of pegylated products for consolidation chemotherapy has not been studied and is not recommended outside clinical trials.
   B. *Acute lymphocytic leukemia (ALL).* In *ALL*, for administration after completion of the first few days of chemotherapy of the initial induction or first postremission course.
   C. *Myelodysplastic syndromes (MDS).* Intermittent administration of CSF may be considered in a subset of MDS patients with severe neutropenia and recurrent infection.
8. *Use in patients receiving radiation therapy.*
   Radiotherapy. In the absence of chemotherapy, therapeutic use of CSFs may be considered in patients receiving radiation therapy alone if pro-longed delays secondary to neutropenia are expected.
9. *Use in older patients.* Prophylactic CSF for patients with diffuse aggres-sive lymphoma aged 65 and older treated with curative chemotherapy (CHOP or more aggressive regimens) should be given to reduce the inci-dence of febrile neutropenia (FN) and infections. (Note. Aside from data available in patients with lymphoma, there is insufficient evidence to sup-port the use of prophylactic CSF in patients solely based on age.)
10. *Use in the pediatric population*
   A. Will almost always be guided by clinical protocols
   B. Primary prophylaxis of pediatric patients with a likelihood of FN
   C. Secondary prophylaxis or therapeutic CSF administration should be limited to high-risk patients. (*Note.* The potential risk for second-ary myeloid leukemia or MDS associated with CSF is a concern in

(*Continued*)

Table 15-1

Clinical Indications for Neutrophil Growth Factors (*Continued*)

children with ALL whose prognosis is otherwise excellent. For these reasons, use of CSF in children with ALL should be with caution.)

11. *Use for radiation injury.* Current ASCO recommendations for the management of patients exposed to lethal doses of total body radiotherapy or accidental total body radiation include the administration of CSF or pegylated G-CSF. This recommendation is based on observation of cases in the Radiation Emergency Assistance Center Training Site in the Radiation Accident Registry Center (REAC/TS registry).

12. *Special comments by ASCO on comparative clinical activity of G-CSF and GM-CSF.* According to ASCO, no guideline recommendation can be made regarding the equivalency of the two colony-stimulating agents, G-CSF and GM-CSF. Further trials are recommended to study the comparative clinical activity, toxicity, and cost effectiveness of G-CSF and GM-CSF.

In addition to the ASCO Guidelines above, CSF agents have other FDA approval or compendia listed indications or orphan drug status including:

1. Chronic administration to reduce the incidence and duration of sequelae of neutropenia (e.g., fever, infections, oropharyngeal ulcers) in symptomatic patients with *congenital neutropenia, cyclic neutropenia, or idiopathic neutropenia.* (FDA approved for Neupogen and included in USPDI for Leukine.)

2. Designated an orphan drug by FDA for the treatment of HIV-infected patients who, in addition, are afflicted with cytomegalovirus retinitis and are being treated with myelosuppressive antiretroviral medication (e.g., ganciclovir; see chart below for off-label compendia).

3. Treatment of moderate to severe aplastic anemia (see chart below for off-label compendia).

4. Treatment for neutropenia associated with HIV infection and antiretroviral therapy (see chart below for off-label compendia).

5. Treatment of drug induced neutropenia (see chart below for off-label compendia).

FDA-approved Indications for CSFs (Package Labeling, 2002–2005)

Indication	Neupogen (filgrastim)	Neulasta (pegfilgrastim)	Leukine (sargramostim)
Use following induction chemotherapy in AML	X		X
Use in mobilization and following transplantation of autologous PBPC	X		X
Use in myeloid reconstitution after autologous or allogeneic (allogeneic not recommended by ASCO) bone marrow transplantation	X		X
Use in bone marrow transplantation failure or engraftment delay			X
To decrease incidence of febrile neutropenia in pts with nonmyeloid malignancies receiving myelosuppressive chemotherapy associated with a clinically significant incidence of febrile neutropenia	X	X	
For chronic administration to reduce the incidence and duration of sequelae of neutropenia in symptomatic pts with congenital neutropenia, cyclic neutropenia, or idiopathic neutropenia.	X		
Orphan drug status. AIDS patients with cytomegalovirus retinitis being treated with ganciclovir	X		

(*Continued*)

Table 15-1 (*Continued*)

Off-label uses listed in compendia (AHFS Online Database, 2005; USPDI Online Database, 2005).

Drug	Indication	Listed in compendia (USPDI or AHFS)
Sargramostim	Chemotherapy-induced neutropenia	USPDI AHFS
Filgrastim	Myeloid engraftment following BMT failure or delay	USPDI
Filgrastim	Myeloid engraftment following hematopoietic stem cell transplant	USPDI
Filgrastim and sargramostim	Neutropenia associated with AIDS	USPDI AHFS
Filgrastim and sargramostim	Myelodysplastic syndromes	USPDI AHFS
Filgrastim and sargramostim	Moderate to severe aplastic anemia	AHFS
Sargramostim	Severe chronic neutropenia (congenital, cyclic, or idiopathic)	USPDI
Filgrastim and sargramostim	Drug-induced neutropenia	USPDI AHFS

Not medically necessary

The use of CSFs is considered *not medically necessary for any of the following*:
1. Routine use in most chemotherapy regimens as prophylaxis; or
2. Receipt of chemotherapy with a risk of febrile neutropenia less than 20% and no significant high risk for complications; or
3. Neutropenic patients who are *afebrile*; or
4. Use as adjunctive therapy to antibiotics in patients with uncomplicated febrile neutropenia, defined as fever less than 10 day duration, no evidence of pneumonia, cellulitis, abscess, sinusitis, hypotension, multiorgan dysfunction, or invasive fungal infection; and no uncontrolled malignancies; or
5. Administration prior to or concurrent with chemotherapy for AML; or
6. Use in relapsed or refractory myeloid leukemia; or
7. Chemo sensitization of myeloid leukemias; or
8. Use to increase the dose intensity of cytotoxic chemotherapy beyond established dosage range for these regimens; or
9. Use in patients receiving concomitant chemotherapy and radiation therapy; particularly involving the mediastinum; or
10. Use either before and/or concurrently with chemotherapy for "priming" effects; or
11. Continued use if no response is seen within 28–42 days (patients who have failed to respond within this time frame are considered nonresponders); or
12. Use in nonchemotherapy-induced infection; or
13. Administration of CSFs to mobilize PBPC after allogeneic PBPC transplant.

Dosage and administration/monitoring

The currently available agents differ in their pharmacokinetic properties. Both sargramostim (Leukine®) and filgrastim (Neupogen®) can be administered intravenously (i.v.) or subcutaneously (SC), whereas pegfilgrastim (Neulasta®) is administered only SC. Pegfilgrastim is a pegylated form of filgrastim developed to allow for less frequent dosing.

Neulasta® is not labeled for use in leukemias, myelodysplasia, and lymphomas as it has not been studied for this indication. The possibility that pegfilgrastim can act as a growth factor for any tumor type cannot be excluded.

(Continued)

Table 15-1

Clinical Indications for Neutrophil Growth Factors (*Continued*)

No data support preferential use of filgrastim or pegfilgrastim in the treatment of febrile neutropenia. Similarly, no data support preferential use of filgrastim or sargramostim in the treatment of AML, mobilization of progenitor cells, or following autologous or allogeneic bone marrow transplant. According to the ASCO, no guideline recommendation can be made regarding the equivalency of the two colony-stimulating agents, G-CSF and GM-CSF (Smith, 2006).

Usual doses: filgrastim 5 μg/kg/day; pegfilgrastim 6 mg once; sargramostim 250 μg/m^2/day.

Toxicities. The acute toxicity associated with G-CSF use is minor. A few patients may experience bone pain. In normal individuals receiving G-CSF to mobilize hematopoietic stem cells, rapid splenic enlargement is possible and rare splenic rupture has occurred. Thus, these patients need to be monitored for abdominal or shoulder pain.

More serious concerns are emerging about long-term effects. First, animal studies have shown that the amount of damage to hematopoietic stem cells by cyclic chemotherapy is increased with the use of colony-stimulating factor support to hasten recovery (6). In addition, at least three studies have reported an increase in the incidence of acute leukemia and myelodysplasia when cancer therapy was supported with G-CSF use compared to the incidence with chemotherapy alone (7–9). The precise mechanism of the G-CSF effect is unclear. Possibly, through its antiapoptotic effects, it keeps damaged cells alive that would normally die. Regardless of mechanism, the twofold increased leukemia/myelodysplasia risk is sufficient to motivate clinicians to use the agent more sparingly and only when indicated, especially when cure is the goal.

GRANULOCYTE-MACROPHAGE COLONY-STIMULATING FACTOR

Granulocyte-macrophage colony-stimulating factor (GM-CSF) is a 127 amino acid glycoprotein (MW 22 kD) encoded by a gene on chromosome 5q31 that acts early and late in myeloid cell development. The GM-CSF receptor has a unique α-chain called CSF2R and shares a β-chain with the IL3 and IL5 receptor. It stimulates the common myeloid progenitor to differentiate toward the granulocyte/monocyte progenitor rather than the erthroid/megakaryocyte progenitor, and it stimulates an increase in all the progeny of the granulocte/monocyte progenitor. It also activates granulocytes, monocytes, and macrophages and promotes the antigen-presenting function of dendritic cells. Like G-CSF, it is produced by macrophages, fibroblasts, and endothelial cells, but unlike G-CSF, GM-CSF is also produced by T cells.

Biologic activity. GM-CSF stimulates the production of all three granulocyte types, neutrophils, eosinophils, and basophils. It increases the number of peripheral blood monocytes and supports the differentiation of monocytes into professional antigen-presenting cells called dendritic cells, an activity that has stimulated its testing as a vaccine adjuvant. GM-CSF also improves target killing by antibody-dependent cellular cytotoxicity. GM-CSF is usually not detectable in the peripheral blood under normal conditions or after the induction of neutropenia. The consequences of its deletion in knockout mice were minor, only a decrease in alveolar macrophages. Thus, GM-CSF is not viewed as a major physiologic regulator of myelopoiesis. Certainly, in its absence, other cytokines are able to stand in for any essential functions it has.

Pharmacology. An intravenously administered dose of GM-CSF (sargramostim) has an α-phase of 5–20 min and a β-phase 1.1–2.4 h. A subcutaneously administered dose has a half-life 1.6–5.8 h. A pegylated version of GM-CSF has been generated but the agent is not approved for use.

Method of administration. Sargramostim is generally given subcutaneously at a dose of 250 μg/m^2/day for all its indications.

Clinical effect. The clinical effects of GM-CSF mimic those of G-CSF to a large degree. Unfortunately, the agents have not been compared head-to-head. However, in general, the magnitude of the beneficial effects seen with GM-CSF and G-CSF are comparable in magnitude (10). No data suggest that the use of either factor improves the response rate, response duration, or overall survival. GM-CSF has also been used as a vaccine adjuvant and appears to be capable of stimulating both antibody and cellular responses to mildly immunogenic proteins such as idiotypic determinants on immunoglobulin molecules (11).

Toxicities. GM-CSF shares the property of G-CSF to induce bone pain in some patients. In general, GM-CSF is associated with more systemic symptoms than G-CSF including more fevers, muscle aches, and fluid retention. Because of their similar effects on neutrophil counts, G-CSF is used more commonly because of the perception that it produces fewer side effects.

ERYTHROPOIETIN

Erythropoietin (EPO) is a 166 amino acid glycoprotein (MW 21kD) encoded by a gene on chromosome 7q21 that regulates erythropoiesis. It is produced mainly in the kidney which senses the level of tissue oxygenation. When levels fall below a certain threshold, hypoxia-inducible factor is produced and acts as a stimulus to produce more EPO. EPO is a hormone that is released by the kidney into the peripheral blood. It binds to the EPO receptor, a 66 kD single-chain molecule expressed on bone marrow erythroid progenitors.

Biologic activity. EPO acts both early and late in red cell production (12). In addition to its effects on the committed erythroid progenitor, it may also exert effects on the early multipotent progenitor cells. EPO suppresses apoptosis and improves the efficiency of red cell production. Additional studies have found that EPO is also produced in neurons and may be involved in protecting hypoxic neurons from cell death (13). Furthermore, EPO appears to exert protective effects on myocardium that has been rendered hypoxic by experimental coronary artery ligation (14). These findings have led to ongoing clinical trials to evaluate the capacity of EPO to protect hypoxic brain and heart.

Pharmacology. An intravenously administered dose of EPO in the form of epoetin has a serum half-life of 4–11 h. Subcutaneous administration leads to a more prolonged and more variable kinetics with a half-life of 9–38 h. Glycosylation can affect the pharmacokinetics greatly. Site-directed mutagenesis was performed to add two N-glycosylation sites producing the product darbepoetin. Its molecular weight is 23% greater than epoetin but the serum half-life is prolonged about threefold. An intravenous injection has a half-life of 18–25 h; a subcutaneous injection has a half-life of 33–49 h.

Method of administration. The usual dose of epoetin in patients with cancer is 100–150 U/kg administered subcutaneously three times weekly. The usual dose of darbepoetin is 200 μg administered once every 2 weeks. No specific level of hemoglobin is used to trigger the intervention. Many physicians intervene when the hemoglobin level falls to 8 g/dl. In the face of cormorbid lung disease or heart disease, a threshold of 10 g/dl may be more appropriate.

Clinical effect. The patients who respond best to EPO have low levels of circulating endogenous EPO and adequate supplies of iron, B12, and folate. In the setting of renal failure, EPO has been very effective at reducing transfusion requirements and improving quality of life. However, in cancer patients, the slow response to EPO has made it difficult to show any influence on the usual efficacy endpoints of response rates, response durations, and survival. Instead, its FDA approval was based on softer quality-of-life data (15, 16). In the absence of complicating factors, a typical patient may get a 1–2 gm/dl increase in hemoglobin over 6–8 weeks of EPO administration. However, an increasing body of data suggests that EPO administration adversely affects the efficacy of concomitantly administered chemotherapy and protects the tumor from chemotherapy-induced killing. Randomized studies in patients with head and neck cancer, lung cancer, and breast cancer have demonstrated poorer response rates and shorter periods of remission in the group of patients receiving chemotherapy or chemotherapy plus radiotherapy together with EPO than in the group of patients receiving the same antitumor treatment without EPO (17). Accordingly, it appears that EPO use should be confined to the palliative care setting and should not be used in patients in whom the goal of therapy is to cure the disease.

Toxicities. EPO is relatively free of toxic symptoms. When the hemoglobin level gets as high as 12 gm/dl, EPO should be stopped because continued use in the setting of hemoglobin levels of 12 gm/dl or above can be associated with hypertension, polycythemia, and thromboembolic disease.

INTERLEUKIN-11

Interleukin-11 (IL11) is a 178 amino acid nonglycosylated protein (MW 23 kD) encoded by a gene on chromosome 19q13 that stimulates thrombopoiesis. Its receptor is a double-chain molecule with a unique α-chain and a second chain called gp130 that it shares with IL6 and leukemia inhibitory factor (LIF). It is produced by bone marrow derived stromal cells, fibroblasts, and epithelial cells. It plays a critical role in placental and fetal development as IL11 receptor knockout mice fail to develop. IL11 appears to be involved in implantation of the embryo into the endometrium.

Biologic activity. IL11 causes the proliferation of hematopoietic stem cells and megakaryocyte precursors and promotes platelet development independent of thrombopoietin. Some evidence suggests that it may also be a growth factor for hybridomas in vitro. IL11 has also been an agent of interest in inflammatory bowel disease because of its therapeutic effects to minimize bowel inflammation probably through inhibitory effects on the production of proinflammatory cytokines, particularly by monocytes/macrophages (18, 19).

Pharmacology. Oprelvekin is administered subcutaneously and has a half-life of about 7 h.

Method of administration. Oprelvekin is administered at a dose of 50 μg/kg/day beginning the day after chemotherapy in a setting where thrombocytopenia is an expected toxicity. The agent is given daily for periods of 10–21 days until the platelet count reaches 50,000/μl. Treatment should be discontinued at least 2 days before the start of the next treatment cycle.

Clinical effect. The administration of oprelvekin to women with breast cancer who had experienced thrombocytopenia in a prior cycle reduced the requirement for platelet transfusion by about 25%. Of the 96% of women who experienced thrombocytopenia with the drugs alone, the need for platelet transfusion was noted in 70% of those who had received oprelvekin (20). A much more exciting possibility for IL11 is its application to inflammatory bowel disease where early clinical testing documented a response rate of over 40% (21).

Toxicities. Oprevelkin may produce fatigue, myalgias, arthralgias, and fluid retention with weight gain. The majority of treated patients have fluid retention. Rare patients develop atrial arrhythmias or syncope.

Other hematopoietic growth factors are being explored for clinical application including stem cell factor, FLT-3 ligand, and thrombopoietin. Currently none of these agents is approved for clinical use.

GROWTH FACTORS

Aside from colony-stimulating factors, most therapeutic strategies that focus on growth factors and their receptors are aimed at blocking the effects of the growth factors. However, growth factors with certain selective properties may be useful in protecting against damage from cancer treatments or in promoting tissue restoration after therapy. A prototype agent is palifermin, keratinocyte growth factor.

Palifermin

Palifermin is a 140 amino acid protein (MW 16.3 kD) that differs from endogenous human keratinocyte growth factor by the removal of the first 23 N-terminal amino acids, which improves the stability of the protein. It is a member of the fibroblast growth factor family (FGF7) and binds to keratinocyte growth factor receptor, one of four receptors in the fibroblast growth factor receptor family. The receptor is expressed on epithelial cells of many tissues including the gastrointestinal tract, breast, genitourinary tract, and skin. It is not expressed on hematopoietic cells. It may have trophic effects on involuted thymi.

Biologic activity. Palifermin is produced by mesenchymal cells in response to epithelial injury. When administered to experimental animals, palifermin increases tissue thickness of the tongue, buccal mucosa, and gastrointestinal tract. When given to mice before and after chemotherapy or radiation, palifermin minimized fatalities and reduced weight loss. Palifermin is capable of enhancing the growth of epithelial-derived tumor cell lines in vitro at concentrations >10 μg/ml (generally more than a log higher than levels achieved clinically).

Pharmacology. The elimination half-life of intravenously administered palifermin is about 4.5 h. Levels do not accumulate with three consecutive daily doses. At least a threefold increase in epithelial cell proliferation was detected in healthy subjects who received 40 μg/kg/day for three days.

Method of administration. Palifermin is given intravenously on three consecutive days before exposure to the toxic regimen (chemotherapy, radiation therapy, or both) and on three consecutive days after treatment at a dose of 60 μg/kg/day. Treatment is given on 6 days.

Clinical effect. Summaries of pivotal clinical trial results are included in the FDA-approved product label (22). Among patients undergoing high-dose therapy and bone marrow transplantation, palifermin reduced duration of grade 3/4 mucositis from 9 days to 3 days, reduced incidence of grade IV mucositis from 62% to 20%, and reduced requirement for pain medication by 60% (23). Furthermore, despite the concern about potential adverse effects on growth of carcinomas, palifermin has been applied to the supportive care of patients with colorectal cancer undergoing fluorouracil-based chemotherapy (24). Oral mucositis was dramatically reduced by the use of palifermin and dose modifications were required in only 14% of the group receiving palifermin compared to 31% of placebo controls. A number of useful supportive measures can further ameliorate the unpleasant consequences of mucositis in patients undergoing cancer treatment (25).

Toxicities. The main toxic effects were grade 3 skin rashes in 3% of patients. Some patients also noted some discoloration of the tongue or mild dysesthesia. Rare patients complained of altered taste. No permanent or life-threatening toxicities were noted.

APPROACHES TO CANCER TREATMENT AND PREVENTION BASED ON ELICITING ANTIGEN-SPECIFIC IMMUNITY

A major goal of oncologists has been to find methods of activating host defenses in the effort to eliminate cancer. The awesome destructive power of the immune system is undeniable given the consequences of its overactivity in conditions like severe rheumatoid arthritis or multiple sclerosis. We also see the antitumor effects of the immune system in graft-vs-tumor effects that are seen in patients undergoing allogeneic bone marrow transplantation. Those positive effects can be boosted and renewed in some patients with donor lymphocyte infusions. However, despite substantial efforts, not many tumor antigen-specific approaches to cancer therapy are active components of our therapeutic armamentarium. We shall briefly review some promising strategies.

Infectious Disease Vaccines

A number of cancers are known to be caused by infectious agents. Epstein–Barr virus causes lymphomas and nasal lymphoepitheliomas. HTLV-I causes adult T-cell leukemia. *Helicobacter pylori* causes gastric lymphoma and probably some gastric adenocarcinomas. The list of potential targets for vaccine development is quite large. The power of this approach is substantial. Liver cancer from hepatitis B is a major health hazard, particularly in Asia. The institution of a mandatory hepatitis B vaccination program in Taiwan in the 1990s reduced the prevalence of chronic hepatitis B infection in children by over 90% (26).

The newest vaccine that should have cancer preventive activity is the quadrivalent vaccine against the human papillomavirus (HPV) called Gardasil. The vaccine is composed of virus-like particles that express the major capsid protein L1 from four HPV types: 16 and 18 that account for about 70% of cases of cervical cancer and 6 and 11 that account for about 90% of venereal warts (27). An aggressive vaccination campaign should eliminate these types from the population. The question then is whether this would translate into fewer cases of cervical cancer and venereal warts or whether other virus types would emerge to take the place of the eliminated ones.

Additional targets for vaccine approaches to cancer prevention that would make a major impact on cancer incidence worldwide should include hepatitis C, Epstein–Barr virus, and *Helicobacter pylori.*

Cancer Vaccines

While cancer prevention by targeting infectious etiologic agents is a clever use of the immune system, the capacity to elicit antitumor immunity in a tumor-bearing host is a challenge we have not yet mastered. The problems are daunting. First, tumor cells are not dramatically different from normal cells; thus, finding a way to attack them uniquely is difficult. One might find a way to activate the immune system that does not distinguish between tumor cells and normal cells. Second, the tumors have undergone several adaptations to protect themselves against host immune attack. They sometimes fail to express major histocompatibility determinants, the molecules through which T cells recognize a target. They erect barriers to penetration by developing high levels of interstitial pressure. Thus, a T cell trying to get into a tumor has to navigate the various natural membrane barriers plus push against a pressure gradient that can be as high or higher than systolic blood pressure. If the cell manages to overcome those odds, tumors can express Fas ligand, which will kill the T cell where it stands. In addition to these serious local barriers to the immune system, tumors make soluble factors that interfere with the antigen-presenting function of dendritic cells, polarize T cells to the less helpful Th2 phenotype (for making antibody) and away from the more helpful Th1 phenotype (for making cytotoxic cells), and alter the signal transduction machinery making the T cells difficult to activate. In short, efforts at activating the immune system of a tumor-bearing host are like whipping a dead horse.

Nevertheless, if we can define the barriers, we may be able to design strategies to overcome them. Many clever approaches are being tested.

Given the apparent success of allogeneic bone marrow transplantation, one idea has been to vaccinate the normal donor against the tumor and adoptively transfer an immune system that may have an even more powerful and specific antitumor effect. Anecdotal reports have been promising (28), but a systematic evaluation of the strategy is needed.

Another strategy to boost the immune response is to perform the immunization during a period of lymphopenia. Several experimental models have documented that vaccine responses are more robust in animals undergoing homeostasis-driven lymphocyte expansion after a lympholytic stimulus (29). Additional data suggest that it would be wise to selectively deplete CD4+ CD25+ regulatory T cells to boost a vaccine response.

Many investigators are focusing more on the composition of the vaccine than on the immunologic environment into which it will be introduced. Accordingly different investigators favor proteins or peptides as antigens; some use DNA that encode the antigenic determinant; some use DNA encoding both the antigen and an adjuvant molecule such as a chemokine; some pulse dendritic cells with peptides, some augment the dendritic cells by introducing genes (for example, GM-CSF) aimed to improve their function. In general, immunologic monitoring of such vaccinations generally shows that tumor-specific T-cell immunity is augmented; but little in the way of an antitumor effect has been seen in cancer-bearing people as a consequence of vaccination strategies.

An exception to this generalization is the work of Bendandi, first at the National Cancer Institute and later at University of Navarre in Spain (11, 30). In one study, idiotype vaccination of patients rendered disease-free by combination chemotherapy was associated with an immune response, as expected; however, in addition, minimal residual disease detected as persistent cells bearing the t(14;18) translocation disappeared from the blood after vaccination. In a second study of follicular lymphoma patients in relapse, multiple vaccinations following conventional chemotherapy produced longer second remissions than first remissions obtained from either similar or the same chemotherapy. These data suggest that idiotype protein given with GM-CSF not only elicits idiotype-specific T cells, but also those T cells are capable of mediating antitumor effects. This is not the same as seeing a tumor mass shrink under the influence of a vaccine. However, additional evidence for an antitumor effect of the cells comes from an analysis of a relapsed patient. The idiotype of the relapsed tumor was altered; thus, the tumor appeared to have escaped the immune surveillance established by the vaccine.

These results point out an additional problem we will have to face down the line; the emergence of tumor variants that evade detection by altering the antigen that we designed our therapy to attack. The implication of this finding is that we should consider multivalent vaccines that are aimed at more than one tumor antigen, if possible.

An additional novel strategy to boost immune effects against tumors is to block the CTLA4 regulatory pathway. CTLA4 is a homologue of CD28 that is upregulated on activated T cells. It binds to costimulatory molecules CD80 and CD86 on dendritic cells 100 times more efficiently than the physiologic ligand CD28 and the effect of its action is to stop the interaction between the T cell and the antigen-presenting cell and turn off the immune response. Two blocking antibodies to CTLA-4 are in clinical trial, ipilimumab (IgG1) and ticilimumab (IgG2). They produce a 15% response rate in metastatic malignant melanoma. However, the toxicity profile suggests a breaking of self-tolerance (31). Toxicities include dermatitis, colitis, uveitis, hepatitis, hypophysitis, arthritis, nephritis, and hyperthyroidism. Additional studies are underway using these antibodies to boost vaccine responses.

We have chosen not to go into more detail about the specialized studies on adoptive cellular therapies. None is ready to become treatments we need to learn how to give in the office, and the field has been associated with claims that have not withstood efforts at repetition. Suffice it to say that adoptive cellular therapy is an active area of investigation and based on the successes of allogeneic hematopoietic stem cell transplantation, it seems likely that some adoptive therapy approach will show efficacy as we learn more about the determinants of response.

REFERENCES

1. Rosenberg SA. Interleukin 2 and the development of immunotherapy for the treatment of patients with cancer. Cancer J Sci Am. 2000; 6(suppl1): S2.
2. McDermott DF. Update on the application of interleukin-2 in the treatment of renal cell carcinoma. Clin Cancer Res. 2007; 13: 720s.
3. Schwartz RN, Stover L, Dutcher J. Managing toxicities of high-dose interleukin 2. Oncology. 2002; 16 (suppl13): 11.
4. Smith TJ, Khatcheressian J, Lyman GH, et al. 2006 update of recommendations for the use of white blood cell growth factors: an evidence-based clinical practice guideline. J Clin Oncol. 2006; 24: 3187.
5. Aapro MS, Cameron DA, Pettengell R, et al. EORTC guidelines for the use of granulocyte-colony stimulating factor to reduce the incidence of chemotherapy-induced febrile neutropenia in adult patients with lymphomas and solid tumors. Eur J Cancer. 2006; 42: 2433.
6. Hornung RL, Longo DL. Hematopoietic stem cell depletion by restorative growth factor regimens during repeated high-dose cyclophosphamide therapy. Blood. 1992; 80: 77.
7. Relling MV, Boyett JM, Blanco JG, et al. Granulocyte colony-stimulating factor and the risk of secondary myeloid malignancy after etoposide treatment. Blood. 2003; 101: 3862.
8. Smith RE, Bryant J, Decillis A, et al. Acute myeloid leukemia and myelodysplastic syndrome after doxorubicin-cyclophosphamide adjuvant therapy for operable breast cancer: the National Surgical Adjuvant Breast and Bowel Project Experience. J Clin Oncol. 2003; 21: 1195.
9. Hershman D, Neugut AI, Jacopson JS, et al. Acute myeloid leukemia or myelodysplastic syndrome following use of granulocyte colony-stimulating factors during breast cancer adjuvant chemotherapy. J Natl Cancer Inst. 2007; 99: 196.
10. Bohlius J, Reiser M, Schwarzer G, Engert A. Granulopoiesis-stimulating factors to prevent adverse effects in the treatment of malignant lymphoma. Cochrane Database Syst Rev. 2004; 1: CD003189.
11. Bendandi M, Gocke CD, Koprin CB, et al. Complete molecular remission induced by patient-specific vaccination plus granulocyte-monocyte colony-stimulating factor against lymphoma. Nat Med. 1999; 5: 1171.
12. Kranz SB. Erythropoietin. Blood. 1991; 77: 419.
13. Brines ML, Ghezzi P, Keenan S, et al. Erythropoietin crosses the blood brain barrier to protect against experimental brain injury. Proc Natl Acad Sci USA. 2000; 97: 10526.

14. Moon C, Krawczyk M, Ahn D, et al. Erythropoietin reduce myocardial infarction and left ventricular functional decline after coronary artery ligation in rats. Proc Natl Acad Sci USA. 2003; 100: 11612.

15. Case DC Jr, Bukowski RM, Carey RW, et al. Recombinant erythropoietin therapy for anemic cancer patients on combination chemotherapy. J Natl Cancer Inst. 1993; 85: 801.

16. Crawford J, Cella D, Cleeland CS, et al. Relationship between changes in hemoglobin level and quality of life during chemotherapy in anemic cancer patients receiving epoetin alfa therapy. Cancer. 2002; 95: 888.

17. http: //www.fda.gov/cder/drug/infopage/RHE/default.htm

18. Du X, Williams DA. Interleukin 11: review of molecular, cell biology and clinical use. Blood. 1997; 89: 3897.

19. Williams DA. Inflammatory cytokines and mucosal injury. J Natl Cancer Inst Monogr. 2001; 29: 26.

20. Isaacs C, Robert NJ, Bailey FA, et al. Randomized placebo-controlled study of recombinant human interleukin-11 to prevent chemotherapy-induced thrombocytopenia in patients with breast cancer receiving dose-intensive cyclophosphamide and doxorubicin. J Clin Oncol. 1997; 15: 3368.

21. Sands BE, Bank S, Sninsky CA, et al. Preliminary evaluation of safety and activity of recombinant human interleukin 11 in patients with active Crohn's disease. Gastroenterology. 1999; 117: 58.

22. http://www.fda.gov/cder/foi/label/2004/125103lbl.pdf

23. Spielberger R, Stiff P, Bensinger W, et al. Palifermin for oral mucositis after intensive chemotherapy for hematologic cancers. N Engl J Med. 2004; 351: 2590.

24. Rosen LS, Abdi E, Davis ID, et al. Palifermin reduces the incidence of oral mucositis in patients with metastatic colorectal cancer treated with fluorouracil-based chemotherapy. J Clin Oncol. 2006; 24: 5183.

25. http://www.nci.nih.gov/cancertopics/pdq/supportivecare/oralcomplications /HealthProfessional/page5

26. Shepard CW, Simard EP, Finelli L, et al. Hepatitis B virus infection: epidemiology and vaccination. Epidemiol Rev. 2006; 28: 112.

27. Lowy DR, Schiller JT. Prophylactic human papillomavirus vaccines. J Clin Invest. 2006; 116: 1167.

28. Kwak LW, Taub DD, Duffey PL, et al. Transfer of myeloma idiotype-specific immunity from an actively immunized marrow donor. Lance. 1995; 345: 1016.

29. Hu HM, Poehlein CH, Urba WJ, Fox BA, Development of antitumor immune responses in reconstituted lymphopenic hosts. Cancer Res. 2002; 62: 2914.

30. Inoges S, Rodriguez-Calvillo M, Zabalegui N, et al. Clinical benefit associated with idiotypic vaccination in patients with follicular lymphoma. J Natl Cancer Inst. 2006; 98: 1292.

31. Korman A, Yellin M, Keler T. Tumor immunotherapy: preclinical and clinical activity of anti-CTLA4 antibodies. Curr Opin Invest Drugs. 2005; 6: 592.

MONOCLONAL ANTIBODIES
IN CANCER TREATMENT

Monoclonal antibodies are used in five different ways in the treatment of human conditions. First, antibodies have a variety of effector mechanisms that focus an array of immunologic agents (complement, various effector cells) on the target to which they bind. Second, antibodies can serve as targeting moieties to specifically deliver diverse killing or inhibitory molecules to a specific site. Third, antibodies can be directed at soluble protein or proteoglycan hormones or cytokines or their receptors to antagonize a particular function such as cell growth, invasion, or migration. Fourth, antibodies can be used as antigens to elicit antitumor responses against immunoglobulin-expressing tumors. Fifth, antibodies can be used to alter the pharmacologic behavior of other substances to either increase or decrease their half-life or alter their distribution (e.g., antibodies to digoxin used to treat digoxin toxicity).

Monoclonal antibody technology was developed in 1975 and has been widely applied in biological sciences since then. The first clinical trial of a monoclonal antibody was performed in 1980 and the first FDA approval of a monoclonal antibody for a cancer indication occurred in 1997. Currently nine monoclonal antibody-based drugs are FDA-approved for therapeutic use; one monoclonal antibody, nofetumomab (NR-LU10, anti-CD56) labeled with technetium-99m is approved for use as an imaging agent in the staging of small cell lung cancer (it will not be discussed here). Both the list of agents and their approved uses are likely to expand.

ANTIBODY STRUCTURE AND FUNCTION

Antibody structure was initially elucidated by using antibodies as probes of other antibodies. Three sets of determinants were defined. *Isotypes* are determinants that distinguish among the main classes of antibodies of a particular species and are defined by antibodies made in different species. Humans have five main heavy chain isotypes (M, G, A, D, E) and two light chain isotypes (κ, λ). *Allotypes* are small sequence differences or allelic differences between immunoglobulins of the same isotype in different individuals within a species and are defined by antibodies made in the same species. *Idiotypes* are antigenic determinants formed by the antigen-combining site of an antibody that distinguish each clonal B-cell product.

Antibodies are generally composed of four chains, two identical heavy chains (M.W. ~50,000 Daltons) and two identical light chains (M.W. ~22–25,000 Daltons). Each chain has a portion with limited sequence variability called the constant region and a portion with extensive sequence variability called the variable region. The heavy and light chains are linked by disulfide bonds and aligned such that the variable regions of the light and heavy chain are adjacent to each other (Figure 16-1) A specific antigen is bound by the antibody in the pocket formed by the heavy and light chains. The contact regions between the antigen and the antibody are usually defined by two or three regions of hypervariability within the variable regions. These are called complementarity-determining regions (CDRs).

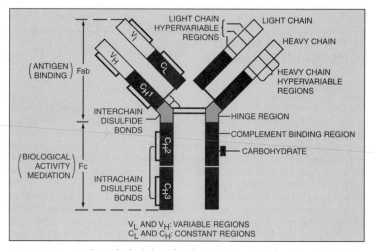

FIGURE 16-1   A schematic depiction of antibody structure and function relationships. (From Wasserman RL, Capra, JD. Immunoglobulins. In MI Horowitz, W Pigman (eds.), "The Glycoconjugates," Academic Press, New York, 1977, p. 323.)

It is possible to generate an antibody of defined specificity that can bind to nearly any biological molecule by immunizing mice and the isolating and immortalizing the B cell that produces the desired antibody. The B cell is then fused to an immunoglobulin nonproducing B-cell line, yielding the monoclonal murine-derived antibodies first used in clinical trials. The efficacy of murine antibodies was found to be limited by several factors. First, murine antibodies cooperate with human effector mechanisms poorly such that important mechanisms like complement fixation and antibody-dependent cellular cytotoxicity were activated weakly or not at all. Second, the human host has developed sophisticated methods to remove animal proteins rapidly from the blood. Therefore, the biological half-life of murine antibodies is short; indeed, much shorter than the biological half-life of human IgG antibodies (~23 days). Third, murine antibodies are themselves immunogenic. Thus, human antimouse antibodies to the therapeutic agent result in even more rapid clearance on repeat administration. Other factors that compromised efficacy of early antibody trials were tumor related. Targets were picked that were suboptimal. The target molecule could be shed into the serum and distract the antibody from reaching the cell producing the target. In some cases, target molecules were down-regulated such that resistance to the therapeutic antibody emerged.

Many of these problems were addressed in a single technical development; the recombinant production of chimeric antibodies that contained the framework and constant regions of human immunoglobulins with the murine-derived antigen binding portion of the molecule (the variable or hypervariable regions). The first of these chimeric antibodies to gain FDA approval and to become widely used clinically was rituximab, an anti-CD20 antibody. The success of rituximab against lymphoid malignancies derived in large measure from the persistence of the company that owned the rights to it. Based on the rather minor antitumor activity of the murine anti-CD20 antibody, a peer-review process would likely have terminated its clinical development. However, the industrial sponsor took the development a step further and generated a chimeric antibody. That final step corrected nearly all of the defects of the murine antibody and pointed the way to other effective antibodies for clinical use.

The nine monoclonal antibodies approved for use in patients with cancer are directed at six different targets, CD20 (rituximab, tositumomab, ibritumomab tiuxetan), epidermal growth factor receptor (cetuximab, panitumumab), HER-2/neu (trastuzumab), CD33 (gemtuzumab ogomycin), vascular endothelial growth factor (bevacizumab), and CD52 (alemtuzumab). Antibodies aimed at dozens of potential targets are in development.

RITUXIMAB (RITUXAN)

CD20, the target of rituximab, is expressed mainly on normal and neoplastic B cells. CD20 is a hydrophobic transmembrane protein of molecular weight 35 kD. CD20 is not expressed on hematopoietic stem cells, pro-B cells or plasma cells, or nonlymphoid tissues. The function of CD20 is unclear; some data have suggested that it functions as a calcium channel. It is not shed or internalized upon antibody binding.

Rituximab is a chimeric IgG1, κ antibody with human constant regions and murine variable regions. Its molecular weight is about 145 kD and it binds CD20 with an affinity of 8 nM. Its antitumor effects are thought to be related to its activation of complement and antibody-dependent cellular cytotoxicity. In addition, signaling through CD20 may activate apoptosis mechanisms. Anti-CD20 improves the antitumor effects of chemotherapeutic agents.

The pharmacokinetics of the agent are influenced by a variety of factors including the tumor burden. Early doses tend to achieve lower serum levels because the tumor and normal B cells bind a larger fraction of an administered dose. The empirically derived treatment schedule is weekly doses of 375 mg/m^2 IV. After the fourth weekly dose, the half-life averages 205 h with a maximum serum concentration of 486 μg/ml. Levels continue to increase with additional weekly administrations. Delivery of rituximab with chemotherapy does not alter its pharmacology. A maximum tolerated dose has not been defined. Doses as high as 500 mg/m^2 are well tolerated. Because of toxicity problems (mainly related to activation of immune effector mechanisms), the drug should be infused at an initial rate of about 50 mg/h.

Toxicities from rituximab are mainly related to the initial infusion. Symptoms generally develop within 30–120 min of starting infusion. In most cases, the symptom complex includes one or more of the following: fever and chills, nausea, pruritus, angioedema, asthenia, headache, bronchospasm, throat irritation, rhinitis, urticaria, myalgia, dizziness, or hypertension. The reactions resolve entirely with either slowing the infusion or temporarily interrupting it. The infusion-related symptoms generally decrease in incidence with each administration from nearly 80% incidence with the first to around 14% with the eighth. Diphenhydramine, acetaminophen, and intravenous fluids are often required to suppress the symptoms. Once symptoms resolve, the administration of rituximab can be reinitiated at about half the rate of the initial infusion. This symptom complex is thought to be largely due to complement activation. The most severe cases can rarely develop adult respiratory distress syndrome, myocardial infarction, ventricular fibrillation, or cardiogenic shock.

Other uncommon problems include the development of tumor lysis syndrome from rapid killing of tumor cells and occasional Stevens–Johnson syndrome with severe mucocutaneous inflammation. When rituximab is administered with chemotherapy, some patients have experienced reactivation of hepatitis B. In general, rituximab is very well tolerated. It only rarely elicits a host antibody response (~1% of patients). The suppression of normal B cells by rituximab is variable in duration depending on the age of the patient and the length of treatment, but most patients recover normal B-cell function within a year of stopping rituximab. No late effects of B-cell suppression have been reported.

Rituximab is effective in nearly all B-cell-derived malignancies that express CD20. It is particularly active when used in combination chemotherapy and has become a component of standard therapy for diffuse large B-cell lymphoma (see the chapter on non-Hodgkin's lymphomas). In addition to its standard use in patients with diffuse large B-cell lymphoma, it is also active in follicular lymphoma, mantle cell lymphoma, chronic lymphoid leukemia, and hairy cell leukemia. It is also being used increasingly to treat autoimmune diseases in which autoreactive antibodies play a pathogenetic role. These include idiopathic thrombocytopenic purpura, thrombotic thrombocytopenic purpura, autoimmune hemolytic anemia, and some cases of pure red cell aplasia.

ALEMTUZUMAB (CAMPATH)

CD52, the target of alemtuzumab, is a 21–28 kD cell surface glycoprotein expressed on normal and malignant B and T cells, NK cells, monocytes, macrophages, a subpopulation of granulocytes, a subpopulation of CD34+ bone marrow cells, and on epididymis, sperm, and seminal vesicle, but not on spermatogonia. Its function is unknown. CD52 does not shed or internalize. Alemtuzumab is an IgG1, κ chimeric antibody with human constant and variable framework regions and rat CDRs. It binds to CD52 with a nanomolar affinity and is thought to act through antibody-dependent cellular cytotoxicity.

Alemtuzumab clearance is nonlinear. Its plasma half-life is much shorter for early doses (11 h) than late doses (6 days) presumably because of the depletion of CD52-bearing cells over time. After 12 weeks of doses, the mean AUC is sevenfold higher than the mean AUC after the first dose. No dosage adjustments are required based on age or sex.

Because of infusion-related toxicity, doses are begun at 3 mg/d administered as a 2 h infusion. When infusion-related toxicities are less than or equal to grade 2, the daily dose is escalated to 10 mg. Once that dose is tolerated, one can advance the dose to 30 mg/d. The usual maintenance dose is 30 mg/d three times a week, usually a Monday–Wednesday–Friday schedule. Weekly doses exceeding 90 mg total are not recommended because of an increased risk of pancytopenia. Dose escalation from 3 mg to 30 mg doses can generally be accomplished in a week.

Like rituximab, alemtuzumab is associated with significant infusion-related toxicity with the first dose, decreasing with subsequent administration. The symptoms include fever, chills, hypotension, shortness of breath, bronchospasm, and rashes. Rarely the symptoms may progress to adult respiratory distress syndrome, cardiac arrhythmias, myocardial infarction, and heart failure. Routine premedication with diphenhydramine 50 mg and acetaminophen 650 mg 30 min before the infusion is recommended.

The next most common serious toxicity of alemtuzumab is immunosuppression. Because of the widespread expression of CD52 on cells involved in host defenses, patients receiving alemtuzumab become severely immunosuppressed and are susceptible to opportunistic infections such as *Pneumocystic carinii*, aspergillosis and other fungal infections, and intracellular pathogens like *Listeria monocytogenes*. The antibody produces profound lymphopenia. CD4+ T-cell counts do not recover above 200/µl for at least 2 months after stopping treatment and full recovery may take more than 1 year. Antiherpes (acyclovir) and antiinfective (bactrim) prophylaxis is recommended and should be continued until lymphocyte recovery. Opportunistic infections may be seen despite prophylaxis. Because of the immune suppression, patients on alemtuzumab who receive blood products should have those products irradiated to prevent graft-vs-host disease. Patients on alemtuzumab should not receive any live vaccines.

The third serious toxicity associated with alemtuzumab is myelosuppression. Neutropenia, anemia, and thrombocytopenia are common, and rarely patients have developed prolonged and occasionally fatal pancytopenia. The mechanism of the cytopenia may be either direct cytotoxicity or autoimmune; idiopathic thrombocytopenic purpura and autoimmune hemolytic anemia have both been documented. Grade 3 or 4 myelosuppression is noted in 50–70% of patients.

Nearly 2% of patients receiving alemtuzumab generate antibodies to it, but no adverse effects on toxicity or response have been documented.

The main clinical use for alemtuzumab has been as a salvage therapy for chronic lymphocytic leukemia that is unresponsive to alkylating agents and nucleosides. It is being tested as salvage therapy for other lymphomas and is particularly promising in the treatment of Tcell lymphomas. It is being tested as an immunosuppressive agent in graft-vs-host disease and other conditions of immune hyperreactivity. It is effective at depleting marrow and peripheral blood collections of T cells in vitro before reinfusing the cells in the setting of allogeneic hematopoietic stem cell transplantation.

BEVACIZUMAB (AVASTIN)

Bevacizumab is an IgG1 recombinant humanized monoclonal antibody that binds to vascular endothelial growth factor (VEGF). The efficacy of the antibody is surprising. Because VEGF is generally secreted locally and acts locally, it would not be expected that a systemically administered antibody to the growth factor itself would achieve relevant concentrations at the sites of production in tissues. The antibody should circulate and be cleared without ever encountering the physiologically relevant VEGF. In general, growth factor receptors make better targets than growth factors themselves because blocking the effects of the ligand at its binding site should be more efficient than attempting to sop up the ligand like a sponge. The proposed mechanism of action of bevacizumab is to prevent the interaction of VEGF with its receptors, Flt-1 and KDR, on the surface of endothelial cells. This should inhibit endothelial cell proliferation and new blood vessel formation and decrease the tumor blood supply. Antiangiogenic drugs also decrease blood vessel permeability, decrease tumor interstitial pressure, and improved delivery of chemotherapy to the tumor.

The half-life of bevacizumab varies according to body weight, sex, and tumor burden; however, the median half-life is around 20 days. The usual dose is 10 mg/kg every 2 weeks. Steady state serum levels are generally reached by 100 days. It is unknown whether doses need to be adjusted in the setting of renal or hepatic impairment.

Toxicities are overall mild in degree if certain features are monitored and certain clinical situations avoided. Bevacizumab can impair wound healing and has led to wound dehiscences and/or perforations and abscesses in 2–4% of patients. If possible, the interval between surgery and initiation of therapy should be 4 weeks. After bevacizumab is administered, elective surgery should be delayed at least 4 weeks, if possible, given the 20 day half-life. A second major side effect is bleeding. Mild bleeding in the form of epistaxis occurs in some patients. However, of greater concern is the risk for major pulmonary or gastrointestinal hemorrhage which has occurred in up to 20% of patients. Active bleeding from the GI tract and hemoptysis are contraindications to bevacizumab use. It should not be used in lung cancer patients with tumor masses that involve the central bronchial airway because of the risk of fatal bronchial hemorrhage. Severe hypertension may also be seen in 7–10% of patients. The drug should be discontinued if the hypertension cannot be readily controlled. Bevacizumab is also associated with proteinuria in up to 20% of patients but less than 1% develop nephrotic syndrome. Bevacizumab may also worsen congestive heart failure, particularly in patients who have received antracyclines or radiation therapy involving the heart. Infusion reactions are uncommon and antibodies to beva-cizumab have not been documented.

Bevacizumab improves outcome in patients with colorectal cancer and is being tested in a large number of other malignancies. Because of the critical and universal role of angiogenesis in cancer biology, bevacizumab is expected to be a useful adjunct to treatment for many types of cancer. Given the success of bevacizumab, antibodies to the VEGF receptor(s) or small molecular weight receptor inhibitors may be equally or even more effective therapies.

TRASTUZUMAB (HERCEPTIN)

Trastuzumab is a humanized IgG1 κ antibody that binds to the extracellular domain of HER-2/neu, a transmembrane tyrosine kinase growth factor receptor in the epidermal growth factor receptor family. The target is a 185 kD protein expressed on the surface of about 25% of breast cancers. Tumors with amplifi-cation of HER-2/neu are generally more refractory to therapy and more aggres-sive in their rate of progression than HER-2/neu-negative tumors. Trastuzumab binding affinity for its target is about 5 nM; it appears to act both by direct tumor growth inhibition and the activation of antibody-dependent cellular cytotoxicity.

The usual method of administration is to give a loading dose of 4 mg/kg intravenously by 90 min infusion followed by a maintenance dose of 2 mg/kg weekly by 30 min infusion. The mean serum half-life is about 6 days. Steady state concentrations are achieved between 16 and 32 weeks of therapy with mean trough levels of 79 µg/ml and peak levels of 123 µg /ml. Some patients with HER-2/neu-positive breast cancers have detectable levels of soluble receptor in the serum; the presence of circulating target delays the achievement of steady state levels by a week or two. The disposition of the antibody is not affected by age or renal function. Coadministration with taxanes results in higher trough levels of the antibody (about 50% higher); other chemotherapeutic agents commonly used in breast cancer do not alter trastuzumab clearance.

Trastuzumab produces a 14% response rate when used as a single agent in metastatic HER-2/neu-positive (at least 2+ by immunohistology) breast cancer. Responses are more common in patients with higher levels of expression. In com-bination with chemotherapeutic agents, trastuzumab improves response rates and survival in patients with metastatic disease and improves disease-free and overall survival in the adjuvant setting. In early breast cancer, addition of trastuzumab to adjuvant chemotherapy reduces recurrence rate by 50% and reduces mortality by 30%. In the setting of metastatic disease, addition of trastuzumab to chemotherapy increases response rates by 18–27%, prolongs disease-free survival by 3–5 months, and improves overall survival by 5–9 months.

Adverse reactions from trastuzumab are generally rare. The usual initial infusion reaction from human antibodies occurs in 40% of patients receiving trastuzumab for the first time. The incidence of diarrhea in patients taking trastuzumab alone is about 25%. Use of trastuzumab with myelotoxic chemotherapy may result in an increase in myelosuppression. The most signifi-cant toxicity from trastuzumab is heart failure. It occurs in about 4% of patients and affects up to 20% of patients in the setting of past or concurrent treatment with anthracyclines. Patients may present with the usual symptoms and signs of heart failure including dyspnea, peripheral edema, and an S3 gallop. Patients being considered for trastuzumab therapy should undergo thorough baseline evaluation of cardiac function including history, physical exam, electrocardio-gram, and an assessment of ejection fraction by echocardiogram or MUGA scan. Advanced age and preexisting cardiac disease increase the risk. Some patients progress to intractable heart failure but most can be effectively managed by discontinuing the trastuzumab and treating the heart failure. Most of these patients experience gradual improvement in cardiac function with time off therapy. In general, trastuzumab is not withheld in patients with mild decreases in ejection fraction who are asymptomatic. Immunogenicity is low; generally <5% of patients make antibodies to trastuzumab.

Small molecular weight inhibitors of HER2/EGFR are in late stages of clinical development and appear to have activity in trastuzumab-resistant patients.

CETUXIMAB (ERBITUX)

Cetuximab is a chimeric human/mouse monoclonal antibody with constant regions of human IgG1 κ origin with murine variable regions that recognize the extracellular domain of the human epidermal growth factor (EGF) receptor. The antibody is thought to work mainly by blocking the EGF receptor and starving the tumor of a needed growth factor. This hypothesis is undermined somewhat by data suggesting that some responding patients have tumors that do not express EGF receptors. EGF receptors are overexpressed in most epithelial malignancies.

The usual method of administration is to give a test dose of 20 mg. Patients then receive a loading dose of 400 mg/m^2 by 2 h infusion followed by weekly administration of 250 mg/m^2 by 1 h infusion. Using this regimen, steady state levels are usually achieved by week 3 with mean peak serum levels being about 200 μg /ml and mean trough serum levels being about 63 μg /ml. Women have about 25% lower clearance rate than men. The half-life is about 5 days (114 h).

Cetuximab was approved for use based on results obtained in patients with metastatic colorectal cancer. In a randomized trial of patients who had previously progressed on irinotecan, cetuximab plus irinotecan produced a 23% overall response rate compared to about 11% for cetuximab alone. Median response duration was about 6 months for cetuximab plus irinotecan. Other single-arm cetuximab trials showed response rates of 9–14% in patients with metastatic colorectal cancer that had progressed following an irinotecan-containing regimen. Although patients were required to have immunohistochemical evidence of EGF receptor expression to be enrolled on these early studies, response did not correlate with either the percentage of positive cells or the intensity of the expression. In a number of other epithelial malignancies, encouraging activity is seen in combination with radiation therapy or chemotherapy in head and neck cancer, nonsmall cell lung cancer, and pancreatic cancer. Investigations are ongoing to assess the role of antibodies to the EGF receptor versus the small molecule inhibitors of EGF receptor signaling such as gefitinib and erlotinib and whether various combinations or sequences of agents may boost response rates.

Upon first exposure, cetuximab produces the same syndrome associated with other humanized monoclonal antibodies including hives, bronchospasm, and hypotension. Severe reactions are encountered in about 3% of treated patients. Slowing the administration rate and use of antihistamines controls most such reactions. Patients with preexisting interstitial lung disease may have a worsening of symptoms with cetuximab. This problem generally emerges between the 4th and 11th doses of antibody. The antibody causes an acneiform rash in nearly 90% of patients, but is severe in grade in about 10%. The lesions can progress to abscesses requiring incision and drainage and sepsis can be a complication. Other mucosal surfaces may also be affected by the antibody including nasal, oral, esophageal, and gastrointestinal. Patients on cetuximab also experience malaise (48%), nausea (29%), fever (27%), constipation or diarrhea (25% each), abdominal pain (26%), and headache (26%). Patients should be followed for the development of hypomagnesemia throughout the course of treatment. Low magnesium levels are detected in about half of treated patients and can progress to dangerous levels with attendant hypocalcemia and hypokalemia if not monitored carefully. Antibodies to cetuximab develop in <5% of patients and do not influence response rates.

PANITUMUMAB (VECTIBIX)

Panitumumab, a second antibody to EGF receptor, is a human IgG2 κ antibody with CDRs of murine origin. Overall it contains a smaller proportion of murine sequences than does cetuximab. Like cetuximab, it acts to block the binding of EGF to its receptor and its antitumor effects are thought to be related to loss of EGF receptor signaling.

The recommended regimen is 6 mg/kg given once every 2 weeks by 1 h infusion. Steady state levels are usually reached by the third dose and mean peak concentrations are 213 μg /ml and mean trough concentrations are 39 μg /ml. The elimination half-life is about 7.5 days. Age, sex, race, renal dysfunction, hepatic dysfunction, and level of EGF receptor staining on tumor cells make no noticeable impact on the pharmacokinetics of panitumomab.

Panitumumab was approved based on an 8% response rate in patients with metastatic colorectal cancer whose tumors expressed EGF receptor and whose disease had progressed on or following treatment containing 5-fluorouracil, oxaliplatin, and irinotecan. The median duration of responses was about 4 months. No relationship was found between level of expression of EGF receptors and response rate or duration.

The toxicity profile is nearly identical to cetuximab and includes the initial infusion reaction, skin toxicity, diarrhea, hypomagnesemia, and a 1% risk of pulmonary fibrosis. Its use together with irinotecan is not recommended because it may increase the incidence of severe diarrhea (58% grades 3–4 in one study). Sunlight exposure may worsen the skin reaction to panitumumab. Antibodies are elicited to panitumumab in <4% of patients and are not associated with any alteration in activity or pharmacokinetics. As the most recently approved antibody for a cancer indication, its activity profile is still actively being defined. There is no reason to suspect that its activity will be substantially different from that of cetuximab.

GEMTUZUMAB OGOMICIN (MYLOTARG)

Gemtuzumab ogomicin is an antibody conjugate. The antibody portion of the molecule is a humanized IgG4 κ antibody that binds to CD33, an adhesion glycoprotein expressed on cells of the myelocytic lineage (but not on pluripotent hematopoietic stem cells or nonhematopoietic cells) and on acute myeloid leukemia cells. The antibody is mainly composed of human sequences with murine CDRs. The antibody is conjugated to calicheamicin, a potent antitumor antibiotic isolated from the bacterium, *Micromonospora echinospora calichensis*. Once the conjugate binds to CD33, it is internalized. The calicheamycin is cleaved away from the antibody and released from the lysosomes intracellularly, and binds DNA in the minor groove to initiate double-strand breaks and cell death.

Gemtuzumab ogomicin is usually administered at a dose of 9 mg/m^2 by 2 h infusion followed by a second dose of 9 mg/m^2 2 weeks later. The elimination half-lives of total and unconjugated calicheamicin are about 45 h and 4 days, respectively, after the first dose and the half-life increases about 50% with the second dose. Clearance is not affected by age, sex, weight, or body surface area.

Gemtuzumab ogomicin is used as a salvage agent in the treatment of acute myeloid leukemia. It was approved for use by the U.S. Food and Drug Administration based on achieving a 26% response rate (13% complete responses) in patients with relapsed acute myeloid leukemia. Response rate and duration of response correlate with the duration of the initial remission. Response rates are 11% for those whose first remission was 6 months or less, 22% for those whose initial remission was 6–12 months, and 35% for those whose first remission was a year or longer. Responding patients survive a median of 1 year following treatment. Response is not influenced by patient age or cytogenetic abnormalities. Because of the many options for younger patients, gemtuzumab ogomicin is often used in patients older than 60 years. It is being assessed for its role in postremission therapy as an alternative to bone marrow transplantation in patients who are not candidates or who lack a suitable donor. It is almost always used as a single agent. Data on combination of gemtuzumab ogomicin with other chemotherapy are limited. The dose is usually reduced to 3 mg/m^2 when it is used together with other chemotherapeutic agents. CD33 is also expressed on the malignant cells of acute promyelocytic leukemia; gemtuzumab ogomicin has been used with all-trans retinoic acid with promising results in pilot studies.

In addition to infusion reactions, gemtuzumab ogomicin causes severe myelosuppression. Delayed recovery of platelet counts is often observed in patients who enter complete remission. Patients with peripheral WBC counts above 30,000/μl are susceptible to serious pulmonary dysfunction from cells blocking the pulmonary vessels. Fever, chills, dyspnea, pulmonary infiltrates, pleural effusions, pulmonary edema, and acute respiratory distress syndrome may occur. The WBC count should be reduced below 30,000/μl (with leukapheresis or hydroxyurea) before starting gemtuzumab ogomicin. The antibody conjugate also increases the risk of developing veno-occlusive disease of the liver. Patients undergoing subsequent hematopoietic stem cell transplantation are at higher risk (15%) than patients not undergoing transplantation (1%). Though rare, the syndrome (rapid weight gain, right upper quandrant pain, hepatomegaly, ascites, hyperbilirubinemia, elevated liver enzymes) can progress to death. Another serious complication of gemtuzumab ogomicin therapy is rapid tumor lysis. Patients with large tumor burdens should receive prophylaxis for tumor lysis syndrome. Like other myelotoxic agents, mucositis, bleeding, and febrile neutropenia may complicate its use. The development of antibodies to gemtuzumab ogomicin is very rare and does not affect the treatment course.

TOSITUMOMAB AND I-131 TOSITUMOMAB (BEXXAR)

Tositumomab is a murine IgG2a λ monoclonal antibody that binds to human CD20 antigen on normal and malignant B cells (see rituximab above). I-131 tositumomab is the same antibody conjugated to I-131, a beta- and gamma-emitting isotope. The physical half-life of the isotope is 8 days. I-131 tositumomab is targeted to CD20 and it kills cells to which it binds and also kills neighboring cells in the vicinity of the cell to which it binds by delivering radiation.

The use of tositumomab and I-131 tositumomab is divided into two stages; the first step is for dosimetry, the second for therapy. Each step involves the sequential administration of tositumomab followed by I-131 tositumomab. The first injection of unconjugated anti-CD20 antibody was demonstrated to saturate the spleen and improve the tumor specificity of the subsequently delivered radiopharmaceutical. In the dosimetry phase, 450 mg of tositumomab is given intravenously over 1 h on day 0. Then a dose of I-131 tositumomab containing 5 mCi of I-131 and 35 mg of tositumomab is infused over 20 min. Dosimetry (by external counting of I-131 radioactivity) and biodistribution measurements are then made within 1 h of infusion, on days 2, 3, or 4 and again on days 6 or 7. Certain criteria are then applied to the biodistribution calculation, and if the biodistribution is acceptable, a therapeutic dose of I-131 tositumomab is calculated. Then sometime between day 7 and day 14, the therapeutic step is begun with an infusion of 450 mg tositumomab over 1 h followed by the calculated dose of I-131 tositumomab to deliver 75 cGy of total body radiation. The dosimetry and therapeutic steps together are a course of therapy and patients do not ever receive more than one course.

The activity of labeled and unlabeled tositumomab was defined mainly in patients with follicular lymphoma. Overall response rates in patients with relapsed follicular lymphoma were 63–68% with 29–33% of the responses defined as complete. Median response duration is about 12–18 months. Some complete remissions appear to be durable.

The main toxicity of unlabeled plus labeled tositumomab is myelosuppression which can be severe. Platelets decrease to less than $50,000/\mu l$ in 53% of patients. Neutrophil counts fall below $1,000/\mu l$ in 63% of patients. Hemoglobin levels fall below 8 gm/dl in 29% of patients. The myelotoxicity is particularly common in the setting of significant marrow involvement with lymphoma; thus, this regimen is not indicated if tumor occupies 25% of more of the marrow space. Febrile neutropenia and other infections were noted in 45% of treated patients. In addition, although patients are pretreated with 3 doses of supersaturated potassium iodide solution, the uptake of radioactive iodine by the thyroid can produce hypothyroidism early on and increase the risk of thyroid cancer years later. The risk of hypothyroidism is about 15% at 4 years. Second malignancies are a problem with this therapy. About 10% of patients develop secondary acute leukemia or myelodysplastic syndrome by 4 years after treatment. In addition, skin, breast, lung, and head and neck cancers may be increased. Other grade 3–4 toxicities are rare. Normal B cells are depleted but this does not lead to hypogammaglobulinemia. About 10% of patients develop human antimurine antibodies, but this is of minor consequence in this group of patients who are unlikely to be exposed to other murine antibodies.

IBRITUMOMAB TIUXETAN (ZEVALIN)

Ibritumomab tiuxetan is a murine IgG1 κ antibody chelated to yttrium-90, a beta-emitting isotope. Ibritumomab binds to human CD20 with an affinity of about 14–18 nM. Tiuxetan is the chelating agent that attaches yttrium-90 to exposed amino groups in lysines and arginines in the antibody sequence. Ibritumomab tiuxetan is used as a salvage regimen for the treatment of CD20-expressing B-cell malignancies.

Like I-131 tositumomab, the ibritumomab tiuxetan therapeutic regimen consists of two steps: dosimetry followed by therapy. Dosimetry is performed by injecting unlabeled rituximab (250 mg/m^2) followed by 5 mCi of indium-111-labeled ibritumomab tiuxetan (containing 1.6 mg of antibody) over 10 min to assess biodistribution of the label. If the biodistribution shows too much lung, renal, or bowel uptake, the therapeutic dose is not given. However, if the biodistribution of the In-111 compound is acceptable, 7–9 days after dosimetry dose, the patient receives a therapeutic dose of 250 mg/m^2 rituximab followed by 0.4 mCi/kg of ibrituximab tiuxetin labeled with Y-90 over 10 min. The physical half-life of the isotope is just under 3 days and the mean half-life of Y-90 activity in the blood iss 30 h.

The efficacy of ibritumomab tiuxetan appears similar to that of I-131 tositumomab.

Patients who have impaired bone marrow reserve (prior hematopoietic stem cell transplantation, radiation to more than 25% of marrow, current low platelet or neutrophil counts) have been treated with ibritumomab tiuxetan at a lower specific activity (0.3 miCi/kg) with response rates of 67% and median response durations of 12 months.

The most common toxicity of ibritumomab tiuxetan therapy is myelosuppression. In initial studies, platelet counts less than 50,000/µl were noted in 61% of patients and neutrophil counts less than 1000/µl were seen in 57% of patients. The risk of severe thrombocytopenia and neutropenia increased to 75% in patients whose platelet counts were between 100K and 150K at the start of treatment. Median time to nadir is 7–9 weeks and median duration of cytopenias is 3–5 weeks. The duration of the myelosuppression complicates subsequent therapeutic decisions. As would be expected, myeloid malignancies and myelodysplasias have been noted in patients surviving more than a year. Gastrointestinal symptoms (nausea, vomiting, abdominal pain, diarrhea) occur in 10% of patients. Human antimouse antibodies or human antichimeric protein antibodies develop in about 4% of cases. Normal Bcells are eliminated but recover after 12–16 weeks. Hypogammaglobulinemia is not a clinically significant sequela. A general problem with the radiopharmaceuticals (both I-131 and Y-90) is the long-term compromise of marrow function. Patients who receive these therapies are not easily treated with subsequent courses of myelotoxic drugs because of the long-term loss of physiologic reserve in the hematopoietic system.

REFERENCES

1. Rastetter W, Molina A, White CA. Rituximab: expanding role in therapy for lymphomas and autoimmune diseases. Annu Rev Med. 2004; 55: 477–503.
2. Ravandi F, O'Brien S. Alemtuzumab. Expert Rev Anticancer Ther. 2005; 5: 39–51.
3. Gordon MS, Cunningham D. Managing patients treated with bevacizumab combination therapy. Oncology. 2005; 69(suppl 3): 25–33.
4. Plosker GL, Keam SJ. Trastuzumab: a review of its use in the management of HER2-positive metastatic and early-stage breast cancer. Drugs. 2006; 66: 449–475.
5. Chong G, Cunningham D. The role of cetuximab in the therapy of previously treated advanced colorectal cancer. Semin Oncol. 2006; 32(suppl 9): S55–S58.
6. Saif MW, Cohenuram M. Role of panitumumab in the management of metastatic colorectal cancer. Clin Colorectal Cancer. 2006; 6: 118–124.
7. Fenton C, Perry CM. Gemtuzumab ozogomicin: a review of its use in acute myeloid leukaemia. Drugs. 2005; 65: 2405–2427.
8. Friedberg JW, Fisher RI. Iodine-131 tositumomab (Bexxar): radioimmunoconjugate therapy for indolent and transformed B-cell non-Hodgkin's lymphoma. Expert Rev Anticancer Ther. 2004; 4: 18–26.
9. Gordon LI: Practical considerations and radiation safety in radioimmunotherapy with yttrium-90 ibritumomab tiuxetan (Zevalin). Semin Oncol. 2003; 30(suppl 17): 23–28.

Matthew R. Smith

BISPHOSPHONATES

INTRODUCTION

Bisphosphonates are potent inhibitors of osteoclast-mediated bone resorption. Bisphosphonates are used to treat benign diseases associated with excessive bone resorption, including osteoporosis and Paget's disease. Bisphosphonates are also an important part of the management for many cancer patients. Bisphosphonates are the treatment of choice for hypercalcemia of malignancy. They decrease the risk of skeletal complications for patients with multiple myeloma and patients with bone metastases from breast cancer, prostate cancer, and other solid tumors. In addition, bisphosphonates may prevent development of bone metastases in women with high-risk primary breast cancer.

Pamidronate disodium (Aredia®) and zoledronic acid (Zometa®) are marketed for metastatic bone disease in the United States (Table 17-1). Clodronate (Ostac®) and ibandronate (Bondronat®) are marketed for oncology in other countries but not in the United States.

Table 17-1

Bisphosphonates for Metastatic Bone Disease in the United States

Generic name	Trade name	Dose and schedule	Approved indications in oncology
Pamidronate disodium	Aredia®	90 mg IV (over 2–4 h) every 3–4 weeks	• Hypercalcemia • Multiple myeloma • Metastatic breast cancer
Zoledronic acid	Zometa®	4 mg IV (over 15 min) every 3–4 weeks	• Hypercalcemia • Multiple myeloma • Any solid tumor with bone metastases

PHARMACOLOGY

Bisphosphonates are synthetic analogs of pyrophosphate characterized by a phosphorus–carbon–phosphorus backbone that renders them resistant to hydrolysis (Figure 17-1). The R_1 and R_2 carbon side chains determine their pharmacology. Most bisphosphonates contain a hydroxyl group at the R_1 position that confers high-affinity binding to calcium phosphate. The R_2 side chain determines antiresorptive potency. Bisphosphonates with a primary amino group at R_2 (pamidronate and alendronate) are approximately 100-fold more potent than

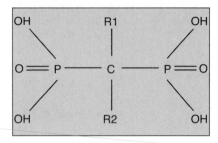

FIGURE 17-1 General structure of bisphosphonates.

etidronate, a first-generation bisphosphonate. Bisphosphonates with a secondary or tertiary amino group at R_2 (ibandronate, risedronate, and zoledronic acid) are among the most potent bisphosphonates, with approximately 10,000-fold greater in vitro potency than etidronate.

Bisphosphonates are adsorbed to calcium phosphate (hydroxyapatite) crystals in bone. Approximately one-half of an intravenously administered dose accumulates in the skeleton. Bisphosphonates preferentially bind to sites of active bone remodeling. Bisphosphonates become biologically inactive after they are incorporated into quiescent bone, and repetitive administration appears to be required to maintain inhibition of bone resorption.

Bisphosphonates are not metabolized. They are eliminated by renal excretion. Bisphosphonates are poorly absorbed. Bioavailability is less than 1% after oral administration. Bisphosphonates bind calcium and calcium-containing foods, beverages, and medications alter drug absorption. Oral administration may be associated with gastrointestinal toxicity.

Bisphosphonates inhibit osteoclast-mediated bone resorption by several mechanisms. Etidronate and clodronate are metabolized to cytotoxic analogs of adenosine triphosphate. More potent nitrogen-containing bisphosphonates (risedronate, pamidronate, zoledronic acid) inhibit farnesyl diphosphate synthase, a key enzyme in the mevalonate pathway, and decrease prenylation of essential GTP-binding proteins.

The most common adverse event for intravenous bisphosphonates is an acute phase reaction, a transient flu-like syndrome of fever, arthralgias, and myalgias starting within 24 h after treatment. Hypocalcemia is also common, but is rarely associated with symptoms. Supplemental calcium (500–1,000 mg daily) and vitamin D (400 IU daily) should be prescribed to reduce the risk of symptomatic hypocalcemia. Parenteral vitamin D should be considered for patients with known vitamin D deficiency or in the rare case of refractory hypocalcemia.

Bisphosphonates have potential renal toxicity related to total drug dose and rate of intravenous administration. Treatment is not recommended for patients with creatinine clearance less than 30 ml/min. Dose reductions are recommended for patients with estimated creatinine clearance between 30 and 60 mL/min. Serum creatinine should be monitored before each treatment.

Zoledronic acid and other bisphosphonates are also associated with increased risk of osteonecrosis of the jaw. Most but not all patients who develop osteonecrosis of the jaw have preexisting dental problems. Excellent oral hygiene, baseline dental evaluation for high-risk individuals, and avoidance of invasive dental surgery during therapy are recommended to reduce risk of this condition.

CLINICAL USES IN ONCOLOGY

Hypercalcemia

Hypercalcemia of malignancy results primarily from increased release of calcium from bone. In the presence of bone metastases, calcium is released from the skeleton by local osteoclast-mediated bone destruction. Hypercalcemia of malignancy may also result from tumor secretion of parathyroid hormone related protein (PTHrP). PTHrP causes hypercalcemia by osteoclast activation and decreased renal calcium excretion. Many malignancies produce PTHrP, including breast cancer, squamous cell carcinoma, renal cell carcinoma, multiple myeloma, and some types of lymphoma. In addition, 1,25-dihydroxyvitamin D lymphoma syndrome and ectopic hyperpararthyroidism are rare causes of hypercalcemia of malignancy.

Intravenous bisphosphonates are by far the most effective agents for patients with hypercalcemia of malignancy (1). In the United States, pamidronate and zoledronic acid are the agents of choice for treatment of mild to severe hypercalcemia of malignancy in the United States. Most patients have normal serum calcium levels within several days after treatment, and responses last for 1–4 weeks. In randomized controlled trials, intravenous zoledronic acid and ibandronate achieve higher rates and duration of normocalcemia than pamidronate, although these differences are relatively small.

Prevention of Skeletal Complications

Skeletal complications are a major cause of morbidity for patients with bone metastases. Bone metastases are associated with pain, fractures, spinal cord or nerve root compression, and hypercalcemia.

Bone metastases are often described as osteoblastic or osteolytic based on their radiographic appearance. Osteoblastic and osteolytic bone lesions represent two extremes of a spectrum, however, and osteoclast number and activity are increased in most bone metastases including typical osteoblastic metastases from prostate cancer (2). Pathological activation of osteoclasts appears to play a central role in most disease-related skeletal complications.

Bisphosphonates decrease risk of skeletal complications across all tumor types. Pamidronate and zoledronic acid, for example, decrease the incidence of skeletal complications in patients with multiple myeloma or breast cancer with bone metastases (3, 4). Zoledronic acid also decreases the risk of skeletal complications in patients with bone metastases from prostate cancer, lung cancer, and other solid tumors (5, 6). While bisphosphonates have a well-established role in supportive care of patients of patients with bone metastases, considerable uncertainty remains about the optimal timing, schedule, and duration of bisphosphonates for prevention of skeletal complications.

Prevention of Bone Metastases

The establishment of bone metastases involves reciprocal interactions between tumor cells and metabolically active bone (7). Development and progression of bone metastases involve tumor cell adhesion to bone, invasion, new blood vessel formation, and proliferation. Preclinical studies suggest that bisphosphonates inhibit each of these steps.

Three randomized controlled trials have evaluated the effect of clodronate on development of bone metastases on women with high-risk primary breast cancer (8). In two of the three studies, clodronate significantly reduced the incidence of new bone metastases. Additional studies are ongoing to evaluate the role of bisphosphonates as adjuvant therapy for breast cancer and other malignancies.

REFERENCES

1. Stewart AF. Clinical practice. Hypercalcemia associated with cancer. N Engl J Med. 2005; 352(4): 373–379.
2. Roodman GD. Mechanisms of bone metastasis. N Engl J Med. 2004; 350(16): 1655–1664.
3. Berenson JR, Hillner BE, Kyle RA, et al. American Society of Clinical Oncology clinical practice guidelines: the role of bisphosphonates in multiple myeloma. J Clin Oncol. 2002; 20(17): 3719–3736.
4. Hillner BE, Ingle JN, Chlebowski RT, et al. American Society of Clinical Oncology 2003 update on the role of bisphosphonates and bone health issues in women with breast cancer. J Clin Oncol. 2003; 21(21): 4042–4057.
5. Saad F, Gleason DM, Murray R, et al. A randomized, placebo-controlled trial of zoledronic acid in patients with hormone-refractory metastatic prostate carcinoma. J Natl Cancer Inst. 2002; 94(19): 1458–1468.
6. Rosen LS, Gordon D, Tchekmedyian S, et al. Zoledronic acid versus placebo in the treatment of skeletal metastases in patients with lung cancer and other solid tumors: a phase III, double-blind, randomized trial–the Zoledronic Acid Lung Cancer and Other Solid Tumors Study Group. J Clin Oncol. 2003; 21(16): 3150–3157.
7. Mundy GR. Metastasis to bone: causes, consequences and therapeutic opportunities. Nat Rev Cancer. 2002; 2(8): 584–593.
8. Dando TM, Wiseman LR. Clodronate : a review of its use in the prevention of bone metastases and the management of skeletal complications associated with bone metastases in patients with breast cancer. Drugs Aging. 2004; 21(14): 949–962.

FEBRILE NEUTROPENIA

INTRODUCTION

Immune-compromised state refers to a change of the host defense systems which confer an increased susceptibility to infection. Neutropenia remains the major defect of the defense systems predisposing to severe infections. Fever in a neutropenic patient should be considered a medical emergency as it has been demonstrated that a delay in specific therapy is associated with up to a 70% mortality (1). In this chapter, we present the medical approach to fever in neutropenic patients by analyzing the predisposing factors, pathogenesis, diagnosis, and treatment.

DEFINITION

Fever in a neutropenic patient is usually defined as a single temperature of >38.3°C (101.3°F), or a sustained temperature >38°C (100.4°F) for more than 1 h. It has to be considered that neutropenic patients may experience clinical deterioration in the absence of fever and that concomitant steroid treatment may also conceal a fever.

Among neutropenic patients, two factors are associated with the increased risk of infection:

- Neutrophil count. The risk increases when the neutrophil count is below $1 \times 10^9/l$. The risk of infection increases further in patients with neutrophil counts of less than $0.1 \times 10^9/l$ neutrophils.
- Duration of neutropenia. A low-neutrophil count and a protracted neutropenia ($0.5 \times 10^9/l$ for 10 days) are major risk factors for infection. A duration of neutropenia of more that 5 weeks is associated with an incidence of infection close to 100%.

Despite this, neutropenic patients remain a heterogeneous population that needs additional parameters that help to define the real risk of infection and tailor a more specific approach for each patient in this category. The risk factors for infection associated with neutropenia include advanced age, poor performance or nutritional status, low baseline and first-cycle nadir blood cell counts, and high-dose chemotherapy. Significant predictors for death, bacteremia, and length of hospital stay include advanced age, hematologic malignancies, disease burden, high fever, and low blood pressure on admission, pneumonia, and single or multiorgan dysfunction.

PATHOGENESIS

A number of predisposing factors other than neutropenia play a role in increasing the risk of infections in neutropenic patients with fever:

- Chemotherapy
- Intravenous or implanted devices
- Hypogammaglobulinemia (i.e., chronic lymphocytic leukemia, multiple myeloma, splenectomy)
- Defects in cell mediated immunity (ALL, NHL, HD, therapy with fludarabine)

- Glucocorticoid therapy
- Disruption of normal anatomic structures.

Chemotherapy not only affects the number of neutrophils, but also impairs chemotaxis and phagocytosis. Either chemotherapy or radiotherapy-associated mucositis may affect the normal mucosal barrier, predisposing to bacteremia.

The existence of an impairment in neutrophil function preceding chemotherapy as in patients with myelodysplastic syndromes or in the presence of bone marrow failure due to tumor cell invasion predisposes to severe infection or death after chemotherapy.

Indwelling catheters and implanted devices pose a significant risk as they can allow access of skin flora directly into blood or subcutaneous tissues or represent a foreign body which bacteria can successfully colonize and infect. Immune defects associated with specific primary cancers may further impair the defense system as in hypogammaglobulinemia associated with CLL or multiple myeloma. Splenectomy predisposes to infection with encapsulated organisms such as pneumococcus or meningococcus.

An increased risk of infection has been observed in patients with Hodgkin's disease as the result of a defect in cell mediated immunity. Patients with ALL, central nervous system tumors, and patients treated with glucocorticoids are also at increased risk of infections.

ETIOLOGY OF INFECTIONS IN FEBRILE NEUTROPENIA ASSOCIATED PATHOGENS

Bacteria

About 65% of neutropenic patients with fever have infection (Table 18-1). In this group of patients, aerobic gram-negative bacilli represented the most frequent isolates. In the past *Pseudomonas aeruginosa* was the most frequent isolate responsible for septic shock and severe pneumonia, and empirical therapy regimens were designed to include antipseudomonal antibiotics. Over the past 20 years, gram-positive bacteria have become the most frequent pathogens isolated from patients with febrile neutropenia. More aggressive chemotherapeutic regimens, widespread use of indwelling catheters, and antibiotic prophylaxis have contributed to the trend toward gram-positive infections.

Fungi

It has been demonstrated that up to 20% of patients with neutropenia may experience an invasive mycosis and this risk is further increased in patients with hematologic malignancies (2) (Table 18-1).

Risk factors for fungal superinfection include:

- greater than 7 days of profound neutropenia
- use of quinolones as antibacterial prophylaxis
- presence of a central venous catheter
- persistence of fever after 3 days of antibiotic therapy (3).

Superficial and invasive candidiasis and invasive aspergillosis represent the most common infections. *Candida albicans* represents the most common fungal isolate in neutropenic patients followed by *C. tropicalis, C. glabrata, and C. parapsilosis.* The use of fluconazole as prophylactic therapy has been associated with an increased frequency of *C. krusei.*

Invasive aspergillosis may be due to *Aspergillus fumigatus, A. terreus, A. flavus, and A. niger.* Invasive aspergillosis is associated with a mortality rate approaching 80% in bone marrow transplantation patients with febrile neutropenia (4). The two most common sites of invasive disease are the lungs and

Table 18-1

Organisms Causing Infection in Neutropenic Patients

Specific sites of infection	Agents
Bacteremia	Gram-positive bacteria - Coagulase negative Staph - Streptococci Gram-negative bacteria - Escherichia coli - Enterobacter - Klebsiella - Pseudomonas aeruginosa
Skin and soft tissues	Localized infections - S. aureus, S. pyogenes More extensive involvement - Varicella zoster - Herpes simplex - Candida, Malassezia Opportunistic pathogens - Atypical mycobacteria - Aspergillus Noncutaneous source - P. aeruginosa - S. aureus - Aeromonas hydrophila - Vibrio spp. - C. septicum - Klebsiella pneumoniae - Histoplasma capsulatum - C. immitis

Lungs	Bacteria
	   Pneumococcus, Pseudomonas,
	   Enterobacteriacee, Legionella
	Fungi
	   Candida, Aspergillus, Fusarium sp
	Viruses
	   Influenza, parainfluenza, RSV,
	   CMV, HSV
	Protozoa
	   Pneumocystis carinii, Toxoplasma,
	   Cryptococcus, Strongyloides

Indwelling catheters	Bacteria
	   Coagulase-neg. Staph, S. aureus
	   Gram-neg. bacilli
	Fungi
	   Candida

Gastrointestinal tract	Upper tract
	   HSV, candida
	Lower tract
	   C. difficile, C. septicum,
	   P.aeruginosa, enteric gram-neg.,
	   anaerobes, E.coli,

Sinuses	Gram-pos., Aspergillus

the sinuses. Prolonged fever and nodular pulmonary infiltrates resistant to antibiotic therapy often represent the only clues to the diagnosis of invasive aspergillosis. A finding of nodular lesions surrounded by a low-attenuation area ("halo sign") may be evident at a chest CT scan. Isolation from culture or histological detection of *Aspergillus* establishes the definitive diagnosis.

Fusariosis, Trichosporon beigelii, Blastoschizomyces capitatus, Saccharomyces cerevisiae, and *Malassenzia furfur* represent other emerging fungi.

EVALUATION

The initial evaluation of a febrile and neutropenic patient should include a detailed history and physical examination. Symptoms and signs of inflammation may be minimal or even absent in patients with severe neutropenia. A thorough physical examination should be performed, with particular attention to the skin, mucus membranes, sinuses, oropharynx, lung, abdomen, perirectal area, surgical sites, and intravenous lines. In the neutropenic patient, the response to bacterial infection may be misleading, with only minimal erythema and rash, and often without signs associated with cellulitis or abscess formation. All indwelling catheters should be carefully inspected. Lines should also be assessed for any malfunction as poor flow may be a sign of an infected clot.

The examination should include inspection of the perianal area. A digital rectal examination (and rectal temperatures) should generally be avoided. Stool softeners should also be given to patients to avoid hard stools or impaction. Patients should be reassessed daily as new sites of infection can become apparent even 72 h after the initial therapy. In addition, as the neutrophil count rebounds, symptoms and signs of an infection may become evident.

LABORATORY STUDIES

A basic evaluation should include a complete blood cell count with differential measurement of serum levels of creatinine, urea nitrogen, SGOT, SGPT, bilirubin, and electrolytes. Specimens should be obtained immediately for the microbiology laboratory, including two or more blood cultures from the device lumen and from a peripheral vein. Blood cultures should be repeated for persistent fevers.

A sample of sputum may be included in the microbiologic evaluation if the patient can produce it. Culture of urine samples is indicated if signs of symptoms of urinary tract infection do exist, in the presence of urinary catheter or if urinalysis is abnormal.

Lumbar puncture is not recommended as a routine procedure but should be considered if symptoms suggest a CNS infection.

Chest radiographs should be performed even in the absence of pulmonary infection. Of note is the fact that high-resolution CT scan can be considered in the evaluation of febrile patients as it has been found that the procedure can reveal pneumonia even in the presence of a normal chest radiography.

If localizing signs or symptoms are present, other tests should be considered such as skin aspiration or biopsy for culture, stool for culture, and imaging of the CNS, sinuses, and abdomen.

TREATMENT

Treatment options for patients with febrile neutropenia include antimicrobial agents and Granulocyte-Colony Stimulating Factor (G-CSF). Antibiotics are usually administered empirically, but should always include appropriate coverage for suspected or known infections (Figure 18-1).

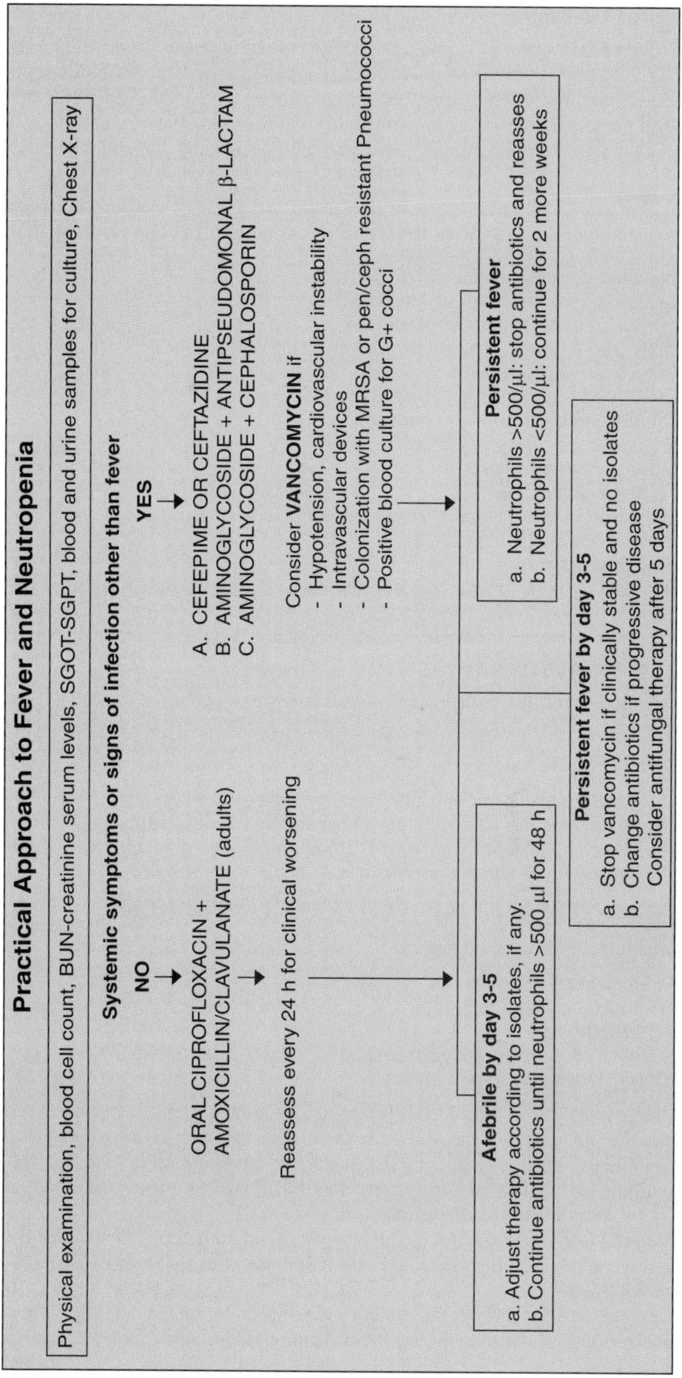

Practical Approach to Fever and Neutropenia

Physical examination, blood cell count, BUN-creatinine serum levels, SGOT-SGPT, blood and urine samples for culture, Chest X-ray

Systemic symptoms or signs of infection other than fever

NO

ORAL CIPROFLOXACIN +
AMOXICILLIN/CLAVULANATE (adults)

Reassess every 24 h for clinical worsening

YES

A. CEFEPIME OR CEFTAZIDINE
B. AMINOGLYCOSIDE + ANTIPSEUDOMONAL β-LACTAM
C. AMINOGLYCOSIDE + CEPHALOSPORIN

Consider **VANCOMYCIN** if
- Hypotension, cardiovascular instability
- Intravascular devices
- Colonization with MRSA or pen/ceph resistant Pneumococci
- Positive blood culture for G+ cocci

Afebrile by day 3-5

a. Adjust therapy according to isolates, if any.
b. Continue antibiotics until neutrophils >500 μl for 48 h

Persistent fever by day 3-5

a. Stop vancomycin if clinically stable and no isolates
b. Change antibiotics if progressive disease
   Consider antifungal therapy after 5 days

Persistent fever

a. Neutrophils >500/μl: stop antibiotics and reasses
b. Neutrophils <500/μl: continue for 2 more weeks

FIGURE 18-1 Practical approach to fever and neutropenia.

Empirical Therapy

Initial management requires evaluation of the patient to define low or high risk of severe infections (Table 18-2). In high-risk patients, several antibiotic regimens have been proposed as initial empirical therapy in febrile neutropenia but none has demonstrated a clear superiority(5). All regimens have been designed to provide coverage against gram-negative bacilli, especially *P. aeruginosa*.

Table 18-2

Criteria Favoring a Low Risk Profile of Patients with Febrile Neutropenia

- Absolute neutrophil count of $\geq 0.1 \times 10^9/1$
- Absolute monocyte count of $\geq 0.1 \times 10^9/1$
- Normal findings on a chest radiograph
- Nearly normal results of hepatic and renal function tests
- Duration of neutropenia of <7 days
- Resolution of neutropenia expected in <10 days
- No intravenous catheter-site infection
- Early evidence of bone marrow recovery
- Malignancy in remission
- Peak temperature of <39°C
- No neurological or mental changes
- No appearance of illness
- No abdominal pain
- No shock, hypoxia, pneumonia or other deep-organ infection, vomiting, or diarrhea

SINGLE-DRUG THERAPY

- Extended-spectrum cephalosporins: ceftazidime or cefepime
- Carbapenem: imipenem or meropenem

TWO-DRUG THERAPY

- Antipseudomonal penicillin plus an aminoglycoside: piperacillin or ticarcillin or mezlocillin plus gentamycin or tobramycin or amikacin.
- Antipseudomonal penicillin plus a fluoroquinolone: piperacillin or ticarcillin or mezlocillin plus ciprofloxacin.

TWO-DRUG THERAPY (ABOVE) PLUS GLYCOPEPTIDES

- Vancomycin, in selected patients:
  - Catheter related infections
  - Colonization with penicillin and cephalosporin-resistant pneumococci or MRSA
  - Growth of gram-positive cocci pending final identification
  - Hemodynamic instability.

A large number of clinical trials performed over the past 30 years have failed to prove the superiority of one antibiotic regimen over others in the management of febrile neutropenia. A patient's risk factors and history, clinical evaluation, the hypothetical source of infection, and the local frequency of specific pathogens should drive the decision.

The antibiotic regimen should still provide broad empirical coverage for the possibility of other pathogens unlike the treatment strategy in most immunocompetent hosts.

Aminoglycosides such as gentamicin and antipseudomonal penicillins represented the conventional therapy for neutropenic patients prior to the advent of fluoroquinolones and third generation cephalosporin. The advantages of dual therapy over single-drug treatment include synergy against aerobic gram-negative bacilli and reduced risk of resistant strain selection. Nephrotoxicity and ototoxicity associated with aminoglycoside therapy represent the major concern. Toxicity can be minimized by careful monitoring of serum levels and by administering aminoglycoside once a day.

Quinolone-based combinations with beta-lactams represent an option for empirical therapy in patients not treated prophylactically with quinolones (5). The next stage corresponds to the development of third- and fourth-generation cephalosporins. In particular, antipseudomonal cephalosporins including ceftazidime and cefepime have potent activity against aerobic gram-negative bacilli including *P. aeruginosa*, and have activity against gram-positive cocci. The effectiveness of ceftazidime led to the introduction a modified monotherapy in which an aminoglycoside was given for the first 72 h and then discontinued if cultures were negative for aerobic gram-negative bacilli (6).

Monotherapy with a carbamenem is particularly effective in febrile neutropenia of unknown origin in patients who had received prophylactic antibiotics (7, 8). In subgroup analyses, meropenem also appeared to be superior to ceftazidime in patients with severe neutropenia (ANC 100 cells/µl) and in bone marrow transplant recipients (7).

One concern about monotherapy is the possibility that an alarming increase in the frequency of antibiotic resistant pathogens would be predicted to occur and may eventually reduce the efficacy of this strategy (8).

Vancomycin in Empirical Therapy

There is no clear evidence that addition of vancomycin to empirical therapy affects morbidity or mortality. Addition of vancomycin should be considered in patients suffering from hypotension, mucositis, skin or catheter site infection, or have a history of MRSA colonization, or have recent quinolone prophylaxis (Figure 18-1) (9, 10). When vancomycin is added to empirical therapy at the initiation of treatment, subsequent discontinuation of the antibiotic should be considered in the presence of negative blood cultures. The risk of acquiring VRE is cited as another reason for avoiding empirical vancomycin use.

Therapy in Low-Risk Patients with Neutropenia

Prospective studies have identified patients with fever and neutropenia at low risk for medical complications. These patients have solid tumors, no underlying immunocompromise, and an expected short duration of neutropenia of 5 days or less: in these patients it appears safe to use an oral rather than parenteral therapy (11) (Table 18-2). Comparison of the oral regimen consisting of ciprofloxacin and amoxicillin-clavulanate against intravenous ceftriaxone plus amikacin demonstrated equal efficacy in patients with microbiologically documented infections (12). Oral antibiotic therapy requires very accurate selection of neutropenic patients with a low-risk profile.

Empirical Antifungal Therapy in Febrile Neutropenia

In view of the finding that up to one-third of patients with fever and neutropenia persisting for more than 7 days develop systemic *Candidal or Aspergillus* infection, empirical treatment with an antifungal drug can be considered, in particular when neutropenia is not expected to resolve within a few days. Diagnostic steps, including fungal isolator blood cultures and chest CT, should precede the commencement of antifungal therapy.

Antifungal therapeutic options include amphotericin B, lipid formulations of amphotericin B, fluconazole, itraconazole, voriconazole, and caspofungin. Amphotericin B has been the standard of antifungal therapy in febrile neutropenia.

When used as lipid formulation, amphotericin causes a lesser incidence of infusion-related fever, chills or rigors, and nephrotoxicity (13). Among azoles, fluconazole has limited activity against *Aspergillus* species and some nonalbicans *Candida* species, and it is generally not recommended for empirical therapy. Intravenous followed by oral itraconazole was found to be as effective as amphotericin B in febrile neutropenic patients (14). Itraconazole should not be used in patients with an estimated creatinine clearance below 30 ml/min and this azole should not be administered for more than 14 days.

Results of three clinical trials assessing the activity of voriconazole, a new azole and capsofungin, and a new echinocandin, have demonstrated their efficacy in the treatment of invasive fungal infections. In one study, voriconazole was superior to liposomal amphotericin B only with respect to documented breakthrough fungal infections, infusion-related toxicity, and nephrotoxicity (15). In another trial, the efficacy of caspofungin in the prevention of breakthrough infections and resolution of fever was superior to liposomal amphotericin B (16). Caspofungin also cured more documented baseline fungal infections than did liposomal amphotericin B. Considering the available evidence, voriconazole and caspofungin both appear to be suitable, and perhaps preferable, alternatives to conventional liposomal amphotericin B as empirical antifungal therapy in patients with persistent fever and neutropenia.

Hematopoietic Growth Factor (HGF)

Both the Infectious Diseases Society of America and the American Society of Clinical Oncology do not support the routine use of growth factors in febrile neutropenic patients. G-CSF has been reported to decrease the duration of neutropenia, fever, and hospitalization but without significant impact on mortality (17). Therapy with G-CSF may be considered to be appropriate in critically ill patients with prolonged neutropenia.

Antibacterial and Antifungal Prophylaxis

There is no consensus to recommend antimicrobial prophylaxis for all afebrile neutropenic patients. A prophylactic strategy should diminish the attack rate and delay the time to the onset of an infectious complication, but it does not eliminate the risk of infection. The goal would be to provide protection during the period of neutropenia and mucositis. In general, the use of prophylactic antibiotic therapy is not recommended for cancer patients undergoing chemotherapy. Trimethoprim-sulfamethoxazole (TMP-SMZ) or quinolones can be considered in patients with hematologic cancer, since they are at higher risk compared to neutropenic patients with solid tumors. Vigorous infection-control practices and careful monitoring for the emergence of resistant organisms should accompany any prophylactic program.

REFERENCES

1. Rubin RH, Ferraro MJ. Understanding and diagnosing infectious complications in the immunocompromised host. Current issues and trends. Hematol Oncol Clin North Am. 1993; 7(4): 795–812.
2. Bodey G, Bueltmann B, Duguid W, et al. Fungal infections in cancer patients: an international autopsy survey. Eur J Clin Microbiol Infect Dis. 1992; 11(2): 99–109.
3. Nucci M, Colombo AL, Spector N, Velasco E, Martins CA, Pulcheri W. Breakthrough candidemia in neutropenic patients. Clin Infect Dis. 1997; 24(2): 275–276.
4. Marr KA, Patterson T, Denning D. Aspergillosis. Pathogenesis, clinical manifestations, and therapy. Infect Dis Clin North Am. 2002; 16(4): 875–894, vi.

5. Bliziotis IA, Michalopoulos A, Kasiakou SK, et al. Ciprofloxacin vs an amino-glycoside in combination with a beta–lactam for the treatment of febrile neutropenia: a meta–analysis of randomized controlled trials. Mayo Clin Proc. 2005; 80(9): 1146–1156.

6. Donowitz GR, Maki DG, Crnich CJ, Pappas PG, Rolston KV. Infections in the neutropenic patient—new views of an old problem. Hematology (Am Soc Hematol Educ Program). 2001: 113–139.

7. Freifeld AG, Walsh T, Marshall D, et al. Monotherapy for fever and neutropenia in cancer patients: a randomized comparison of ceftazidime versus imipenem. J Clin Oncol. 1995; 13(1): 165–176.

8. Raad, II, Escalante C, Hachem RY, et al. Treatment of febrile neutropenic patients with cancer who require hospitalization: a prospective randomized study comparing imipenem and cefepime. Cancer. 2003; 98(5): 1039–1047.

9. Paul M, Borok S, Fraser A, Vidal L, Leibovici L. Empirical antibiotics against Gram-positive infections for febrile neutropenia: systematic review and meta-analysis of randomized controlled trials. J Antimicrob Chemother. 2005; 55(4): 436–444.

10. Vardakas KZ, Samonis G, Chrysanthopoulou SA, Bliziotis IA, Falagas ME. Role of glycopeptides as part of initial empirical treatment of febrile neutropenic patients: a meta-analysis of randomised controlled trials. Lancet Infect Dis. 2005; 5(7): 431–439.

11. Koh A, Pizzo PA. Empirical oral antibiotic therapy for low risk febrile cancer patients with neutropenia. Cancer Invest. 2002; 20(3): 420–433.

12. Kern WV, Cometta A, De Bock R, Langenaeken J, Paesmans M, Gaya H. Oral versus intravenous empirical antimicrobial therapy for fever in patients with granulocytopenia who are receiving cancer chemotherapy. International Antimicrobial Therapy Cooperative Group of the European Organization for Research and Treatment of Cancer. N Engl J Med. 1999; 341(5): 312–318.

13. Walsh TJ, Finberg RW, Arndt C, et al. Liposomal amphotericin B for empirical therapy in patients with persistent fever and neutropenia. National Institute of Allergy and Infectious Diseases Mycoses Study Group. N Engl J Med. 1999; 340(10): 764–771.

14. Boogaerts M, Winston DJ, Bow EJ, et al. Intravenous and oral itraconazole versus intravenous amphotericin B deoxycholate as empirical antifungal therapy for persistent fever in neutropenic patients with cancer who are receiving broad-spectrum antibacterial therapy. A randomized, controlled trial. Ann Intern Med. 2001; 135(6): 412–422.

15. Walsh TJ, Pappas P, Winston DJ, et al. Voriconazole compared with liposomal amphotericin B for empirical antifungal therapy in patients with neutropenia and persistent fever. N Engl J Med. 2002; 346(4): 225–234.

16. Walsh TJ, Teppler H, Donowitz GR, et al. Caspofungin versus liposomal amphotericin B for empirical antifungal therapy in patients with persistent fever and neutropenia. N Engl J Med. 2004; 351(14): 1391–1402.

17. Hughes WT, Armstrong D, Bodey GP, et al. 2002 guidelines for the use of antimicrobial agents in neutropenic patients with cancer. Clin Infect Dis. 2002; 34(6): 730–751.

19

ANEMIA

INTRODUCTION

Anemia is defined as a decrease in the red blood cell mass circulating in the bloodstream, and derives from an imbalance in the production and loss of erythrocytes. Symptoms and signs associated with anemia result from impaired oxygen delivery to the tissues. Common symptoms include fatigue, malaise, weakness, dyspnea on exertion, and chest pressure. Patients may manifest additional overt signs such as pallor, tachycardia, impaired mentation, high-output congestive heart failure, shock, and death. The WHO organization criteria define anemia as being present in women with hemoglobin less than 12 g/dl and men with hemoglobin less than 13 g/dl.

Among patients with cancer, anemia is a prevalent complication of both the disease and its treatment. Nearly 50% of patients have laboratory evidence of anemia at the time of diagnosis with cancer. With hematologic malignancies, anemia is coincident in as many as 70% of patients. Cancer patients at particular increased risk for anemia are those with a low hemoglobin before the diagnosis of cancer, those with lung or gynecologic cancers, and those receiving platinum-based therapy (1). Due to the prevalence of anemia with cytotoxic chemotherapy, grading systems have been established to standardize reporting of myelosuppression in clinical studies and to guide clinical decision-making. The grading system offered by the National Cancer Institute is presented in Table 19-1 (2).

Anemia decreases quality of life in cancer patients (3). The correlation between fatigue and hemoglobin levels is particularly strong, establishing fatigue as a modifiable risk factor for clinical trials of transfusion or erythropoietins (EPOs). A negative impact of anemia on cancer patient survival has been reported, though it is unclear whether anemia is a truly independent risk factor (4). Because anemia in the cancer patient is frequently multifactorial, the appropriate diagnostic evaluation and therapeutic interventions must be individualized to fit the cause, the severity of anemia, and the clinical setting. However, for the majority of patients, the two major available therapeutic tools are packed red blood cell transfusions and EPO.

Table 19-1

NCI Grading System for Anemia

Grade	Severity	Hemoglobin (g/dl)
0	Normal	12.0–16.0 (women)
		14.0–18.0 (men)
1	Mild	10.0–WNL
2	Moderate	8.0–10.0
3	Severe	6.5–7.9
4	Life threatening	<6.5

WNL: within normal limits.

ERYTHROPOIESIS

Red cell production is a tightly regulated process. In the marrow, hematopoietic stem cells (HSCs) differentiate into committed erythroid progenitors in response to growth factors, cytokines, and stromal cells. The common myeloid progenitor gives rise to a megakaryocyte/erythroid progenitor, and under the influence of EPO, red cells are generated. After nuclear extrusion in the marrow, immature red cells called reticulocytes are released into the circulation. The reticulocytes retain some ribosomes and mRNA that are generally destroyed after the first day in the circulation. The resulting cell is a mature red blood cell. The marrow produces more than a million erythrocytes per second, compensating for the normal 1% daily loss. EPO, a glycoprotein hormone secreted by the kidney (and to a lesser extent by the liver) in response to hypoxia, is primarily responsible for the pace of red cell production provided that the HSC is normal and adequate supplies of iron are available.

Dietary iron is absorbed in the duodenum and proximal jejunum by apical transporters on enterocytes. The recommended daily allowance (RDA) of iron for adults is 18 mg per day. Absorbed iron then passes across the gut basement membrane into the circulation where it binds transferrin and enters the liver, the primary storage site. Particularly relevant in patients with cancer and systemic inflammatory diseases is the production of hepcidin by the liver and other cells, which impairs iron reutilization by increasing duodenal crypt cell and macrophage iron retention and down-regulating iron transporters (5). Elevated hepcidin levels in patients with cancer may impair erythropoiesis. Transferrin receptors on erythrocytic precursors mediate iron uptake. Red cell production, like other processes that require DNA synthesis, also requires adequate vitamin B12 and folate. Dietary folate derives from leafy vegetables and animal products. The RDA of folate for adults is 50 μg per day. Dietary folate, mainly in the form of 5-methyltetrahydrofolate, is absorbed in the jejunum, exhibits significant enterohepatic recirculation, and ultimately enters HSCs by the reduced folate receptor. It is stored in the liver and other tissues as a polyglutamated derivative, and released as needed into the circulation. Dietary cobalamin is derived from animal products. The RDA of cobalamin is 2 μg per day. The first step in cobalamin absorption requires splitting the dietary vitamin from binding proteins in food through the action of acid and pepsin in the stomach. This step is followed by additional proteolysis by pancreatic enzymes, binding of the free cobalamin to intrinsic factor (a glycoprotein secreted by the stomach), and receptor-mediated internalization in the ileum. Medications that impair gastric acid secretion and atrophic gastritis can impair the essential process of splitting vitamin B12 from food binders and interfere with intrinsic factor production.

Under normal circumstances, an erythrocyte circulates for 120 days. Thereafter, red cells are removed from circulation by tissue macrophages of the reticuloendothelial system (RES). Heme-bound iron is recycled and stored as ferritin and hemosiderin in the liver, spleen, and bone marrow. Iron stores may be mobilized by release into the plasma and oxidation by ceruloplasmin. Important additional tissues contribute to red cell homeostasis, such as endothelial and serum control of hemostasis and cardiorenal maintenance of plasma volume.

DIAGNOSTIC EVALUATION

The diagnostic evaluation of anemia aims to identify etiologies upon which treatment can be based. A detailed history provides important insights into the pace of development of anemia, and informs the interpretation of laboratory studies. The evaluation of anemia requires a detailed family history, as well as consideration of the family's ethnic, racial, and geographic origins, which may suggest parasites, sickle cell inheritance or thalassemia, or pernicious anemia as causes of anemia. As patients with cancer are frequently treated with agents that cause oxidative stress, glucose-6-phosphate dehydrogenase deficiency with drug-induced hemolysis may become a relevant diagnostic consideration, particularly in patients of Mediterranean origin.

Laboratory evaluation serves to quantify the degree of anemia and the immediate risk posed by the red cell deficit. The hemoglobin concentration in whole blood is routinely used to define anemia. The physiologic reserve of the patient may play a dominant role in the level of symptoms associated with a particular hemoglobin level. The time frame over which the anemia developed and the presence of concurrent illness all influence the degree of symptoms for a particular level of hemoglobin.

Laboratory evaluation of peripheral blood and, if necessary, bone marrow usually yields the cause of anemia. A careful review of the blood smear may reveal morphologic clues useful in confirming the underlying etiology (see below). A complete blood count with differential is obtained to determine if additional hematopoietic lineages are affected. Measurement of the serum creatinine is used to rule out renal failure as a contributing cause or complication. The red cell indices, such as mean corpuscular volume and mean corpuscular hemoglobin, differentiate microcytic anemia from megaloblastic anemia. Among microcytic anemias, the red cell distribution width (RDW) distinguishes between iron deficiency (wide RDW) and thalassemia (narrow RDW). Iron studies (iron, ferritin, and total iron binding capacity) are useful to differentiate iron-deficiency anemia from the anemia of chronic disease. Examination of the stool for occult blood is essential to rule out chronic gastrointestinal bleeding.

Additional studies may diagnose specific etiologies. Reticulocytosis, elevation of serum lactate dehydrogenase and indirect bilirubin, and depressed serum haptoglobin suggest hemolysis. Serum free hemoglobin or urinary hemosiderin reflect intravascular hemolysis. A positive direct antiglobulin (Coombs) test confirms autoimmune hemolytic anemia. In patients with macrocytic anemia, measurement of red blood cell folate levels and plasma homocysteine indicate the presence of folate deficiency, while serum methylmalonic acid and cobalamin are measured to establish B12 deficiency anemias. Low-serum levels of thyroxine or testosterone may also contribute to anemia. In patients with multilineage cytopenias, refractory anemia or those with malignancies commonly metastatic to bone, a bone marrow aspirate and biopsy and cytogenetics may establish tumor replacement (myelophthisis) or treatment-related myelodysplasia as the cause.

CLASSIFICATION OF ANEMIA IN PATIENTS WITH CANCER

Anemia can be classified as either relative or absolute. Relative anemia occurs with increases in plasma cell volume, such as with volume overload or pregnancy. Absolute anemia reflects a true decrease in the red cell mass. Causes of anemia in the cancer patient may be ascribed to three fundamental processes:

Decreased red cell production (*the dominant factor in anemia in cancer patients*)

- Myelosuppression due to chemotherapy or radiation therapy is the most common etiology of anemia in the cancer patient. Multiagent, dose-intense or dose-dense regimens of nonselective cytotoxins are the most likely causes. Regimens employing cisplatin, taxanes, or alkylating agents are often implicated. Cycles of common regimens lead to progressive anemia, with incomplete recovery between cycles. The anemia is typically normocytic or macrocytic with a low-reticulocyte index.

- Replacement of the normal bone marrow elements by malignancies such as lymphoma, multiple myeloma, or leukemia, and less commonly by solid tumors such as metastatic prostate or breast cancer may lead to anemia. In such patients, progressive, normocytic anemia is accompanied by a low-reticulocyte index. Rarely, in such cases, the peripheral blood smear contains early precursors of both the myeloid and erythroid lineages (a leukoery-throblastic response).

- Abnormal stem cell function or impairment in maturation can cause an anemia of underproduction of red cells, as with aplastic anemia, pure red cell aplasia, myelodysplastic syndrome, or acute leukemia. Myelodysplasia is an infrequent sequel of chronic alkylating agent therapy or combined modality therapy with radiation therapy and chemotherapy. A macrocytic anemia with a low-reticulocyte index may be present. The bone marrow examination typically demonstrates dysplastic, immature myeloid and erythroid forms, and abnormal cytogenetics.

- Due to compromised nutritional status, malabsorption, treatment-related anorexia, and the hypermetabolic demands of the neoplastic process, cancer patients may manifest folate and/or vitamin B-12 deficiency anemia. In the absence of concurrent iron deficiency, both will result in a macrocytic or megaloblastic anemia with depressed reticulocyte index and elevated plasma homocysteine. Functional iron deficiency may result from blood loss or prolonged EPO use, requiring oral or intravenous supplementation.

- Reduced endogenous EPO levels are reported in cancer patients with anemia in the absence of other obvious causes (6). A normocytic anemia with low reticulocytes is seen on the peripheral smear. Renal impairment may contribute to decreased EPO production as a consequence of the malignancy (i.e., multiple myeloma) or therapy (i.e., cisplatin). Serum EPO level may confirm the diagnosis, but is rarely needed to guide the therapeutic intervention.

- Inflammatory cytokines, such as tumor necrosis factor alpha, interleukin-1, interleukin-6, and interferon gamma, may be increased in cancer patients as a consequence of tissue destruction, inflammation, or tumor secretion, and may suppress erythropoiesis.

Increased red cell destruction (rare in cancer patients)

- Autoimmune hemolytic anemia is observed occasionally in B-cell lympho-proliferative disorders, such as chronic lymphocytic leukemia and non-Hodgkin's lymphoma. Fludarabine or allogeneic stem cell transplantation may unveil or exacerbate autoimmune anemias. A Coombs test will usually identify a warm agglutinin; other findings are an elevated LDH and depressed haptoglobin. Brisk hemolysis may result in an elevated indirect bilirubin and critically low hemoglobin. The extent of marrow involvement and timing of myelosuppressive therapy will affect the degree of reticulocytosis. Here, effective treatment should include supportive measures, immunosuppressive therapy (i.e., glucocorticoids, intravenous immunoglobulin, or rituximab), and agents targeting the underlying disease.

- Microangiopathic hemolytic anemia occasionally accompanies gastrointestinal malignancies, immunosuppression with cyclosporine or tacrolimus, or exposure to chemotherapeutic agents such as gemcitabine and mitomycin C. Chronic disseminated intravascular coagulopathy can manifest as a mild to moderate anemia.

- Hypersplenism, characterized by increased red cell destruction in the absence of a positive Coombs test, may accompany hematologic malignancies, especially lymphomas. Portal hypertension may lead to a normocytic anemia due to splenic pooling. Patients with significant, refractory hypersplenism may respond well to splenectomy.

Blood loss

- Acute and chronic blood loss is a frequently presenting problem in patients with gastrointestinal and genitourinary malignancies. Disease or chemotherapy-related thrombocytopenia may contribute to the risk of bleeding. Brisk hemorrhage due to tumor erosion into medium and large blood vessels may be life threatening, as observed in locally advanced head and neck or pancreatic cancer. Acute intratumoral hemorrhage is uncommon, but described in hepatocellular carcinoma, sarcoma, metastatic melanoma, and other rapidly proliferative, bulky solid tumors. Unusual causes of life-threatening tumor hemorrhage include bleeding from cavernous hemangioma, splenic hemangiosarcoma, and tumors metastatic to the ovary. Bevacizumab is associated with hemorrhage occasionally, particularly in patients with lung cancer.
- Chronic hemorrhage is a frequent complication of gastrointestinal tumors and gynecologic tumors, in particular endometrial cancer. Often, blood loss is surreptitious and manifests as an iron-deficiency anemia.

INTERVENTION

The adverse consequences of cancer-related anemia warrant intervention appropriate to symptoms and comorbidities. The variable causes of anemia in the cancer patient require specific, directed therapies. Rapid identification of the cause(s) of anemia should prompt the appropriate intervention to correct causes of blood loss, hemolysis, clotting defects, or other reversible processes. Most offten, however, no specific and reversible cause is identified other than therapy and the anemia of chronic illness. To replenish red cell mass, two interventions are most often considered: red blood cell transfusion and recombinant EPO.

Transfusion of red blood cells acutely alleviates the symptoms of anemia. However, transfusion is not without risk. Though extremely rare, complications of blood transfusion include volume overload, infection (bacterial, HIV, CMV, HBV, HCV, HTLV), acute transfusion reactions, iron overload, transfusion-related acute lung injury, and allo-immunization. Unless the donor cells are irradiated, there is a risk that donor lymphocytes could induce fatal graft-vs-host disease. Nonetheless, with acute or severe anemia, transfusion may prove life-saving. Under less emergent conditions, the decision to restore red cell mass through transfusion or the use of EPO requires clinical judgment. Evidence-based guidelines for transfusion have been published by a number of organizations, and their conclusions are consistent with a large study that compared restrictive versus liberal transfusion in the critically ill (7). For reasons that remain largely undefined, efforts to keep hemoglobin levels near normal in patients with acute illness are actually associated with poorer overall survival. Without evidence of severe cardiac disease, it is appropriate to restrict transfusion to those patients with a hemoglobin less than 7 g/dl, maintaining levels between 7 and 9 g/dl. The rate of transfusion depends on the severity of symptoms related to hypoxia (dyspnea, fatigue, changes in mental status, tachycardia, angina), taking care to avoid acute fluid overload.

Initially marketed for anemia in advanced renal disease, recombinant EPO was approved by the United States FDA for the treatment of cancer-related anemia in 1993 based on quality-of-life endpoints. The two commercially available preparations of recombinant EPO in the United States are epoetin alpha (Epogen, Amgen; Procrit, Ortho Biotech) and darbepoetin alpha (Aranesp, Amgen). Recombinant epoetin alpha is almost identical to the endogenous human glycoprotein, EPO, differing importantly in glycosylation of key residues that prolong half-life. Darbepoetin alpha differs from endogenous EPO at five amino acid residues, allowing for hypoglycosylation and an even more prolonged serum half-life.

Modest clinical efficacy of epoetin alpha and darbepoetin alpha has been established in pivotal, placebo-controlled, registration studies of patients with solid and hematologic malignancies (8–10). Epoetin alpha and darbepoetin alpha demonstrate comparable efficacy in cancer-related anemia. Epoetin alpha was initially studied as a three-time weekly formulation in FDA registration studies. Subsequent clinical trials have established the safety and activity of weekly, high-dose treatment. Weekly epoetin alpha (40,000 units, adjusted in subsequent doses according to the increase in hemoglobin) and darbepoetin alpha every two weeks (200 mcg, adjusted) are equally effective (11).

In these and subsequent studies, a consistent, small positive effect has been observed in hemoglobin levels, diminished transfusion requirement and quality of life, though the response develops slowly over several weeks. Evidence-based guidelines have been established and, in general, a consensus has been reached that EPO can produce a symptomatic benefit, but various guideline-developing groups differ in their target hemoglobin. Quality of life data support an upper boundary hemoglobin of 12 g/dl (12). However, data have begun to raise the question of whether EPO might protect tumors against therapeutic interventions like radiation therapy and chemotherapy.

An increased risk of adverse complications such as hypertension, venous thromboembolism, and cardiovascular events is reported with recombinant EPO. An international placebo-controlled study of epoetin alpha in patients with metastatic breast cancer was terminated early due to an unexpected, increased recurrence rate and mortality in the treatment arm (13). A study of epoetin beta (NeoRecormon, Roche), approved in Europe for cancer-related anemia, illustrated increased thrombotic and cardiovascular events among treated patients (14). Six clinical studies have generated data suggesting that EPO is associated with increased risk of cancer recurrence, cancer progression, or death.

For example, the Danish Head and Neck Cancer Study Group trial (DAHANCA 10) compared radiotherapy-to-radiotherapy plus darbepoetin alpha (target hemoglobin 14.0–15.5 g/dl) in the treatment of advanced head and neck cancer. Three-year locoregional control and overall survival were both worse in patients treated with darbepoetin alpha (http://conman.au.dk/dahanca). A double-blind study of 989 patients treated with darbepoetin alpha (target hemoglobin 12 g/dl) or placebo failed to demonstrate a favorable effect of darbepoetin on red cell transfusion requirements. However, patients treated with darbepoetin demonstrated an increase in mortality. A similar study of weekly epoetin alpha (40,000IU; target hemoglobin 12–14 g/dl) in anemic patients with lung cancer was closed prematurely due to increased mortality in treated patients. Median time to death was 68 days with ESA versus 131 days with placebo. Accordingly the FDA has issued a boxed warning for EPO products (http://www.fda.gov/cder/drug/infopage/RHE/default.htm).

EPOs are not approved for use in cancer patients not receiving chemotherapy. EPO is being evaluated clinically for its capacity to limit the size of strokes and myocardial infarcts through its action to protection of hypoxic cells from cell death. It is possible that this protective effect on dying cells will be beneficial in some settings but detrimental in patients with cancer. Until the issue is better defined, the use of EPO might wisely be confined to those settings where it is a component of palliative care. Its use as a component of curative regimens is undefined and potentially harmful.

REFERENCES

1. Barrett-Lee PJ, Ludwig H, Birgegard G, et al. Independent risk factors for anemia in cancer patients receiving chemotherapy: results from the European Cancer Anaemia Survey. Oncology. 2006; 70: 34–48.
2. Groopman JE, Itri LM. Chemotherapy-induced anemia in adults: incidence and treatment. J Natl Cancer Inst. 1999; 91: 1616–1634.

3. Cella D. The functional assessment of cancer therapy-anemia (FACT-An) scale: a new tool for the assessment of outcomes in cancer anemia and fatigue. Semin Hematol. 1997; 34: 13–19.

4. Caro JJ, Salas M, Ward A, Goss G. Anemia as an independent prognostic factor for survival in patients with cancer: a systemic, quantitative review. Cancer. 2001; 91: 2214–2221.

5. Nemeth E, Ganz T. Regulation of iron metabolism by hepcidin. Annu Rev Nutr. 2006; 323–342.

6. Miller CB, Jones RJ, Piantadosi S, Abeloff MD, Spivak JL. Decreased erythropoietin response in patients with the anemia of cancer. N Engl J Med. 1990; 322: 1689–1692.

7. Hebert PC, Wells G, Blajchman MA, Marshall J, Martin C, Pagliarello G, Tweeddale M, Schweitzer I, Yetisir E. A multicenter, randomized, controlled clinical trial of transfusion requirements in critical care. Transfusion requirements in critical care investigators, Canadian Critical Care Trials Group. N Engl J Med. 1999; 340: 409–417.

8. Case DC Jr, Bukowski RM, Carey RW, et al. Recombinant human erythropoietin therapy for anemic cancer patients on combination chemotherapy. J Natl Cancer Inst. 1993; 85: 801–806.

9. Hedenus M, Adriansson M, San Miguel J, et al. Efficacy and safety of darbepoetin alfa in anaemic patients with lymphoproliferative malignancies: a randomized, double-blind, placebo-controlled study. Br J Haematol. 2003; 122: 394–403.

10. Vansteenkiste J, Pirker R, Massuti B, et al. Double-blind, placebo-controlled, randomized phase III trial of darbepoetin alfa in lung cancer patients receiving chemotherapy. J Natl Cancer Inst. 2002; 94: 1211–1220.

11. Glaspy J, Vadhan-Raj S, Patel R, Bosserman L, Hu E, Lloyd RE, Boccia RV, Tomita D, Rossi G. Randomized comparison of every-2-week darbepoetin alfa and weekly epoetin alfa for the treatment of chemotherapy-induced anemia: the 20030125 Study Group Trial. J Clin Oncol. 2006; 24: 2290–2297.

12. Crawford J, Cella D, Cleeland CS, Cremieux PY, Demetri GD, Sarokhan BJ, Slavin MB, Glaspy JA. Relationship between changes in hemoglobin level and quality of life during chemotherapy in anemic cancer patients receiving epoetin alfa therapy. Cancer. 2002; 95: 888–895.

13. Leyland-Jones B. Breast cancer trial with erythropoietin terminated unexpectedly. Lancet Oncol. 2003; 4: 459–460.

14. Henke M, Laszig R, Rube C, et al. Erythropoietin to treat head and neck cancer patients with anaemia undergoing radiotherapy: randomised, double-blind, placebo-controlled trial. Lancet. 2003; 362: 1255–1260.

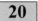

CANCER AND COAGULOPATHY

INTRODUCTION

The association between cancer and thrombosis was first proposed by Armand Trousseau (Figure 20-1) when he recognized the condition of *thrombophlebitis migrans*, as a forewarning of occult malignancy (1). In 1865, he remarked, "Should you, when in doubt as to the nature of an affection of the stomach, should you when hesitating between chronic gastritis, simple ulcer, and cancer, observe a vein become infected in the arm or leg, you may dispel your doubt, and pronounce in a positive manner that there is a cancer ..." (1). Although the association of hemostatic disorders and cancer has been studied extensively over the past 100 years, venous thromboembolism (VTE), defined herein as pulmonary embolus (PE) or deep vein thrombosis (DVT), remains a major cause of morbidity and mortality in cancer patients.

This chapter will explore the pathogenesis of thrombosis in cancer as well as the epidemiology and risk factors. This review will also focus on the current diagnostic and management strategies for VTE in cancer patients and the challenges of antithrombotic therapy in this population. Finally, new diagnostic and therapeutic developments in this area will be addressed.

PATHOGENESIS

The precise pathophysiological mechanisms of thrombosis in cancer patients are incompletely understood and likely involve multiple factors including tumor cells, the hemostatic system, inherited and acquired thrombophilia, and exogenous contributors such as chemotherapy and radiotherapy (2). Tumors contribute to thrombosis through the production of tissue factor and cancer procoagulant, two well-studied procoagulant factors. Tumor cells can also induce platelet activation and aggregation through secretion of proteases. Tumor-related release of various cytokines, growth factors and proteases including tumor necrosis factor α (TNFα), interleukin 1β, and vascular endothelial growth factor (VEGF) contributes not only to angiogenesis and inflammation, but also to the activation of the hemostatic system. Furthermore, tumor cells interact directly with the host blood vessels, endothelial cells, leukocytes, and monocytes. These many and varied interactions lead to both a direct and indirect activation of the clotting system, an increase in thrombin generation, and ultimately a hypercoagulable state.

EPIDEMIOLOGY

Venous thrombosis is a common complication in patients with cancer. Although the exact incidence of VTE in cancer patients is unknown, it occurs in approximately 15%, with reports ranging from 4% to 30% (3, 4). These numbers likely underestimate the problem as VTE often causes no symptoms. In addition, if symptoms are present, they are often nonspecific or attributed to a patient's underlying malignancy.

Certain malignancies exhibit high rates of VTE such as hematological malignancies and neoplasms of the pancreas, gastrointestinal tract, ovary, brain, colon, kidney, lung, and prostate. However, it is unclear if the high rates are due

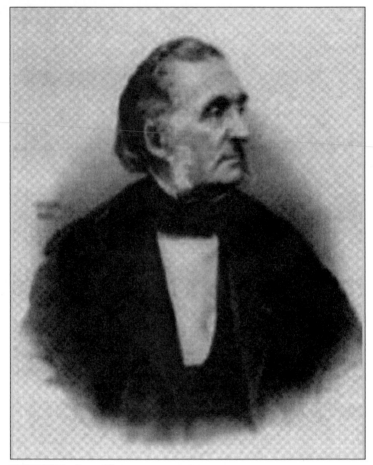

FIGURE 20-1 Armand Trousseau.

to the underlying properties of particular cancers or merely reflect the high prevalence of certain cancers. Nevertheless, it is well documented that cancers diagnosed at the same time as an episode of VTE are more likely to have distant metastases and lower survival rates (4, 5). One study showed that cancer patients with VTE had a 1 year survival of 12% as compared to 36% in cancer patients without VTE (5). Similarly, patients who develop VTE within a year after a cancer diagnosis are more likely to have advanced stage and poorer prognosis when compared to analogous cancer patients without VTE (5). A study of over 235,000 cancer patients showed that after adjusting for age, race, and stage of disease, VTE at the time of or within 1 year of cancer diagnosis was a significant predictor of death within that year (4). It also appears that cancer patients with VTE are two to three times more likely to have recurrent VTE and two to six times more likely to experience hemorrhagic complications from anticoagulant therapy than noncancer patients with VTE (6, 7). These findings clearly indicate that VTE may be more aggressive and difficult to treat in cancer patients than in noncancer patients.

The association between cancer and thrombosis is further supported by the many studies, suggesting that an idiopathic VTE is often associated with occult cancer. Approximately 10% of patients who present with an idiopathic or unprovoked VTE are diagnosed with cancer within the next 1–2 years (8). These provocative findings raise the unanswered question as to whether all patients with idiopathic VTE should undergo extensive cancer screening. The SOMIT study attempted to address this matter (9). Patients with an idiopathic VTE were randomized to either extensive or nonextensive cancer screening and followed for 24 months. Subjects in the extensive screening arm seemed to have a shorter delay in the diagnosis of cancer, their cancers were detected at earlier stages, and they had a lower cancer-related mortality (9). Unfortunately, this trial was stopped prematurely due to recruitment issues leaving these conclusions unsubstantiated. Thus, current recommendations are to provide age appropriate cancer screening for patients who present with idiopathic VTE, and any additional testing should be driven by what is discovered in a thorough history and physical examination. However, given the SOMIT observations, albeit underpowered, future studies evaluating extensive cancer screening for patients with idiopathic VTE are needed.

RISK FACTORS

Many inherited and acquired risk factors are associated with the development of VTE and are listed in Table 20-1. Cancer patients may have additional risk factors related to their malignancy including surgery, immobilization, chemotherapy, some forms of hormone therapy, and the presence of indwelling central venous catheters (CVC). Without appropriate prophylaxis, cancer patients have twice the risk of developing postoperative DVT and three times the risk of developing a fatal PE than patients without cancer (10). Long-term immobilization, often due to lengthy hospital stays, also increases the risk of developing VTE.

Tamoxifen, estrogen, thalidomide, L-asparaginase, and VEGF inhibitors are a few of the cancer therapies associated with high rates of thromboembolic complications, especially when used in combination with other chemotherapeutic agents. In a trial involving over 2,600 women with early stage breast cancer, the incidence of developing VTE was 0.2% with placebo and 0.9% with tamoxifen (11). Another trial involving women with advanced stage breast cancer showed that the incidence of VTE was 2.6% with tamoxifen alone versus 13.6% with tamoxifen plus chemotherapy (12). Similarly, in studies involving multiple myeloma, treatment with thalidomide alone had a risk of 2%. The risk increased to 33% with the addition of chemotherapy (13). Cancer patients who receive either cytotoxic or immunosuppressive therapy have a 6.5-fold increased risk of developing a VTE when compared to noncancer patients, and a twofold increased risk compared to cancer patients not receiving chemotherapy (14). Furthermore, venous thrombosis, and in particular, cortical sinus thrombosis, is a frequent complication of L-asparaginase treatment, and it is related to inhibition of the synthesis of anticoagulant factors, protein C and protein S.

CVC are another common risk factor for VTE. These devices are commonplace among cancer patients who require long-term chemotherapy. The reported incidence of catheter-related thrombosis ranges from 5% to 75%, and this wide range likely reflects the distinct types of malignancy, the kind of catheter used, and the duration of its implantation (15). In addition, the complications associated with CVC-related thrombosis can result in loss of catheter function, postphlebitic syndrome of the upper extremity, PE, and even mortality. There have been major efforts to identify disease management approaches to decrease the risk of VTE with CVC, and these mechanisms are discussed in Prevention section of this chapter.

Table 20-1
___

Risk Factors for Venous Thromboembolism (VTE)*
___

- Inherited
  - Antithrombin deficiency
  - Protein C deficiency
  - Protein S deficiency
  - Factor V Leiden
  - Prothrombin G20210A
  - Dysfibrinogenemias
- Environmental
  - Smoking
  - Prolonged air travel
- Treatment-related
  - Hormonal (estrogens, tamoxifen)
  - Chemotherapy (bevacizumab, thalidomide)
  - Central venous catheterization
  - Surgery
  - Heparin-induced thrombocytopenia
  - Immobilization
- Comorbid states and diseases
  - Malignancy
  - Advanced age
  - Prior thrombotic event
  - Prolonged immobilization, paresis
  - Pregnancy and the postpartum period
  - Obesity
  - Major trauma
  - Congestive heart failure
  - Antiphospholipid antibody syndrome
  - Myeloproliferative disorders (e.g., essential thrombocytosis, polycythemia vera)
  - Inflammatory bowel disease
  - Paroxysmal nocturnal hemoglobinuria
  - Nephrotic syndrome
___

* Applies to cancer and noncancer patients.

CLINICAL MANIFESTATIONS

Cancer patients can present with a wide range of thromboembolic events. The two most commonly recognized are DVT and pulmonary embolism (PE). However, symptoms and signs may result from migratory thrombophlebitis, nonbacterial thrombotic endocarditis, disseminated intravascular coagulopathy (DIC), thrombotic microangiogaphy, and arterial thrombosis. Cancer patients may also present with multiple clinical sequelae as was originally reported in 1977 by Sack et al in a review of 182 cases of neoplasia associated with alterations in blood coagulation (16). Figure 20-2 is an expansion of the original Venn diagram created by Sack et al which represents the interrelations between the various clinical phenomena. Discussion of all these clinical presentations is beyond the scope of this chapter and, therefore, only DVT and PE will be presented in detail.

Patients with DVT may experience complaints of leg pain, swelling, tenderness, discoloration, venous distension, or a palpable cord. Nonspecific symptoms of PE include dyspnea, tachypnea, tachycardia, pleuritic chest pain, cough, and wheeze. Signs may include hemoptysis, hypotension, syncope,

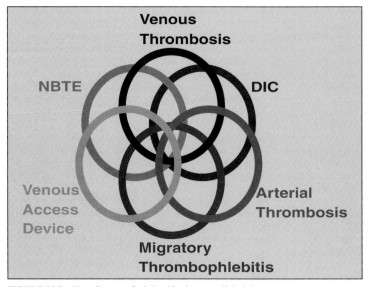

FIGURE 20-2   Venn diagram of relationships between clinical signs.

coma, pleural effusion, or pulmonary infiltrates. Each of these clinical features can be a manifestation of other cardiac or pulmonary processes, such as pneumonia or heart failure, making the diagnosis of PE difficult.

The consequences of DVT and PE are many and include acute morbidity or even death. Some of the short- and long-term complications due to thrombotic events consist of extension of the clot, embolization, postthrombotic syndrome, pulmonary hypertension, and recurrent VTE. Furthermore, there may be significant morbidity associated with long-term anticoagulation or with placement of an inferior vena cava (IVC) filter. The psychological stress and fear that patients face when suffering from a thromboembolic event must also be appreciated. Moreover, the presence of VTE or its complications may cause delays in chemotherapy or other treatments, which may have considerable consequences for the patient. Lastly, VTE can be the cause of death as was shown in one autopsy-based study where one out of every seven cancer deaths in the hospital was due to PE (17). Over 60% of those who died of a PE had either limited metastatic or local disease indicating a reasonable chance of prolonged survival if not for the fatal PE (17).

DIAGNOSIS OF VTE

Diagnosing VTE in cancer patients, as in other patients, may be difficult. The signs and symptoms of VTE are often variable and nonspecific, and available diagnostic tests have varying sensitivities and specificities. Moreover, commonly employed models for predicting the probability of VTE have limited value in cancer patients because of the significant additional risk factors at play. Ultimately, a diagnosis requires a combination of modalities.

If VTE is clinically suspected, a common first test is the D-dimer, which reflects the degradation product of cross-linked fibrin. This test is highly sensitive, but not specific (18). Because it is elevated in a variety of situations including malignancy, acute VTE, underlying lung abnormalities, recent surgery, hospitalization, and aging, the primary value of the D-dimer test is a negative result, which constitutes strong evidence against significant thrombosis (18). If the D-dimer test is positive, additional diagnostic tests should be performed.

Duplex venous ultrasound (US) imaging, the most widely available modality for diagnosing DVT, is highly sensitive for detecting proximal vein thrombosis but less so for detecting calf vein clots. Therefore, if a patient presents with symptoms suggestive of a calf vein thrombosis, but has a negative US test, a repeat test at 3–5 days may be warranted, especially if symptoms persist and no alternative diagnosis has been established. If the US is inconclusive, magnetic resonance imaging (MRI) of the lower extremities is usually definitive.

If PE is suspected, a variety of imaging tests may aid in making the diagnosis, including lung radionuclide scans (VQ), spiral computed tomography (CT), pulmonary angiography, MRI and magnetic resonance angiography (MRA). Although pulmonary angiography has been the gold standard, it is invasive and often unavailable or impractical and, therefore, has been replaced by CT angiography.

VQ scans, formerly a frequently used diagnostic tool, are now employed only when there is a contraindication to CT scans with contrast, such as renal failure or iodine allergy. VQ scans are helpful when they are either positive or negative, but their results are often inconclusive or confounded by underlying lung abnormalities.

The spiral CT or computerized tomographic angiography (CTA) is highly sensitive for large emboli. Multidetector scanners are able to visualize the sub-segmental arteries effectively. Simultaneous imaging of the lower extremities, which is helpful in identifying an associated DVT, can further increase the diagnostic sensitivity of CTA. Moreover, the spiral CT may help identify alternative etiologies for a patient's symptoms if a PE is not identified.

One of the newest diagnostic tools to diagnose PE, MRI/MRA of the chest, has been incompletely evaluated and standardized. Currently studies are underway to assess its accuracy and safety.

TREATMENT

The management of VTE in cancer patients is a challenge due to the frequent presence of a hypercoagulable state, physical obstructions to blood flow, patient immobility, and the general impression that these patients are relatively resistant to anticoagulant therapy. This section will outline current treatment recommendations for both the acute and long-term treatment of VTE in cancer patients based on the seventh American College of Chest Physicians (ACCP) Conference guidelines and Journal of National Comprehensive Cancer Network (JNCCN) (10, 19, 20).

Acute Treatment

The initial treatment for DVT and PE are similar. There are three options for anticoagulation: unfractionated heparin (UFH), low-molecular weight heparin (LMWH), and fondaparinux sodium. LMWH is a fragment of UFH and exerts its anticoagulant effect through antifactor Xa and antithrombin activities. It is cleared from plasma by metabolism in the liver, and a small portion is excreted in the urine. LMWH has largely replaced the use of UFH as the initial treatment for VTE because of its similar efficacy, superior safety profile, and pharmacokinetic advantages that allow for once or twice daily subcutaneous administration without laboratory monitoring, lower risk of complications such as heparin-induced thrombocytopenia (HIT) or heparin-induced osteoporosis, and potential for outpatient treatment. LMWH, a weight based therapy, may need to be episodically monitored in two particular situations: in patients who are at the extremes of body weight or in those suffering from renal failure, the latter situation because of LMWH clearance by renal excretion. This monitoring involves measuring the antifactor Xa activity 3–4 h after subcutaneous injection with a therapeutic goal of 0.5–1.3 U/ml.

If a patient requires a short-acting initial anticoagulant or one that needs to be carefully monitored, is anticipating an invasive procedure, or has a contraindication to LMWH such as severe renal failure, UFH is the favored treatment. UFH, a glycosaminoglycan, exerts its anticoagulant effect at several steps in the formation of fibrin clots. Specifically, when combined with antithrombin III, it inactivates activated factor X and inhibits the conversion of prothrombin to thrombin. UFH is metabolized in the liver and can be reversed with the antidote, protamine sulfate, if necessary. However, unlike LMWH, UFH is usually given intravenously and needs to be monitored frequently, and the dose must be adjusted with the use of nomograms to maintain an activated partial thromboplastin time (aPPT) of 1.5–2.5 times the normal.

A third anticoagulant option is the synthetic pentasaccharide, fondaparinux sodium, which works by indirectly inhibiting factor Xa. It has similar efficacy and safety for the initial treatment of PE and DVT as UFH or LMWH. It is an attractive medication because of its once daily subcutaneous administration and linear pharmacokinetic profile. In addition, it does not cause a syndrome akin to HIT to date. However, it cannot be reversed and its 17 h half-life makes it an unreasonable option in patients who require a short-acting therapy. In addition, because fondaparinux is excreted unchanged in the urine, monitoring is essential in patients with mild or moderate renal insufficiency, and the medication is contraindicated in patients with severe renal failure.

Other options for the initial treatment of DVT and PE that are not anticoagulants include thrombolytic therapy, thromboendarteretomy, and IVC filters. The use of thrombolytics is controversial in DVT and currently should be considered only for patients with massive iliofemoral thrombosis and at risk for limb gangrene (19). A recent meta-analysis has helped clarify the use of thrombolytics for the initial treatment of PE (21). While there was no overall benefit of thrombolytics in terms of recurrent PE or death, patients who were hemodynamically unstable (systolic blood pressure <90–100 mmHg) had a significantly lower rate of recurrent PE and death, but a significantly higher rate of major bleeding (21). The use of thrombolytics has also been considered in patients who are hemodynamically stable but exhibit evidence of severe right ventricular dysfunction. Results thus far are not definitive.

Thrombolytic drugs in current use include tissue-type plasminogen activator (t-PA), urokinase, and streptokinase. T-PA, the most commonly used of the group, is given as a 100 mg infusion over 2 h, followed by heparin. In patients refractory to t-PA, one should consider the presence of a saddle embolus, which might require thromboendarterectomy.

IVC filters are another option for the initial treatment of VTE. They are primarily used in patients with recurrent DVT or PE on anticoagulation, or in patients at high risk of bleeding on anticoagulation. There is little published evidence to document an improvement in outcome after their use. Moreover, if necessary, removable filters are preferred.

Long-Term Treatment

Similar to the initial treatment for VTE, the long-term treatment for VTE in cancer patients can be complicated by the concomitant need for chemotherapy, hormone therapy, invasive procedures, or CVCs. In addition, cancer patients have higher rates of recurrent VTE and bleeding with traditional anticoagulant therapy than noncancer patients, which adds a further challenge to their management. For many years, the long-term treatment recommendation for VTE in cancer patients was similar to that of the general population, the vitamin K antagonist (VKA), warfarin (Coumadin). After the initiation of UFH, LMWH or fondaparinux, warfarin is started on day 1 and adjusted to maintain an INR of 2–3. Given the slow onset of action, there needs to be a 5–7 day overlap between the two medications.

Although warfarin has the advantage of being an oral medication, it has significant disadvantages. It requires regular laboratory monitoring, has significant drug interactions because of its cyp 3A4–dependent metabolism, and is influenced by nutritional status. Fortunately, several trials have shown that LMWH is an attractive alternative.

A randomized controlled trial (RCT) demonstrated a clear benefit to LMWH compared with warfarin in cancer patients for long-term treatment or secondary prophylaxis after VTE (22). After 6 months of therapy, cancer patients who received LMWH had a significantly lower rate of recurrent VTE (9%) than those who received warfarin (17%), with no difference in the rates of bleeding (Figure 20-3). In addition, a post hoc analysis of the patients with non-metastatic solid tumors revealed a survival advantage in the LMWH group. Twelve month cumulative mortality in this population was 20% in the LMWH group versus 36% in the warfarin group (23).

The mechanism by which anticoagulants may decrease cancer mortality is not clear. However, in the past decade, multiple trials have suggested a survival advantage in cancer patients receiving LMWH as compared to UFH or warfarin for treatment or prevention of VTE (22). Interestingly, the survival advantages were not solely attributable to decreases in the rate of fatal pulmonary emboli. Three trials studying the value of LMWH in patients without VTE found a significant survival advantage in patients who received LMWH versus placebo (24–26). Confirmatory trials are underway.

LMWHs are thus the most attractive antithrombotic choice for the long-term treatment or secondary prophylaxis in cancer patients. Appropriately, the

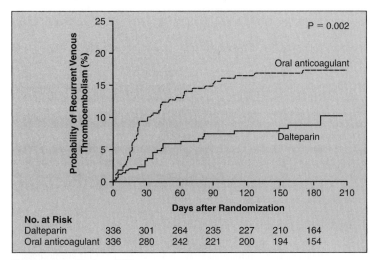

FIGURE 20-3 Recurrent VTE.
Kaplan–Meier estimates of the probability of symptomatic recurrent VTE among cancer patients who were randomized to secondary prophylaxis with dalteparin vs warfarin treatment for acute VTE (22). (From Lee AY, Levine MN, Baker RI, et al. Low-molecular-weight heparin versus a coumarin for the prevention of recurrent venous thromboembolism in patients with cancer. N Engl J Med. 2003; 349: 146–53. Copyright © 2003. Massachusetts Medical Society. All rights reserved.)

ACCP and JNCCN guidelines recommend LMWH for the first 3–6 months of long-term anticoagulant therapy for cancer patients with VTE (19).

The duration of long-term treatment of acute VTE in cancer patients has not been clearly established. For noncancer patients, in whom the inciting factor has been removed, the recommendation is to treat for 3–6 months. However, in patients with idiopathic VTE, where the inciting factor is unknown and may still exist, two trials have demonstrated decreased recurrence with prolonged anticoagulation beyond 3 months (27, 28). Patients with active cancer are similar to patients with idiopathic VTEs. Thus, current ACCP and JNCCN guidelines recommend anticoagulant therapy indefinitely or until the cancer is resolved (19, 20).

Complications of Treatment

The treatment of VTE in cancer patients is not without morbidity. Potential complications include bleeding, HIT, heparin-induced osteoporosis, or warfarin or heparin-induced skin necrosis. In two trials involving the use of warfarin, patients with cancer had a clinically and statistically significant increase in the overall incidence of major bleeding compared with noncancer patients: 12.4% and 13.3 per 100 patient-years in patients with cancer versus 4.9% and 2.1 per 100 patient-years in patients without cancer (6, 7). Importantly, the use of LMWH has not been associated with an increased risk of bleeding when compared to warfarin, and some evidence even suggests a decreased risk (22). In addition, treatment doses of fondaparinux have the same or fewer bleeding episodes as compared to LMWH (29).

In addition to bleeding, there is a 3% risk of HIT with UFH and 1% risk with LMWH (30). Skin necrosis due to heparins or warfarin is another infrequent but serious complication. Skin necrosis presents first with erythema then purpura and hemorrhage, and eventually necrosis (Figure 20-4). Specific complications

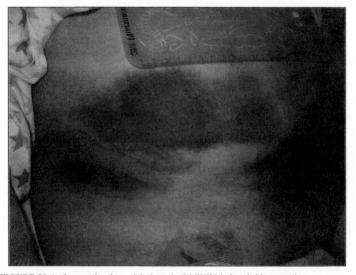

FIGURE 20-4   Low-molecular-weight heparin (LMWH) induced skin necrosis.
The ecchymosis seen superiorly and the adjacent indurated, erythematous plaques with central purpura and necrosis are abdominal sites of LMWH injection. (Photo courtesy of Dr. David Kuter, MD, D.Phil, MGH.)

are associated with therapeutic devices, including an increased risk of DVT with IVC filters, and an increased risk of infection with CVCs.

PREVENTION

Because of the high rate of VTE in cancer patients, primary prophylaxis has become a major area of interest. This section will briefly discuss preventive strategies associated with surgery, hospitalization, chemotherapy, and CVC.

Surgery

Cancer patients have a twofold higher risk of developing a postoperative DVT and threefold higher risk of fatal PE than noncancer patients undergoing similar procedures (10, 31, 32). Trials have led to the conclusion that antithrombotic therapy can reduce the rate of postoperative PE and clinical DVT when comparing LMWH or UFH with no treatment.

Additional studies have shown a significant reduction in postoperative VTE in cancer patients who receive prophylaxis beyond their hospitalization. The ENOXACAN II trial found a 60% reduction in the rate of VTE in cancer patients who received extended LMWH prophylaxis (up to 30 days) after their abdominal or pelvic surgery versus those who received prophylaxis only during their hospital stay (approximately 6-10 days) (33).

Other anticoagulants have also been investigated in this setting. The PEGA-SUS trial compared fondaparinux to LMWH and found no difference in the rates of postoperative VTE or bleeding in the general population (34). However, in a post hoc analysis of cancer patients, there was a statistically significant reduction in VTE in the fondaparinux group (4.7%) but not the LMWH group (7.7%) (34). Further studies are needed to confirm this finding. However, it is likely that anticoagulant therapy reduces the postoperative risk of VTE in cancer.

Occasionally, cancer patients may have a contraindication to anticoagulant therapy. In these situations, mechanical forms of prevention can be employed such as pneumoboots or TEDS stockings. However, the efficacy of these measures has not been established by rigorous trials.

Detailed and specific recommendations for prophylactic anticoagulation in cancer patients undergoing surgical procedures can be found in the ACCP guidelines (10).

Hospitalizations

Cancer patients who are immobile or bedridden with an acute medical illness or because of cancer-related morbidity are at increased risk of developing VTE. In a study in which the vast majority of patients had cancer, the risk of VTE was reduced by 41% in the patients whose physicians received a computer generated alert reminding them to provide VTE prophylaxis (35). The ACCP and JNCCN recommend that these "high risk" immobilized and hospitalized cancer patients receive VTE prophylaxis, either a LMWH such as dalteparin (5,000 U subcutaneously (sc) everyday (qd)), enoxaparin (40 mg sc qd), or tinzaparin (4,500 U sc qd); or UFH (5,000 U sc three times daily); or fondaparinux (2.5 mg sc qd) (10, 20). For patients with a contraindication to anticoagulant prophylactic therapy, graduated compression stockings or pneumatic compression boots can be used as alternatives.

Chemotherapy

High rates of VTE are associated with the use of chemotherapy. The value of thromboprophylaxis has been studied in a trial involving metastatic breast cancer patients (36). Over 300 women were randomized to chemotherapy plus or minus warfarin. There was an 85% relative risk reduction of VTE (4.4% versus 0.66%) in the warfarin group with no difference in bleeding rates (36). Despite these significant findings, thromboprophylaxis has not been adopted as standard practice. The reasons may be related to the difficulties associated with the use of warfarin, especially given the low absolute risk of VTE in the control group (4.4%), a hesitancy to extrapolate the findings to other tumors, or a paucity of confirmatory trials. Further investigation is clearly needed.

Central Venous Catheters

There have been major efforts to decrease catheter-related clotting and its complications with prophylactic anticoagulation. The majority of studies have shown no benefit (37, 38). Current ACCP guidelines state that low-dose warfarin or LMWH to prevent thrombosis related to long-term indwelling CVCs in cancer patients is not warranted (10).

NEW DEVELOPMENTS

In view of the limitations and side effects associated with the current antithrombotic therapies, better treatments are needed for cancer patients who have unique risks and comorbidities. There is a particular need for longer acting, oral agents that have few drug interactions, do not depend on nutritional status, and do not require monitoring. The oral direct thrombin inhibitor, ximelagatran, was initially a promising new contender. However, its use was halted when it was discovered to be associated with abnormal liver function tests in up to 13% of patients (39). Current trials are examining the safety and efficacy of longer acting pentasaccharides, oral thrombin inhibitors, and oral factor Xa inhibitors. In addition, future studies will address some of the unanswered questions in this population such as ideal duration of treatment and the role of thromboprophylaxis. Lastly, the evidence linking the use of LMWH to increases in cancer survival in both patients with and without VTE is compelling and is presently being explored further.

CONCLUSION

VTE in cancer patients is a challenging clinical problem. The pathogenesis is complex and multifactorial, and the additional risk factors for cancer patients are often unavoidable. Diagnosing VTE has become more successful and easier with newer noninvasive modalities. The practice of providing extensive screening to identify occult malignancies in patients who present with an idiopathic VTE is intriguing and needs to be explored further. The treatment for VTE can often be difficult and risky, especially given the unique risk factors such as chemotherapy, hormonal therapy and CVCs, and the comorbidities that are often associated with cancer patients. Moreover, the complications that are related to both VTE and their therapy can cause significant morbidity and even mortality in cancer patients.

LMWH has become a valuable tool for preventing and treating VTE and may have independent beneficial effects on the progression of cancer. Thromboprophylaxis in patients undergoing surgery or hospitalization appears safe and may be effective in lowering the risk of VTE although additional studies are needed to determine the utility of thromboprophylaxis in conjunction with chemotherapy or hormonal therapy.

Given all the limitations and challenges associated with cancer patients and the current available therapies, it is clear that better, safer, and easier treatments are urgently needed. In order to discover these much needed novel treatments, well-designed prospective RCTs specifically for cancer patients are required.

REFERENCES

1. Trousseau A. Phlegmasia alba dolens. Clin Med l'Hotel-Dieu Paris. 1865; 3: 654–712.
2. Falanga A, Rickles FR. Pathophysiology of the thrombophilic state in the cancer patient. Semin Thromb Hemost. 1999; 25: 173–182.
3. Deitcher SR. Cancer–related deep venous thrombosis: clinical importance, treatment challenges, and management strategies. Semin Thromb Hemost. 2003; 29: 247–258.
4. Chew HK, Wun T, Harvey D, Zhou H, White RH. Incidence of venous thromboembolism and its effect on survival among patients with common cancers. Arch Intern Med. 2006; 166: 458–464.
5. Sorensen HT, Mellemkjaer L, Olsen JH, Baron JA. Prognosis of cancers associated with venous thromboembolism. N Engl J Med. 2000; 343: 1846–1850.
6. Hutten BA, Prins MH, Gent M, Ginsberg J, Tijssen JG, Buller HR. Incidence of recurrent thromboembolic and bleeding complications among patients with venous thromboembolism in relation to both malignancy and achieved international normalized ratio: a retrospective analysis. J Clin Oncol. 2000; 18: 3078–83.
7. Prandoni P, Lensing AW, Piccioli A, et al. Recurrent venous thromboembolism and bleeding complications during anticoagulant treatment in patients with cancer and venous thrombosis. Blood. 2002; 100: 3484–8.
8. Prandoni P, Lensing AW, Buller HR, et al. Deep-vein thrombosis and the incidence of subsequent symptomatic cancer. N Engl J Med. 1992; 327: 1128–33.
9. Piccioli A, Lensing AW, Prins MH, et al. Extensive screening for occult malignant disease in idiopathic venous thromboembolism: a prospective randomized clinical trial. J Thromb Haemost. 2004; 2: 884–9.
10. Geerts WH, Pineo GF, Heit JA, et al. Prevention of venous thromboembolism: the Seventh ACCP Conference on Antithrombotic and Thrombolytic Therapy. Chest. 2004; 126: 338S–400S.
11. Fisher B, Costantino J, Redmond C, et al. A randomized clinical trial evaluating tamoxifen in the treatment of patients with node-negative breast cancer who have estrogen-receptor-positive tumors. N Engl J Med. 1989; 320: 479–84.
12. Pritchard KI, Paterson AH, Paul NA, Zee B, Fine S, Pater J. Increased thromboembolic complications with concurrent tamoxifen and chemotherapy in a randomized trial of adjuvant therapy for women with breast cancer. National Cancer Institute of Canada Clinical Trials Group Breast Cancer Site Group. J Clin Oncol. 1996; 14: 2731–7.
13. Zangari M, Barlogie B, Anaissie E, et al. Deep vein thrombosis in patients with multiple myeloma treated with thalidomide and chemotherapy: effects of prophylactic and therapeutic anticoagulation. Br J Haematol. 2004; 126: 715–21.
14. Heit JA, Silverstein MD, Mohr DN, Petterson TM, O'Fallon WM, Melton LJ, III. Risk factors for deep vein thrombosis and pulmonary embolism: a population-based case-control study. Arch Intern Med. 2000; 160: 809–15.
15. Rosovsky RP, Kuter DJ. Catheter-related thrombosis in cancer patients: pathophysiology, diagnosis, and management. Hematol Oncol Clin North Am. 2005; 19: 183–202, vii.
16. Sack GH, Jr., Levin J, Bell WR. Trousseau's syndrome and other manifestations of chronic disseminated coagulopathy in patients with neoplasms: clinical, pathophysiologic, and therapeutic features. Medicine (Baltimore). 1977; 56: 1–37.
17. Shen VS, Pollak EW. Fatal pulmonary embolism in cancer patients: is heparin prophylaxis justified? South Med J. 1980; 73: 841–3.
18. Stein PD, Hull RD, Patel KC, et al. D-dimer for the exclusion of acute venous thrombosis and pulmonary embolism: a systematic review. Ann Intern Med. 2004; 140: 589–602.
19. Buller HR, Agnelli G, Hull RD, Hyers TM, Prins MH, Raskob GE. Antithrombotic therapy for venous thromboembolic disease: the Seventh ACCP

Conference on Antithrombotic and Thrombolytic Therapy. Chest. 2004; 126: 401S–428S.

20. Wagman LD, Baird MF, Bennett CL, et al. Venous thromboembolic disease. Clinical practice guidelines in oncology. J Natl Compr Cancer Netw. 2006; 4: 838–69.

21. Wan S, Quinlan DJ, Agnelli G, Eikelboom JW. Thrombolysis compared with heparin for the initial treatment of pulmonary embolism: a meta-analysis of the randomized controlled trials. Circulation. 2004; 110: 744–9.

22. Lee AY, Levine MN, Baker RI, et al. Low-molecular-weight heparin versus a coumarin for the prevention of recurrent venous thromboembolism in patients with cancer. N Engl J Med. 2003; 349: 146–53.

23. Lee AY, Rickles FR, Julian JA, et al. Randomized comparison of low molecular weight heparin and coumarin derivatives on the survival of patients with cancer and venous thromboembolism. J Clin Oncol. 2005; 23: 2123–9.

24. Altinbas M, Coskun HS, Er O, et al. A randomized clinical trial of combination chemotherapy with and without low-molecular-weight heparin in small cell lung cancer. J Thromb Haemost. 2004; 2: 1266–71.

25. Kakkar AK, Levine MN, Kadziola Z, et al. Low molecular weight heparin, therapy with dalteparin, and survival in advanced cancer: the fragmin advanced malignancy outcome study (FAMOUS). J Clin Oncol. 2004; 22: 1944–8.

26. Klerk CP, Smorenburg SM, Otten HM, et al. The effect of low molecular weight heparin on survival in patients with advanced malignancy. J Clin Oncol. 2005; 23: 2130–5.

27. Kearon C, Ginsberg JS, Kovacs MJ, et al. Comparison of low-intensity warfarin therapy with conventional-intensity warfarin therapy for long-term prevention of recurrent venous thromboembolism. N Engl J Med. 2003; 349: 631–9.

28. Ridker PM, Goldhaber SZ, Danielson E, et al. Long-term, low-intensity warfarin therapy for the prevention of recurrent venous thromboembolism. N Engl J Med. 2003; 348: 1425–34.

29. Buller HR, Davidson BL, Decousus H, et al. Fondaparinux or enoxaparin for the initial treatment of symptomatic deep venous thrombosis: a randomized trial. Ann Intern Med. 2004; 140: 867–73.

30. Warkentin TE. Heparin-induced thrombocytopenia: pathogenesis and management. Br J Haematol. 2003; 121: 535–55.

31. Huber O, Bounameaux H, Borst F, Rohner A. Postoperative pulmonary embolism after hospital discharge. An underestimated risk. Arch Surg. 1992; 127: 310–3.

32. White RH, Zhou H, Romano PS. Incidence of symptomatic venous thromboembolism after different elective or urgent surgical procedures. Thromb Haemost. 2003; 90: 446–55.

33. Bergqvist D, Agnelli G, Cohen AT, et al. Duration of prophylaxis against venous thromboembolism with enoxaparin after surgery for cancer. N Engl J Med. 2002; 346: 975–80.

34. Agnelli G, Bergqvist D, Cohen AT, Gallus AS, Gent M. Randomized clinical trial of postoperative fondaparinux versus perioperative dalteparin for prevention of venous thromboembolism in high-risk abdominal surgery. Br J Surg. 2005; 92: 1212–20.

35. Kucher N, Koo S, Quiroz R, et al. Electronic alerts to prevent venous thromboembolism among hospitalized patients. N Engl J Med. 2005; 352: 969–77.

36. Levine M, Hirsh J, Gent M, et al. Double-blind randomised trial of a very-low-dose warfarin for prevention of thromboembolism in stage IV breast cancer. Lancet. 1994; 343: 886–9.

37. Reichardt P, Kretzschmar A, Biakhov M, et al. A phase III randomized, double-blind, placebo-controlled study evaluating the efficacy and safety of daily low-molecular-weight heparin (dalteparin sodium, Fragmin) in preventing catheter-related complications (CRCs) in cancer patients with central venous catheters (CVCs). Proc Am Soc Clin Oncol. 2002; 21: 369a.

38. Verso M, Agnelli G, Bertoglio S, et al. Enoxaparin for the prevention of venous thromboembolism associated with central vein catheter: a double-blind, placebo-controlled, randomized study in cancer patients. J Clin Oncol. 2005; 23: 4057–62.

39. Fiessinger JN, Huisman MV, Davidson BL. S. Ximelagatran vs low-molecular-weight heparin and warfarin for the treatment of deep vein thrombosis: a randomized trial. J Am Med Assoc. 2005; 293: 681–9.

METABOLIC EMERGENCIES IN ONCOLOGY

TUMOR LYSIS SYNDROME

Definition

Tumor lysis syndrome is a collection of metabolic derangements secondary to the release of tumor cell contents into the extra-cellular space (see Table 21-1). We distinguish tumor lysis syndrome, a clinically significant entity requiring active management, from tumor destruction that is associated with minor changes in electrolyte concentrations. Clearly this represents a continuum.

Tumor lysis syndrome can occur spontaneously in rare, highly proliferative tumors but usually occurs 6–72 h following initiation of antitumor therapy. There are case reports suggesting even brisker onset with the use of novel targeted therapies. It is most frequently associated with cytoxic therapy but can occur after embolization, radiation, or corticosteroids. Tumor lysis syndrome can also occur more distantly from treatment and following surgery. There is a proposed definition and grading system for laboratory and clinical tumor lysis syndrome, but it has not been widely adopted (see Table 21-2) (1).

Incidence and Risk Factors

Clinically significant tumor lysis syndrome is estimated to occur in less than 8% of at-risk patients but 40% or more may have laboratory evidence of biochemical tumor cell destruction (1, 2).

There are both tumor-related risk factors for tumor lysis syndrome, as well as patient specific risks (1, 3). Tumor specific risks include a large burden, a high-proliferative rate, or a highly treatment sensitive tumor (see Table 21-3). Tumor lysis syndrome occurs most commonly in the hematologic malignancies. The specific diseases that have a substantial risk of tumor lysis syndrome include acute lymphocytic leukemia, high-grade lymphomas, particularly Burkitts, acute myelogenous leukemia and rarely in chronic lymphocytic leukemia, and multiple myeloma (1, 2). Tumor lysis syndrome is rare in solid tumors, with breast cancer and small cell lung cancer comprising the most common reports (1–3).

Patient comorbidities may increase the risk of tumor lysis syndrome. Decreased urinary flow or dehydration, chronic renal insufficiency or frank renal failure, acidic urine, or preexisting hyperuricemia are all risk factors for tumor lysis syndrome development (1, 3).

Table 21-1

Features of Tumor Lysis Syndrome

- Hyperkalemia
- Hyperuricemia
- Hyperphosphatemia
- Hypocalcemia
- Metabolic acidosis and
  renal failure

Table 21-2

Cairo and Bishop Definition and Grading Classification of Tumor Lysis Syndrome

	Laboratory TLS*	Grade 0	Grade I	Grade II	Grade III	Grade IV	Grade V
Uric acid	≥476 mmol/l or 25% IFB	LTLS −	LTLS +	LTLS +	LTLS +	LTLS +	LTLS +
Potassium	≥6.0 mmol/l or 25% IFB						
Phosphorous	≥2.1 mmol/l in children or ≥1.45 mmol/l in adults or 25% IFB						
Calcium	≤1.75 mmol/l or 25% DFB						
Creatinine	Not defined	≤1.5 ULN	1.5 × ULN	>1.5–3.0 × ULN	>3.0–6.0 × ULN	>6.0 × ULN	Death
Cardiac arrhythmia/sudden death	None	None	No intervention indicated	Nonurgent intervention indicated	Symptomatic and incompletely or device controlled	Life threatening	Death
Seizure	None	None	None	One seizure or well controlled by anticonvulsants or infrequent focal motor seizures not interfering with ADL	Seizure with altered consciousness, poorly controlled or generalized seizure despite intervention	Prolonged, repetitive, or difficult to control seizures	Death

* LTLS or laboratory tumor lysis syndrome is alterations in the above values on two different measurements within 3 days before or 7 days after initiation of cyto-toxic therapy and assumes a patient has or will receive adequate hydration and a hypouricemic agent.

IFB: Increase from baseline.
DFB: Decrease from baseline.
ULN: Upper limit of normal (all creatinine values are assumed to be age and gender specific).

Table 21-3

Risk Factors for Tumor Lysis Syndrome

	Low risk	Intermediate risk	High risk
Tumor type	Breast, small cell lung cancer	CML, Hodgkins	High grade lymphoma, Burkitt, ALL, AML
Tumor burden			
WBC count			$>50 \times 10\ 9/l$, high blast count
LDH	<200 U/l		>400 U/l
Other			Extensive bone marrow involvement Bulky disease
Treatment intensity			Cisplatin, etoposide, rituximab ionizing radiation, fludarabine, IT MTX, paclitaxel, interferon alpha
Tumor treatment sensitivity	Low		High
Baseline renal function	Normal	Renal insufficiency	Renal failure
Other			Renal infiltration by disease
Baseline serum uric acid	<10 mg/dl		
Other			
Hydration	Euvolemic	Euvolemic	Dehydrated
Serum pH			Acidic
Urine pH	Alkaline		Acidic
Urine output	High		Low
Calcium-phosphorus product			>70

Hemodialysis and death are more common among those with tumor lysis syndrome and, accordingly, costs are estimated to be 10 times higher in those with tumor lysis injury, with hemodialysis and intensive care contributing the most to these costs (2).

Mechanisms

PURINE CATABOLISM The major contributing element in the pathophysiology of tumor lysis syndrome is hyperuricemia caused by the release of nucleic acids (purines), which are catabolized to uric acid, leading to elevated plasma urate levels (see Figure 21-1). Elevated uric acid levels can overwhelm the excretory capacity of the renal tubules particularly in the presence of an acidic pH and low urine flow. Crystalline obstruction of the renal tubules, uric acid nephropathy, renal failure, and uremia may result. Renal failure may also occur due to volume depletion and changes in autoregulation within the kidney.

INTRACELLULAR ION RELEASE Other intracellular ions are released, including potassium and phosphorus. Hyperkalemia, potentially leading to cardiac arrhythmias, and exacerbated by renal failure, is one of the most potentially morbid complications of tumor lysis syndrome.

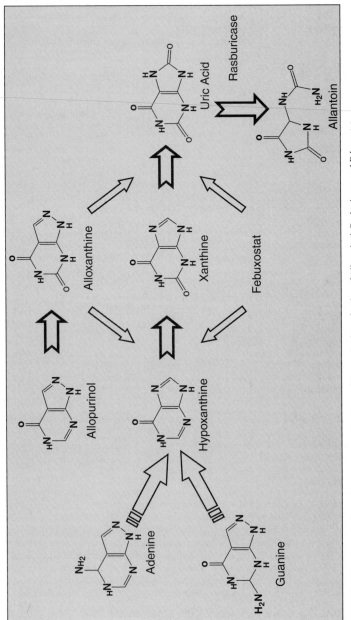

FIGURE 21-1   Uric acid formation via purine catabolism and the mechanism of action of Allopurinol, Rasburicase, and Febuxostat.

Intracellular phosphorous, which may be overproduced in malignant cells, is also released, renally excreted, and may precipitate as calcium phosphate in the renal tubules, leading to hypocalcemia, metastatic calcification, intrarenal calcification, nephrocalcinosis, nephrolithiasis, and obstructive uropathy.

Hypocalcemia is generally due to precipitation of calcium phosphate in the soft tissues and kidneys during periods of hyperphosphatemia and inappropriately low levels of 1,25-dihydroxyvitamin D3. This can be clinically associated with tetany and cardiac arrythmias.

Clinical Presentation

The clinical presentation of tumor lysis syndrome is characterized by the symptoms of the individual electrolyte imbalances and resultant renal failure (see Table 21-4).

Differential Diagnosis

The differential diagnosis of tumor lysis syndrome is limited. Injuries to large structures such as ischemic limb or rhabdomyolysis can replicate the varied clinical and laboratory presentations of tumor lysis syndrome but should be clinically apparent. The other laboratory abnormalities may be present to some extent in patients with renal insufficiency from any cause (see Table 21-5).

Diagnosis

As there is no agreed upon definition or classification system for tumor lysis syndrome, outlining diagnostic criteria is not possible, nor is delineating a clear distinction between laboratory values and clinically relevant tumor lysis syndrome. As described above, Cairo and Bishop (2004) have attempted to put forth a diagnostic and classification scheme that is outlined in Table 21-2 and is currently being evaluated (1).

Table 21-4

Clinical Signs and Symptoms of Tumor Lysis Syndrome

- Nausea, vomiting, diarrhea, lethargy
- Edema and fluid overload, including congestive heart failure and pulmonary edema
- Muscle cramps, paresthesias, tetany
- Acute renal failure or uremia
    - Hematuria, flank pain, hypertension, acidosis, oliguria
- Cardiac arrhythmia, hypotension, syncope
- Confusion, hallucinations, seizures
- Death

Table 21-5

Differential Diagnosis of Tumor Lysis Syndrome

- Tumor infiltration of kidneys or ureters
- Drug associated renal toxicity
- Acute renal failure secondary to other causes
    - Acute tubular necrosis
- Sepsis
- Keto or lactic acidosis
- Parathyroid or thyroid disease
- Hemolysis, rhabdomyolysis, crush injuries or ischemic limb

Prophylaxis and Monitoring

See Table 21-6 for an overview of the following discussion (1, 4, 5). In patients at high risk of developing tumor lysis syndrome, the decision to delay therapy must be weighted against the risks of tumor lysis syndrome, but in any case prophylactic measures should be instituted. Drugs that contribute to electrolyte abnormalities are nephrotoxic, or block uric acid, or potassium excretion should be stopped.

HYDRATION AND DIURESIS   The mainstay of prevention is aggressive hydration and diuresis, with individuals receiving 2–4 times usual maintenance fluids or 3–6 l/m^2/day. Clearly these fluids should not initially include potassium, calcium, or phosphate unless the patient is severely depleted. If the patient is not hypovolemic but is oligo or anuric, diuretics such as furosemide (or mannitol, particularly if furosemide fails) may be used to maintain an appropriate urine output with the following as goals: urine specific gravity should be <1.010 and urine output >150–250 ml/h. Furosemide diuresis may also decrease serum potassium levels. Dosing of diuretics is patient dependent and may be intermittent or continuous.

Traditionally, recommendations have also suggested alkalinization of urine. However this has become more controversial due to the increased risk of urinary xanthine and calcium phosphate deposition, fluid overload, and metabolic alkalosis. If using this method, classical recommendations have included: urine pH >7.0 prior to, during, and for 2 days posttreatment, and sodium bicarbonate as tablets or as an additive to IV fluids (50–100 mEq/l fluid).

ALLOPURINOL   Allopurinol, a xanthine analog that is converted to alloxanthine and acts as a competitive inhibitor of xanthine oxidase, reduces the production of uric acid and the incidence of related obstructive uropathy (see Figure 21-1). It does not reduce uric acid already present and leads to lower urate levels over days. In addition, Allopurinol may result in xanthine nephropathy and calculi due to accumulation of xanthine and hypoxanthine which are renally excreted and may precipitate in alkaline urine.

Usual dosing of Allopurinol is 2 mg/ m^2/day or 600–800 mg/day orally, 12 h to 3 days prior to initiation of chemotherapy (or 200–400 mg/m^2/day IV, 24–48 h prior to initiation of chemotherapy; maximum dose 600 mg/day if unable to take orally). Allopurinol should be renally dosed in those patients with preexisting renal insufficiency or failure.

Allopurinol also reduces the degradation of other purines including 6-mercaptopurine (6-MP) and azothioprine, and therefore these drugs should be dose reduced by 50–70% when used with Allopurinol (1).

RASBURICASE   Rasburicase (Elitek) is a recombinant urate oxidase that converts uric acid to allantoin, a more soluble compound, which is then renally excreted (see Figure-21-1) (4). Usual dosing is 0.05–0.20 mg/kg IV over 30 min for 1–7 days and does not require renal dosing. Side effects include anaphylaxis or hypersivity reactions (bronchospasm, hypoxemia) in 5% of those who receive this drug. In addition, patients may form antibodies to this drug, the significance of which is currently unknown. Rasburicase should not be used in patients with G-6PD deficiency as hemolytic anemia and methemoglobinemia may occur.

FUTURE PROPHYLAXIS

Febuxostat   Febuxostat is a nonpurine selective inhibitor of xanthine oxidase used for prevention of gout, which may have future applications for tumor lysis syndrome (see Figure 21-1) (5). Febuxostat is metabolized via glucuronide formation and oxidation in the liver and has been studied at doses of 80 and

Table 21-6

Overview of Tumor Lysis Prophylaxis and Treatment

	Prophylaxis	Treatment — Moderate or asymptomatic	Severe or symptomatic
Hyperkalemia	• Avoid potassium supplements, including dietary sources • Avoid drugs that increase serum potassium	• Sodium polystyrene sulphonate (15 g orally 1–4×/day or as a retention enema, 30–50 g rectally every 6 h)	• Insulin (0.1 u/kg) and D5W IV • Sodium bicarbonate (1 mEq/kg) • Loop diuretics • Inhaled beta-agonist • Calcium gluconate 10% (500mg–2g) • Hemodialysis or hemofiltration
Hyperuricemia	• Stop drugs that inhibit uric acid excretion • Hydration 2–3 days prior to treatment • Allopurinol • Rasburicase • Febuxostat?	• Hydration (3–6 l/m²) and diuresis • ±Alkalinize urine	• Allopurinol (2/m²/day or 600–800 mg/day orally or 200–400 mg/m(2)/day IV maximum dose 600 mg/day in adults) • Rasburicase (0.15 or 0.2 mg/kg/day IV over 30 min for 1–7 days) • Hemodialysis or hemofiltration
Renal failure	• Stop nephrotoxic drugs • Hydration	• Renally dose medications • Monitor fluid status • Aggressive fluid and electrolyte management • Aggressive uric acid and phosphate management	• Hemodialysis or hemofiltration
Hyperphosphatemia	• Avoid phosphate and calcium supplements including dietary sources	• Aluminum hydroxide or carbonate (500 to 1,800 mg, 3–6x/day between meals) or aluminum carbonate (2 cap/tabs or 12 ml suspension 3–4x/day with meals)	• Insulin and dextrose as above • Hemodialysis or hemofiltration
Hypocalcemia		• None	• *Calcium gluconate 50–100 mg/kg IV

* Not recommended.

120 mg orally per day for urate levels greater than 8 mg/dl in individuals with normal renal and liver function in a noninferiority trial comparing Febuxostat to Allopurinol. Further investigation in a population of patients at risk for tumor lysis syndrome is required.

MONITORING   Monitoring for tumor lysis involves twice daily serum electrolytes (more frequently if the patient is at high risk or clinically unstable), and at least daily urinary pH and spot uric acid to creatinine ratio (value should be >1.0), evaluation of volume status (including daily weights, blood pressure, and examination looking for edema, pleural effusions, and ascites), and serum WBC count, LDH, ionized or corrected calcium, and calcium phosphorus product.

ECG changes associated with hyperkalemia include widening of the QRS complex (late manifestations include a sine wave appearance, ventricular arrhythmias, or asystole) and peaked T-waves, while hypocalcemia is associated with a long QT secondary to a prolonged ST segment.

Treatment

HYPERKALEMIA   Hyperkalemia treatment can be divided into treatment for moderate or asymptomatic hyperkalemia and those for severe or symptomatic hyperkalemia (see Table 21-6).

For asymptomatic or moderate hyperkalemia, oral sodium polystyrene sulphonate (Kayexalate), an exchange resin, is the primary treatment (15 g orally one to four times daily as a slurry in water or 70% sorbitol or as a retention enema, 30–50 g rectally every 6 h as a warm emulsion in 100 ml aqueous vehicle (sorbitol or D20W), retained for 30–60 min in adults).

For severe cases, Kayexalate in addition to insulin and dextrose, sodium bicarbonate (1 mEq/kg, repeated as needed based on blood gas values), loop diuretics, inhaled beta-agonists, and, in extreme examples, calcium gluconate or chloride is appropriate. For calcium gluconate the dosage is 2–4 mg/kg of a 10% solution, repeated at 10 min intervals as necessary. Calcium chloride is reserved for emergency situations. Hemodialyis or hemofiltration should also be considered.

HYPERURICEMIA AND RENAL FAILURE   Hyperuricemia should be treated either with Allopurinol or Rasburicase. Rasburicase may be superior (4). Hemodialysis or hemofiltration may be necessary.

Renal failure requires aggressive fluid, electrolyte, and uric acid management along with close monitoring for indications requiring hemodialysis or hemofiltration. Hemodialysis indications may include fluid overload, metabolic acidosis, electrolyte disturbances that are recalcitrant to the treatments outlined above, uremia and hypertension.

HYPERPHOSPHATEMIA   Hyperphosphatemia is treated with oral aluminum hydroxide (adult dosing: 500–1,800 mg, three to six times daily between meals) or aluminum carbonate (two capsules or tablets or 12 ml suspension three to four times daily with meals). Insulin and dextrose as administered in hyperkalemia can also be given. Severe or symptomatic cases should receive hemodialysis or hemofiltration.

HYPOCALCEMIA   Moderate or asymptomatic hypocalcemia usually does not require treatment and the risks of treatment may outweigh the benefits. In severe cases, calcium gluconate 500mg–2g (10% solution) IV in adults at a rate not to exceed 1.5 ml/min can be used but may lead to calcium phosphate precipitation resulting obstructive uropathy or metastatic calcification. In an emergency situation, calcium chloride should be used for hyperkalemia or hypocalcemia at 2–4 mg/kg of a 10% solution, repeated at 10 min intervals as necessary.

HYPONATREMIA

Incidence and Risk Factors

Hyponatremia is a common electrolyte abnormality, occurring in 1–40% of elderly and/or hospitalized patients (6–8). Increasing age is a risk factor for hyponatremia (8). In cancer patients, hyponatremia may be due to primary or metastatic disease, cancer-related medical interventions or complications, usually via the syndrome of inappropriate antidiuretic syndrome (SIADH), as well as other causes (6, 9). This section will focus primarily on the diagnosis and treatment of SIADH-related hyponatremia in the setting of malignancy.

The greatest risk for malignancy-related hyponatremia is among lung cancer patients, particularly small cell lung cancer. However, head and neck cancers, leukemia, and mediastinal cancers have also been implicated, along with limited reports in a number of other cancers (7, 9).

Hyponatremia can occur following stem cell transplantation (7). Of the 40% of transplant patients who developed hyponatremia in Kobayashi's study, more than 11% were due to SIADH. Risk factors for SIADH in this population were younger age, HLA mismatched or unrelated donor, cord blood transplant, and GVHD prophylaxis with methylprednisolone.

The relationship between malignancy-related hyponatremia, the extent of cancer, response to antitumor treatment and prognosis has not been fully elucidated (7, 9).

Mechanisms

Hyponatremia can be characterized by varying levels of osmolality (see Table 21-7) (10, 11). Hypotonic hyponatremia, the most common form, is caused by abnormal retention of water with varying amounts of fluid intake (see Table 21-8). Retention of water occurs because the ability of the kidneys to excrete fluid has been impaired or overwhelmed. Edema of the central nervous system is the most concerning consequence of hyponatremia (10, 12).

Other uncommon causes of hypotonic hyponatremia, not included in Table 21-8, include excessive water intake either orally (as in polydipsia) or via absorption of sodium-free fluids (irrigant solutions, enemas) or reset osmostat syndrome; the later is a subset of SIADH (6, 10, 11).

Table 21-7

Types of Hyponatremia with Mechanism and Representative Causes

Hypotonic hyponatremia
Extracellular fluid may be decreased (hypovolemic), euvolemic (dilutional), or increased
  May be hypoosmolar or not depending upon etiology

Isotonic hyponatremia
Shift of water to an isotonic extracellular space Mannitol

Hypertonic hyponatremia
Shift of water to a hypertonic extracellular space Solutes other than sodium, e.g., hyperglycemia

Pseudohyponatremia
Presence of other osmoles in the extracellular space
  Hypertriglyceridemia
  Paraproteinemia

Table 21-8

Causes and Treatment of Hypotonic Hyponatremia by Extracellular Fluid Volume, Total Body Water, and Sodium Stores

Decreased extracellular fluid	Normal extracellular fluid	Increased extracellular fluid

Renal sodium losses
  Diuretics
  Osmotic diuretics
  Adrenal disease
  Salt-wasting
  Tubular or keto acidosis
Other sodium losses
  GI losses
  Bleeding
  Insensible and third space Losses
	Thyroid or adrenal disease
	SIADH
	  Cancer related CNS
	
	  Pulmonary disease
	  Mechanical ventilation
	
	Drugs
	  SSRIs, tricyclics
	  Carbamazepine
	  ACE inhibitors
	  Thiazide, loop and osmotic diuretics
	  Morphine, NSAIDs
	Other
	  Pain, nausea, HIV
	  Decreased solutes
	Postoperative state
		Cirrhosis
		Congestive Heart Failure
		Renal failure
		Nephrotic syndrome
		Pregnancy

Treatment • Sodium stores are decreased • Total body water is decreased (hypovolemic) • Volume and sodium deficit must be corrected	• Sodium stores are normal • Total body water may be slightly increased • Treat the underlying condition/etiology. May include fluid restriction and/or hypertonic saline	• Sodium stores are increased • Total body water is increased (hypervolemic) • Treat the underlying condition. May include loss of water

MECHANISM OF SIADH   SIADH occurs because of paraneoplastic or ectopic production of antidiuretic hormone (ADH) or arginine vasopressin (AVP). AVP binds to the V2 vasopressin receptor (V2R), a G protein-coupled receptor, in the collecting duct and the ascending limb of the loop of Henle. This leads to increases in intracellular cyclic AMP (c-AMP) that in turn leads to increased water permeability, inappropriate water retention, and, therefore, hyponatremia and hypo-osmolality (9). Patients with this syndrome may exhibit inappropriate thirst (6).

Normally, AVP or V2 vasopressin is produced in the supraoptic and paraventricular nuclei of the hypothalamus and transported down the neurohypophysis, or posterior lobe of the pituitary gland, where it is released into the blood stream when cardiovascular baro- and osmoreceptors signal that blood pressure or plasma volume are too low or plasma osmolality is too high (6, 9). AVP then acts on the kidney as described above, to retain water and concentrate urine and may have a direct, pressor effect on arteries and arterioles.

However, the etiology of malignancy-associated hyponatremia may not be due only to ectopic production of AVP (see Tables 21-7 and 21-8). Consideration should be given to other causes of hyponatremia or SIADH, as this will affect treatment.

Clinical Presentation

See Table 21-9 (6, 8, 10–12).

Differential Diagnosis

See Tables 21-7, 21-8, 21-10, and 21-11 (6–11).

Diagnosis

Variable definitions for hyponatremia are used and make comparison of cases difficult. In this chapter, hyponatremia is defined as serum sodium concentration below 135 mmol/l (this is consistent with our institutional range, 135–145 mmol/l, of serum sodium). Diagnostic testing is based upon the hypothesized cause of hyponatremia. For SIADH, the diagnosis should also be based on the criteria in Table 21-12 (6, 9). AVP level need not be checked.

Prophylaxis and Monitoring

There is no prophylaxis for hyponatremia other than to anticipate electrolyte abnormalities, actively replete electrolyte losses, and avoid drugs that induce hyponatremia.

Treatment

GENERAL COMMENTS   Treatment of the underlying disease is the most important therapy. For SIADH tumor response is correlated with resolution of

Table 21-9

Clinical Signs and Symptoms of Hyponatremia

- Difficulty concentrating, headache, confusion, personality changes, lethargy
- Anorexia, impaired taste, nausea, vomiting, diarrhea
- Muscle cramps, weakness, fatigue
- Incontinence and oliguria
- Depressed deep tendon reflexes, seizure, coma, cerebral edema/uncal herniation and death

Table 21-10

Differential Diagnosis of Malignancy-Associated Hyponatremia

- Primary or metastatic disease causing:
  - Adrenal insufficiency and steroid withdrawal
  - Thyroid disease
  - Hepatic dysfunction and ascites
  - CNS involvement (stroke, mass, meningitis)
  - Pulmonary disease (including infection) and positive pressure ventilation
  - Renal disease and obstructive uropathy
- Chemotherapeutic agents
  - Vincristine, vinblastine, cyclophosphamide, and cisplatin are most common
  - Nephrotoxicity
- Fluids and parenteral nutrition
- Pain (and drugs used to treat pain—opiates, acetaminophen), nausea and vomiting, diarrhea, bleeding

Table 21-11

Clinical Features and Response to Clinical Challenges by Type of Hyponatremia

	Primary polydipsia	Hypovolemic	Reset osmostat	SIADH
Urine osmolality	<100 mOsm/kg	>100 mOsm/kg	<100 mOsm/kg	>100 mOsm/kg
Urine sodium	≤20-40 mmol/l	≤20-40 mmol/l	20-40 mmol/l	≥20-40 mmol/l
FE Na	>1%	<1%	>1%	>1%
Water excretion	Normal	Impaired	Normal	Impaired
ADH level	Low	High	Low, normal	High
Serum urea and urate levels	Decreased	Increased	Normal	Decreased
Response to 0.9% saline administration				
Serum Na		>5 mmol/l increase	Depends on osmostat level. Can concentrate urine if above.	No change
FE Na		<0.5% increase		>0.5% increase
Following normalization of hyponatremia				
Serum urate				Normalizes
Urine urate				Normalizes
Response to water loading			Able to dilute urine	Unable to dilute urine

*Hyponatremia is not necessary for a diagnosis of cerebral salt wasting, although they often present together.

Table 21-12

Diagnostic Factors Suggesting Syndrome of Inappropriate Antidiuretic Hormone (SIADH)

- Serum sodium <134 mmol/l
- Serum osmolality <275 mOsm/kg
- Urine osmolality >300 mOsm/kg or greater than serum pecific gravity may also be elevated
- Urine sodium >40 mmol/l (although not necessarily)
- Serum glucose and albumin should be normal
- Serum creatinine and BUN as well as urine urate are generally low

hyponatremia (9). If other factors, such as drugs, diet, or free water consumption are worsening the condition, appropriate adjustments should be made.

Hypokalemia is often present with hyponatremia and correction of hypokalemia will increase serum sodium either via osmotic shifts of sodium and free water or urinary losses. Administration of potassium therefore must be taken into account (see the formula below). Hyperkalemia, without obvious cause, in the presence of hyponatremia warrants consideration of adrenal insufficiency (11).

Treatment of hypotonic hyponatremia is dependent upon the cause, severity, chronicity, and presence or absence of symptoms (10). In general, correction of hyponatremia, regardless of etiology, should not exceed 0.5 mM/h or more than 10–15 mEq/l in 24 h unless severe symptoms are present (seizures, coma). In severe cases with acute onset of hyponatremia, rates of correction of 1–3 mM/h have been recommended for short periods (8, 10, 12).

Treatment of SIADH

The initial approach to mild, asymptomatic hyponatremia is fluid restriction to 500–800 ml/day or a negative water balance (6, 8–10).

Symptomatic or moderate to severe hyponatremia will likely require hypertonic saline administration. Isotonic saline should not be used in SIADH. The formula below can assist in determining the expected rise in serum sodium to a given quantity of fluid repletion (10):

Change in serum sodium = ((Fluid sodium + fluid potassium) – serum sodium) / (total body water + 1).

See Table 21-13. Total body water (TBW) is 0.6 in men and children, 0.5 for women. These values are slightly lower for older individuals. Based on the goal rate of change, the rate of fluid administration can be calculated.

Another method to determine the amount of saline necessary is to calculate the patient's sodium deficit and then the amount and rate of fluid administration needed to correct this deficit using the formula below:

Sodium deficit = TBW × weight (in kgs) × (desired serum sodium – current serum sodium).

The desired serum sodium is generally 120–125 mmol/l as correction to strictly normal levels of serum sodium via hypertonic saline is generally not necessary or desirable (6, 8, 10).

Diuresis (with furosemide) may be used to maintain appropriate volume status and to inhibit sodium chloride reabsorption in the kidney and thereby aid in sodium correction, but should be used cautiously to avoid overly rapid correction. Serum sodium should be monitored every 2 h initially and adjustments made accordingly.

Table 21-13

Fluid Choice for Correction of Hyponatremia

Fluid	mmol/l of sodium	Extracellular fluid distribution (%)
3% NaCl	513	100
0.9% NaCl	154	100
Ringer's lactate	130	97
0.45% NaCl	77	73

Salt supplementation (high-salt diet, salt tablets), loop diuretics, and water restriction are employed in the long-term management for SIADH once severe hyponatremia has been corrected.

DRUG THERAPIES   Demeclocycline, a tetracycline antibiotic that can block AVP activation of renal c-AMP, induces a state of nephrogenic diabetes insipidus. It can be given as 600–1200 mg/day in two–three divided doses if the above methods fail or cannot be tolerated. It should be renally and hepatically dosed. Photosensitivity, nausea, and nephrotoxicity may occur and it may take days to see a response (6, 8–10). Lithium, urea, and fludrocortisone are other medications that have been used in refractory cases (9).

FUTURE THERAPIES   New therapies including AVP receptor antagonists are being created, but are not yet widely available (6, 8, 12). They cause loss of water without loss of electrolytes and are targeted toward use in congestive heart failure, SIADH, and cirrhosis.

Treatment of Other Causes of Hyponatremia

Initial techniques for mild, hypervolemic hyponatremia includes both fluid and salt restriction. Further treatment must be based on the underlying etiology of the hyponatremia.

Patients who have hypovolemic hyponatremia with sodium loss may benefit from larger volumes of 0.9% sodium chloride initially, especially if blood pressure is low. However, these patients must be monitored closely as they approach euvolemia, as they tend to excrete water more rapidly than sodium as the impetus for ADH release declines, leading to more rapid sodium correction.

Reset osmostat, which is a special case of SIADH, presents as a mild, stable hyponatremia that generally does not require correction and is best treated by treating the underlying condition.

Treatment of hypertonic hyponatremia should be directed at the underlying cause.

Treatment Complications

A feared complication of overrapid sodium repletion is cerebral myelinolysis (8, 10, 12). This condition has been described most in the pons where it presents as a rapidly progressive weakness of limbs combined with dysarthria, dysphagia, seizures, and death occurring 2–6 days after correction, with CT and MRI evidence developing 6–10 days after clinical symptoms (12). Hepatic failure, hypokalemia, and malnutrition increase the risk of myelinolysis (10, 12).

HYPERCALCEMIA

Incidence and Risk Factors

Normal values for serum calcium levels are population, laboratory, and laboratory machinery specific. However, one author defined moderate hypercalcemia as total serum calcium (adjusted for albumin) greater than 12 mg/dl and severe as greater than 14 mg/dl (13). At our institution normal values for serum calcium are 8.5–10.5 mg/dl and for ionized calcium are 1.14–1.30 mmol/l.

Hypercalcemia may occur in as many as 30% of cancer cases (13, 14). Among solid tumors, breast, nonsmall cell lung cancer, squamous cell, head and neck, and renal cancers are highest risk; while in liquid tumors, multiple myeloma and lymphoma are highest risk (13–15). Hypercalcemia is uncommonly seen in other solid malignancies, such as colon, prostate, and small cell lung cancer.

The risk for hypercalcemia is determined by the histology and location of the cancer, the duration of illness, and the site of metastases (13, 14). Risk of death is reported to be higher in individuals with malignancy-associated hypercalcemia (13, 16).

Mechanisms

Normally PTH and vitamin D act on bone, kidney, and gut to maintain serum calcium levels. Hypercalcemia occurs when either intestinal absorption of calcium increases, bone resorption increases, renal reabsorption increases, or release of tumor-related humoral factors leads to increased serum calcium levels that exceed renal excretion. The two most common causes of malignancy-associated hypercalcemia are local, osteolytic activity of tumor cells and humoral hypercalcemia of malignancy (13). These two etiologies represent a continuum of malignancy-related pathology.

OSTEOLYTIC HYPERCALCEMIA   Osteolytic hypercalcemia comprises 20% of cases and is usually due to breast cancer, myeloma, and lymphoma usually in the presence of bone disease (13–15). Release of osteoclast activating factors including lymphotoxin, IL-1 alpha, TGF alpha and beta, TNF alpha, and IL 6 have been identified, among others (14, 15). In osteolytic hypercalcemia, phosphate is usually normal, while $1,25(OH)_2$ vitamin D_3, intestinal reabsorption of calcium and PTH are low, and renal clearance of calcium is increased (14).

HUMORAL HYPERCALCEMIA OF MALIGNANCY   The other 80% of hypercalcemia cases are due to humoral hypercalcemia via parathyroid hormone related protein (PTHrP) and are usually associated with squamous cell cancers, renal, breast, ovarian, or endometrial cancers and HTLV-associated lymphomas (13–15). Release of PTHrP appears to contribute to osteolysis locally and systemically by increasing osteoclast activity and therefore bone resorption.

Due to close homology with PTH at the amino-terminal end, PTHrP can also stimulate distal tubular calcium reabsorption and prevent proximal tubular phosphate transport, with calcium reabsorption being the most important mechanism (14, 15). In addition, PTHrP likely aids in development and progression of bone metastases and growth of cancer cells. PTHrP and severity of hypercalcemia are associated with worse prognosis (16).

Humoral hypercalcemia should be considered when PTH levels are low, when metastases are absent, and when metabolic alkalosis with low chloride and high bicarbonate concentrations are present. In addition, $1,25-(OH)_2$ vitamin D_3 and phosphorus levels are generally low, while urinary c-AMP concentrations and renal calcium clearance are high (14).

OTHER MECHANISMS OF HYPERCALCEMIA   There are further rare causes of malignancy-associated hypercalcemia that represent a small fraction of cases. These are included in Table 21-14 (13, 14).

Clinical Presentation

The symptoms of hypercalcemia can be remarkably protean with effects on numerous organ systems (see Table 21-15). The presence or absence of symptoms is dependent upon individual patient factors such as severity, chronicity, preexisting mental status, age, concomitant sedatives, or narcotics (13, 14).

Differential Diagnosis

The most frequent causes of hypercalcemia are cancer, primary hyperparathyroidism, and vitamin D intoxication (see Table 21-16).

Diagnosis

Ideally ionized calcium would be drawn given variations in calcium level by albumin level and the presence of calcium-binding immunoglobulins (13). If

Table 21-14

Rare Causes of Hypercalcemia in Malignancy

1,25-dihydroxyvitamin D (calcitriol) secreting cancers
- Rare, usually lymphomas, with extrarenal production
- Tumor cells increase the conversion of 25(OH)D3 to 1,25(OH)2D3, causing increased osteoclastic bone resorption and intestinal absorption of calcium
- PTH and urinary c-AMP are low, with increased urinary calcium excretion and GI absorption

Primary hyperparathyroidism
- Can coexist with PTHrP, in which case, both PTH and PTHrP are elevated. Incidence of copresentation may be 15% and occur most in breast, colon and lymphoma
- In addition, there are rare ectopic PTH secreting tumors
- Leads to increased renal tubular, GI calcium reabsorption, osteoblastic activity, and metabolic acidosis
- In isolated primary hyperparathyroidism, 1,25(OH)2 vitamin D3 is high

Drugs
- Administration of estrogen or antiestrogens (such as tamoxifen) in the presence of bone metastases has been associated with hypercalcemia

Table 21-15

Clinical Signs and Symptoms of Hypercalcemia

• Neurologic	Anxiety, depression, confusion, psychosis and hallucinations, somnolence and coma, hyporeflexia
• Cardiac	QT interval shortening, bradycardia, prolonged PR intervals, widened T waves, arrhythmia
• Gastointestinal	Nausea and vomiting, constipation, anorexia, pancreatitis, peptic ulcer disease
• Renal	Polyuria and dypsia, acute and chronic renal insufficiency, with chronic hypercalcemia: distal renal tubular acidosis, nephrolithiasis, nephrogenic diabetes insipidus
• Musculoskeletal	Weakness or fatigue

Table 21-16

Differential Diagnosis for Hypercalcemia

- Primary or tertiary hyperparathyroidism, thyrotoxicosis
- Hypervitaminosis D or A, increased calcium intake (milk alkali), total parenteral nutrition
- Drugs: lithium, thiazide diuretics, theophylline toxicity
- Granulomatous diseases including sarcoidosis, Paget's, acromegaly
- Acute renal failure
- Rhabdomyolysis, immobilization
- Pheochromocytoma, adrenal insufficiency
- Familial hypocalciuric hypercalcemia

total serum calcium levels are used, one should consider correcting for albumin level via the following formula (13):

$$\text{Corrected Ca} = \text{measured Ca} + 0.8 \times (4.0 - \text{measured albumin}).$$

In addition to calcium, serum electrolytes, phosphorus, BUN and creatinine, PTH, and PTHrP (as well as SPEP, UPEP, free serum kappa and lambda light chains, and Bence Jones proteins if myeloma is suspected) are often measured in malignancy-associated hypercalcemia. The presence of bone metatstases on radionucleide imaging may also help confirm the diagnosis. Distinguishing between rare causes of malignancy-related hypercalcemia and other causes usually requires further testing, such as vitamin D levels, thyroid function tests, fasting calcium to creatinine urine ratio, chest x-ray, and serum ACE levels.

Prophylaxis and Monitoring

The incidence of hypercalcemia may be falling due to the use of bisphosphonates; however there have been no controlled studies verifying this assumption.

There are no clear guidelines for the frequency of calcium monitoring. However, it should be based, at least in part, on the expected length of efficacy of any treatment rendered. For instance, for bisphosphonates, the treatment effect generally lasts a month or less. Measurement of serum or ionized calcium, urea and other electrolytes, albumin, volume status including urine output, and mental status are typical.

Treatment

The primary treatment of malignancy-associated hypercalcemia is directed toward the underlying cancer. However, Table 21-17 summarizes treatments frequently used as temporizing measures (adapted from Stewart 2005).

FIRST-LINE TREATMENTS

Hydration and Diuresis Mild hypercalcemia can be treated with saline hydration, and when appropriate, diuresis. Most patients with hypercalcemia are severely dehydrated due to calcium's effect on the kidney's ability to concentrate urine (as in nephrogenic diabetes insipidus) and decreased intake (14). Isotonic saline is used to improve renal blood flow and encourage calcium excretion via exchange for sodium in the renal distal tubule and is the mainstay of treatment. Attention must be paid to volume overload and electrolyte abnormalities. Loop diuretics (furosemide) may be used to help block renal calcium reabsorption while the patient remains volume replete.

Table 21-17

Treatment for Malignancy-Related Hypercalcemia

First line	Dose	Side effects	Second line	Dose	Side effects
Hydration	200–500 ml/h IV normal saline	Volume overload, electrolyte abnormalities	Calcitonin	4–8 IU/kg/day IM or SQ in divided doses Q6–12 h, may need to be given with steroids to avoid side effects	Nausea, flushing, tachyphylaxis, hypersensitivity
Diuresis	Dose by volume status and prior exposure to diuretics				
Bisphosphonates	Pamidronate 30 mg mild HC, 60–90 mg severe HC IV over 2 h in saline or D5W	Renal failure, leukopenia	Gallium nitrate	100–200 mg/m^2 IV over 24 h for 5 days	Nephrotoxicity, pleural effusion and pulmonary infiltrates, optic neuritis
	Zoledronate 4 mg IV over 15 min in saline or D5W 8 mg dosing for relapsed or refractory HC	Renal failure, osteonecrosis			
Dialysis		Hypotension	Plicamycin	25 µg/kg per dose given over 4–6 h in saline. A second dose may be given in 2 days	Renal insufficiency, hepatitis, thrombocytopenia, nausea and vomiting, coagulopathy
			Steroids*	1 mg/kg/day or 40–60 mg/day prednisone for no more than 10 d	Hyperglycemia, GI bleeding, myopathy, infections, confusion, hypertension

*For vitamin D secreting lymphomas.

174

Bisphosphonates   Most cases of hypercalcemia will require further treatment to decrease bone resorption, specifically bisphosphonates. Bisphosphonates are pyrophosphate analogs that inhibit bone resorption via osteoclasts but do not affect renal tubular absorption. They may also have an effect indirectly via osteoblasts (14). They require days to work and their effect generally last from 20–30 days. In the United States, two are available: pamidronate and zoledronate. Outside the United States, ibandronate and clodronate are also used.

Typical dosing for pamidronate is 30 mg IV for mild and 60–90 mg IV for severe hypercalcemia infused over 2 h in 50–200 ml of saline or D5W. Pamidronate can be used synergistically with calcitonin. Zoledronate dosing is 4 mg IV over 15 min in 50 ml saline or D5W for most cases of hypercalcemia, although lower doses are used in patient with some degree of renal impairment. The 8 mg dose is not FDA approved due to significant drug side effects and in studies was recommended only for relapsed or refractory hypercalcemia (17). Serum PTHrP levels greater than 12 are associated with a less robust response to treatment and more frequent recurrence of hypercalcemia with Pamidronate (15). Zoledronate appears to be the more potent bisphosphonate (17).

Dialysis   Dialysis is available for severe hypercalcemia with acute or chronic renal failure when other treatments cannot be used or are ineffective. However initiation of dialysis is best reserved for cases in which there are effective treatments for the underlying malignancy.

Supportive Measures and Follow-Up   All patients with hypercalcemia should have efforts made toward removal of exogenous calcium (including TPN, supplements, diet), discontinuation of medications that decrease calcium excretion or reduce renal blood flow (like thiazide diuretics, NSAIDs), and increased mobilization or physical activity (13).

In patients with hypercalcemia, oral phosphate administration can be used to limit oral calcium bioavailability and can make correction of hypercalcemia easier (13). Usual dosing is 1–2 g per day orally after meals in divided doses but must be monitored in patients with preexisting renal dysfunction or high serum phosphorus levels. Due to potential side effects, intravenous phosphorus is not recommended.

In cases in which no further cancer treatment can be offered, thought should be given to withholding or withdrawing treatment for hypercalcemia. If neurological depression predominates and other symptoms are not significant (anxiety, gastrointestinal distress), withholding treatment may be preferable and should be discussed with the patient and/or the patient's health care proxy and family.

Follow-up for hypercalcemia usually includes periodic calcium measurement and bisphosphonate administration.

SECOND-LINE TREATMENTS   Second-line treatments include calcitonin, gallium nitrate, mithromycin, and steroids. Calcitonin also acts by increasing urinary calcium and can be used synergistically with bisphophonates. Gallium nitrate increases bone formation, but the long infusion and side effects temper its use.

Mithramycin/plicamycin is an inhibitor of DNA-dependent RNA synthesis that decreases cell-mediated bone resorption by killing osteoclasts. It also has significant side effects. Corticosteroids likely decrease intestinal calcium absorption and inhibit osteoclast-mediated bone resorption and are best used in cases of increased $1,25(OH)_2$ vitamin D_3 or if the malignancy is responsive to steroids as a treatment as well (such as lymphoma), given the attendant side effects.

FUTURE THERAPIES   New therapies under investigation include humanized anti-PTHrP antibodies and inhibitors of the receptor activator of nuclear factor-kB (RANK) and its ligand (RANKL) system (14). RANK and the associated ligand lead to osteoclast formation, activation and survival, and bone resorption. Recombinant osteoprotegrin, a decoy receptor for RANKL, humanized RANKL antibodies and fusion proteins for RANK and RANKL are being studied for their ability to bind and prevent the above actions (14, 18–20).

REFERENCES

1. Cairo M, Bishop M. Tumor lysis syndrome: new therapeutic strategies and classification. Br J Haematol. 2004; 127: 3–11.
2. Annemans L, Moeremans K, Lamotte M, et al. Incidence, medical resource utilization and costs of hyperuricemia and tumor lysis syndrome in patients with acute leukaemia and non-Hodgkin's lymphoma in four European countries. Leuk Lymphoma. 2003; 44(1): 77–83.
3. Kalemkerian G, Darish B, Varterasian ML. Tumor lysis syndrome in small cell carcinoma and other solid tumors. Am J Med. 1997; 103: 363–367.
4. Goldman SC, Holcenberg JS, Finkelstein JZ, et al. A randomized comparison between Rasburicase and Allopurinol in children with lymphoma or leukemia at high risk for tumor lysis. Blood. 2001; 97: 2998–3003.
5. Becker MA, Schumacher HR, Wormann RL, et al. Febuxostat compared with Allopurinol in patients with hyperuricemia and gout. N Engl J Med. 2005; 353: 2450–2461.
6. Baylis P. The syndrome of inappropriate antidiuretic hormone secretion. Int J Biochem Cell Biol. 2003; 35: 1495–1499.
7. Kobayashi R, Iguchi A, Nakajima M, et al. Hyponatremia and syndrome of inappropriate antidiuretic hormone secretion complicating stem cell transplantation. Bone Marrow Transplant. 2004; 34: 975–979.
8. Miller M. Hyponatremia and arginine vasopressin dysregulation: mechanisms, clinical consequences and management. J Am Geriatr Soc. 2006; 54: 345–353.
9. Shapiro J, Richardson G. Hyponatremia of malignancy. Crit Rev Oncol/Hematol. 1995; 18: 129–135.
10. Adrogue HJ, Madias NE. Hyponatremia. N Engl J Med. 2000; 342(21): 1581–1589.
11. Milionis HJ, Liamis GL, Elisaf MS. The hyponatremic patient: a systematic approach to laboratory diagnosis. Canad Med Assoc J. 2002; 166(8): 1056–1062.
12. Gross P, Reimann D, Henschkowski J, Maxwell D. Treatment of severe hyponatremia: conventional and novel aspects. J Am Soc Nephrol. 2001; 12: S10–14.
13. Stewart A. Hypercalcemia associated with cancer. N Engl J Med. 2005; 352: 373–379.
14. Clines GA and Guise TA. Hypercalcaemia of malignancy and basic research on mechanisms responsible for osteolytic and osteoblastic metastasis to bone. Endocrine Relat Cancer. 2005; 12: 549–83.
15. Rankin W, Grill V, Martin TJ. Parathyroid hormone-related protein and hypercalcemia. Cancer. 1997; 80: 1564–71.
16. Truong NU, Edwardes MD, Papavasiliou V, Goltzman D, Kremer R. Parathyroid hormone-related peptide and survival of patients with cancer and hypercalcemia. Am J Med. 2003; 115: 115–21.
17. Major P, Lortholary A, Hon J, et al.. Zolendronic acid is superior to pamidronate in the treatment of hypercalcemia of malignancy: a pooled analysis of two randomized, controlled clinical trials. J Clin Oncol. 2001; 19(2): 558–67.
18. Oyajobi, BO, Anderson DM, Traianedes K, Williams PJ, Yoneda T, Mundy GR. Therapeutic efficacy of a soluble receptor activator of nuclear factor kb-IgG Fc fusion protein in suppressing bone resorption and hypercalcemia in a model of humoral hypercalcemia of malignancy. Cancer Res. 2001; 61: 2572–78.

19. Morony S, Warminton K, Adamu S, Asuncion F, Geng Zhaopo, Grisanti Mario. The inhibition of RANKL causes greater suppression of bone resorption and hypercalcemia compared with bisphosphonates in two models of humoral hypercalcemia of malignancy. Endocrinology. 2005; 146(8): 3235–3243.
20. Sato K, Onuma E, Yocum R, Ogata E. Treatment of malignancy-associated hypercalcemia and cachexia with humanized anti-parathyroid hormone-related protein antibody. Semin Oncol. 2003; 30(S16): 167–173.

PAIN MANAGEMENT

INTRODUCTION

Cancer causes pain. Although studies give varying results, even the most conservative studies report that at least 20% of patients have pain at diagnosis or in the advanced stages of their illness. Numerous studies show that clinicians often undertreat cancer pain and that undertreated pain causes undue burdens on patients and their families. Clinicians may underestimate how much pain patients feel, or not be facile in pain management techniques that have the potential to greatly improve a patient's quality of life. Patients' misconceptions about pain medications also contribute to inadequate pain management. Patients' may be reluctant to take pain medications for fear of addiction or worry that requiring pain medication indicates that death is imminent. Patients at particular risk for undertreatment include women, minorities, the poor, and the old (1).

PAIN ASSESSMENT

With simple treatments, more than 80% of patients can have their pain controlled (2). The first step in devising a pain management plan requires the patient to characterize the pain. It is helpful to distinguish neuropathic pain, which patients will characterize as burning, sharp, or shooting, from visceral and somatic pains, which are dull and aching. In a cancer patient, pain is usually caused by chemotherapy, radiation therapy, or tumor recurrence (3). Understanding the origin of the pain aids in the development of the appropriate pain management plan. Pain from bony metastases, for example, may require an NSAID or radiation; whereas pain from a local recurrence outside of the bone may require only opioids.

The next step is to assess the baseline level of pain using simple, validated methods such as visual analog scales, numerical scales (for example, from 1 to 10), or pictoral scales (faces, circles of different colors). Many clinicians are unaware that patients with chronic pain will often lack physiologic signs which may indicate pain. Patients with chronic pain rarely show signs of sympathetic arousal such as tachycardia or hypertension. Patient self-report is the gold standard of pain assessment.

THE EXPERIENCE OF PAIN

A patient's experience of pain is not limited to the physical sensations that they experience. Depression, anxiety, and existential distress can all exacerbate a patient's perception of and ability to cope with pain. Because psychosocial and spiritual factors play such a large role in a clinician's ability to treat pain, it is critical to include assessment of these factors when developing a comprehensive pain management plan. The comprehensive clinical assessment should therefore include:

- Psychological, social, financial, and spiritual sources of coping and of distress.
- An assessment of mood disorders: screen for and treat depression and anxiety.
- Evaluating how the patient and family are coping with the illness.

Table 22-1

A Step-by-Step Approach to Cancer-Pain Management

		Severe pain or pain persisting/increasing Potent opioid agent—morphine, hydromorphone, oxycodone, fentanyl, methadone ±nonopioids ±adjuvants and interventions (intrathecal device)
	Moderate pain or pain persisting/increasing Mild opioids—codeine, hydrocodone, tramadol, oxycodone ±nonopioids ±adjuvants	
Mild pain Acetaminophen or NSAIDS ±adjuvants (gabapentin, XRT)		

Source. Modified with permission from (4).

TREATMENT

The goal of treatment is to adequately manage the pain while trying to minimize toxicity. The WHO analgesic ladder (4) (Table 22-1) is a validated step-by-step approach that provides 88% of cancer-pain patients with adequate analgesia (3).

The ladder begins with acetaminophen and NSAIDs because they have minimal side effects. When prescribing acetaminophen, use caution in patients with heavy alcohol use as even therapeutic doses (4 g/day) can precipitate severe hepatotoxicity. Patients with stable chronic liver disease can take acetaminophen at therapeutic doses. Use NSAIDs with caution in patients with renal impairment. Overall, no NSAID works better than any other. However, individual patients may do best with a particular NSAID.

Starting Short-Acting Opioids

For moderate pain or pain that persists despite NSAIDS or acetaminophen, the next step is the initiation of short-acting opioids in conjunction with NSAIDs or acetaminophen. Consider the patient's preferences and experience when choosing an opioid, and avoid codeine except in a patient who has used it with success. Short-acting opioids are dosed every 3–4 h and delivered via the least invasive route that works, preferably oral.

Starting Long-Acting Opioids

For a patient with intermittent pain, short-acting opioids may suffice. However, for a patient with continuous pain or with a combination of continuous and intermittent worsening pain, the next step is to begin long-acting opioids.

Choosing the appropriate long-acting opioid dose requires multiple steps. First, determine the total daily dose required to provide adequate analgesia. Second, choose the long-acting preparation. Commonly morphine or oxycodone is used in a short-acting preparation and both have long-acting preparations that are inexpensive and well tolerated. The total daily dose of short-acting opioid can be directly converted to long-acting opioid. For example, a patient requiring 5 mg of oxycodone every 3 h is taking a total of 40 mg of oxycodone in a 24 h period. This patient may be started on 20 mg of long-acting oxycodone every 12 h. The appropriate dose for breakthrough pain is 10–20% of the total daily opioid dose.

Table 22-2

Recommended Initial Dosing Intervals (7)

Drug	Onset (Min)	Peak effect (min)	Duration of analgesia (h)
Morphine			
Oral, IR	15–60	30–60	4
Oral, SR			
Avinza			24
Kadian			12–24
MS Contin			8–12
Oramorph			8–12
Oxycodone			
Oral, IR	10–15	30–60	4
Oral, SR (Oxycontin)			8–12
Hydromorphone			
Oral, IR	15–30	30–60	4
Intravenous	1–2	5–20	4
Fentanyl			
Oral transmucosal	5–15	20–30	1–2
Transdermal (patch)		12 h	48–72
Intravenous	<1	5–15	0.5–1

Table 22-3

Opioid Equianalgesic Table (mg) (8)

Hydromorphone (Dilauded)		Morphine		Oxycodone	
IV	Oral	IV	Oral	Oral	IV
1.5	7.5	10	30	20	n/a

(Fentanyl transdermal patch 25 mcg/h = 50 mg oral morphine.)

In this case, that would be approximately 5–10 mg of oxycodone every 3–4 h as needed for pain (Table 22-2). Alternatively, if the patient requires a different opioid, it is possible to determine the correct dose using equianalgesic tables (Table 22-3). When converting a patient from one opioid to another, it is important to account for incomplete cross-tolerance by decreasing the dose of the new opioid by 25–50%. Patients will often require a lower dose of the new opioid because their bodies are not as efficient at metabolizing the new opioid.

Case Example

A 45-year-old women with breast cancer metastatic to her ribs presents to clinic and describes aching pleuritic chest pain that is worse with movement. For pain she takes 4 mg of oral hydromorphone (Dilauded) every 6 h around the clock. She complains that her pain medication wears off, and she is frequently in pain. What are the problems with her pain management? How do you convert her to a long-acting opioid and what breakthrough dose do you give?

Her first problem is that she is not taking an adjuvant that would minimize the toxicity of the opioid. Start an adjuvant medication such as acetaminophen or an NSAID. An NSAID would be a good choice in this patient because NSAIDs are particularly effective for bone metastases. If this works, she could take less opioid.

Her second problem is that with her persistent pain, her current dosing interval of 6 h is too long: the short-acting opioid has worn off in 4 h. She could take it more frequently, but every 4 h dosing is cumbersome and interrupts sleep. She needs a long-acting opioid. Since hydromorphone has no long-acting formulation, switch her medication to long-acting oxycodone (Oxycontin), long-acting morphine (MS Contin), or transdermal fentanyl. Of these choices, transdermal fentanyl is more difficult to titrate in a patient who is requiring multiple changes in dosing. Oxycodone and morphine, in their respective doses, are similarly effective and easy to titrate. Here is the procedure for changing her medication from oral hydromorphone to long-acting oral morphine:

1. Calculate her 24 h short-acting opioid dose:
   4 mg hydromorphone $\times$ 4 doses/24 h = 16 mg/24 h.
2. Look up the equianalgesic conversion from oral hydromorphone to oral morphine:
   Hydromorphone 7.5 mg oral = morphine 30 mg oral.
3. Set up an equation to convert the dose:
   Hydromorphone 7.5 mg = morphine 30 mg.
   Hydromorphone 16 mg/24 h = morphine X mg/24 h.
   Solve for X
   X = 64 mg morphine in 24 h.
4. Reduce this dose by 25–50% due to incomplete cross-tolerance between the old and new opioids. Choosing the lower reduction of only 25%, the final dose is computed as follows:
   0.25 $\times$ 64 mg = 16 mg reduction.
   64 mg $-$ 16 mg = 48 mg oral morphine in 24 h.
5. Divide the 24 h total into divided doses. Long-acting morphine can be given q 8 or q 12. Note: these medications should *not* be dosed TID, but rather q 8 h to ensure adequate analgesia and to decrease sedation. For this example, the q 8 h dosing is 48 mg/3 = roughly 15 mg long-acting morphine every 8 h.

Breakthrough Dosing

All long-acting opioids must be paired with an appropriate dose of short-acting medication in the event that the patient experiences breakthrough pain. The usual dose for breakthrough pain is 10–20% of the total 24 h dose. Opioids prescribed for breakthrough pain may be safely dosed as often as every 1–2 h. Short-acting opioids that are orally dosed reach peak analgesic effect at 1 h and last no more than 4 h. In this example, the patient is taking 45 mg of oral long-acting morphine per day. An appropriate dose for breakthrough pain would be 10–20% of the total daily long-acting dose or 5–10 mg every 4 h as needed.

Taking excessive doses of breakthrough medication can be a symptom of poorly controlled pain. Ideally a patient would not need more than two to three breakthrough doses over 24 h. If a patient requires more frequent dosing, the long-acting dose may be too low. To calculate the increase in the long-acting dose, add up the total amount of breakthrough medication taken in 24 h and convert it to the appropriate amount of the long-acting formulation that the patient is already taking. In this example, if your patient consistently took 5 mg of morphine every 4 h for breakthrough pain, the 24 h total (30 mg) should be given instead as long-acting morphine. Her previous dose of morphine 15 mg q 8 h could be increased to 30 mg in the morning and evening and 15 mg in the afternoon.

Safety

Care must be taken when dosing opioids in elderly patients or in those with hepatic or renal insufficiency as they will be more sensitive to the medication and experience side effects such as sedation at lower doses. Start at a low dose and increase slowly. The key to safe and competent pain management is assessment and frequent reassessment. Also, watch for delirium and sedation in patients taking concomitant benzodiazepines. Delirium can improve with a slight reduction in the opioid. While respiratory depression is a concern with opioids, it is always preceded by sedation, which is your early warning to decrease the opioid gently.

Side Effects

Common side effects of opioids include nausea, vomiting, sedation, and constipation. Nausea and sedation usually resolve within 1 week. However, patients who drive should not drive for 2 weeks after beginning a long-acting opioid or for one to 2 weeks after a change in their regimen. This waiting period gives patients time to become tolerant to the sedative effect of the opioid. In most cases no psychoimpairment remains 2 weeks after the change in the opioid dose. Constipation, unlike other side effects, does not attenuate with long-term use. Therefore all patients on opioids require a bowel regimen that includes a stimulant laxative (e.g., senna 2 tab po BID) and stool softener (e.g., docusate (colace) 100 mg po BID).

DIFFICULT-TO-CONTROL PAIN

Even with standard pain control, some patients still suffer. Patients with severe pain may need rapid titration of opioid medications; for protocols, see the NCCN guidelines on adult cancer pain (www.nccn.org). When pain is difficult to control, consider the following etiologies: neuropathic pain, incident pain, tolerance, addiction, somatization, and (the most frequent) undermedication.

- *Neuropathic pain*. Treat with effective adjuvants such as gabapentin (start 300 mg PO qhs and increase gradually to 300–600 mg PO TID, max 3,600 mg/day) or tricyclic antidepressants (nortriptyline 10 mg PO qhs and increase to therapeutic dose). Methadone, which blocks opioid and NMDA receptors, may also be helpful.
- *Incident pain* (such as before dressing changes or planned activity). Provide quick-onset, short-acting analgesia with an extra dose of short-acting opioid (use the breakthrough dose, 10–20% of the daily opioid dose). For incident pain due to bony metastases, consider adjuvants such as NSAIDS (ibuprofen 600–800 mg PO TID) or radiation treatment.
- *Tolerance*. Consider increasing the opioid dose or changing the opioid.
- *Psychological addiction*. It is rare in cancer patients treated with narcotics (5), but patients who have a history of substance abuse have a higher risk (6).
- *Somatization*. Consult the psychiatry, pain, or palliative-care services.

TRANSDERMAL FENTANYL PATCH

Transdermal fentanyl, a long-acting fentanyl preparation available in a patch, is changed every 48–72 h. It is ideal for patients who have trouble taking oral medication, due to nausea, difficulty swallowing, or gastrointestinal tract dysfunction. Fentanyl, a lipophile, diffuses into the fat of the skin and then into the bloodstream, so place the patch over an area of the body with subcutaneous fat such as the abdomen, upper arm, or buttocks. The patch is not an effective initial treatment for severe pain because at least 12 h are required to build enough drug in the fat reservoir to establish adequate blood levels. Frequent rescue dosing is needed for the first 12–24 h until the fentanyl accumulates. Because the patches need a reservoir of subcutaneous fat, they are not recommended for

Table 22-4

Guidelines for Immediate Discontinuation of Opioid and Rotation to Methadone (9)

Morphine dose	Ratio to convert to methadone
<100 mg/24 h	1 mg of methadone for every 3 mg of morphine (1:3)
101–300 mg/24 h	1:5
301–600 mg/24 h	1:10
601–800 mg/24 h	1:12
801–1,000 mg/24 h	1:15
>1,000 mg/24 h	1:20

patients who weigh less than 110 lb or for older cachectic patients. In contrast, febrile patients may have increased absorption and suffer possible toxicity.

METHADONE

Rotation to methadone is complex because methadone has a long half-life, accumulates in the fat stores, and it potency increases when a patient is taking another opioid. Methadone can be up to 10 times more powerful in patients on high doses of opioids than in patients who are opioid naive or on lower doses (Table 22-4). Contact a pain or palliative-care specialist for assistance when converting to methadone.

Oversedation

Opioid respiratory depression is due to generalized CNS depression. Therefore when respiratory depression is due to an overdose of opioids, it is always preceded by somnolence. Respiratory depression due to opioids does not commonly occur in patients on a stable dose of opioids unless the patient is experiencing alterations in metabolism or excretion of the drug or has been given another sedating medication such as benzodiazepines. Therefore, if sedation does occur, it is important to evaluate for a change in renal or hepatic function. In the sedated but clinically stable patient, initial management includes discontinuation of the opioid, supplemental oxygen, and efforts to arouse the patient. For significant respiratory depression, dilute 0.4 mg naloxone into 10 cc of normal saline and administer 1 cc every 1–2 min until the respiratory rate is satisfactory. The clinical goal is to reverse the respiratory depression without reversing the analgesic effect of the opioid. Beware that too rapid infusion of naloxone may precipitate a pain crisis in a patient on chronic opioids.

CONCLUSION

Effective management of cancer pain requires a systematic approach that includes assessment of symptoms, aggressive pharmacologic and nonpharmacologic treatment (relaxation exercises, massage, cognitive-behavioral therapy, and exercise), and education of the patient and family about how to achieve optimal pain control. Involve specialty services when your patient does not respond to standard treatments.

REFERENCES

1. American Pain Society. "Guideline for the Management of Cancer Pain in Adults and Children," American Pain Society, Glenview, IL, 2005.
2. Zech DF, Groud S, Lynch J, et al. Validation of world health organization guidelines for cancer pain relief: a 10-year prospective study. Pain. 1995; 63: 65–76.
3. Portney RK, Lesage P. Management of cancer pain. Lancet. 1999; 353: 1695–700.
4. WHO Expert Committee on Cancer Pain Relief and Active Supportive Care. "Cancer Pain Relief and Palliative Care: Report of a WHO Expert Committee," World Health Organization, Geneva, 1990.
5. Schug SA, Zech D, Grond S, et al. A long-term survey of morphine in cancer pain patients. J Pain Symptom Manage. 1992; 7: 259–66.
6. Passik SD, Kirsh KL, Donaghy KB, et al. Pain and aberrant drug-related behaviors in medically ill patients with and without histories of substance abuse. Clin J Pain. 2006; 22: 173–181.
7. Omoigui, S. "Pain Drugs Handbook," 2nd edition, Blackwell Science, Malden, MA, 1999.
8. American Pain Society. "Principals of Analgesic Use in the Treatment of Acute Pain and Cancer Pain," American Pain Society, Glenview, IL, 2003.
9. Ayonrinde OT, Bridge DT. The rediscovery of methadone for cancer pain management. Med J Aust. 2000; 173(10): 536–540.

COMPREHENSIVE END-OF-LIFE CARE

INTRODUCTION

Comprehensive end-of-life (EOL) care is an essential component of oncology. While we aim to cure as many cancer patients as possible, many of them ultimately die of their disease. Our role as physicians includes guiding patients and their families through the EOL. One of the most difficult challenges of oncology is the balance between maintaining hope and preparing patients for death. In many areas in oncology, we face this task daily. Overcoming this challenge requires skills in communication, symptom management, and knowledge of the services available in the community.

END-OF-LIFE CARE COMMUNICATION

Overview

Like other components of medical care, communication in EOL care is a skill, which must be learned and practiced. Clinicians should be proficient in EOL communication in order to lead patients and their families through discussions regarding goals of care.

One of the largest challenges we face is the dichotomy between cure and palliation. Traditionally, these goals have been viewed as mutual exclusive. Much of this historical division is based on the reimbursement system in the United States. Medicare covers curative therapies and the hospice benefit covers palliative therapies. Clinicians have tended to follow this model of care and have not focused on palliation and EOL communication until all life-prolonging options have been exhausted. However, cancer patients and their families benefit greatly from receiving palliative therapies, communication regarding the goals of care, and psychosocial support throughout the course of their illness.

How should we guide conversations in making EOL care decisions? The first step in EOL care communication is to set an appropriate environment. The clinician should ask the patient who he or she would like present in the discussion. He or she should arrange a quiet, private setting and ensure there is ample sitting room for all participants. The clinician should be well prepared for the meeting and know the basic information about the patient's disease, prognosis, and options. The conversation should start with the clinician establishing what the patient and family know about their illness. The clinician can then build on the patient's illness understanding by clarifying realistic goals and addressing unrealistic expectations. Once the clinician and patient establish the goals of care, decision-making on how to achieve these goals should follow. This model can be used for communicating bad news, discussing advanced care planning, and shifting toward palliative care (1).

Discussing Prognosis

A patient's understanding of his prognosis may directly impact his decision-making at the end of life. Patients who overestimate their survival may choose life-prolonging therapies or invasive procedures rather than supportive care. Patients must have a clear understanding of the utility of therapies on their life expectancy and quality of life in order to make appropriate choices (2). The study to understand prognoses and preferences for risks of treatment (SUP-PORT) was one of the largest and broad reaching efforts to understand patient's preferences for outcomes based on their understanding of prognosis (3). The initial report revealed that the physicians caring for seriously ill hospitalized patients did not know their patients preferences for care. An analysis focusing only on patients with metastatic colon cancer or nonsmall cell lung cancer revealed that patient's overly optimistic prognostic estimates led them to choose medically futile therapies (4). Therefore, it is essential that patients with life-threatening cancers receive full prognostic disclosure from their clinicians.

Advanced Care Planning and Code Status Discussions

Advanced care planning (ACP) is the process by which patients describe their preferences for future care. ACP is essential for any patient with a life-threatening illness. It is an important step to ensure that patient's wishes are clearly documented if they are unable to express these wishes themselves.

Written advanced directives are the basis of advanced planning and serve two main roles. First, they can provide guidance regarding the aggressiveness of care a patient would desire at the time of a life-threatening event (living will). Second, they can identify a health care proxy (durable power of attorney for health care) to communicate a patient's wishes if he or she are unable to do so themselves. It is important that the designated health care proxies understand that their role is to provide decisions based on what the patients would want in that particular situation, not what they would choose.

Advanced directive should only be utilized when patients are unable to directly participate in decision-making about their care. While advanced directives can be helpful as a catalyst to discussions about current goals of care, they are not detailed enough to assist with many of the issues for terminal cancer patients. Advanced directives are not the same as do-not-resuscitate (DNR) orders. DNR is an order written by a clinician to formalize a certain set of preferences. The living will documents a preference, but is not an order. In addition, many of the terms used in a living will are ambiguous and require interpretation in the context of the current medical situation.

Initial discussions about ACP and code status should begin early in the course of disease in patients with terminal conditions. Once patients have already become ill, it can be difficult for them to think clearly about EOL care preferences. It is also challenging for the family members to be more objective about a patient's goals when he or she is ill or hospitalized. By beginning these dialogues early in the illness and revisiting them periodically, the idea of talking about death and dying and EOL care preferences is normalized (5).

Maintaining Hope

One of the most difficult tasks in oncology is maintaining hope while preparing for inevitable death. Patients often want to continually focus on the next treatment and avoid conversations about transitioning to a palliative approach. When physicians join in with their patients in focusing exclusively on hope, they may miss the opportunity to appropriately prepare patients and their families for death. While the two seem mutually exclusive, hoping for the best while at the same time preparing for the worse is probably the most effective strategy for dealing with patients with life-threatening illnesses.

It is useful to help our patients redirect unrealistic hopes for a cure toward other important goals as their diseases progress. Once death is inevitable, we should encourage our patients to hope for quality times with their loved ones, time for goodbyes and to bring closure to their lives, and for a peaceful death. Regardless of our efforts to redirect their focus, some patients will continue to express hope for a cure or further treatments for their cancer. Dr. Quill writes about the statement "I wish things were different" (6). This allows physicians to empathize with the patient and support their hopes, while acknowledging the realities of their prognosis.

PALLIATIVE AND HOSPICE CARE

Palliative Care

Palliative care teams consist of clinicians with expertise in the management of dying patients. The team usually includes a specially trained nurse and physician and often social workers, chaplains, and pharmacists. Palliative care teams can assist with symptom management, ACP, psychosocial support for patients and families, and spiritual and existential suffering. While the majority of hospitals in the United States do not have palliative care services, hospice organizations are increasingly including palliative care. Medicare allows for a hospice medical director to do a single home palliative consultation prior to hospice enrollment.

Hospice

The Medicare Hospice Benefit began in 1982 as part of the Tax Equity and Fiscal Responsibility Act. Hospice is an essential resource for terminal cancer patients. Hospice programs consist of interdisciplinary teams who offer comfort and dignity to patients and their families. They provide education and counseling for families and offer bereavement programs after death. The only entry criterion for cancer patients is that both the referring physician and the hospice director certify that the patient is terminally ill with a life expectancy of less than 6 months. While hospices will not provide life-prolonging therapy, it is not necessary for patients to be DNR.

All Medicare-certified hospices are required to provide four levels of care: routine home care, continuous home care, respite care, and inpatient care (7). However, 80% of patient care days must take place within the home. Routine home care includes nursing care, home health aides, social work, chaplains, and home therapists. Hospice provides the majority of the costs for prescription drugs related to the terminal illness and all durable medical equipment. Due to the capitated reimbursement program, hospices are limited in the amount of aggressive measures that can provide.

Bridge Programs

Bridge programs provide many of the services offered by hospice but eligibility is not limited by a prognosis of less than 6 months or an agreement to abstain from life-prolonging therapies. Bridge programs allow cancer patients to receive some degree of specialty nursing care while receiving anticancer therapy. They also provide for a smooth transition to hospice when the patient chooses to defer additional life-prolonging therapies.

SYMPTOM MANAGEMENT AT THE END OF LIFE

Symptoms at the End of Life

While palliation of symptoms is of utmost importance in all cancer patients, it becomes paramount in dying patients. With high-quality palliative care, most patients can have a good and peaceful death. Pain is a common symptom in dying patients and must be aggressively managed at all times. Pain management in cancer patients is another chapter, as are mood disorder and fatigue. Two other prevalent symptoms in terminal patients are dyspnea and delirium.

Dyspnea, an uncomfortable awareness of breathing, is very common in end stage cancer patients. Even patients without pulmonary involvement of their cancer can experience dyspnea at the end of life. Dyspnea cannot be measured, and it does not correlate with hypoxia, so it is important to ask patients if their breathing is uncomfortable. The mainstay of therapy for dyspnea is opioids. The relief of dyspnea is not related to respiratory drive suppression, so opioids will not hasten death (8).

The majority of terminal cancer patients experience some alteration in their mental status (9). In the last few days of life, many cases of delirium are not reversible. Correctable causes of agitation include medication side effects, pain, and bladder distention. Symptomatic management of delirium includes sedating agents such as benzodiazepines or neuroleptics.

Syndrome of Imminent Death

In the days immediately prior to death, nearly all patients go through a recognizable pattern of symptoms. It is important for clinicians to identify imminent death so that they can provide appropriate symptom management for patients and education for families. For example, while most clinicians are familiar with Cheyne–Stokes respirations and mottled extremities, family members are not. It is vital that family members know what to expect during the dying process. Since, this education process can be difficult and time consuming for clinicians, it may be necessary to seek the assistance of the palliative care team.

Patients can be "actively dying" for days or weeks, depending on their underlying health status. Some of the early changes include decreasing oral intake and increasing time in bed or sleeping. Patients will then become more difficult to arouse or be awake for only brief periods throughout the day. At this time patients may develop the "death rattle" when sleeping. This noisy breathing results from pooled oral secretions, which are not cleared due to loss of the swallowing reflex. In the last stages of active death, patients will enter a coma and have an altered respiratory pattern. They will develop mottled extremities as their cardiac output declines.

Caring for Dying Patients

Caring for an actively dying patient requires that clinicians regularly evaluate for the presence of new symptoms and review the medical list. As patients become more ill, they may be unable to take oral medications. Nonessential drugs, which are not contributing to comfort, should be discontinued. Clinicians should also ensure that unnecessary monitoring and procedures are discontinued at this time. It is also important that they continually communicate and educate patient's families about the process and therapies. It is important that patient's families have no uncertainties or unanswered questions about the care process.

REFERENCES

1. Morrison RS, Meier DE. Clinical practice. Palliative care. N Engl J Med. 2004; 350(25): 2582–2590.
2. Fried TR, Bradley EH, Towle VR, Allore H. Understanding the treatment preferences of seriously ill patients. N Engl J Med. 2002; 346(14): 1061–1066.
3. The SUPPORT Principal Investigators. A controlled trial to improve care for seriously ill hospitalized patients. The study to understand prognoses and preferences for outcomes and risks of treatments (SUPPORT). J Am Med Assoc. 1995; 274(20): 1591–1598.

4. Weeks JC, Cook EF, O'Day SJ, et al. Relationship between cancer patients' predictions of prognosis and their treatment preferences. J Am Med Assoc. 1998; 279(21): 1709–1714.

5. Back AL, Arnold RM, Quill TE. Hope for the best, and prepare for the worst. Ann Intern Med. 2003; 138(5): 439–443.

6. Quill TE, Arnold RM, Platt F. "I wish things were different": expressing wishes in response to loss, futility, and unrealistic hopes. Ann Intern Med. 2001; 135(7): 551–555.

7. Herbst L. Hospice care at the end of life. Clin Geriatr Med. 2004; 20(4): 753–765, vii.

8. Mazzocato C, Buclin T, Rapin CH. The effects of morphine on dyspnea and ventilatory function in elderly patients with advanced cancer: a randomized double–blind controlled trial. Ann Oncol. 1999; 10(12): 1511–1514.

9. Lawlor PG, Gagnon B, Mancini IL, et al. Occurrence, causes, and outcome of delirium in patients with advanced cancer: a prospective study. Arch Intern Med. 2000; 160(6): 786–794.

DEPRESSION, ANXIETY, AND FATIGUE

INTRODUCTION

Depression, anxiety, and fatigue are frequent complications of cancer and cancer treatment. Although fatigue can be caused by depression and anxiety, it is a separate symptom that often does not have psychological origins.

An estimated one-third of all people with cancer experience psychosocial distress. Psychosocial distress encompasses both psychiatric disorders as well as emotional states that do not meet full criteria for psychiatric illnesses. Depression, anxiety disorders, and adjustment disorders are the most common psychiatric disorders in cancer patients. Delirium, however, may be more prevalent in hospitalized cancer patients, affecting almost 25%.

REACTION TO DIAGNOSIS OF CANCER

A diagnosis of cancer can elicit a variety of emotions, including sadness, anxiety, anger, and fear. These symptoms usually are not part of a psychiatric illness. People may have difficulty sleeping, loss of appetite, anxious thoughts about their cancer, poor concentration, and low mood. These symptoms can persist for 3 weeks after diagnosis. Usually by 4 weeks after diagnosis, people have their coping mechanisms in place and the depressive and anxiety symptoms have resolved. Unless the psychological symptoms are severe or are markedly impairing functioning, the diagnosis of a psychiatric disorder is usually reserved during the first 4 weeks after diagnosis, while people are reacting and coping with learning they have cancer.

DEPRESSION

Depression can be used to describe a symptom, feeling sad, as well as a serious illness, major depressive disorder (MDD). MDD is associated with poor quality of life, worse adherence to treatment, longer hospital stays, greater desire for death, suicide, and, possibly, increased mortality (1).

Prevalence

Reports of the prevalence of MDD in people with cancer have varied widely, but the majority falls within the range of 10–25%. Similarly, the majority of reports of clinical levels of depressive symptoms, not necessarily MDD, in people with cancer are within the range of 10–15% (2).

Diagnosis

The diagnosis of MDD is made by using a set of diagnostic criteria that include having a persistently low mood and five of the following symptoms for at least 2 weeks: sleep disturbance; loss of interest or anhedonia (inability to experience pleasure); feelings of hopelessness, helplessness, or guilt; low energy; poor concentration; appetite disturbance; psychomotor retardation/agitation; and suicidal ideation. Because many of these symptoms overlap with cancer and cancer treatments, substitutive criteria have been proposed, such as the Endicott criteria which substitute four psychological symptoms in place of four of the more physical symptoms in the standard criteria. The inclusion of physical symptoms that could be related to cancer or cancer treatment in making the diagnosis of MDD remains controversial and the different sets of criteria may not yield markedly different results (3).

Differential Diagnosis

In making a diagnosis of MDD it is important to evaluate possible medical contributions to low mood and to consider the differential diagnosis. Untreated pain, hypothyroidism, and medications such as corticosteroids and certain chemotherapies (alpha interferon, pemetrexed, and procarbazine) may contribute to MDD. The differential diagnosis includes:

- *Adjustment disorder*. Low mood has been present for less than 2 weeks or there are less than five of the symptoms needed for the diagnosis of MDD. Adjustment disorders are usually in response to a negative event. Treatment usually focuses on symptoms such as sleep disturbance, and antidepressants are usually not prescribed unless the symptoms persist or there is significant impairment in functioning.
- *Delirium* (mood symptoms and cognitive impairment or psychotic symptoms). In delirium there is a generalized impairment of cognition, waxing and waning severity of symptoms, sleep–wake disturbance, language impairment, and psychotic symptoms, especially visual hallucinations and paranoid delusions. Agitation does not need to be present and in fact, one subtype of delirium, hypoactive delirium, presents with social withdrawal and inactivity, which is often mistaken for MDD. Addressing the underlying cause and the use of antipsychotics, not antidepressants, are the treatment for delirium.
- *Fatigue*. Fatigue may be difficult to tease apart from MDD because of overlapping symptoms. Anhedonia may be the best distinguishing factor for MDD. Severe hopelessness and suicidal ideation are usually less frequent in fatigue.
- *Anxiety*. Tearfulness and depressed mood when worries are about bad things happening, like disease progression or cancer recurrence can be anxiety. In this case the low mood is not persistent and is usually triggered by the anxious thoughts. However, anxiety and MDD often occur together.
- *Personality disorders*. Personality disorders can present with depressed mood, but the mood symptoms are not usually constant and persistent. Mood changes are usually triggered by a perceived injury or threat of abandonment. People with personality disorders can have difficulties maintaining stable social support and a history of self-harmful behaviors like cutting. Although antidepressants and other psychotropic medications may be useful in managing specific symptoms, the treatment of personality disorders is primarily behavioral.
- *Apathy*. Apathy is a neurological symptom that can also look like MDD and it is associated with a lesion in the frontal or temporal lobes. There is little spontaneous action or speech; responses are delayed, short, slowed, or absent, and it is usually associated with cognitive impairment and older age. Stimulants and dopaminergic medications may be helpful.

Treatment

Treatment for MDD consists of antidepressants and/or psychotherapy. Severe cases of MDD, especially those with wasting because of MDD, may be treated with electroconvulsive therapy. Although complementary treatments such as herbal preparations, acupuncture, and massage are available, there is currently little data on their efficacy for treating MDD in cancer patients. Suicidal ideation should be assessed and, if present, a referral to a mental health professional should be made.

ANTIDEPRESSANTS   Antidepressants are commonly used to treat MDD comorbid with cancer (Table 24-1). Antidepressants should be selected with potential side effects in mind. Side effects can be a negative in terms of tolerability, but a positive in terms of helping with accompanying symptoms such as sleep disturbance and poor appetite. Some of the selective serotonin reuptake inhibitors (SSRIs) (fluoxetine, fluvoxamine, and paroxetine) and buproprion may interfere with the metabolism of commonly used medications in oncology because of their effects on cytochrome P450 2D6 system (4). Antidepressants usually take 4–8 weeks to see full benefit, but some patients may show signs of improvement earlier. Antidepressants should be continued for 9–12 months after remission of depressive symptoms if this has been the person's first episode. Patients with recurrent MDD should continue the medication longer in order to lessen the chances of recurrence.

Stimulant medications may be beneficial for MDD in medically ill patients, but there is little evidence to support this practice. Stimulants, such as methylphenidate and dextroamphetamine, may lift mood, increase appetite, and improve fatigue. Effects of stimulants are usually seen within 1 week.

PSYCHOTHERAPY   Psychotherapy often needs to take a flexible approach because of medical morbidity and the demands of cancer treatment. Referrals should be made to trained therapists with experience in working with medically ill patients, if possible. Because issues around coping with cancer are often the focus, certain short-term therapies that target current life stresses and strengthen coping skills, such as cognitive–behavioral therapy, may be beneficial. Similar to antidepressants, these short-term therapies may still take weeks to see improvement.

ANXIETY

Less literature exists on anxiety in people with cancer than MDD. Anxiety can also be used to describe an emotional experience, feeling nervous, and also to refer to set of psychiatric disorders. Anxiety becomes a psychiatric disorder when it leads to functional impairment. Several kinds of anxiety disorders are seen in people with cancer, such as phobias, panic disorder, generalized anxiety disorder, and post-traumatic stress disorder (PTSD), as well as some presentations of anxiety that do not fit into the current diagnostic system, like persistent anxiety around cancer recurrence.

Prevalence

The presence of clinical levels of anxiety in people with cancer has been estimated to be as high as 30%, but the rates of the specific anxiety disorders is lower: panic disorder 6–7%, generalized anxiety disorder 5%, and PTSD 2% (5).

Diagnosis

- *Phobia.* A phobia is an extreme anxiety about a specific thing that leads to avoidance. Common phobias in medical settings include needles, blood, and confined spaces. Although the use of anxiolytic medication, like lorazepam, before entering a phobic situation may be helpful, the primary treatment is behavioral therapy.
- *Panic.* Panic is a constellation of physical symptoms (shortness of breath, palpitations, chest pain, abdominal discomfort, nausea, headache, and numbness/tingling) along with anxious cognitions, such as, "I am dying," or "I need to get out of here immediately." Panic attacks are recurrent, unexpected, and usually last less than 30 min. Panic usually first presents in early adulthood and onset late in life is unusual. Pulmonary emboli, which can have similar symptoms, can be misdiagnosed as a panic attack.

Table 24-1

Selected Antidepressants Commonly Used in Cancer Patients

Medication	Beneficial for these comorbid symptoms	Potential for drug interactions	Side effects	Starting dose	Dose range
Selective serotonin reuptake inhibitors (SSRIs)					
Escitalopram (Lexapro)	Anxiety, Hot flashes	Low	Nausea, anxiety, insomnia, headache, sexual dysfunction	10 mg qd	10–20 mg qd
Citalopram (Celexa) Sertraline (Zoloft)	Same as above, also available as liquids		Same as above but more GI side effects	20 mg qd 25–50 mg qd	20–40 mg qd 50–200 mg qd
Serotonin–norepinepherine reuptake inhibitors (SNRIs)					
Venlafaxine (Effexor)	Neuropathic pain, hot flashes	Low	Nausea, constipation, sedation, insomnia, increased blood pressure	25 mg bid-tid; 37.5–75 mg qd of extended release capsule (XR)	75–300 mg per day
Duloxetine (Cymbalta)	Neuropathic pain Hot flashes	Moderate: substrate for CYP 1A2+ 2D6; inhibitor of CYP 2D6	Nausea, anorexia, constipation, sedation, insomnia	20 mg bid	20–30 mg bid
Tricyclics					
Nortriptyline (Pamelor)	Inexpensive, diarrhea, sleep problems; neuropathic pain	Moderate: substrate for CYP 1A2+ 2D6	Constipation, orthostatic hypotension, sedation, dry mouth, cardiac conduction, confusion	10–25 mg qh	25–150 mg qh (dosed by serum level)
Newer generation antidepressants					
Mirtazapine (Remeron)	Least GI side effects, sleep problems, anorexia, available in dissolving tablet	Low	Sedation, weight gain	15 mg qh	15–45 mg qh
Buproprion (Wellbutrin, Zyban)	Fatigue, Least sexual side effects	Moderate: Inhibitor of CYP 2D6	Tremor, insomnia, restlessness, lowers seizure threshold	100 mg bid	200–450 mg per day

- *Generalized anxiety disorder.* Generalized anaxiety disorder is unrealistic and excessive worry for at least 6 months that is accompanied by motor tension, autonomic hyperactivity, or excessive vigilance.
- *PTSD.* PTSD is a constellation of symptoms that persist months after a traumatic event. Symptoms include nightmares, flashbacks, avoidance behaviors related to the trauma, and hypervigilance. Although having cancer can be thought of as "traumatic," the specific event is usually a particular point in time, such as waking up intubated and restrained in an intensive care unit.

Treatment

Similar to MDD, anxiety is treated with medications, psychotherapy, or both.

MEDICATIONS   Benzodiazepines are first line treatment of anxiety because of their quick onset of action. Benzodiazepines should be selected on the basis of their half-lives and duration of action. Short-intermediate acting lorazepam may be useful for situational anxiety around receiving a MRI, while longer acting clonazepam may be useful for preventing panic attacks throughout the day. In patients with impaired hepatic function, lorazepam, oxazepam, and temazepam are preferred because they undergo glucuronide conjugation. Side effects include sedation, ataxia, disinhibition, and confusion, especially in the elderly. Benzodiazepines can cause dependence and withdrawal, which is more likely with the shorter acting ones, like alprazolam.

Low-dose antipsychotic medications, once called major tranquilizers, can also be useful for the immediate treatment of anxiety. They may be used for anxiety resistant to benzodiazepines or in people in whom benzodiazepines should be avoided, such as someone who developed confusion from a benzodiazepine or someone with serious substance abuse. Atypical antispsychotics, such as olanzapine and quetiapine may be better both in terms of effect and side effects.

Antidepressants are effective for the treatment of anxiety disorders, but do not provide immediate relief. Higher doses and longer duration of treatment may be required compared to the treatment of MDD. Additional medications, like benzodiazepines, may be needed for more immediate relief while waiting at least 4 weeks for effects.

PSYCHOTHERAPY   Short-term targeted therapies that include increasing distress tolerance and strengthening coping skills, identifying cognitive distortions and catastrophizing, and systematic desensitization may be particularly beneficial. Other techniques such as distraction, relaxation exercises, and visualization are also helpful.

FATIGUE

Fatigue is the most commonly reported symptom in people with cancer and it is the symptom that causes the most functional impairment (6). Fatigue can be present at any time of the cancer trajectory. It may be the presenting symptom at the time of cancer diagnosis, occur during treatment, and persist into survivorship in some people. More is being learned about the physiologic mechanisms of fatigue related to cancer, but there are often identifiable causes that can be treated. Although psychiatric disorders, especially MDD and anxiety, can contribute to fatigue, they are often not present.

Prevalence

Reports on the rate of fatigue in people affected by cancer vary widely because of differing measures of fatigue and heterogeneous populations. It is estimated that 60–90% of patients have fatigue (7, 8).

Diagnosis

Fatigue is diagnosed by history. There are validated instruments for the measurement of fatigue, like the functional assessment of chronic illness therapy—fatigue scale (FACIT-F). Because questionnaires may not be feasible in busy clinical settings, the NCCN recommends screening for fatigue at visits with a one-item, 0–10 scale, similar to screening for pain, with, 0 being "no fatigue" and 10 being "the most severe fatigue." Scores of 4 or greater are recommended to have further evaluation.

Evaluation should consist of identifying any possibly modifiable causes of fatigue such as anemia, pain, sleep disturbance (insomnia, difficulty staying asleep, and sleep apnea), emotional distress (MDD and anxiety), poor nutrition, inactivity/deconditioning, medications and chemotherapies that cause fatigue (for example, gemcitabine, corticosteroids, narcotics, antiemetics, and beta-blockers), and other medical conditions such as hypothyroidism, hypogonadism, adrenal insuffiency, hypercalcemia, hepatic failure, and cardiovascular or pulmonary compromise. Fatigue can also be a side effect of radiation therapy. The time course of the onset of fatigue is also important in trying to identify possible causes as well as detecting preexisting fatigue in people with fibromyalgia and chronic fatigue syndrome.

Treatment

The primary treatment for fatigue is addressing the contributing factors described above. Persistent fatigue may be treated with stimulants, exercise, and behavioral interventions.

STIMULANTS   Stimulants, such as methylphenidate, dextroamphetamine, and modafinil, are commonly used in the clinical treatment of fatigue. Open label trials have suggested benefit, but randomized, placebo-controlled trials are needed to evaluate their efficacy. Stimulants may also help with mood, concentration, and appetite. Stimulants may raise blood pressure and heart rate and should be used with caution in patients with cardiac disease. Common side effects include constipation, sleep disturbance, anxiety, and anorexia, which is usually seen at higher doses.

EXERCISE   Several studies have demonstrated the benefit of exercise for fatigue in people with cancer (9). A physical therapist can design an exercise program, containing both strength training and cardiovascular, that is appropriate for a person with physical limitations from cancer or cancer treatments. For medically complicated patients, exercise might best be done in a cardiovascular or pulmonary rehabilitation center.

BEHAVIORAL INTERVENTIONS   Behavioral interventions have focused on energy conservation, prioritizing activities and delegating if possible, problem solving around difficulties caused by the fatigue, improving organizational skills, and trying to maximize functioning through careful observation of symptoms and planning activities around them.

REFERENCES

1. Richardson J, Sheldon D, Krailo M, et al. The effect of compliance with treatment on survival among patients with hematologic malignancies. J Clin Oncol. 1990; 8: 356–364.
2. Pirl WF. Evidence report on the occurrence, assessment, and treatment of depression in cancer patients. JNCI Monogr. 2004; 32: 32–390.
3. Kathol RG, Mutgi A, Williams J, et al. Diagnosis of major depression in cancer patients according to four sets of criteria. Am J Psychiatry. 1990; 147: 1021–4.

4. Kalash GR. Psychotropic drug metabolism in the cancer patient: clinical aspects of management of potential drug interactions. Psycho-oncology. 1998; 7: 307–320.

5. Kadan-Lottick NS, Vanderwalker LC, Block SD, Zhang B, Prigerson HG. Psychiatric disorders and mental health service use in patients with advanced cancer: a report from the coping with cancer study. Cancer. 2005; 104: 2872–2881.

6. Curt CA, Breitbart W, Cella D, Groopman JE, Horning SJ, et al. Impact of cancer-related fatigue on the lives of patients: new findings from the Fatigue Coalition. Oncologist. 2000; 5: 353–360.

7. Vainio A. Prevalence of symptoms among patients with advanced cancer: an international collaborative study. Symptom Prevalence Group. J Pain Symptom Manag. 1996; 12: 3–10.

8. Lawrence DP, Kupelmick B, Miller K, Devine D, Lau J. Evidence report on the occurrence, assessment, and treatment of fatigue in cancer patients. JNCI Monogr. 2004; 32: 40–50.

9. Ahlberg K, Ekman T, Gaston-Johansson F, Mock V. Assessment and management of cancer-related fatigue in adults. Lancet. 2003; 362: 640–650.

RESPIRATORY EMERGENCIES

Oncologic respiratory emergencies are remarkably common, and pulmonary complications are a primary cause of death in patients with malignancies. Lung cancer is the leading cause of cancer death in the United States, resulting in more deaths per year than the next four leading causes of cancer death combined, and the lungs and pleura are a frequent site of metastasis for most solid tumors. Dyspnea, defined as the subjective sensation of shortness of breath, is an ominous symptom in the cancer patient. In a review of cancer patients presenting to an emergency department with dyspnea, the median survival overall was only 12 weeks, and the median survival for lung cancer patients with dyspnea (37% of the total population) was only 4 weeks (1). While pulmonary complication are often the final terminal event in many patients with advanced cancer, respiratory emergencies and complications can also present a grave risk to life and/or quality of life in patients who still have the opportunity to achieve meaningful survival. Therefore, a working knowledge of the diagnostic and treatment approaches for these patients is critical.

The differential diagnosis for dyspnea in the oncology patient is broad and is outlined in Table 25-1. Usually, the diagnosis is directly related to the malignancy

Table 25-1

Causes of Dyspnea in Oncology Patients

Pulmonary causes

Airway obstruction/atelectasis due to tumor
Diffuse parenchymal metastases/lymphangitic carcinomatosis
Pleural effusion/pleural tumor
Pneumonia
    Community acquired, hospital acquired, postobstructive, aspiration, atypical,
        fungal, viral
Radiation pneumonitis/fibrosis
Drug-induced lung toxicity
Pneumothorax
Chronic obstructive pulmonary disease/asthma

Cardiovascular causes
Pericardial effusion/tamponade
Congestive heart failure
Myocardial infarction/Angina
Pulmonary embolism
Superior vena cava syndrome

Metabolic/systemic causes
Anemia
Metabolic acidosis
Hypersensitivity reaction
Overwhelming carcinomatosis

Other
Massive ascites
Anxiety

---

or its treatment. However, with improving therapies for malignancy, cancer patients are also at increasing risk for dyspnea caused by comorbid conditions that are unrelated though potentially exacerbated by their malignancies.

The approach to the dyspneic patient includes a rapid initial evaluation to ascertain risk of impending respiratory failure. Pertinent information from history involves determination of the type and stage of malignancy as well as the variety and timing of any antineoplastic treatments. Additional critical information includes the acuity of the onset of dyspnea and the presence of associated symptoms such as chest pain, fevers, cough, hemoptysis, palpitations, facial swelling, extremity edema, and syncope or presyncope. On physical examination, the presence of tachycardia and hypotension are essential to note as are the respiratory rate, oxygen saturation, and the presence or absence of a pulsus paradoxus. Deviation of the trachea must be noted along with an appreciation of any inspiratory stridor. A careful examination of the heart and lungs must be performed and the presence of any edema or ascites noted. Initial evaluation should include a complete blood count, a chemistry panel with a calculated anion gap, a chest x-ray, and potentially an arterial blood gas if the patient appears at risk for impending respiratory failure or if an acid/base abnormality may exist.

PULMONARY MALIGNANCY CAUSING DYSPNEA

It is remarkable how much of the lung parenchyma can be inhabited by diffuse metastases without causing dyspnea in a patient with otherwise healthy lungs. Therefore, multiple pulmonary metastases as a cause of new onset or worsening dyspnea in a cancer patient are a diagnosis of exclusion. Lymphangitic spread of tumor diffusely within the lungs is more likely to cause shortness of breath, and progressive pleural tumor as in the case of mesothelioma can also lead to increasing dyspnea. The treatment of choice in all of these cases is effective antineoplastic treatment. Depending upon the type of malignancy and the degree of prior treatment, such therapy may or may not exist. If there are no such options, palliative treatments including narcotics, oxygen, and hospice referral are appropriate.

AIRWAY OBSTRUCTION

Tumors within or surrounding a central airway (larynx, trachea, or proximal bronchus) can present with rather sudden onset of dyspnea or respiratory distress as tumor growth and/or secretions cause obstruction. In the case of very central tumors at the level of the trachea or carina, this represents a true emergency. Extrathoracic airway tumors present with inspiratory stridor. Atelectasis on imaging can be seen with more distal tumors. Surgical resection of the malignancy as a treatment option is usually reserved for those patients who can be approached with curative intent: laryngectomy in patients with squamous cell carcinoma of the larynx, tracheal resections in patients with primary tracheal tumors, and pulmonary resections in patients with localized primary bronchogenic carcinomas of the central airway.

In most cases of airway obstruction, surgery is not a treatment option either because of the degree of local invasion from the primary tumor or because of widely metastatic disease. In these cases, palliative treatments are appropriate. External beam radiation is the least invasive approach, and this can frequently be successful in cases of nonlife-threatening, partial airway obstruction, but radiation has limited efficacy in reestablishing patency of completely obstructed airways. In cases of life-threatening tracheal obstructions, tracheostomy may be required. For lower airway tumors, interventional bronchoscopic techniques can be particularly

Table 25-2

Interventional Bronchoscopic Approaches to Open Airways

- Mechanical debridement
- Laser treatment
- Photodynamic therapy
- Endobronchial brachytherapy
- Balloon dilatation
- Stent placement

valuable (2) (Table 25-2). Such techniques include mechanical debridement, laser therapy, endobronchial brachytherapy, and photodynamic therapy, all of which require intrinsic endobronchial tumor. If a tumor is causing stenosis by extrinsic airway compression, balloon dilatation and stent placement are potential options. External beam radiation and/or chemotherapy may be able to prevent restenosis following bronchoscopic procedures.

PULMONARY EMBOLISM

Pulmonary embolism is incredibly common in patients with malignancies. As discussed in the coagulapathy chapter, there are several aspects of malignancy that predispose patients to clots—immobility, surgical procedures, and the hypercoagulability of malignancy and chemotherapy. Pulmonary embolism is the one diagnosis that absolutely must be in the forefront of the minds of any clinicians treating cancer patients with dyspnea because:

- It is so common.
- It is a potentially rapidly fatal condition in patients who may otherwise have a reasonably long survival.
- Patients frequently do not present in a typical fashion.
- It can be notoriously difficult to positively diagnose or to rule out pulmonary embolism with absolute certainty.
- It is very treatable.

All patients with active malignancy or patients on chemotherapy have at least one risk factor for pulmonary embolus. This diagnosis should be considered in any such patient who is short of breath or who is experiencing chest pain. Supporting symptoms and signs include hypoxia, tachycardia, and lower extremity edema, but *none* of these symptoms is reliably present. It is critical to keep in mind that a normal oxygen saturation does not rule out pulmonary embolism, nor does a normal pulse rate, particularly in a patient taking beta-blockers. Some patients with pulmonary emboli may experience hemoptysis. Patients may even be entirely asymptomatic; incidentally noted pulmonary emboli are commonly visualized on thoracic CT scans of cancer patients.

Diagnosis of pulmonary embolism can be difficult. Ventilation/perfusion scans are unlikely to be definitive in patients with lung masses or previous thoracic surgery or radiation. A d-dimer, which can essentially rule out pulmonary embolism when negative, is typically not helpful in cancer patients because the d-dimer is frequently positive in cancer patients regardless of the presence of PE. Therefore, it has become common practice to immediately perform CT angiography in cancer patients in whom PE is suspected (3). This approach has the additional advantage of also contributing to the detection of other potential causes of dyspnea if PE is ruled out: pericardial effusion, pneumonitis, pneumonia, and progressive pulmonary malignancy. CT angiography can, however, miss subsegmental pulmonary emboli. The sensitivity of CT angiography for PE is

53–100%, while the specificity is 83–100% (4). Pulmonary angiography current-ly remains the gold standard for diagnosis of pulmonary emboli.

The preferred treatment for pulmonary embolism is immediate anticoagula-tion. There is frequently concern that brain metastases represent a contra-indication to anticoagulation, though the risk of bleeding for most brain metastases is fairly low. An exception to this includes metastases secondary to melanoma, renal cell carcinoma, and choriocarcinoma which do carry a bleeding risk. If a patient does have a true contra-indication to anticoagulation, then a filter in the inferior vena cava is a reasonable treatment option. It must be remembered, however, that the filter itself can form a nidus for clots, and the cancer patient with a known pul-monary embolus who is not anticoagulated remains at very high risk for deep venous thromboses within the legs which can lead to substantial morbidity.

PLEURAL EFFUSION

Pleural effusions in cancer patients are usually malignant in etiology, but other potential causes include congestive heart failure, pulmonary embolus, parap-neumonic effusions, and hypoalbuminemia. Lung cancer, breast cancer, and lymphoma are the most common causes of malignant effusions. Dyspnea results from compression of the lung. Thoracentesis can be diagnostic as well as ther-apeutic. Hemorrhagic and exudative effusions are very likely to be malignant in etiology, and fluid should be sent for cytology to determine whether malignant cells are present.

Invariably, malignant pleural effusions recur if the patient is left untreated. Chemotherapy-naïve patients with chemosensitive tumors (breast cancer, small cell lung cancer, lymphoma) are best treated with chemotherapy following initial percutaneous drainage of fluid. Patients with chemo-resistant tumors likely will require either a pleurodesis procedure or a pleural catheter. A pleu-rodesis procedure (sclerosis) can be performed through the placement of a chest tube. This allows for drainage of the effusion and reexpansion of the lung with resultant appostition of the visceral and parietal pleura. A sclerosant (doxycycline, bleomycin, or talc, most commonly) can then be instilled through the chest tube and thereby cause an inflammatory reaction which leads to fusion of the visceral and parietal pleurae and obliteration of the potential space in which effusions occur. Pleurodesis is effective in approximately 80% of cases of malignant pleural effusions and generally requires inpatient hospi-talization. Talc insufflation during video-assisted thoracic surgery can also be utilized to induce sclerosis. An alternative approach to chemical pleurodesis involves the placement of a small tunneled catheter into the pleural space. This can be intermittently drained when the effusion accumulates. This approach does not require full reexpansion of the lung and can generally be performed on an outpatient basis. In addition, the catheter itself frequently induces an inflammatory reaction and ultimately leads to pleurodesis.

TREATMENT-RELATED LUNG DAMAGE

Interstitial pneumonitis, at times progressing to pulmonary fibrosis, is a potential side effect of many antineoplastic treatments including cytotoxic chemotherapy (bleomycin), molecularly target agents such as the epidermal growth factor recep-tor inhibitors (gefitinib and erlotinib), and thoracic radiation. A list of the antineo-plastic agents associated with pulmonary toxicity is noted below (Table 25-3). Chemotherapeutic agents can also cause a hypersensitivity reaction with severe bronchospasm. Pneumonitis due to radiation generally occurs 1–3 months following treatment, and the risk increases with increasing treatment dose and volume of treated lung, and with the concurrent use of chemotherapy.

Table 25-3

Antineoplastic Agents Known to Cause Pulmonary Toxicity

Bleomycin
Gemcitabine
Cyclophosphamide
Methotrexate
Cytarabine
Mitomycin-C
Carmustine
Procarbazine
Busulfan
Paclitaxel
Docetaxel
Gefitinib
Erlotinib

In general, the management for all treatment-related lung toxicities is to stop the offending agent. Hypersensitivity reactions are best managed through administration of antihistamines and strreoids. In cases of pneumonitis, oxygen may be required in hypoxic patients, and steroids can be beneficial, though frequently a prolonged course with a slow taper is required. Prophylaxis for pneumocystis for patients on prolonged steroids should be considered.

PNEUMONIA

Pneumonia in combination with malignancy is frequently a lethal combination. In fact, in the Pneumonia Severity Index, "neoplastic disease" (defined as any cancer except basal- or squamous-cell cancer of the skin that was active at the time of pneumonia presentation or diagnosed within one year of presentation) weighs as heavily in predicting mortality as an arterial pH <7.35 and counts more toward predicting mortality than altered mental status, respiratory rate $\geq$30/min, or systolic blood pressure <90 mm Hg (5).

While oncology patients are clearly at risk for community acquired and atypical pneumonias, many are also immunocompromised due to the neoplastic disease, chemotherapy, or steroid usage and are therefore also at risk for fungal pneumonia and pnumocystis carinii. Due to altered mental status, tumor involving neurologic and/or muscular structures, vocal cord paralysis, or even profound generalized weakness, cancer patients are also at high risk for aspiration. Tumors within the bronchi can also lead to a postobstructive pneumonia. A high index of suspicion for a diagnosis of pneumonia and the broad type of pathogens that represent potential etiologies are critical to the successful management of pneumonia in cancer patients.

HEMOPTYSIS

Hemoptysis in cancer patients can be a simple nuisance or can represent a life-threatening emergency. Lung cancer is by far the most common malignancy to cause hemoptysis, and approximately 50% of lung cancer patients develop some degree of hemoptysis during their disease course. Usually hemoptysis is minor, resulting from a vascular endobronchial tumor oozing blood, but it can also be a result of infection or pulmonary infarction. Thoracic radiation can usually palliate minor tumor hemoptysis by causing tumor regression and coagulation of the vasculature.

Massive hemoptysis (defined as >600 ml in 24 h) in the cancer patient generally results from tumor or fungal invasion into the bronchial arteries or, less commonly, into the pulmonary arteries. Invasion of tumor into the central vasculature is a potential cause of sudden, catastrophic, fatal hemoptysis. A small percentage (approximately 3%) of lung cancer patients die of massive hemoptysis as part of the natural disease course, and most of these patients have squamous cell carcinoma (6). Bevacizumab, a monoclonal antibody against the vascular endothelial growth factor that shows promise in improving the overall survival of patients with advanced lung cancer, increases the risk of massive, fatal hemoptysis. It is therefore contraindicated in patients with squamous histology.

Early treatment of invasive fungal infections is a critical component of preventing hemoptysis in these patients. In cases of massive hemoptysis, immediate airway control through intubation and placement of the bleeding lung down has the best chance for producing a successful outcome. Bleeding may be manageable through bronchoscopic attempts at coagulation, catheter-directed embolization of a feeding bronchial artery, or, in the rare appropriate patient, surgical resection of the bleeding portion of the lung. In spite of any intervention, however, massive hemoptysis in the setting of malignancy is usually fatal (7).

PERICARDIAL TAMPONADE

Pericardial tamponade in cancer patients is most commonly caused by malignant involvement of the pericardium. However, thoracic radiation can also cause a reactive pericardial effusion that may progress to tamponade. Patients most commonly present with a sensation of dyspnea, frequently with associated lower extremity edema. On examination, they are usually tachycardic and may be hypotensive. A pulsus paradoxus of greater than 10 mm Hg is usually present in true tamponade, and frequently this is apparent on palpation of the peripheral pulses (8). Neck veins are usually elevated. Hypovolemia, however, may lead to extreme hypotension without respiratory variation, and therefore a pulsus paradoxus may not be detectable, and the patient also may not have substantial edema or distended neck veins. Chest x-ray may sometimes reveal an enlarged cardiac silhouette, but this only occurs in cases of particularly large effusions. Patients with tamponade do not normally experience pulmonary edema, and therefore the lungs are usually clear on examination and chest x-ray, and while patients invariably experience dyspnea, they are rarely hypoxic.

The diagnosis of tamponade is confirmed by echocardiogram. The pericardial effusion causes right ventricular diastolic collapse, and the filling of the cardiac chambers varies with respiration, respiratory variation. The only appropriate treatment for pericardial tamponade is urgent drainage of the pericardium, usually performed by a needle in the cardiac catheterization laboratory. Pending definitive drainage, it is critical to support the patient with intravenous fluids and to not diurese. Patients with malignant tamponade frequently develop recurrences. A hole cut into the pericardium, commonly termed a pericardial window, allows for outflow of the accumulating pericardial fluid and thereby reduces the risk of recurrent tamponade. Chemical sclerosing procedures, similar to those used for pleural effusions, can also be performed in the pericardium.

SUPERIOR VENA CAVA SYNDROME

Superior vena cava syndrome is a constellation of symptoms, usually facial swelling and flushing with dyspnea, resulting from obstruction of the superior vena cava. Usually tumor causes the obstruction, most commonly lung cancer, although lymphomas and germ cell tumors are also potential offenders.

Classically, SVC syndrome has been regarded as an oncologic emergency requiring immediate external beam radiation. However, unless a mediastinal tumor mass is also causing tracheal obstruction, fatalities attributable to SVC syndrome are distinctly uncommon. Chemotherapy rather than radiation may well be the most appropriate first-line treatment for some malignancies causing SVC syndrome. Therefore, it is critical that prior to initiating treatment, a pathologic evaluation of the malignancy must be performed. Steroids should be avoided prior to biopsy because these can partially treat a lymphoma and thereby make full pathologic characterization difficult to impossible. If it has been determined that the tumor causing SVC obstructing is unlikely to respond to chemotherapy or radiation or that more rapid palliation is required, placement of an SVC stent may be beneficial. It is also important to remember that not all cases of SVC syndrome in cancer patients are due to obstruction by tumor; thrombus formation, frequently around intravenous catheters or pacemaker wires, can also lead to SVC obstruction, and these should be treated by anticoagulation and/or removal of the thrombogenic nidus.

RESPIRATORY FAILURE

Many of the above diagnoses can ultimately lead to respiratory failure where the patient is incapable of maintaining oxygenation or ventilation sufficient to support life without mechanical support. While there may be a temptation for the patient, their loved ones, or their physicians to prolong life through any necessary means, rarely do patients with active malignancy and respiratory failure survive to breathe on their own. Ideally, physicians should discuss the futility of mechanical ventilation and patient preferences for care with their advanced-cancer patients well before the urgent circumstance of respiratory failure arises. Circumstances do not always allow for this. It is also important to remember, however, that some cases of respiratory failure in cancer patients are reversible, and in these cases mechanical ventilation may be appropriate. For example, patients with respiratory failure due to a particularly chemotherapy-sensitive malignancy (lymphoma, germ cell tumors, and small cell lung cancer) can be treated with chemotherapy while on a ventilator and survive to extubation, and may even achieve long-term survival.

REFERENCES

1. Escalante CP, Martin CG, Elting LS, et al. Dyspnea in cancer patients. Etiology, resource utilization, and survival-implications in a managed care world. Cancer. 1996; 78(6): 1314–1319.
2. Seijo LM, Sterman DH. Interventional pulmonology. N Engl J Med. 2001; 344(10): 740–749.
3. Wittram C, Maher MM, Yoo AJ, Kalra MK, Shepard JA, McLoud TC. CT angiography of pulmonary embolism: diagnostic criteria and causes of misdiagnosis. Radiographics. 2004; 24(5): 1219–1238.
4. Rathbun SW, Raskob GE, Whitsett TL. Sensitivity and specificity of helical computed tomography in the diagnosis of pulmonary embolism: a systematic review. Ann Intern Med. 2000; 132(3): 227–232.
5. Fine MJ, Auble TE, Yealy DM, et al. A prediction rule to identify low-risk patients with community–acquired pneumonia. N Engl J Med. 1997; 336(4): 243–250.
6. Miller RR, McGregor DH. Hemorrhage from carcinoma of the lung. Cancer. 1980; 46(1): 200–205.
7. Jean-Baptiste E. Clinical assessment and management of massive hemoptysis. Crit Care Med. 2000; 28(5): 1642–1647.
8. Spodick DH. Acute cardiac tamponade. N Engl J Med. 2003; 349(7): 684–690.

26	Karen Ballen

MYELOID MALIGNANCIES

ACUTE MYELOGENOUS LEUKEMIA

Etiology and Epidemiology

Acute myelogeneous leukemia (AML) is a disease of older people, with a median age in the sixth decade. Approximately 10,000 new cases of AML are diagnosed in the United States each year. AML is more frequent in men and in higher socioeconomic groups. Most cases of AML are idiopathic. However, AML is being seen more frequently in survivors of other cancers, as a result of chemotherapy and radiotherapy. Alkylating agents, such as melphalan and chlorambucil, can give rise to therapy-related AML, with a median time of onset of 5–7 years, and is associated with abnormalities in chromosomes 5 and 7. Epipodophyllotoxins, such as etoposide, can also cause therapy-related AML, with a median time of onset of 2–3 years, and is associated with abnormalities of chromosome 11. Myelodysplastic syndrome and myeloproliferative disorders, such as polycythemia vera and myelofibrosis, can also progress to AML. The risk of leukemia is 20-fold higher in patients with Down's syndrome (1).

- Most cases are idiopathic
- May arise from prior chemotherapy, radiotherapy, or myelodysplastic syndrome, or myeloproliferative disorders

Pathophysiology

Acute leukemia is a clonal disease involving stem cells. The myeloid cells in patients with AML do not mature normally, creating an excess number of myeloblasts. The proportion of blasts cells in S-phase (undergoing DNA synthesis) or in mitosis is lower than in normal bone marrow blasts. The myeloblasts eventually "take over" the normal cells in the bone marrow, resulting in hematopoietic insufficiency. The cell population can be predominantly eosinophils, basophils, monocytes, erythrocytes, megakaryocytes, or neutrophils or combinations of these cells. Single cells can demonstrate lineage infidelity and express lymphoid markers.

Diagnosis

The presentation of AML can be subtle with many patients presenting with days to weeks of nonspecific symptoms of fatigue, shortness of breath, and bleeding. A complete blood count, examination of the peripheral blood smear, and bone marrow aspirate and biopsy are essential in establishing the diagnosis of acute leukemia. The myeloblasts have distinct nucleoli, scant cytoplasm, and azurophilic granules. The characteristic Auer rods are formed by azurophilic granules within lysosomes. Histochemical stains can be helpful; for example, acute monocytic leukemia can be differentiated using a nonspecific esterase stain. Immunophenotyping by flow cytometry now helps to establish a definitive diagnosis and distinguish AML from acute lymphoblastic leukemia. CD33 is positive in approximately 75% of patients with AML, CD13 is positive in approximately 70% of patients with AML, and CD14 is positive in more than 50% of the monocytic and myelomonocytic subtypes.

- History and exam: Fatigue, shortness of breath, pallor, petechiae, occasionally splenomegaly, flow murmur. Skin, gum, and CNS lesions seen in monocytic variants.
- Laboratory: White blood cell count may be normal, high or low, anemia, thrombocytopenia. Examination of the peripheral blood smear mandatory and may show immature cells.
- Definitive diagnosis: Bone marrow aspirate and biopsy with flow cytometry, histochemical stains, cytogenetics, genetic markers (fms-like tyrosine kinase, flt-3). Definition of AML: >20% myeloblasts in peripheral blood or bone marrow

Treatment

Treatment of AML involves remission induction and postremission therapy. Induction chemotherapy for AML has not changed in the last 10 years. The mainstay of induction chemotherapy is 3 days of an anthracycline, such as idarubicin 12 mg/m^2/day, and 7 days of cytosine arabinoside therapy 100–200 mg/m^2. Experimental trials are underway to assess the addition of a third chemotherapy agent etoposide, addition of the proteosome inhibitor bortezomib, or addition of an oral antagonist to flt-3.

After remission is achieved, consolidation chemotherapy is given for 2–4 months, usually with high doses of cytosine arabinoside, in doses of 3 g/m^2/bid on days 1, 3, and 5 of therapy for 3–4 cycles. The landmark study performed by the Cancer and Leukemia Group B (CALGB) showed superior survival to the high dose ara-c regimen compared to lower doses; overall survival was 46% at 4 years in the high-dose ara-c group(2). There is no role for maintenance therapy for patients with AML (3).

Patients with a high risk of relapse, such as patients with complex cytogenetic abnormalities or secondary AML, should be considered for either allogeneic or autologous stem cell transplantation in first remission. Disease-free survival for patients with AML in first remission receiving an allogeneic transplant from a fully matched sibling donor is 70%. However, the transplant-related mortality is 20%. Disease-free survival for patients with AML receiving autologous transplants in first remission is 50% with a 5% transplant-related mortality. Results are worse for patients in second or subsequent remission with approximately 30% disease-free survival (see Chapter 37).

Elderly patients or patients with significant comorbidities do not tolerate induction chemotherapy well. Elderly patients are more likely to have poor risk cytogenetics and a history of myelodysplasia. Patients under the age of 70 with a good performance status should be considered for induction chemotherapy (4, 5). Older frail patients may be treated with supportive care approaches including hydroxyurea (6). Gefitinib is also being studied for the treatment of elderly patients with AML based on preclinical studies showing its capacity to induce myeloid differentiation in myeloid leukemia cells.

The majority of patients with AML relapse but the optimal treatment for relapsed AML has not been defined. Relapsed AML is not curable with standard chemotherapy. Patients who relapse more than 1 year after their initial therapy can be treated with idarubicin and cytosine arabinoside again. Patients who relapse within 1 year after their first induction are treated with different agents such as mitoxantrone and etoposide. Once a second remission is achieved, these patients should be considered for allogeneic or autologous stem cell transplantation:

- Induction chemotherapy with idarubicin and cytosine arabinoside
- Consolidation chemotherapy with high-dose cytosine arabinoside
- Stem cell transplantation for patients at high risk of relapse or for patients in complete remission 2

Complications

Both AML and the treatment of AML pose several life-threatening complications. The death rate from complications of induction therapy is approximately 10%. Leukostasis is more common with a blast count >100,000 and is characterized by pulmonary infiltrates, visual changes, and CNS bleeding. The treatment consists of intravenous fluids, hydroxyurea to lower the white blood count, and leukapheresis.

Infection is the most common cause of death in patients with AML. Patients are functionally neutropenic even if their white blood count is high. Gram positive infections such as staphylococcus and streptococcus have become the most common bacterial infections; gram negative infections, however, may be more immediately life threatening. The risk of dying from untreated gram negative sepsis is 20% within the first 24 h. The use of quinolones for prophylaxis has created the emergence of resistant gram negative organisms. Candida and aspergillus are the most common fungal infections. Aspergillus should be considered in patients with nodular or cavitary pneumonias. All febrile patients with AML should be presumed to have an infection and treated with broad spectrum antibiotics, such as cefepime.

Tumor lysis syndrome occurs because of the rapid destruction of tumor cells. The syndrome can progress to acute renal failure. Intravenous fluids, allopurinol, and alkalinization of the urine should be started before the start of chemotherapy. The recombinant urate oxidase rasburicase abruptly lowers the uric acid level and is being compared to allopurinol in a randomized study (7).

Bleeding is usually related to thrombocytopenia, and patients should receive prophylactic platelet transfusions for platelets counts below $10 \times 10^9/l$.

Disseminated intravascular coagulation is most commonly seen with acute promyelocytic leukemia (see below) but can also be seen with non-M3 variants of AML, particularly the monocytic variants. Treatment involves replacement of clotting factors with fresh frozen plasma and repletion of fibrinogen with cryoprecipitate.

Leukemic meningitis occurs in less than 10% of adult AML patients at the time of diagnosis, more frequently in patients with the monocytic variants of AML. Lumbar punctures should not be performed at the diagnosis of AML unless there is clinical suspicion (headache, change in mental status) for CNS disease. Leukemic meningitis is treated with intrathecal therapy such as methotrexate 12 mg given via lumbar puncture twice weekly until the CNS clears.

Leukostasis. Intravenous fluids, hydroxyurea to lower white blood count, leukapheresis, avoid red blood cell transfusions which increase viscosity

- Bleeding: transfuse irradiated, filtered platelets for platelet count <10,000
- Infection: treat fever presumptively as infection, and start with broad spectrum gram negative coverage
- Tumor lysis syndrome: preventive measures with allopurinol, IV hydration with bicarbonate

Table 26-1

Cytogenetic Abnormalities in the Myeloid Leukemias

Cytogenetics	Disease	Molecular marker	Prognosis
T (8;21)	AML		Good
T (15;17)	APML	PML–RAR-alpha	Good
Inversion 16	AML		Good
Normal	AML		Intermediate
–5	AML		Poor
–7	AML		Poor
11q23	AML	MLL	Poor
T (9;22)	CML	Bcr-abl	Poor prognosis for ALL

Prognosis

The overall 5 year survival for patients with AML is 25%. For patients over the age of 60, the 5 year survival is less than 10%. Patients between 60 and 70 years old, with a performance status of 0 or 1, primary AML, and no cytogenetic abnormalities have an overall survival rate of greater than 20% at 3 years. Patients under the age of 60 experience a 5 year survival of 40%. Remission is achieved in the majority of patients, but relapse is common, particularly in older patients. Older age, complex cytogenetic abnormalities, and secondary AML are poor prognostic factors. Cytogenetics can help define prognostic categories and determine who should receive more aggressive post-remission therapy, such as bone marrow transplantation (Table 26-1). Patients with the t (8;21) or inv 16 mutation have a more favorable prognosis. Patients with abnormalities of chromosomes 5 or 7 or complex (>3) cytogenetic abnormalities have a worse prognosis. Approximately 40% of adult AML patients have normal cytogenetics at diagnosis and have an intermediate prognosis. Molecular markers are now being used to determine prognosis in this group of patients; for example, mutations in flt-3 connote a poor prognosis and nucleophosmin gene mutations denote a favorable prognosis (8).

ACUTE PROMYELOCYTIC LEUKEMIA

Etiology and Epidemiology

Acute promyelocytic leukemia (APML) is a rare disease, with only 1,000 new cases per year in the United States. Most cases are idiopathic.

Pathophysiology

The breakpoint on chromosome 15 in APML occurs at the PML transcription unit and on chromosome 17, the retinoic acid receptor alpha gene is involved. A chimeric PML–RAR-alpha gene product is created. This breakpoint is associated with the dramatic response of APML to all trans-retinoic acid (ATRA) therapy.

Diagnosis

It is critical to make the diagnosis of APML quickly since the treatment is different than other subtypes of AML. Characteristic morphology is the presence of promyelocytes with intense azurophilic (red) granules. Many of the cells will have Auer rods. The nucleus is often bilobed or kidney shaped. However, in the microgranular variant of APML, the granules can be very small and difficult to see on Wright stain. The diagnosis of APML can be made by cytogenetics revealing the classic t (15;17) translocation. Molecular diagnostics can confirm the breakpoint of PML–RAR-alpha; this test can also be helpful to determine minimal residual disease after treatment. The white blood count is often lower in patients with APML than in the other subtypes of AML.

- History and physical with careful attention to bleeding and thrombosis
- Laboratory: CBC, Chemistry panel, uric acid, LDH, PT, PTT, DIC screen. Bone marrow with specimen for cytogenetics and molecular diagnostic studies for PML–RAR-alpha

Treatment

It is important to start therapy for APML promptly; 5% of patients with APML die before a diagnosis can be made. If a cytogenetic diagnosis is not available within 24 h and the diagnosis of APML is suspected, APML treatment should be started (9). The treatment consists of induction with ATRA given orally; chemotherapy, such as daunorubicin 50 mg/m^2/day for 4 days and ARA-C 100 mg/m^2/day for 7 days, begins 3–4 days after ATRA. The French APML trial reported a complete remission rate of 92% and a relapse rate of 6% with the ATRA plus chemotherapy approach. ATRA rapidly corrects the coagulation defects in APML. Consolidation therapy over 2–3 months is also ATRA based, usually with an antracycline. Two randomized studies have documented a benefit from ATRA maintenance therapy, given either intermittently or continuously. Some centers have shown a benefit to the addition of oral methotrexate and 6 mercaptopurine to ATRA maintenance therapy (10).

Elderly patients can be treated with ATRA alone or ATRA in combination with arsenic. Gemtuzumab (Mylotarg) also has efficacy in this setting.

Arsenic is the treatment for relapsed APML. Arsenic is administered as a daily intravenous infusion over 35 days. Approximately 50% of patients with relapsed APML will achieve a molecular remission after arsenic therapy. Electrolyte replacement and frequent EKG monitoring for prolonged QTc are part of routine monitoring during arsenic therapy. For relapsed patients a regimen of arsenic to achieve a second remission followed by autologous stem cell transplant for PCR negative patients will cure an additional 60% of relapsed patients (11).

- Start induction promptly with ATRA followed by anthracycline-based chemotherapy
- Consolidation chemotherapy with ATRA and anthracycline ± arsenic
- Maintenance therapy with ATRA ± 6 MP and MTX
- Relapsed patients: arsenic followed by autologous SCT

Complications

Tumor lysis, infection, bleeding, and leukostasis can occur with APML, as with the other AML variants. Bleeding is more common in APML; 40% of patients with APML present with low fibrinogens. Disseminated intravascular coagulation can present with thrombotic events such as stroke or bleeding, including CNS bleeds. Prompt treatment for disseminated intravascular coagulation includes cryoprecipitate, fresh frozen plasma, and platelets as necessary. The use of heparin is controversial in this setting.

APML has the unique potential complications of ATRA syndrome and DIC. ATRA syndrome occurs within the first few days of ATRA administration and is associated with a rapid rise in the WBC, fever, weight gain, and shortness of breath with pulmonary infiltrates. ATRA syndrome can be treated by promptly starting dexamethasone 10 mg twice daily. Severe cases require temporary discontinuation of ATRA. ATRA can be used safely in consolidation and maintenance even for patients who develop ATRA syndrome during induction.

A rare complication of ATRA therapy is pseudotumor cerebri, characterized by increased intracranial pressure, headaches, nausea, and visual changes. This complication is more common in children, and is treated by discontinuation of ATRA and diuretics such as mannitol.

- ATRA syndrome—high WBC, pulmonary infiltrates—treat with defamethasone
- To prevent bleeding, transfuse cryoprecipitate to fibrinogen >100, fresh frozen plasma to PT <15, platelets to platelet count >10 × 10^9/l
- Prompt (<24 h) initiation of therapy to avoid potentially fatal complications of DIC and bleeding

Prognosis

APML has the most favorable prognosis of all the acute leukemias in adults. Ninety percent of patients will achieve complete molecular remission after induction and consolidation therapy. Marrows performed at 10–14 days after chemotherapy will often be cellular; therefore, unlike other AML subtypes, the bone marrow can be assessed 4–5 weeks postchemotherapy. The majority of patients will have molecular evidence of disease after induction therapy; the European Program for the Study and Treatment of Hematological Malignancies (PETHEMA) group and American Intergroup studies have failed to find any correlation between postinduction PCR results and survival. After consolidation therapy molecular testing should be negative. Conversion from negative to positive PML–RAR-alpha is a harbinger of hematologic relapse. Approximately 70% of patients will be long-term survivors. For those patients who do relapse, arsenic reinduction followed by autologous stem cell transplant for PCR negative patients will cure an additional 60% of patients.

CHRONIC MYELOGENEOUS LEUKEMIA

Etiology and Epidemiology

Chronic myelogeneous leukemia (CML) is a clonal myeloproliferative disorder. The median age at diagnosis is 50 years. There is no particular socioeconomic, gender, or racial predisposition. The cause of CML is unknown.

Pathophysiology

CML was one of the first human cancers associated with a chromosomal abnormality, the translocation 9;22 or Philadelphia chromosome. This translocation creates a novel fusion gene, bcr-abl, which expresses an activated tyrosine kinase. CML develops when a single, pluripotential hematopoietic stem cell acquires the Philadelphia chromosome carrying the bcr-abl fusion gene, and creates a Ph positive clone with a proliferative advantage over normal hematopoietic cells. The uncontrolled kinase activity of the bcr-abl takes over the functions of the normal ABL enzyme, causing unregulated cellular proliferation and resistance to apoptosis.

Diagnosis

Most patients with CML, particularly in the stable phase (<5% myeloblasts in the bone marrow), are asymptomatic. An elevated WBC may be noted on a routine physical. Patients in accelerated phase (5–20% marrow blasts) may have night sweats, adenopathy, and splenomegaly. The blast crisis (>20% marrow or blood blasts) has similar presentation to acute leukemia above. The blood smear and bone marrow in CML will show an abundance of cells in all stages of maturation. The definitive diagnosis can be made by the presence of the bcr-abl translocation in the blood or bone marrow, determined by PCR analysis.

- Positive bcr-abl in blood or marrow diagnostic of CML
- Chronic phase: high WBC, often asymptomatic, <5% blasts, low LAP score
- Accelerated phase: may be symptomatic, 5–20% blasts
- Blast crisis: 70% myeloid, 30% lymphoid, like acute leukemia, >20% blasts

Treatment

The treatment for CML has changed dramatically since the approval of imatinib (Gleevec) in 2002 (12). Imatinib is a tyrosine kinase inhibitor that blocks the kinase activity of bcr-abl, and inhibits the proliferation of Philadelphia chromosome positive progenitors. Chronic phase disease is treated with imatinib at a dose of 400 mg/day. A randomized study is ongoing comparing 400 mg to 800 mg daily of imatinib. Approximately 95% of chronic phase patients receiving imatinib will have a complete hematologic response, 74% cytogenetic response, and 39% molecular response (13). Eighty-six percent of patients who achieve a complete cytogenetic response do so within 3 months. After 2 years, CML progresses in 3% of patients with a major cytogenetic response (<35% Philadelphia positive metaphases) and 12% of patients without a major cytogenetic response (14). Side effects of imatinib include nausea, rashes, headache, diarrhea, fluid retention, and cytopenias.

Allogeneic stem cell transplantation is now reserved for very young patients (under age 30), for patients who do not attain a molecular remission on imatinib, or for patients in accelerated or chronic phase. Cure rates of 70% have been reported, with either related or unrelated donors. However, the 100 day transplant-related mortality is 15–20% (see Chapter 37). A significant advance in the transplantation field is the recognition over the past 10 years that leukemia control is dependent on an allogeneic graft-versus-leukemia effect, first demonstrated in CML patients. Patients with graft-versus-host disease, particularly chronic graft-versus-host disease, have a lower risk of relapse, and patients who relapse after allogeneic transplantation can be cured by donor lymphocyte infusions.

There are several drugs in clinical trial for patients with CML who are intolerant to or resistant to imatinib. These drugs are tyrosine kinase inhibitors that have been shown in preliminary studies to induce a response in imatinib refractory patients. Dasatinib is a second-generation tyrosine kinase inhibitor that has activity in most kinds of imatinib resistant CML, except for those patients with the T315I mutation.

- Initial therapy with imatinib at 400 mg daily
- Allogeneic stem cell transplantation for patients with imatinib resistance or accelerated/blast crisis
- Nontransplant candidates who do not respond to imatinib 400 mg daily, consider trial of newer tyrosine kinase inhibitors, or increase imatinib to 800 mg daily

Prognosis

The prognosis for patients with CML has changed since the introduction of imatinib. The landmark IRIS study (a randomized study comparing interferon and cytosine arabinoside) resulted in complete cytogenetic response in 74% of the imatinib patients and 9% in the interferon group (13). Patients who achieve a complete cytogenetic remission and a 3-log reduction in bcr-abl transcript have a progression-free survival of 100% at 2 years. Patients who do not achieve a complete cytogenetic remission after 12 months of imatinib therapy had an 85% progression-free survival at 2 years. Deletions of chromosome 9q are associated with shorter survival.

Summary

Considerable advancement has been made in the diagnosis and treatment of the myeloid leukemias. In APML, the discovery of the PML–RAR-alpha translocation led to the development of directed therapy using retinoic acid. The cure rate is over 70% for patients with APML treated with retinoic acid-based regimens. Patients with CML are now able to take a pill, imatinib, and avoid or postpone the morbidity and mortality of allogeneic transplantation. Discovery of molecular lesions and targeted drugs in the leukemias serves as a paradigm for treatment of other malignancies.

REFERENCES

1. Lowenberg B, Downing JR, Burnett A. Acute myeloid leukemia. N Engl J Med 1999; 341: 1051–1062.

2. Farag S, Ruppert AS, Mrozek K, et al. Outcome of induction and postremission therapy in younger adults with acute myeloid leukemia with normal karyotype: a Cancer and Leukemia Group B study. J Clin Oncol. 2005; 23: 482–493.

3. National Comprehensive Cancer Network. Acute myeloid leukemia: clinical practice guidelines in oncology. J Compr Cancer Netw. 2003; 4: 520–539.

4. Anderson JE, Kopecky KJ, Willman CL, et al. Outcomes after induction chemotherapy for older patients with acute myeloid leukemia is not improved with mitoxantrone and etoposide compared to cytarabine and daunorubicin: a Southwest Oncology Group study. Blood. 2002; 100: 3869–3872.

5. Rowe JM, Neuberg D, Friedenberg W, et al. A Phase 3 study of three induction regimens and of priming with GM-CSF in older adults with acute myeloid leukemia: a trial by the Eastern Cooperative Oncology Group. Blood. 2004; 103: 479–85.

6. Estey EH. How I treat older patients with AML. Blood. 2000;96:1670–1673.

7. Jeha S, Kantarjian H, Irwin D, et al. Efficacy and safety of rasburicase, a recombinant urate oxidase in the management of malignancy-associated hyperuricemia in pediatric and adult patients: final results of multicenter compassionate use trial. Leukemia. 2005; 19: 34–38.

8. Schnittger S, Schoch C, Kern W, et al. Nucleophosmin gene mutations are predictors of favorable prognosis in acute myelogeneous leukemia with a normal karyotype. Blood. 2005; 106: 3733–3739.

9. Sanz MA, Tallman MS, Lo-Coco F. Tricks of the trade for the appropriate management of newly diagnosed acute promyelocytic leukemia. Blood. 2005; 105: 3019.

10. Sanz MA, Martin G, Gonzalez M, et al. Risk-adapted treatment of acute promyelocytic leukemia with all-trans-retinoic acid and anthracycline monotherapy: a multicenter study by the PETHEMA group. Blood. 2004; 103: 1237–1243.

11. Tallman MS, Nabhan C, Feusner JH, et al. Acute promyelocytic leukemia: evolving therapeutic strategies. Blood. 2001; 99: 3554–3558.

12. Goldman JM, Melo JV. Chronic myeloid leukemia—advances in biology and new approaches to treatment. N Engl J Med. 2003; 349: 1451–1464.

13. Hughes TP, Kaeda J, Branford S, et al. Frequency of major molecular responses in imatinib or interferon alpha plus cytarabine in newly diagnosed chronic myelogeneous leukemia. N Engl J Med. 2003; 349: 1423–1432.

14. Kantarjian H, Sawyers C, Hochhaus A, et al. Hematologic and cytogenetic responses to imatinib mesylate in chronic myelogeneous leukemia. N Engl J Med. 2002; 346: 645–652.

27	Dan L. Longo

HODGKIN'S DISEASE

Hodgkin's disease is a clonal lymphoid malignancy mainly confined to lymph nodes and lymphoid organs. For the period 1960–1963, 5 year survival from Hodgkin's disease was 40%; for the period from 1989 to 1993, 5 year survival had increased to 86%.

EPIDEMIOLOGY

About 7,500 new cases are diagnosed in the United States each year (roughly 2.9 per 100,000 population) (1). Males are affected somewhat more often than females (M:F 1.4:1). Hodgkin's disease accounts for about 11% of all lymphomas and is about half as common as multiple myeloma. It has a bimodal age distribution with the first peak in the late 20s and a second peak in late life. The etiology is unknown. Farmers, wood workers, and meat workers are at somewhat increased risk. A minor increased risk is associated with an HLA linkage dysequilibrium. Hodgkin's disease can complicate the genetic disease, ataxia telangiectasia, and occurs at increased frequency in patients with AIDS. An identical twin of an affected person is at 99-fold increased risk of developing the disease. Some geographic clusters have been noted and molecular studies have implicated Epstein–Barr virus in the pathogenesis of some cases, particularly cases in Central and South America and patients with mixed cellularity histology (2) (see below).

PATHOLOGY

Two major forms of Hodgkin's disease are recognized: classical Hodgkin's disease accounts for 95% of cases and nodular lymphocyte predominant Hodgkin's disease accounts for 5% (3). Classical Hodgkin's disease is divided into four histologic subtypes: nodular sclerosis (70% of cases), mixed cellularity (20% of cases), lymphocyte rich (3–5% of cases), and lymphocyte depleted (<2% of cases). As diagnostic methods have improved, cases of lymphocyte depleted Hodgkin's disease have declined both because some cases were actually other lymphoma entities and because earlier diagnosis has made the entity more rare.

The malignant cell of Hodgkin's disease is the Reed–Sternberg cell; it has different forms in distinct histologic subtypes. In classical Hodgkin's disease, it is usually derived from a follicular center B cell that has clonally rearranged its immunoglobulin genes but does not transcribe them. Thus, no tumor immunoglobulin molecules are detected. From a clinical perspective, the distinction between classical Hodgkin's disease and nodular lymphocyte predominant Hodgkin's disease is critical because the entities differ in natural history and in standard approach to treatment. The distinction between subsets of classical Hodgkin's disease is not technically difficult, but carries little impact as the natural history and management are not affected by the subset diagnosis.

Immunophenotypic studies define differences between classic and nodular lymphocyte predominant Hodgkin's disease (see Table 27-1). All forms of

Table 27-1

Immunophenotype of Malignant Cells in Hodgkin's Disease

	Classical Hodgkin's disease	Nodular lymphocyte predominant Hodgkin's disease
CD30	+	−
CD15	+	−
EMA	−	+
CD45	−	+
CD20, CD79	±	+
J Chain	−	+

Hodgkin's disease share three histologic features: effacement of the normal lymph node architecture; infiltration with a broad range of normal-appearing cells including reactive T cells, plasma cells, histiocytes, neutrophils, eosinophils, and stromal cells (the malignant cells are usually 3% or less of the total cells in an enlarged node); and presence of the characteristic neoplastic cells.

Nodular sclerosis Hodgkin's disease is the most common form in the United States and is slightly more common in women than men and in the younger age group. The disease grows in nodules separated by bands of collagen fibrosis and the Reed–Sternberg cell is the "lacunar" variant. The name derives from a fixation artifact that causes the cytoplasm to retract leaving a single or multilobed nucleus surrounded by a clear area.

Mixed cellularity Hodgkin's disease grows in a diffuse pattern and has a florid inflammatory cell background. Reed–Sternberg cells are usually binucleated with prominent nucleoli that give the cell an "owl's eyes"-like appearance.

Nodular lymphocyte predominant Hodgkin's disease is characterized by the lymphocyte and histiocyte (L&H) Reed–Sternberg cell variant that is also called a popcorn cell because of a lobulated nuclear contour that resembles popcorn. The cell expresses B-cell markers, surface immunoglobulin, often expresses epithelial membrane antigen (EMA), and cytoplasmic J chains. Unlike the Reed–Sternberg cell in classic Hodgkin's disease, it is CD30 and CD15 negative. The T cells that cluster around the neoplastic cells often express CD57, a natural killer cell marker and the tumor nodules contain a vague meshwork of CD21+ follicular dendritic cells.

GENETICS

Unlike other lymphoid malignances, Hodgkin's disease does not have a characteristic genetic lesion. The cells are aneuploid; Reed–Sternberg cells contain two–eight copies of individual chromosomes (3). A variety of genetic abnormalities have been noted, but none recurs in different cases at high frequency. Cells may contain mutant p53. Evidence for Epstein–Barr virus is noted in 30–60% of cases, varying with the technique used to detect it. It is commonly present in a clonal episome; however, the only consistent viral gene expressed in the cells containing the EBV genome is LMP1. Its role in the genesis or maintenance of the malignant cells is undefined.

CLINICAL FEATURES OF CLASSICAL HODGKIN'S DISEASE

Patients usually present with painless adenopathy localized to the neck. The mediastinum is involved in the majority of patients (~2/3), occasionally with large masses. When the mediastinal shadow is greater than 1/3, the greatest chest diameter on PA chest radiograph, the mediastinal involvement is considered massive. B symptoms are present in 20–25%. The disease tends to start in cervical nodes (left side more commonly than right) and march to contiguous lymph node groups. The first intraabdominal site is most often the spleen. Because the spleen has no afferent lymphatics, spleen involvement implies hematogenous spread. The liver is never involved unless the spleen is involved. Involvement of Waldeyer's ring or epitrochlear nodes is rare. Extranodal involvement is also unusual; when present, bone marrow, liver, lung, pleura, and pericardium are the most commonly involved sites.

In patients with B symptoms, the pattern of the fever may be intermittent. Pel–Ebstein fever describes a pattern in which fever is noted more or less continuously for 1 or 2 weeks followed by afebrile periods of similar duration. However, Pel–Ebstein fevers are unusual. When present, fever tends to occur every evening and breaks while the patient is sleeping giving rise to drenching night sweats.

Pruritis is common, but is not a B symptom. Patients occasionally experience pain in involved lymph nodes upon ingesting alcohol. This is thought to be due to alcohol-induced degranulation of eosinophils. A wide range of symptoms may be noted based on the direct effects of the tumor or paraneoplastic syndromes from tumor products. These symptoms are listed in Table 27-2.

Patients with AIDS who develop Hodgkin's disease are more likely to have mixed cellularity histology and to have extranodal involvement (2/3 of cases).

CLINICAL FEATURES OF NODULAR LYMPHOCYTE PREDOMINANT HODGKIN'S DISEASE

Patients are predominantly male, in the 30–50 year age group, and usually present with localized peripheral adenopathy involving the cervical, axillary, or inguinal nodes. Mediastinal, spleen, or bone marrow involvement are rare.

DIAGNOSIS AND STAGING

The diagnosis depends on an excisional lymph node biopsy. Needle aspiration is an inadequate diagnostic procedure in a patient with undiagnosed lymphadenopathy. Once a diagnosis is made, a variety of tests are performed to define the extent of disease and the presence or absence of factors that affect prognosis (see Table 27-3). As a result of the testing, the patient is assigned a stage of disease based upon the Cotswolds modification of the Ann Arbor staging classification (see Table 27-4) (4). Because of the orderly progression of Hodgkin's disease from one lymph node-bearing site to the contiguous node-bearing site, the staging system is an anatomic-based system. However, improvements in treatment over the last 30 years have changed the role of staging in patient management. Stage no longer affects prognosis as primary treatment leads to the cure of about 80% or greater of all patients at all stages of disease. Clinical features other than stage of disease may affect prognosis (Table 27-5).

Most patients receive systemic chemotherapy either alone or as part of a combined modality treatment program. Accordingly, the need for precise pathologic staging and exploratory laparotomy has vanished. This change in practice has served to reduce the acute surgical morbidity and mortality risk of the staging laparotomy and to avoid the increased risk of infection associated with splenectomy. Thus, the current state-of-the-art in staging evaluation is to perform clinical staging tests and to include systemic therapy in the management of all patients.

The most poorly evaluated common site of disease is the paraaortic lymph nodes. Bipedal lymphography is more sensitive and specific than abdominal CT in detecting paraaortic node involvement; however, the skill to perform lymphatic channel cannulation is disappearing from radiology departments and, unfortunately, the test is not widely available. However, the widespread use of

Table 27-2

Clinical Manifestations of Hodgkin's Disease

Findings at presentation
   Adenopathy, most often cervical
   Mediastinal mass
   Splenomegaly (in 25%)
Symptoms
   Fever, unexplained weight loss, night sweats
   Pruritis
   Alcohol-induced pain in enlarged lymph nodes
   Bone pain (rare)
   Pericardial effusion or tamponade (rare)
   Pleural effusion
Laboratory findings
   Granulocytosis
   Thrombocytosis
   Eosinophilia
   Elevated erythrocyte sedimentation rate
   Elevated alkaline phosphatase
Paraneoplastic syndromes
   Dermatologic
      Nodular prurigo
      Ichthyosis
      Psoriaform lesions
      Erythema nodosum
      Dermatomyositis
      Linear IgA bullous dermatosis
      Leukocytoclastic vasculitis
      Toxic epidermal necrolysis
   Renal and metabolic
      Nephrotic syndrome
      Hypercalcemia
      Hypoglycemia
      Lactic acidosis
   Neurologic
      Brachial plexopathy
      Guillian–Barre syndrome
      Sensory ganglionitis
      Acute cerebellar degeneration
      Stiff-man syndrome
      Ophelia syndrome

systemic treatment has resulted in no apparent cost in survival as a consequence of inaccurate abdominal staging.

TREATMENT

Primary Treatment of Nodular Lymphocyte Predominant Hodgkin's Disease

Patients with localized disease are often managed with involved-field radiation therapy (5). The disease may have long periods of remission punctuated by intermittent relapses that do not appear to affect overall survival. The natural history is quite prolonged with survival that is generally as good or better than classical Hodgkin's disease. Patients with advanced stage disease are usually

Table 27-3

Recommended Staging Evaluation in Patients with Hodgkin's Disease

Mandatory procedures
  Excisional biopsy of an involved lymph node
  History with attention to B symptoms
  Physical examination, record bidimensional dimensions of adenopathy, splenomegaly
  Laboratory tests
    CBC, differential count, platelet count
    Chemistry panel, liver and renal function tests
    Erythrocyte sedimentation rate
  Radiographic tests
    PA and lateral chest radiograph
    Abdominal and pelvic computed tomography (CT)
    Bipedal lymphogram (not widely available, yet the best test for paraaortic nodes)
  Bilateral bone marrow biopsies and aspirates
  Nuclide imaging
    PET scan or gallium scan

Procedures useful under certain circumstances
  Thoracic computed tomography if chest radiograph abnormal (of minimal value if chest x-ray normal)
  Liver biopsy if there is evidence of splenic or hepatic involvement
  Bone scan if bone pain is present
  Echocardiography if pericardial disease is suspected

Table 27-4

Staging Classification for Hodgkin's Disease

Stage	Definition
I	Involvement of a single lymph node region or structure (e.g., spleen)
II	Involvement of two or more lymph node regions on the same side of the diaphragm
III	Involvement of lymph node regions or structures on both sides of the diaphragm
IV	Involvement of extranodal site(s) beyond that designated as 'E,' more than one extranodal deposit at any location, any involvement of liver or bone marrow
A	No symptoms
B	Unexplained weight loss >10% of body weight in last 6 months Unexplained fever >38°C in the previous month Recurrent drenching night sweats in the previous month
X	Bulky disease: ≥10 cm maximal diameter of a nodal mass, mediastinal mass >1/3 chest diameter
E	Localized solitary involvement of extralymphatic tissue except liver and bone marrow: if this is the only site of disease, it is stage IE By limited direct extension from a known nodal site Single-discrete site proximal to a regional involved nodal site (IIE)

Table 27-5

Prognostic Factors in Various Settings

Early stage disease
B symptoms
Massive mediastinal involvement

Advanced stage disease
Serum albumin <4 g/dl
Hemoglobin <10.5 g/dl
Male sex
Age >45 years
Stage IV disease
Leukocytosis >15,000/mm^3
Lymphcytopenia <600/mm^3 or <8% of total white count

Once treatment has begun
Disease progression through treatment
Failure to achieve a complete response
Persistent PET-positive disease after cycle 2 or 3

After relapse
Short duration of initial remission
B symptoms
Multiple relapses

managed like patients with classical Hodgkin's disease (see below). About 3–5% of patients may undergo histologic progression to diffuse large B-cell lymphoma that is derived from the same malignant clone that gave rise to the Hodgkin's disease. Such lymphomas are usually responsive to combination chemotherapy and patients are often are put into long-term complete remission.

Primary Treatment of Classical Hodgkin's Disease

Combination chemotherapy is the cornerstone of Hodgkin's disease treatment. ABVD combination chemotherapy appears to have the best overall efficacy with the least acute and chronic toxicity (6, 7). Clinical staging followed by six cycles of ABVD chemotherapy is certainly a reasonable management approach. Controversy surrounds the use of radiation therapy in the management of Hodgkin's disease. Many have taken the approach that a shorter course of chemotherapy together with mantle-field or extended-field radiation therapy should further improved disease control. While combined modality therapy does somewhat lower the risk of relapse in previously involved lymph nodes, combined modality therapy has not been demonstrated to improve overall survival in early stage (8) or advanced stage disease (9). A key component to assess the impact of treatment is to measure both acute and chronic toxicities.

Radiation therapy to the mediastinum is associated with a threefold increased risk of *fatal* myocardial infarction (10) and an increased risk of second malignancies in as many as 30% of patients within 30 years of treatment (11). By contrast, randomized comparisons between ABVD versus ABVD plus radiation therapy have not demonstrated significant differences in outcome (12). In the range of doses used to treat Hodgkin's disease, no convincing evidence has been obtained of a dose response curve such that lower doses of radiation therapy are less likely to produce late fatal complications. Thus, it is safest to reserve radiation therapy only for the subset of patients who need it to optimize control of their disease.

Who, then, needs radiation therapy? About 5–12% of patients treated with six cycles of ABVD chemotherapy will not achieve a complete response. This subset of patients benefits from the use of radiation therapy to convert the partial response to a complete response. Patients with low volume residual disease have a very high rate of conversion to durable complete response. Patients with larger volume residual disease have about a 50% chance of achieving a durable remission. The small group of patients who have a tumor that grows in the face of chemotherapy have a poor prognosis and should be managed with salvage chemotherapy, see below.

Other patients might also benefit from added radiation therapy. Some data suggest that the persistence of PET-positive disease after two or three cycles of chemotherapy may identify patients at risk of relapse if managed with chemotherapy alone. In one series, 80% of patients had no residual PET-positive disease after two cycles of therapy; among the 20%, who had residual PET positivity, 2/3 of those patients relapsed (13). Thus, while prospective trials need to be performed, it should be possible to define criteria that permit the use of radiation therapy in the subset of patients who have the greatest need for its therapeutic effects while protecting the 80% or so of patients who do well without exposing them to the late toxicities of radiation therapy.

Other regimens have been advocated including Stanford V (14) and BEACOPP (15). Stanford V is a combined modality regimen that involves administering radiation therapy to 100% of patients. It should be kept in mind that it takes 20–30 years to assess the late complications from radiation therapy. Comments about technical advances that should lower the risks are meaningless until a lower risk is actually demonstrated. No one has demonstrated any therapeutic radiation technique that is not associated with late second malignancies. BEACOPP is a multidrug alkylating agent based regimen that is said to be superior to COPP/ABVD based on a randomized clinical trial. However, BEACOPP is highly myelotoxic and likely to have an unacceptable late toxicity profile, including secondary leukemia and myelodysplasia, especially because 75% of the patients also received involved-field radiation therapy. Efforts to improve treatment outcome by combining the active agents into 7-, 8-, or 10-drug regimens have not demonstrated clear superiority over ABVD alone.

Salvage Treatment

High-dose chemotherapy with autologous hematopoietic stem cell transplantation is the cornerstone of salvage therapy for patients with Hodgkin's disease who relapse or who experience progression during remission induction. The likelihood of success is related to the initial remission duration (16). Those whose initial remission lasted more than 12 months may have a 75–80% of achieving a durable second remission. Initial remissions shorter than 12 months identify a group of patients that have about a 40–50% chance of achieving a second durable remission. Patients with progressive disease during induction chemotherapy generally have a 20% or less chance of attaining durable remission.

Salvage treatment is administered in two phases; first a conventional dose regimen to achieve major reduction in tumor bulk and promote mobilization of hematopoietic stem cells into the peripheral blood followed by high-dose therapy with stem cell support. The choice of the conventional dose regimen is usually based on the original remission duration.

In general, patients who experience long initial remissions remain sensitive to the drugs that induced the first remission. However, alkylating agent based regimens like MOPP (17) or ChlVPP (18) may offer some advantage over a second course of ABVD in the setting of resistant disease (7) as the mechanisms of resistance to natural products like vinblastine and doxorubicin do not appear to influence alkylating agent based killing. Patients with initial remissions lasting less than 1 year should receive an alkylating agent based conventional dose salvage regimen. Patients who experienced progressive disease on ABVD may respond to MOPP or MOPP-like regimens. However, a newer regimen with novel agents such as ESHAP (etoposide, methylprednisolone, high-dose cytarabine, cis-platin) (19) may be more effective. One has considerable freedom of choice in selecting the conventional dose regimen. The goal is to achieve as close to a complete response as possible before embarking on the high-dose chemotherapy regimen. Patients entering the high-dose therapy phase with the lowest tumor bulk generally have the highest likelihood of attaining a durable remission.

A number of myeloablative regimens have been employed in the salvage treatment of Hodgkin's disease including BEAM (20), CVB (21), and high-dose melphalan (22) (see Chapter 36 High-Dose Chemotherapy). One has not been convincingly shown to be better than the others. It is important that the treating physician has experience using the regimens at these high doses. Doses and schedules of all the regimens are provided in Table 27-6.

Table 27-6

Treatment Programs for Hodgkin's Disease

Primary treatment programs
ABVD
        Doxorubicin 25 mg/m^2 IV days 1, 15
        Bleomycin 10 U/m^2 IV days 1, 15
        Vinblastine 6 mg/m^2 IV days 1, 15
        Dacarbazine 375 mg/m^2 IV days 1, 15
        28 day cycle
MOPP
        Nitrogen mustard 6 mg/m^2 IV days 1, 8
        Vincristine 1.4 mg/m^2 IV days 1, 8 (NO cap at 2 mg; dose
           reduction for motor, not sensory, neuropathy)
        Procarbazine 100 mg/m^2 PO days 1–14
        Prednisone 40 mg/m^2 PO days 1–14
        28 day cycle
ChlVPP
        Chlorambucil 6 mg/m^2 (10 mg maximum) PO days 1–14
        Vinblastine 6 mg/m^2 (10 mg maximum) IV days 1, 8
        Procarbazine 100 mg/m^2 PO days 1–14
        Prednisone 40 mg/m^2 PO days 1–14
        28 day cycle
Stanford V
        Nitrogen mustard 6 mg/m^2 IV on weeks 1, 5, and 9
        Doxorubicin 25 mg/m^2 IV on weeks 1, 3, 5, 7, 9, and 11
        Vinblastine 6 mg/m^2 IV on weeks 1, 3, 5, 7, 9, and 11
        Vincristine 1.4 mg/m^2 (capped at 2 mg) IV on
           weeks 2, 4, 6, 8, 10, and 12
        Bleomycin 5 U/m^2 IV on weeks 2, 4, 6, 8, 10, and 12
        Etoposide 60 mg/m^2 IV on days 1 and 2 of weeks 3, 7, and 11
        Prednisone 40 mg/m^2 PO every other day weeks 1–10
        12 weeks of therapy followed by radiation therapy to 36 Gy
BEACOPP
        Bleomycin 10 U/m^2 IV day 8
        Etoposide 100 mg/m^2 IV days 1–3
        Doxorubicin 25 mg/m^2 IV day 1

(Continued)

Table 27-6 (*Continued*)

BEACOPP (*Continued*)
  Cyclophosphamide 650 mg/m^2 IV day 1
  Vincristine 1.4 mg/m^2 (2 mg maximum) IV day 8
  Procarbazine 100 mg/m^2 PO days 1–7
  Prednisone 40 mg/m^2 PO days 1–14
  21 day cycles
Escalated BEACOPP
  Bleomycin 10 mg/m^2 IV day 8
  Etoposide 200 mg/m^2 IV days 1–3
  Doxorubicin 35 mg/m^2 IV day 1
  Cyclophosphamide 1250 mg/m^2 IV day 1
  Vincristine 1.4 mg/m^2 IV day 8
  Procarbazine 100 mg/m^2 PO days 1–7
  Prednisone 40 mg/m^2 PO days 1–14
  G-CSF SC from d*
  21 day cycles
Conventional-dose salvage programs
If ABVD was the initial treatment program, MOPP or ChlVPP should be the
  initial salvage regimen
If MOPP or ChlVPP was the initial treatment program, ABVD should be the
  initial salvage regimen
CR or good PR should be followed by high-dose therapy and autologous
  hematopoietic stem cell transplantation
If disease fails to respond or progresses through the initial salvage regimen
ASHAP
  Doxorubicin 10 mg/m^2/day continuous IV infusion days 1–4
  Methylprednisolone 500 mg/day IV days 1–5
  Cisplatin 25 mg/m^2/day continuous IV infusion days 1–4
  Cytosine arabinoside 1.5 g/m^2 IV day 5
  2–3 28 day courses and then high-dose therapy with transplant
Mini-BEAM
  Carmustine 60 mg/m^2 IV day 1
  Etoposide 75 mg/m^2 IV days 2–5
  Cytarabine 100 mg/m^2 IV q12h days 2–5
  Melphalan 30 mg/m^2 IV day 6
  2–3 28 day cycles and then high-dose therapy with transplant
If patient relapses after high-dose therapy with autologous hematopoietic
  stem cells, consider allogeneic transplant
If bone marrow donor is unavailable, useful palliative regimens include
  single agents
Vinblastine 4–6 mg total dose IV weekly
Gemcitabine 1,000 mg/m^2 IV days 1, 8 every 4 weeks
High-dose salvage and marrow ablative preparative programs
CBV
  Carmustine 300 mg/m^2 IV day-6
  Cyclophosphamide 1,500 mg/m^2/d IV days$-6,-5,-4,-3$
  Etoposide 125 mg/m^2 IV q12h days$-6,-5,-4$
  Stem cells on day 0
BEAM
  Carmustine 300 mg/m^2 IV day-6
  Etoposide 200 mg/m^2 IV days$-5,-4,-3,-2$
  Cytarabine 200 mg/m^2 IV q12h days$-5,-4,-3,-2$
  Melphalan 140 mg/m^2 IV day-1
  Stem cells on day 0

The consequence of this overall approach to treatment is cure of about 85–90% of the patients. However, some patients will not obtain a durable remission after high-dose therapy with stem cell support. It is important to keep in mind that it is still possible to provide palliation in such patients with the judicious use of single-agent chemotherapy. For example, weekly low-dose vinblastine (23) is extremely effective at controlling disease progression at doses that are not myelosuppressive. Anecdotes of prolonged survival with such palliative approaches foster a spirit of continuing to explore novel treatment options. Gemcitabine (24) has activity in patients with refractory disease. In addition, new approaches are in development including exploitation of the expression of CD30 on the tumor cells by agonistic antibodies and immunotoxins. For the subset of patients with matched sibling donors, allogeneic bone marrow transplantation is also an option and mini-transplants are being evaluated as an experimental approach.

Long-Term Follow-Up

About half of the patients destined to relapse will do so in the first year after treatment, and nearly all the relapses occur within 5 years of treatment. While it is common to follow patients every few months for the first couple of years gradually extending the interval between visits, there is no evidence that careful surveillance detects relapses sooner or that treatment outcome of those relapses is improved by the careful surveillance. Most relapses are detected by the patients themselves.

The point of routine follow-up of treated patients is not just monitoring for relapse but also monitoring for early and late toxicities of the disease and its treatment (25). Patients treated for Hodgkin's disease have an increased risk of secondary non-Hodgkin's lymphoma, often diffuse large B-cell lymphomas involving the gastrointestinal tract. As this complication seems to occur with equal frequency regardless of the treatment approach, it is thought to be a feature of the underlying disease. Patients also remain at infectious disease risk for up to a year after their treatment. This problem has been greatly ameliorated by the omission of splenectomy from staging workups and the decline in the use of splenic radiation therapy. Chemotherapy regimens each have their own special concerns. ABVD treatment must be monitored for bleomycin-related pulmonary dysfunction using diffusion tests, and bleomycin should be withheld if the diffusing capacity declines greater than 25%. The doses of doxorubicin are generally below the level that is associated with cardiac dysfunction, but patients need to be queried regarding exercise tolerance and fatigue. Alkylating agent based regimens (MOPP, ChlVPP, BEACOPP) induce infertility and, when used together with radiation therapy, increase the risk of developing acute leukemia and/or a myelodysplastic syndrome. The absolute risk is about 3%, and returns to zero if no marrow damage has appeared within 10 years of treatment (26). The alkylating agent based regimens also induce premature menopause; while this may somewhat reduce the risk of breast cancer, it increases the risk of osteoporosis.

Radiation therapy can produce xerostomia, dental caries, dysgeusia, and hypothyroidism, and can accelerate atherosclerosis with a threefold increased risk of fatal myocardial infarction. It also increases the risk of second malignancies in or adjacent to the treatment fields. The risk of second cancers begins to appear about 5 years after treatment and increases steadily for at least 30 years. A woman treated with mediastinal radiation therapy at age 25 years has a 30% absolute risk of developing breast cancer by age 55 years, compared to a 3% risk for an age-matched control. It is important that patients be informed of the risk and that healthy behaviors be encouraged including frequent surveillance. Women who received chest radiation therapy might benefit from breast cancer chemoprevention with tamoxifen or an aromatase inhibitor, but studies confirming a benefit have not yet been undertaken. In addition, lung cancers, sarcomas, melanomas, and thyroid cancers also occur with increased frequency after radiation therapy.

REFERENCES

1. Jemal A, Murray T, Ward E, et al. Cancer statistics 2005. CA Cancer J Clin. 2005; 55: 10–30.
2. Mueller NC, Grufferman S. Epidemiology of Hodgkin's disease. In P Mauch, JO Armitage, V Diehl (eds.), "Hodgkin's Disease," Lippincott Williams and Wilkins, Philadelphia, 1999, p. 61.
3. Stein H, Delsol G, Pileri S, et al. Hodgkin lymphoma. In ES Jaffe, NL Harris, H Stein, et al. (eds.), "World Health Organization Classification of Tumors; Pathology and Genetics; Tumours of Haematopoietic and Lymphoid Tissues," IARC Press, Lyon, 2001, p. 237.
4. Lister TA, Crowther D, Sutcliffe SB, et al. Report of a committee convened to discuss the evaluation and staging of patients with Hodgkin's disease: Cotswolds meeting. J Clin Oncol. 1989; 7: 1630–1636.
5. Diehl V, Sextro M, Franklin J, et al. Clinical presentation, course, and prognostic factors in lymphocyte-predominant Hodgkin's disease and lymphocyte-rich classical Hodgkin's disease; report from the European Task Force on Lymphoma Project on Lymphocyte-Predominant Hodgkin's disease. J Clin Oncol. 1999; 17: 776–783.
6. Bonadonna G, Zucali R, Monfardini S, et al. Combination chemotherapy of Hodgkin's disease with adreiamycine, bleomycin, vinblastine, and imidazole carboxamide versus MOPP. Cancer. 1975; 36: 252–259.
7. Canellos GP, Anderson JR, Propert KJ, et al. Chemotherapy of advanced Hodgkin's disease with MOPP, ABVD, or MOPP alternating with ABVD. N Engl J Med. 1992; 327: 1478–84.
8. Specht L, Gray RG, Clarke MJ, Peto R. Influence of more extensive radiotherapy and adjuvant chemotherapy on long-term outcome of early-stage Hodgkin's disease: a meta-analysis of 23 randomized trials involving 3,888 patients. International Hodgkin's Disease Collaboratorive Group. J Clin Oncol. 1998; 16: 830–43.
9. Loeffler M, Brosteanu O, Hasenclever D, et al. Meta-analysis of chemotherapy versus combined modality treatment trials in Hodgkin's disease. International Database on Hodgkin's Disease Overview Study Group. J Clin Oncol. 1998; 16: 818–29.
10. Hancock SL, Tucker MA, Hoppe RT. Factors affecting late mortality from heart disease after treatment of Hodgkin's disease. J Am Med Assoc. 1993; 270: 1949–55.
11. Travis LB, Hill D, Dores GM, et al. Cumulative absolute breast cancer risk for young women treated for Hodgkin lymphoma. J Natl Cancer Inst. 2005; 97: 1428–37.
12. Straus DJ, Portlock CS, Qin J, et al. Results of a prospective randomized clinical trial of doxorubicin, bleomycin, vinblastine and dacarbazine (ABVD) followed by radiation therapy (RT) versus ABVD alone for stages I, II and IIIA nonbulky Hodgkin disease. Blood. 2004; 104: 3483–9.
13. Hutchings M, Loft A, Hansen M, et al. FDG-PET after two cycles of chemotherapy predicts treatment failure and progression-free survival in Hodgkin lymphoma. Blood. 2006; 107: 52–9.
14. Bartlett NL, Rosenberg SA, Hoppe RT, et al. Brief chemotherapy, Stanford-V, and adjuvant radiotherapy for bulky or advanced-stage Hodgkin's disease. J Clin Oncol. 1995; 13: 1080–9.
15. Diehl V, Franklin J, Hasenclever D, et al. BEACOPP, a new dose-escalated accelerated regimen, is at least as effective as COPP/ABVD in patients with

advanced-stage Hodgkin's lymphoma: interim report from a trial of the German Hodgkin's Lymphoma Study Group. J Clin Oncol. 1998; 16: 3810–21.

16. Longo DL, Duffey PL, Young RC, et al. Conventional-dose salvage combination chemotherapy in patients relapsing with Hodgkin's disease after combination chemotherapy: the low probability for cure. J Clin Oncol. 1992; 10: 210–8.

17. DeVita VT Jr, Simon RM, Hubbard SM, et al. Curability of advanced Hodgkin's disease with chemotherapy. Long-term follow-up of MOPP-treated patients at the National Cancer Institute. Ann Intern Med. 1980; 92: 587–95.

18. Dady PJ, McElwain TJ, Austin DE, et al. Five years' experience with ChlVPP: effective low-toxicity combination chemotherapy for Hodgkin's disease. Br J Cancer. 1982; 45: 851–9.

19. Aparicio J, Segura A, Garcera S, et al. ESHAP is an active regimen for relapsing Hodgkin's disease. Ann Oncol. 1999; 10: 593–5.

20. Gribben JG, Linch DC, Singer CR, et al. Successful treatment of refractory Hodgkin's disease by high-dose combination chemotherapy and autologous bone marrow transplantation. Blood. 1989; 73: 340–4.

21. Jagannath S, Dicke KA, Armitage JO, et al. High-dose cyclophosphamide, carmustine, and etoposide and autologous bone marrow transplantation for relapsed Hodgkin's disease. Ann Intern Med. 1986; 104: 163–8.

22. Stewart DA, Guo D, Sutherland JA, et al. Single-agent high-dose melphalan salvage therapy for Hodgkin's disease: cost, safety, and long-term efficacy. Ann Oncol. 1997; 8: 1277–9.

23. Little R, Wittes RE, Longo DL, Wilson WH. Vinblastine for recurrent Hodgkin's disease following autologous bone marrow transplant. J Clin Oncol. 1998; 16: 584–8.

24. Santoro A, Bredenfeld H, Devizzi L, et al. Gemcitabine in the treatment of refractory Hodgkin's disease: results of a multicenter phase II study. J Clin Oncol. 2000; 18: 2615–9.

25. Bookman MA, Longo DL: Concomitant illness in patients treated for Hodgkin's disease. Cancer Treat Rev. 1986; 13: 77–109.

26. Blayney DW, Longo DL, Young RC, et al. Decreasing risk of leukemia with prolonged follow-up after chemotherapy and radiotherapy for Hodgkin's disease. N Engl J Med. 1987; 316: 710–4.

NON-HODGKIN'S LYMPHOMA

Non-Hodgkin's lymphomas (NHLs) are a heterogeneous group of lymphoid malignancies that differ greatly in clinical presentation, prognosis, and response to therapy. An estimated 63,190 new cases of NHL were diagnosed in the United States in 2007, making this the sixth most common malignancy in men and fifth most common in women. Since the 1970s, the incidence rate of NHL has doubled for unclear reasons. Because of the significant cure rate of some lymphoid malignancies, NHL will only account for 18,600 deaths in 2007.

Each of the NHLs has characteristic clinical presentations and often overlapping, but distinct, therapies. The two most common types of NHL, diffuse large B-cell lymphoma and follicular lymphoma (FL), account for nearly 2/3 of the cases and will be considered first, and the rarer B-cell lymphomas will then be briefly summarized followed by the T- and NK-cell lymphomas, which are also rare. The incidence of the various subtypes of NHL derived from a worldwide survey is shown in Table 28-1.

DIFFUSE LARGE B-CELL LYMPHOMA

Diffuse large B-cell lymphoma (DLBCL) is the most common histological subtype of NHL, accounting for approximately 30–45% of all cases. The annual incidence of 3–5/100,000 adults has steadily increased over the past decade. If DLBCL is untreated, survival is measured in terms of months; however, with modern combination chemotherapy, a majority of patients achieve durable remissions. For the majority of patients, no clear risk factors can be identified. A minority of patients will develop DLBCL after years of struggling with a more indolent lymphoma such as FL or chronic lymphocytic leukemia (CLL). In FL, the risk of histologic transformation is about 5–7% per year.

Table 28-1

Incidence of Non-Hodgkin's Lymphomas

B-cell neoplasms	88%	
	Diffuse large B-cell lymphoma	31%
	Follicular lymphoma	22%
	MALT lymphoma	8%
	CLL/SLL	7%
	Mantle cell lymphoma	6%
	Mediastinal large B-cell lymphoma	2%
	Nodal marginal zone lymphoma	2%
	Burkitt/Burkitt-like lymphoma	3%
	Splenic marginal zone lymphoma	<1%
T-cell neoplasms	12%	
	Peripheral T-cell NOS	4%
	Anaplastic large cell lymphoma	2%
	Precursor T-LBL	2%
	Nasal NK/T-cell lymphoma	1%

In CLL, histologic progression to DLBCL is called Richter's transformation, and occurs in about 5% of patients. Other documented risk factors for DLBCL include HIV disease (see below), coexistent autoimmune disease, and the use of immunosuppressive medications.

Patients with DLBCL usually present with symptoms of a rapidly enlarging nodal mass, most commonly in the neck or in the abdomen, and/or "B" symptoms—fevers, drenching night sweats, or weight loss (Table 28-2). Local complications can arise depending on the anatomic site of presentation and can cause medical emergencies such as superior vena cava (SVC) syndrome, airway compromise from extrinsic compression, and spinal cord compression. DLBCL shares the Ann Arbor staging system (Table 28-3) with other lymphomas. Originally developed for Hodgkin's disease, it applies poorly to DLBCL, because it does not share the biologic features of Hodgkin's disease of spread to contiguous nodal anatomic sites. Approximately 25% of patients will present with stage 1 disease and 50% will present with extensive disease (stage III or IV) at diagnosis. Thirty percent of all patients will present with evidence of extranodal disease but bone marrow involvement is found in only 10–20%. Initial evaluation should include:

- A thorough physical exam with attention to nodal areas and assessment of performance status
- Laboratory studies including a CBC with differential, LDH, uric acid, calcium, liver function tests as well as an HIV test
- Imaging studies including at least CT scans of the neck, chest, abdomen, and pelvis (PET scans are routinely performed at most institutions as well)
- Assessment of ejection fraction with echocardiography or nuclear medicine (to assess eligibility to receive cardiotoxic anthracyclines)

Table 28-2

B Symptoms

• Unexplained fever >38°C
• Drenching night sweats
• Unintentional weight loss >10% of body weight over 6 months or less

Table 28-3

Ann Arbor Staging System

• Stage I – involvement of single LN region or single extralymphatic organ or site (IE)
• Stage II – two or more LN regions on same side of diaphragm alone or with involvement of limited, contiguous extralymphatic organ or tissue (IIE)
• Stage III – involvement of LN regions on both sides of the diaphragm which can include the spleen (IIIS) or limited, contiguous extralymphatic organ or site (IIIE), or both (IIIES)
• Stage IV – diffuse or disseminated foci of involvement of one or more extralymphatic organs or tissues with or without assoicated lymphatic involvement
• Cotswold modifications
– A single extranodal site as only site of disease is IE, not IV.
– Use A or B for the absence of presence of B symptoms
– S is for splenic involvement, H is for hepatic involvement
– X is for bulky disease (>10 cm or >1/3 the intrathoracic diameter of patient if mediastinal mass)

- A bone marrow aspirate and biopsy
- A lumbar puncture in patients with initial sinus, testicular, orbital, epidural disease, bone, or bone marrow involvement or in any patient with focal neurologic symptoms
- Discussion of fertility issues in younger patients

The diagnosis of DLBCL is made by an excisional biopsy of involved tissue. A fine-needle aspirate (FNA) is not adequate. Pathological analysis will usually show large lymphocytes with nuclei greater than twice the size of normal small lymphocyte nuclei, prominent nucleoli, and basophilic cytoplasm. A high-proliferation index is often observed. Malignant cells express the B-cell antigens CD19, CD20, CD22, and CD79a.

Patients are prognostically stratified according to the International Prognostic Index (IPI) (1). The IPI scoring system is based on five clinical factors (each worth 1 point): stage III or IV disease, age >60, elevated serum LDH, ECOG performance status ≥2, and ≥2 extranodal sites of disease. The IPI directly correlates with both disease-free and overall survival (Table 28-4). Rituximab-treated patients were not included in the original IPI and its addition to chemotherapy has produced improved outcome for all prognostic subsets. A modification of the risk groupings has been proposed to account for rituximab effects (2) (Table 28-4).

DLBCL may also be divided into molecular subsets based on gene expression profiling (GEP). Three prognostically important subgroups of DLBCL have been identified; the activated B-cell-like subgroup (worst prognosis), the germinal center B-cell subgroup (best prognosis); and Type 3 (3). The impact of these molecular signatures in the era of rituximab therapy is not defined. Molecular profiling remains an experimental approach to lymphoma nosology, which is not yet ready for clinical application. The role of PET–CT staging is another active area of investigation.

Combination chemotherapy is the mainstay of treatment for patients with DLBCL. Even for patients with localized disease (a single-nodal or extranodal site), historically treated with radiotherapy alone, the addition of chemotherapy improves outcome. One option for localized good risk disease is combined modality therapy with three—four cycles of CHOP chemotherapy (Table 28-5) followed by involved field radiotherapy. Several series have confirmed the high rate of success for such a combined modality regimen, but they have also shown a significant rate of systemic relapse for high-risk disease as defined by clinical

Table 28-4

International Prognostic Index (IPI)

IPI Score	Risk group	5 Year OS (%)	CR rate (%)
0–1	Low risk	73	87
2	Low–intermediate risk	51	67
3	High–intermediate risk	43	55
4–5	High risk	26	44

IPI	Revised risk group	% Patients	5 Year OS (%)
0	Very good	10	94
1,2	Good	45	79
3,4,5	Poor	45	55

Factors (each worth 1 point): age >60, serum LDH above normal, ECOG performance status ≥2, Ann Arbor stage III or IV, number of extranodal disease sites ≥2.

Table 28-5

R-CHOP Chemotherapy Regimen

- Cyclophosphamide 750 mg/m^2 IV on day 1
- Adriamycin (Hydroxydaunorubicin) 50 mg/m^2 IV on day 1
- Vincristine (Oncovin) 1.4 mg/m^2 (max 2 mg) IV on day 1
- Prednisone 100 mg po qd days 1–5
- Rituximab given 375 mg/m^2 IV on day 1
- Cycles are every 21 days

factors such as bulky disease and elevated serum LDH. Thus, using systemic chemotherapy alone (i.e., R-CHOP × six–eight cycles) for these unfavorable patients is a reasonable option as well. In addition, extrapolating from studies in advanced stage disease (see below), rituximab has been incorporated into the treatment of localized disease.

For advanced stage disease, the treatment of choice is R-CHOP (4). The addition of the monoclonal antibody rituximab (humanized murine monoclonal IgG1 antibody directed against CD20) to CHOP chemotherapy significantly improves treatment outcome. In the landmark GELA trial involving patients age 60–80 with advanced stage DLBCL, rituximab improved complete remission and overall survival rates at 2 years by approximately 10–15% in both low-risk and high-risk subgroups. Several studies have since confirmed this benefit in other cohorts of patients with DLBCL. Most data support the use of eight cycles of R-CHOP but many centers restage patients after four cycles, and if the patient has achieved a CR, therapy is stopped after six cycles (the "CR+2" rule).

Only about 1/3 of patients who achieve complete response go on to relapse. Relapse of DLBCL, if it occurs, will usually take place within the first 2 years after achieving remission. If the patient is still able to tolerate aggressive therapy, salvage chemotherapy is employed. Common regimens include ICE, DHAP, and ESHAP (Table 28-6) with the routine inclusion of rituximab (although minimal data support this addition). If patients respond to salvage chemotherapy, high-dose chemotherapy with autologous stem cell rescue is the current standard therapy. The PARMA trial randomized relapsed chemo-sensitive patients to four more cycles of chemotherapy + RT versus RT + intensive chemotherapy followed by autologous stem cell transplant (ASCT) (5). Transplanted patients had better response rates (84% versus 44%), event-free survival (46% versus 12%), and overall survival (53% versus 32%). For patients to be eligible for ASCT, most centers require at least a partial response to salvage chemotherapy. In addition, the benefit of ASCT has not yet been analyzed for patients who received rituximab as part of their initial therapy.

CNS relapse occurs in 2–5% of patients after remission induction with CHOP-based chemotherapy (6). CNS relapse mainly occurs in the setting of

Table 28-6

Some Salvage Chemotherapy Regimens for Relapsed / Refractory DLBCL

- ICE – ifosfamide, carboplatin, etoposide
- DHAP – dexamethasone, high-dose cytarabine, procarbazine
- ESHAP – etoposide, methylprednisolone, cytarabine, cisplatin
- R-EPOCH – infusional etoposide, doxorubicin, and vincristine, with prednisone and cyclophosphamide boluses and rituximab

progressive systemic disease, and occurs most often in patients with bone, bone marrow, testis, orbital, or sinus involvement. The majority of chemotherapy agents, including doxorubicin and vincristine, do not achieve therapeutic levels in the CNS due to the blood–brain barrier. Prognosis is poor with median survival measured in months. Several series have attempted to clarify predictive factors for CNS relapse. In one series, patients with more than one extranodal site of disease and an elevated serum LDH had a 17% risk of CNS relapse. Involvement of the breast, testicles, paranasal sinuses, epidural space, and bone marrow each independently predict a higher rate of CNS relapse. Thus, patients with disease in these locations or with more than one extranodal site of involvement and an elevated LDH level should be given CNS prophylaxis. This can be done with three–four cycles of high-dose systemic methotrexate ($3–3.5 \text{ g/m}^2$ IV) incorporated into combination chemotherapy (usually given on day 14 of a standard cycle of R-CHOP). Intrathecal therapy with methotrexate or cytarabine on day 1 of each cycle of R-CHOP is another option but may be inadequate as leptomeningeal relapse only accounts for ~65% of secondary CNS disease.

Febrile neutropenia is a concern with all myelosuppressive combination chemotherapy regimens. Granulocyte colony stimulating factor (G-CSF) given either as daily injections of filgrastim or a single injection of peg-filgrastim reduces risk, especially for the elderly. Empiric use of G-CSF has never improved response, prevented serious infections, or improved overall survival when treating with a standard CHOP-like regimen in patients with DLBCL. Thus, we incorporate G-CSF into our care in specific situations: (1) delay of chemotherapy due to neutropenia in previous cycles, (2) a past episode of fever and neutropenia complicating therapy, (3) therapy given in a dose-dense manner (R-CHOP at 14 day intervals), (4) preexisting evidence for infection, and (5) elderly patients. Standard recommendations are to allow a 24 h interval between chemotherapy and G-CSF to avoid the theoretical increased risk of early stem cell damage. Similarly, the empiric use of prophylactic antibiotics in between cycles is not recommended. Prophylaxis against *Pneumocystis jiroveci* pneumonia (aka PCP) is commonly recommended when administering treatment regimens containing prolonged glucocorticoid courses, purine analogs, or high-dose chemotherapy courses, although it is often routinely prescribed even when treating with CHOP-like regimens.

Chemotherapy induced anemia is a common occurrence with CHOP-like chemotherapy, especially in the latter cycles of therapy. Anemia may aggravate concurrent comorbidities such as compromised cardiac or pulmonary function. Transfusion of packed RBCs is the preferred method of alleviating anemia complicating lymphoma treatment.

UNCOMMON SUBTYPES OF DIFFUSE LARGE B-CELL LYMPHOMA

Several subtypes of DLBCL warrant specific mention due to their unique characteristics. These include intravascular lymphoma, mediastinal large B-cell lymphoma (MLBCL), primary effusion lymphoma (PEL), and HIV-related DLBCL.

Intravascular large cell lymphoma, previously known as angiotropic large cell lymphoma and malignant angioendotheliomatosis, presents with a constellation of symptoms affecting multiple organs due to vascular occlusion from malignant lymphoid cells (7). This unusual subtype of DLBCL has malignant large lymphocytes entirely contained within the vascular system. Significant delay in diagnosis is the rule in the vast majority of cases due to the variegated and often confusing presentations. The most commonly affected organs are the CNS, kidney, lung, and skin, although all organs are susceptible. Even with modern combination chemotherapy, the prognosis of intravascular lymphoma is quite poor.

MLBCL, which makes up 7% of all DLBCL, commonly presents with signs and symptoms of SVC syndrome, airway compression, and/or pericardial effusions (8). MLBCL occasionally creates diagnostic confusion with classical Hodgkin's lymphoma, nodular sclerosis type, because of the demographics of the patients (female predominance and median age in the 30s) and the small size of routine biopsy specimens in the mediastinum. However, unlike classical Hodgkin's lymphoma, immunophenotypical analysis reveals that the cells of MLBCL express B-cell markers CD20 and CD79a, and express CD30 weakly. Many centers routinely administer consolidative radiotherapy for MLBCL after completion of R-CHOP; however, its value has not been demonstrated in controlled trials. Whether or not radiation therapy is given, long-term survival is seen in 2/3 of patients. While MLBCL is usually restricted to the thorax at diagnosis, it is known for recurrence in unusual extranodal sites such as the liver and kidney.

PEL presents as effusions in body cavities such as the pleural space, peritoneum, or pericardium, in the absence of tumor masses. The majority of cases occur in HIV-positive patients, and the malignant cells usually contain genomic material from both HHV-8 (human herpes virus 8) and EBV (9). Immunophenotypically, these neoplastic B-cells express leukocyte common antigen (CD45), but rarely B-cell markers (CD19, CD20, CD79a). Activation (CD30) and plasma cell-related (CD38, CD138) antigens are usually present, and thus the tumor cells are thought to originate from a lineage destined to become a plasma cell. Although rarely disseminated at presentation, PEL has a poor prognosis even with combination chemotherapy.

HIV disease is a significant risk factor for the development of NHL including DLBCL (9). The relative risk of developing NHL is estimated at 60–200-fold compared to the general population. About 1–3% of all HIV-positive patients will eventually develop NHL. While the advent of HAART has decreased the incidence of opportunistic infections, primary CNS lymphoma, and Kaposi's sarcoma, the effect on systemic NHL is less clear. The most common types of HIV-associated NHL include Burkitt's lymphoma (BL), immunoblastic large cell lymphoma (a DLBCL variant), DLBCL, PEL, and plasmablastic lymphoma of the oral cavity. HIV-associated DLBCL has higher rates of extranodal involvement as well as a more advanced stage (80% present with stage IV) at initial presentation. Stage for stage, HIV-associated DLBCL patients do significantly worse than HIV-negative patients, but by far, the most important prognostic factor in these patients is the CD4+ T-cell count at presentation. Treatment for HIV-associated DLBCL is similar to patients without HIV; however, infusional EPOCH may be more effective than bolus regimens. Furthermore, rituximab should be used with caution in patients with compromised CD4 T-cell counts, given the apparent increased risk for infection. HAART should be initiated before and continued during chemotherapy as it has been shown to reduce the rate of opportunistic infections and may prolong survival as well.

FOLLICULAR LYMPHOMA

FL represents 20–30% of all NHLs and is the second most common NHL after DLBCL. It comprises about 80% of the indolent NHLs. The name follicular is based on the tendency of the tumor to form nodules. The cell of origin is the follicular center B cell. FL is usually a disease of the middle-aged or elderly. Eighty–ninety percent of all cases have the characteristic cytogenetic translocation t(14;18) in which the anti-apoptotic bcl-2 gene is put under the control of the Ig heavy chain promoter on chromosome 14. Importantly, this translocation can also be found in 30% of cases of DLBCL.

Clinically, patients with FL usually present with painless peripheral adenopathy. Large mediastinal masses, CNS involvement, and organ involvement are all uncommon. The majority of patients (70–80%) will present with advanced stage disease, but only 20% will have B symptoms or an elevated serum LDH level. Median survival is in the range of 7–10 years. Although it was believed that cytotoxic therapy did not change the natural history of the disease, recent studies show improving survival over time for patients treated with mono-clonal antibody-based therapies. The 15% of patients with early-stage disease are potentially curable with local radiotherapy. As therapy has become more effective based on incorporation of rituximab into combination chemotherapy regimens like CHOP, a larger fraction of patients achieve complete remissions and those remissions last longer than the median of 2 years that characterized remissions from older regimens. However, it is not yet clear that longer remissions translate into improved overall survival. Patients with FL have a risk (5–7% annually) of transformation into a more aggressive NHL, most commonly DLBCL. This process is usually heralded by rapidly enlarging masses, the onset of systemic symptoms, and a rapidly rising LDH. DLBCL that evolves from previously treated FL is more refractory to treatment than de novo DLBCL.

Like all NHLs, the diagnosis of FL is established by an excisional biopsy. Upon pathological analysis, the gross infiltrate is composed of a mixture of centrocytes (small cleaved or irregular cells) and centroblasts (large noncleaved cells) in a nodular pattern of growth, but with notable crowding of follicles and attenuation of mantle zones. The lymphoma can rarely present as a diffuse infiltrate. The bone marrow, when involved, will show paratrabecular lymphoid aggregates. The neoplastic cells express CD19, CD20, and CD79a and germinal center antigens, CD10 and bcl-6. CD5 is usually not present in FL and distinguishes it from SLL/CLL. Cytoplasmic staining of neoplastic follicle center cells is usually strongly positive for bcl-2, whereas bcl-1 is not expressed in hyperplastic normal germinal center B cells. Histology is graded on a scale from I to III and is based on the number of centroblasts in the biopsy specimen. Grade III FL has a clinical course more akin to DLBCL and usually responds to R-CHOP with durable remissions. Some evidence also suggests that patients with grade II FL may achieve prolonged remission with attempts at curative therapy, but this has not been a universal finding.

For the majority of patients (80–90%) with FL who present with advanced stage disease, prognosis can be stratified according to the Follicular Lymphoma International Prognostic Index (FLIPI) (10). The FLIPI score was defined from a retrospective cohort of over 4,000 patients with FL and defined five adverse prognostic factors: age > 60, stage III/IV, elevated serum LDH level, Hgb < 12 g/dl, and > 4 nodal areas involved (a nodal map was defined). With each factor worth

Table 28-7

Follicular Lymphoma International Prognostic Index (FLIPI)

Risk group	No. of factors	5 Year survival (%)	10 Year survival (%)
Low	0 or 1	91	71
Intermediate	2	78	51
High	3–5	52	36

FLIPI factors (each worth one point): age >60, stage III / IV disease, elevated LDH, hemoglobin <12 g/dl, and >4 nodal areas involved.

one point, three risk groups could be identified correlating with 5 and 10 year survivals (see Table 28-7). While the FLIPI score allows some prediction of prognosis and some means of stratification for use in clinical trials, it still does not give firm indications for treatment. Evidence is accumulating that aggressive treatment, for example, with R-CHOP, is inducing a higher rate of complete remission, the remissions are lasting longer, and the rate of histologic progression appears to be decreased by aggressive treatment. However, no randomized trial has shown that aggressive treatment produces better overall survival than a palliative treatment approach. Therefore, the main indications for treatment for patients with advanced stage grade I/II FL are (1) symptomatic bulky lymphadenopathy or splenomegaly, (2) compromise of organ function from disease, (3) significant B symptoms, (4) significant cytopenias, (5) transformation to a more aggressive NHL, or (6) patient insistence. Many experts make an initial attempt to obtain a durable complete response with a course of R-CHOP or other combination chemotherapy and switch to palliative mode if the patient relapses.

In the absence of cure, the goal of therapy for FL is to achieve the longest possible duration of a treatment-free interval while balancing the potential for toxicity and complications. In general, FL is a chemosensitive disease to either single-agent chemotherapy (such as alkylating agents or purine analogs) or combination regimens (such as CHOP or CVP). Combination regimens appear to offer higher response rates and faster response times, but also carry associated risks of increased toxicity and myelosuppression. Median relapse-free intervals are prolonged with higher intensity regimens, but the first remission is generally the longest and subsequent remissions become gradually shorter as chemoresistance builds.

Rituximab alone produces overall response rates ranging from 50 to 70% with a median response duration of 12–14 months (11). Disease-free intervals can often be prolonged with intermittent maintenance doses of rituximab. Rituximab has also been added to combination chemotherapy regimens. Combinations of either R-CVP or R-CHOP have yielded overall response rates of 80–100% and significant benefits in terms of progression-free survival and overall survival over regimens without rituximab (12,13). Rituximab in combination with fludarabine has comparable results. Rituximab as maintenance therapy in both upfront and relapsed/refractory patients following a response to initial therapy confers significantly longer progression-free and overall survival (14).

There is no agreement on the value of high-dose therapy with ASCT for patients with FL. The lack of consistent benefit may be due to the increase in secondary malignancies such as myelodysplastic syndrome or acute myeloid leukemia. Modern conditioning regimens that omit total body irradiation may have a lower long-term risk of MDS/AML. Some patients achieve durable remissions.

Because of the high transplant-related mortality, allogeneic SCT has only been used for patients whose disease was chemotherapy resistant. T-cell depletion of the graft reduces acute graft-versus-host complications but the long-term benefits of this approach as well as the impact of nonmyeloablative conditioning regimens are unproven. Both ablative and nonablative allogeneic transplants are experimental.

The development of radioimmunotherapy (RIT) has given practitioners another option in the treatment of FL. Currently, two radiolabeled anti-CD20 monoclonal antibodies are approved by the FDA: Yttrium-90 ibritumomab tiuxetan (Zevalin) and Iodine-131 tositumomab (Bexxar). Trials have shown a significant response rate in patients with recurrent disease, including disease resistant to rituximab, with many patients achieving remission, some of which last longer than those obtained from previous treatments. RIT as initial treatment was tested in one study showing a 95% overall response rate (75% CR) in 76 patients treated with I-131 tositumomab and a median progression-free survival of 6 years. Other studies using RIT as part of initial therapy are ongoing with some using RIT as consolidation therapy after initial induction chemotherapy. In addition, RIT is also being added to conditioning regimens before ASCT. Thus far, the toxicities of RIT have been acceptable with hematological effects occurring for approximately 4–8 weeks after therapy due to the radiation effects on the bone marrow. Obstacles to its routine use include the need for a qualified nuclear medicine staff on site, potential injury to hematopoietic stem cells, and concerns over long-term toxicities, especially secondary hematological malignancies. These therapies also make subsequent myelotoxic therapy more difficult to deliver.

In managing patients who display clinical evidence of relapse, biopsy is recommended to exclude histological transformation particularly if suspicion is raised by a rising serum LDH, disproportionate growth in one area, new development of extranodal disease, or new "B" symptoms. Intervention in patients with relapsed FL is dictated by treatment goals. If the duration of the intial remission has been substantial, the same regimen may be given again; however, a shorter duration of remission should be expected. If the remission duration has been only a few months, then using different agents is recommended. If the patient is young and otherwise healthy with a short remission period, consideration can be given to high-dose therapy with autologous or allogeneic stem cell therapies.

The prognosis for previously treated patients with histologic transformation to DLBCL is poor with most series showing a median survival <12 months. Some patients treated with R-CHOP may achieve long-term remissions after consolidation with high-dose chemotherapy and autologous stem cell rescue; 5 year disease-free survivals range from 30 to 60%. However, the low-grade follicular component may reemerge after therapy.

MANTLE CELL LYMPHOMA

Mantle cell lymphoma (MCL) accounts for about 8% of NHL in the Western world. The usual age at diagnosis is between 50 and 70 years with a 3:1 male predominance. Most patients will have advanced stage disease at diagnosis and usually present with involvement of regional lymph nodes, liver, spleen, bone marrow, or peripheral blood. Other sites of extranodal spread include Waldeyer's ring and especially the gastrointestinal tract, in which MCL can manifest as multiple lymphomatous polyps.

The cell of origin is thought to be a mantle zone B cell. The neoplastic cells of MCL have small- to medium-sized nuclei, irregular nuclear contours, and indistinct nucleoli. Involved tissue lacks normal architecture, and is effaced by a monotonous population of neoplastic cells in a vaguely nodular or diffuse arrangement. In lymph nodes, markedly expanded mantle zones may be present. Immunophenotypic analysis will usually show expression of CD20 and CD5, but not CD10 (unlike FL) nor CD23 (unlike SLL/CLL). The hallmark of MCL is overexpression of cyclin D1 (bcl-1) which is usually due to the t(11;14)(q13; q32) translocation. Cyclin D1 promotes progression of cells through the G1–S boundary and is thus thought to contribute to oncogenesis by allowing proliferation. The blastoid variant of MCL is defined pathologically by cells with slightly increased nuclear size, greater chromatin dispersal, and a high mitotic rate (>10 mitotic figures / 10 hpf) and usually portends a more aggressive course and a worse prognosis.

There is no accepted standard therapy for MCL as no prospective randomized trials to date have shown a significant benefit of one regimen over another.

Indeed, even with high overall response rates to combination chemotherapy, relapses are common and the median survival for patients with MCL remains between 3 and 4 years. Occasional patients with low-risk and early-stage MCL will display quite indolent behavior, and watchful waiting and single-agent therapy for these patients are reasonable options especially if the patient is elderly or has other comorbidities.

Common choices for initial therapy include combinations of purine analogs, alkylating agents, and monoclonal antibodies (i.e., R-FCM, R-CHOP). Unlike in DLBCL, the addition of rituximab, while improving overall response rates, has not clearly improved PFS or OS in patients with MCL. If patients are being considered for ASCT, then purine analog-based regimens are not the best choice given their potential for stem cell injury. If the patient is otherwise healthy with a good performance status, then two current approaches seem to offer the highest potential for a prolonged duration of remission. One choice is initial therapy with standard R-CHOP chemotherapy followed by upfront consolidation with high-dose chemotherapy and ASCT. The second option is treatment with the R-hyperCVAD regimen, which includes alternating cycles of high-dose methotrexate and cytarabine, without consolidation with ASCT (15).

Patients with relapsed or refractory disease are occasionally considered for allogeneic stem cell transplant, more recently with nonmyeloablative conditioning regimens. RIT has become another option for patients with MCL. Current trials are attempting to define exactly where RIT should fit on the growing list of choices. Given the poor prognosis of most patients with MCL, novel therapies are an active area of investigation. Small trials have shown encouraging response rates using the proteasome inhibitor bortezomib and mTOR inhibitors in patients with relapsed/refractory disease. Other drugs in early-phase trials include inhibitors of cyclin D1.

BURKITT'S LYMPHOMA

BL is a highly aggressive subtype of NHL, often presenting as rapidly growing extranodal masses or less commonly as acute leukemia. It accounts for 2% of NHL in adults in Europe and North America, whereas it comprises 30–40% of NHLs in children. In the past, the solid tumor phase was classified as small non-cleaved cell lymphoma, and the leukemic phase was labeled L3 acute lymphoblastic leukemia (ALL), but the WHO classification system recognizes these two presentations as a single entity. BL arises in three different patterns: as an endemic disease, sporadically, and in immunodeficient patients. The endemic variant, which is highly associated with EBV infection, occurs mainly in equatorial Africa in children less than 10 years of age and commonly presents with disease in the jaw, face, kidney, and other extranodal sites. Sporadic BL usually presents in young healthy adults, often with large intraabdominal masses, and is much less commonly associated with EBV. Immunodeficient BL often occurs in the setting of HIV disease with seemingly little association with the baseline CD4 T-cell count. About 20–40% of immunodeficient BL is EBV+ and all cases of HIV-associated BL generally have a worse prognosis than disease in patients with competent immunity.

BL requires urgent treatment as rapidly growing masses may have doubling times as short as 24–48 h. Bone marrow (about 30% of cases) and CNS involvement (about 15% of cases) are relatively common. Serum LDH and uric acid levels are routinely elevated, and caution must be exercised as tumor lysis syndrome can occur spontaneously or as a result of initial cytotoxic treatment.

The diagnosis of BL is based on biopsy of an involved area or analysis of peripheral blood if the leukemic phase is present. Typical morphology shows medium-sized cells in a diffuse infiltrative pattern with abundant basophilic cytoplasm, frequent lipid vacuoles, and round monotonous nuclei with clumped chromatin and multiple nucleoli. The classic histologic "starry sky" appearance is due to numerous macrophages ingesting apoptotic tumor cells. Characteristic immunophenotypic findings include positive staining for B-cell markers including CD19, CD20, CD22, CD79a, and the germinal center markers, CD10 and bcl-6. Cells do not express CD5, CD23, TdT, or bcl-2. CD21, the receptor for EBV, will be present if the tumor is EBV related. Ki-67 growth fraction (proliferation index) is always near 100%. The defining genetic abnormality in all cases of BL is overexpression of the c-myc oncogene (16). Eighty percent of cases result from translocation of c-myc from chromosome 8 to chromosome 14 where it falls under the control of the promoter for the immunoglobulin heavy chain. In the remaining 20% of cases, the c-myc gene is translocated to either chromosome 2 or 22 where the genes for κ immunoglobulin λ light chains are located. Overexpression of c-myc induces the transcription of a myriad of genes that regulate the cell cycle, apoptosis, cell growth, cell adhesion, and differentiation.

Some cases of DLBCL morphologically resemble BL and/or possess c-myc overexpression associated with the t(8;14) translocation. The distinction between DLBCL and BL is important because treatment regimens are quite different. Combination chemotherapy for BL is much more intense, with significantly higher risks of acute regimen-related toxicity and infection. The diagnosis of atypical Burkitt's or Burkitt's-like lymphoma is restricted to cases that possess *c-myc* translocation, a growth fraction near 100% and atypical morphology. These patients should be treated with Burkitt's regimens. Otherwise, cases should be classified and treated as DLBCL.

Clinical staging and prognostication for BL is based on several classification schemes. The Ann Arbor staging system is used for most NHLs and Hodgkin's lymphomas. The most common currently used system for BL divides patients into only two subsets: low and high risk (Table 28-8). Low-risk patients have a single site of disease < 10 cm in bulk or a completely resected abdominal lesion and a normal serum LDH level. High-risk disease includes all other patients.

Standard treatment for BL consists of intensive combination chemotherapy given with minimal intervals between cycles. The most significant toxicites are myelosuppression and resulting infection. Prophylaxis for CNS disease is mandatory. Patients who have pathologically proven CNS involvement upon CSF sampling (all patients should have a staging LP) receive additional CNS directed therapy. Prophylaxis against tumor lysis syndrome must be started before the initial course of therapy. Nearly 100% of patients achieve a CR with modern therapy, and most patients remain in remission at 1 year. Overall about 80% of patients are cured. It is difficult to compare different regimens as most studies are single-center cohorts with differences in patient selection, risk stratification, and pathological eligibility. HIV+ patients are treated with the same chemotherapy along with antiretroviral therapy.

The most commonly used regimens include HyperCVAD and the CODOX-M/IVAC or Magrath regimen (Table 28-9) (17). Small studies have not shown consistent differences in efficacy between these regimens. There is no proven role for consolidation therapy.

Table 28-8

High-Risk Versus Low-Risk Staging System for Burkitt's Lymphoma

---

- Low risk – single site of disease <10 cm in diameter or a completely resected abdominal lesion, both with a normal serum LDH level
- High risk – all other patients

Table 28-9

Modified Magrath Regimen for Adult Burkitt's Lymphoma: LaCasce et al. 2004

Regimen A[a] CODOX-M Day	1	2	3	4	5	6	7	8	9	10	11	12	13
Cyclophospharride 800 mg/m²	x	x											
Vincristine[b] 1.4 mg/m²	x							x					
Doxorubicin 50 mg/m²	x												
Melhotrexate 3 gm/m²										x			
Leucovorin											x		
IT Cytarabine 50 mg	x												
IT Methotrexate 12 mg	x												
IT Cytarabine 50 mg			x[c]										
G-CSF[d]			x	x	x	x						x	x
Regimen B[c] IVAC Day	1	2	3	4	5	6	7	8	9	10	11	12	13
Ifosfamide 1500 mg/m²	x	x	x	x	x								
Mesna	x	x	x	x	x								
Etoposide 60 mg/m²	x	x	x	x	x								
Cytarabine 2 gm/m²[e]	x	x	x	x									
IT Methotrexate 12 mg					x								
G-CSF						x	x	x	x	x	x	x	x

[a]Low-risk patients receive 3 cycles of regimen A (A-A-A) High-risk patients receive 4 alternating cycles of regimens A and B (A-B-A-B).

[b]Vincristine maximum 2 mg dose

[c]High-risk only.

[d]ANC <1000 on day 12, restart G-CSF

[e]Cytrabine 2 g/m²q 12 h × 4 doses

The prognosis for relapsed or refractory BL is quite poor. Relapse usually happens within the first 12 months. There is no standard salvage chemotherapy regimen for relapsed or refractory disease. If patients achieve a good response with salvage therapy, consolidation with high-dose chemotherapy followed by autologous stem cell rescue is reasonable, though the benefit of the approach remains undefined.

Improvements are still needed in the treatment of BL as a number of patients relapse and die of their disease. Those with initial bone marrow or CNS involvement are at the highest risk for treatment failure. Because the neoplastic cells in BL express CD20, rituximab has been added to standard regimens (i.e., R-HyperCVAD or R-CODOX-M/R-IVAC), although prospective trials have not yet documented an improved overall survival.

MARGINAL ZONE B-CELL LYMPHOMAS

Mucosa-associated lymphoid tissue (MALT) or marginal zone B-cell lymphomas comprise about 7–8% of all NHLs in the Western world and display a generally indolent course. Marginal zone lymphomas can be classified into three distinct entities: extranodal marginal zone lymphoma (EMZL), splenic marginal zone lymphoma (SMZL), and nodal marginal zone lymphoma (NMZL). Upon immunophenotypical analysis, neoplastic cells from all three types express surface immunoglobulin, CD19, CD20, and CD79a, whereas the usual lack of expression of CD5, CD10, CD23, CD25, and CD103, distinguishes

Table 28-10

Immunophenotype of B-Cell Lymphoproliferative Disorders

Disease	sIg	CD5	CD10	CD19	CD20	CD22	CD23	CD25	FMC7
Chronic lymphocytic leukemia	dim	++	–	++	dim	dim	++	–	–
B-cell prolymphocytic leukemia	+++	–/+	–	++	+++	++	–	–	++
Follicular Lymphoma	++	–	++	++	++	++	–	–	++
Diffuse large B-cell lymphoma	++	–/+	–/+	++	++	++	–	–	+
Hairy cell Leukemia	+++	–	–/+	+++	+++	+++	–	+++	++
Mantle cell lymphoma	++	++	–	++	++	++	–	–	+
Lymphoplasmacytic lymphoma	++	–	–	++	++	++	–	–	+
Marginal zone lymphoma	++	–	–	++	++	++	–	–	+

sIg = surface immunoglobulin; – = not expressed; –/+ = usually not expressed; +/– usually expressed; + to +++ = varying degrees of strength of expression; dim = low level of expression.

them from other B-cell lymphoproliferative disorders (Table 28-10). No marker is specific for marginal zone lymphoma. The diagnosis is often made by the appearance of typical morphology correlated with clinical findings and by exclusion of other disorders. Recurrent cytogenetic abnormalities have been identified in gastric MALT lymphoma including trisomy 3, trisomy 18, t(11;18), t(1;14), t(14;18), and t(3;14). Current research is focusing on their importance in oncogenesis.

MALT lymphoma involves the marginal zone of reactive B-cell follicles and extends into the interfollicular regions, often infiltrating the epithelium of extranodal tissue sites. Invasion of the epithelium will often show characteristic lymphoepithelial lesions, a hallmark of MALT lymphoma, defined as clusters of three or more marginal zone cells with distortion or destruction of the epithelium, often with eosinophilic degeneration of epithelial cells. Cellular morphology can be varied and may take on a marginal zone (centrocyte-like), monocytoid, or plasmacytic appearance. Occasional large cells may be present, but if noted in solid or sheet-like proliferations, the diagnosis should be DLBCL, and the patient should be treated accordingly.

From a pathophysiological standpoint, MALT lymphomas are fascinating because they frequently occur in the setting of underlying chronic inflammation, usually caused by autoimmune or infectious etiologies (Table 28-11). Examples include *Helicobacter pylori* induced chronic gastritis, Sjogren's syndrome, Hashimoto's thyroiditis, *Chlamydia psittaci* infection, and *Campylobacter jejuni* infection. The gastrointestinal tract is the most common site of MALT lymphoma while other sites of involvement include the lung, head and neck, ocular adnexa, breast, skin, and thyroid. The majority of cases of MALT lymphoma will present with localized disease, found usually because of local symptoms. Regional XRT can often confer years of treatment-free benefit or even cure, while advanced symptomatic disease should be treated with systemic chemotherapy regimens similar to those used for other indolent NHLs.

Table 28-11

Infectious/Autoimmune Associations with Lymphoma

- *Helicobacter pylori* → primary gastric MALT lymphoma or DLBCL
- *Chlamydia psittaci* → ocular adnexal MALT lymphoma
- *Borrelia burgdorferi* → cutaneous MALT lymphoma
- *Hepatitis C virus* → splenic marginal zone lymphoma
- *Campylobacter jejuni* → immunoproliferative small intestinal disease (IPSID or α heavy chain disease)
- Sjogren's syndrome → extranodal MALT lymphoma or DLBCL
- Hashimoto's thyroiditis → extranodal MALT lymphoma or DLBCL
- Gluten enteropathy → intestinal T-cell lymphoma

Transformation to a higher grade NHL, usually DLBCL, should be suspected if there is an acute change in local or systemic symptoms.

Gastric MALT lymphoma is the most common type of MALT lymphoma and its development is associated with *Helicobacter pylori* infection in 70–90% of cases. Initial infection results in the accumulation of B-cell follicles in the gastric mucosa, which is normally devoid of organized lymphoid tissue. Oncogenesis is not through antigen induced activation and proliferation of *H. pylori*-specific postgerminal center B cells. Rather, it is thought that *H. pylori* stimulates the infiltrating CD4+ helper T cells. These T cells then drive B cell proliferation secondarily. The proliferating cells then acquire additional chromosomal lesions that bring about *H. pylori*-independent growth and more aggressive disease.

For early-stage gastric disease *H. pylori* eradication alone can bring about complete histological regression in 50–80% of cases (18). Disease that is deeply invasive, involves regional lymph nodes or possesses t(11; 18)(q21; q21) translocation responds poorly to antibiotics. Patients with relapsed/refractory or locally advanced disease are usually treated with radiation therapy. It should be noted that most patients will have PCR-detectable disease upon monitoring after therapy has been completed, but it is unclear if this warrants additional therapy.

Ocular adnexal MALT lymphomas account for about 50% of all ocular lymphoproliferative disorders. High rates of *Chlamydia psittaci* infection have been found in some but not all series. A small series has even shown clinically significant responses to anti-Chlamydia treatment with doxycycline therapy. The diagnosis of ocular MALT lymphoma often requires complete excision of the tumor. Regardless, full staging studies including an orbital MRI should be performed to document the extent of disease. Most patients receive radiotherapy for localized disease. Other options include single-agent chemotherapy, rituximab, anti-Chlamydia therapy, and a watch-and-wait policy. Unlike higher grade ocular NHLs, CNS prophylaxis is unnecessary.

SMZL usually affects patients older than 50. Patients typically present with significant splenomegaly and peripheral lymphocytosis while peripheral lymph node or extranodal involvement outside of the bone marrow is quite uncommon. Autoimmune hemolytic anemia (AIHA) can occur and one-third of patients will also have a monoclonal gammopathy (usually IgM) on serum electrophoresis. A peripheral blood smear will often show the presence of villous lymphocytes, which have characteristically short polarized cytoplasmic projections. Morphological examination of splenectomy specimens demonstrates a population of small lymphocytes that surround and replace the splenic white pulp germinal centers and merge with an outer marginal zone of small- to medium-sized cells. Bone marrow biopsy will often show a nodular interstitial infiltrate; an intrasinusoidal pattern of invasion, although characteristic, is less common. In the absence of splenectomy, morphologic and immunophenotypical analysis of peripheral blood or bone marrow, along with the typical clinical presentation, can support a diagnosis of SMZL.

Ten–forty percent of patients with SMZL are positive for hepatitis C (HCV) infection. The mechanism of oncogenesis of HCV is unclear, but hypotheses include direct infection of B cells leading to eventual transformation, or more likely, persistent antigenic stimulation leading to clonal proliferation. While HCV infection does not seem to influence overall prognosis, SMZL regression after antiviral treatment has been reported. Screening for HCV infection has become standard for patients diagnosed with SMZL.

Prognosis for SMZL is good with a median survival around 10 years; only a small number of patients display an aggressive course. Lower albumin levels, higher LDH levels, and lower hemoglobin levels predict higher risk disease. Symptoms and/or significant cytopenias prompt initial therapy, often splenectomy, which can yield a prolonged treatment-free benefit. There is no proven advantage for adjuvant chemotherapy after splenectomy, though this is a subject of current investigation. If patients are unable to tolerate splenectomy or require treatment afterwards, chemotherapy with alklyating agents, purine analogs, or rituximab produces significant rates of response. Lastly, if HCV infection is diagnosed, antiviral treatment should be considered.

NMZL is a rare NHL that is diagnosed when typical marginal zone lymphoma cells are seen in involved lymph nodes without evidence of extranodal or splenic disease. NMZL typically presents with local lymphadenopathy, usually in the cervical regions. NMZL has two morphological subtypes: one that resembles extranodal MZL and one that appears more similar to splenic MZL. Occasional biopsies of FL will show areas of apparent NMZL, but in these cases, the diagnosis is FL with marginal zone differentiation. Given the rarity of NMZL, large prospective series do not exist, but the prognosis does appear to be relatively good with median survival times measured in years. Indications for treatment are cytopenias and symptoms, and recommendations for therapy include local radiation for early-stage disease and either single-agent or combination chemotherapy (alkylating agents, purine analogs, rituximab) for advanced disease states.

LYMPHOMAS OF NK- OR T-CELL ORIGIN

Anaplastic Large Cell Lymphoma

Anaplastic large cell lymphoma (ALCL), T/null cell type, is a rare disease, accounting for <5% of NHL, though comprising a larger fraction of cases of NHL in pediatric populations. In general, ALCL occurs as two distinct clinical syndromes; primary cutaneous ALCL (PCALCL) and systemic ALCL, which have very different natural histories, responses to therapy, and prognoses. Systemic ALCL is important to consider because of the diagnostic confusion in certain cases. Although mediastinal disease is less frequent than in Hodgkin's lymphoma, some cases of ALCL may be confused with classical Hodgkin's lymphoma due to the presence of a large mediastinal mass in a young adult composed of CD30+ Reed–Sternberg-like cells with some surrounding sclerosis and inflammation (see below). Other cases may be interpreted initially as primary mediastinal B-cell lymphoma due to patient demographics and variable CD30 expression.

PCALCL is classified under the new WHO-EORTC category of CD30+ lymphoproliferative disorders of the skin. It is generally considered an indolent disorder with 10 year survival usually at 85% or better, even in the 10–15% who develop systemic ALCL in the local lymph nodes draining the affected areas of the skin. Immunophenotypically, PCALCL differs from systemic ALCL in usually being CLA+ (cutaneous lymphocyte antigen), EMA- (epithelial membrane antigen), and rarely expressing ALK (anaplastic lymphoma kinase). Treatment is usually localized such as local radiotherapy or excision. Low-dose systemic methotrexate has been used in refractory cases.

Systemic ALCL is classified as a moderately aggressive NHL, akin to DLBCL (19). Patients commonly present with advanced stage disease with systemic symptoms. Pathologically, the "hallmark" cells of ALCL are large with pleomorphic kidney- or horseshoe-shaped nuclei and abundant cytoplasm. Some forms with prominent nucleoli may resemble Reed–Sternberg cell variants, but the eosinophilic, inclusion-like nucleoli of Reed–Sternberg cells are generally absent. Despite the presence of background, nonneoplastic inflammatory cells, eosinophils are not a prominent feature and the malignant cells of ALCL are usually more numerous and form clusters or sheets in contrast to Reed–Sternberg cells and variants in most cases of Hodgkin's lymphoma. The immunophenotype is usually one of mature activated T cells, generally positive for HLA-DR and CD25, and variably positive for CD45 and the T-cell antigens CD2, CD3, CD4, CD43, and CD45RO. Importantly, CD30 is positive, while CD15 is negative. The malignant T cells often lack one or more pan-T-cell antigen, usually CD3, CD5, or CD7. The rare null cell type does not express T-cell antigens, but will have TCR rearrangement by PCR. Forty–sixty percent of patients have the t(2;5)(p23;q35) translocation, resulting in constitutive ALK expression. ALK expression carries critical prognostic implications with a 5 year overall survival of 80–90% in ALK+ cases versus 30–40% in ALK- cases (20).

Systemic ALCL is treated with anthracycline based combination chemotherapy—that is, CHOP-like regimens—based on extrapolations from data from patients with DLBCL. Rituximab is not indicated because the tumor cells do not express CD20. There have been no large randomized prospective clinical trials investigating the treatment of ALCL. Relapsed disease is usually treated with salvage chemotherapy followed by consolidation with high-dose chemotherapy and autologous stem cell rescue. The use of autologous transplant as consolidation therapy in first remission for patients with ALK negative disease is a subject of current investigation. Specific inhibitors of ALK and agents targeting CD30 are being developed for treatment of ALCL.

Other T- and NK-Cell Lymphomas

Aside from ALCL, the other T- and NK-cell lymphomas are rare entities making up in total less than 7% of all lymphomas. The WHO (2001) and WHO-EORTC cutaneous lymphoma (2005) classifications divide these entities into a precursor hematologic neoplasm and 14 mature T- or NK-cell neoplasms. The mature entities are further subdivided into neoplasms with predominantly leukemic or disseminated disease, cutaneous disease, nodal disease, and other extranodal disease. These entities are briefly summarized in Table 28-12.

In general, the T- and NK-cell lymphomas show significant geographic diversity. While they represent a small fraction of lymphomas in the United States, they are much more common in Asia. It is unclear whether this represents the prevalence of specific genetic factors that may predispose to the development of these diseases or whether it is due to differential exposure to viruses that may play a role in pathogenesis (HTLV-1, etc.).

Table 28-12

Subsets of T-cell Neoplasms

Disease category	Phenotype	Genetics	Presentation	Therapy	Notes
Precursor					
CD4+/CD56+ hematodermic neoplasm (Blastic NK-cell Lymphoma)	CD56, 4, 43, 123+ CD2, 3, –	TCR germline	Skin +/– nodal sites	ALL-like regimens Limited data	Rapidly fatal Cutaneous-only presentations may do better
Leukemic					
T-cell PLL	CD2, 3, 7+, Tdt– 4+/–, 8–/+	inv(14)	HSMG, adenopathy	Nucleoside analogs, Campath, CHOP	Rapidly fatal Coexpression of CD4 and 8 with absence of TdT likely diagnostic
T-cell LGL	CD3, TCRαβ, 8+ CD4-	TCRβ rearranged	Severe neutropenia, splenomegaly	Immunosuppressives (MTX, steroids, CyA), G-CSF	Indolent, Associated with autoimmune disease - RA
Aggressive NK-cell leukemia	CD2, 56+ Surface CD3–	TCR germline Clonal episomal EBV	Fever, constitutional symptoms	Combination chemotherapy	Rapidly fatal More prevalent in Asians and younger pts EBV associated
ATLL	CD2, 3, 5+ CD4+/–, 8–/+, CD7– CD30+/–	Causally linked to HTLV-1 which is clonally integrated in all cases	Adenopathy and cutaneous presentation Hypercalcemia	Combination chemotherapy with antiviral therapy	Fatal with some indolent cases, Endemic in Japan, Caribbean and Central Africa

(Continued)

241

Table 28-12 (Continued)

Subsets of T-cell Neoplasms

Disease category	Phenotype	Genetics	Presentation	Therapy	Notes
Cutaneous					
MF	CD2, 3, 4, 5+, TCRβ+ CD7, 8–	TCR rearranged	Scaly eruptions -> limited patches -> infiltrated plaques	Stage dependent Topical therapies and UV common	Very indolent but stage dependent Most common cutaneous T-cell NHL
Sezary Syndrome	CD2, 3, 4, 5+, TCRβ+ CD8–	TCR rearranged Complex karyotype frequent	Cutaneous, adenopathy, peripheral blood	Topical therapies, UV Photopheresis Ontak Targretin	Aggressive Considered a variant of MF
PCALCL	CD4+, CD30+ Granzyme+ Variable loss of CD2, 3, ± 5 ALK–	TCR rearranged t(2; 5)–	Slight male predominance Limited to skin at presentation	Stage-dependent local XRT	Indolent Overlap with LP Can spontaneously remit
LP	CD4+, CD8– CD30 ± ALK–	TCR rearrangement in ~50%	Cutaneous spontaneously remitting nodules	For large lesions: low-dose MTX PUVA	Very indolent Treatment does not impact natural history and is reserved for symptomatic pts
Nodal					
AILT	CD3+, CD4+ cells with variable CD10 coexpression; expanded CD21+	EBV+ B-cells	Adenopathy, HSMG, rash B symptoms Hypergammag	Combination chemotherapy	Fatal

(Continued)

Table 28-12 (Continued)

Disease category	Phenotype	Genetics	Presentation	Therapy	Notes
Nodal (*Continued*)			lobulinemia Edema		
PTCL-U	FDC; arborizing HEVs CD4 > 8+ CD30 ±	TCR rearranged Complex karyotype frequent	Nodal and cutaneous disease; can also be extranodal	Combination chemotherapy Auto-BMT sometimes suggested	Likely represents an agglomeration of undescribed subtypes
ALCL			Discussed seperately		
Extranodal Nasal	CD2+, 56+ Surface CD3− Granzyme+, perforin+	TCR germline Clonal episomal EBV	Nasal obstruction but can disseminate quickly B symptoms	Combination chemotherapy + IFRT for limited stage disease, combination chemotherapy if disseminated	Variable prognosis "lethal midline granuloma" More common in Asia, Mexico, South America EBV associated
Enteropathy	CD3+, 7+ CD8 ±, CD4−, 5−; small cell variant: CD8+, 56+	HLADQA1*0501, HLADQB1*0201 TCRβ rearranged	Solitary or multiple GI mucosal masses	Combination chemotherapy	Fatal Highly associated with celiac disease
Hepatosplenic	CD3, TCRδ1+, CD56± TCRαβ, 4, 8−	TCRγ rearranged Isochromo some 7q	HSMG without adenopathy Thrombocytopenia, anemia and leukocytosis	Combination chemotherapy	Fatal Responds to initial therapy but relapses Younger patients More common in immuno-suppressed following solid organ transplantation (*Continued*)

Table 28-12 (*Continued*)

Subsets of T-cell Neoplasms

Disease category	Phenotype	Genetics	Presentation	Therapy	Notes
Extranodal (*Continued*) Subcutaneous Panniculitis	CD3, 8+ Granzyme+ Perforin+	TCR rearranged	Multiple subcutaneous nodules, extremities and trunk	Combination chemotherapy	Indolent but progressive once nodal Can be complicated by hemophagocytic syndrome

PLL (prolymphocytic leukemia), LGL (large granular leukemia), ATLL (acute T-cell leukemia/lymphoma), MF (mycosis fungoides), PCALCL (primary cutaneous anaplastic large cell lymphoma), LP (lymphomatoid papulosis), AILT (angioimmunoblastic T-cell lymphoma), PTCL-U (peripheral T-cell lymphoma, unspecified), Nasal (Extranodal NK/T-cell lymphoma, nasal type), Enteropathy (Enteropathy-type T-cell lymphoma), Hepatosplenic (Hepatosplenic T-cell lymphoma), subcutaneous panniculitis (subcutaneous panniculitis-like T-cell lymphoma) HSMG (hepatosplenomegaly), FDC (follicular dendritic cell networks), HEV (high endothelial venule), CyA (cyclosporine), MTX (methotrexate), G-CSF (granulocyte colony stimulating factor), EBV (Epstein–Barr virus), IFRT (involved field radiotherapy).

REFERENCES

1. A predictive model for aggressive non-Hodgkin's lymphoma. The International Non-Hodgkin's Lymphoma Prognostic Factors Project. N Engl J Med. 1993; 329: 987–994.
2. Sehn LH, Berry B, Chhanabhai M, et al. The revised International Prognostic Index (R-IPI) is a better predictor of outcome than the standard IPI for patients with diffuse large B-cell lymphoma treated with R-CHOP. Blood 2007; 109: 1857-1861.
3. Rosenwald A, Wright G, Chan WC, et al. The use of molecular profiling to predict survival after chemotherapy for diffuse large-B-cell lymphoma. N Engl J Med. 2002; 346: 1937–1947.
4. Coiffer B, Lepage E, Briere J, et al. CHOP chemotherapy plus rituximab compared with CHOP alone in elderly patients with diffuse large-B-cell lymphoma. N Engl J Med. 2002; 346: 235–42.
5. Philip T, Guglielmi C, Hagenbeek A, et al. Autologous bone marrow transplantation as compared with salvage chemotherapy in relapses of chemotherapy-sensitive non-Hodgkin's lymphoma. N Engl J Med. 1995; 333: 1540–5.
6. Van Besien K, Ha CS, Murphy S, et al. Risk factors, treatment and outcome of central nervous system recurrence in adults with intermediate-grade and immunoblastic lymphoma. Blood. 1998; 91: 1178–84.
7. Ferreri AJ, Campo E, Seymour JF, et al. Intravascular lymphoma: clinical presentation, natural history, management and prognostic factors in a series of 38 cases with special emphasis on the 'cutaneous variant.' Br J Haematol. 2004; 127: 173–83.
8. Van Besien K, Kelta K, Bahaguna P. Primary mediastinal B-cell lymphoma: a review of pathology and management. J Clin Oncol. 2001; 19: 1855–64.
9. Navarro WH, Kaplan LD. AIDS-related lymphoproliferative disease. Blood. 2006; 107: 13–20.
10. Solal-Celigny P, Roy P, Colombat P, et al. Follicular lymphoma international prognostic index. Blood. 2004; 104: 1258–65.
11. Colombat P, Salles G, Brousse N, et al. Rituximab (anti-CD20 monoclonal antibody) as single first-line therapy for patients with follicular lymphoma with a low tumor burden: clinical and molecular evaluation. Blood. 2001 97: 101–106.
12. Marcus R, Imrie K, Belch A, et al. CVP chemotherapy plus rituximab compared with CVP as first-line treatment for advanced follicular lymphoma. Blood. 2005; 105: 1417–23.
13. Hiddemann W, Kneba M, Dreyling M, et al. Frontline therapy with rituximab added to the combination of cyclophosphamide, doxorubicin, vincristine, and prednisone (CHOP) significantly improves the outcome for patients with advanced-stage follicular lymphoma compared with therapy with CHOP alone: results of a prospective randomized study of the German Low-Grade Lymphoma Study Group. Blood. 2005; 106: 3725–32.
14. van Oers MH, Klasa R, Marcus RE, et al. Rituximab maintenance improves clinical outcome of relapsed/resistant follicular non-Hodgkin lymphoma in patients both with and without rituximab during induction: results of a prospective randomized phase 3 intergroup trial. Blood. 2006; 108: 3295–3301.
15. Romaguera JE, Fayad L, Rodriguez MA, et al. High rate of durable remissions after treatment of newly diagnosed aggressive mantle-cell lymphoma with rituximab plus hyper-CVAD alternating with rituximab plus high-dose methotrexate and cytarabine. JC Clinl Oncol. 2005; 23: 7013–23.
16. Hecht JL and Aster JC. Molecular biology of Burkitt's lymphoma. J Clin Oncol. 2000; 18: 3703–21.
17. Lacasce A, Howard O, Lib S, et al. Modified magrath regimens for adults with Burkitt and Burkitt-like lymphomas: preserved efficacy with decreased toxicity. Leuk Lymphoma. 2004; 454: 761–7.

18.   Bertoni F and Zucca E. State-of-the-art therapeutics: marginal-zone lymphoma. J Clin Oncol. 2005; 23: 6415–20.
19.   Falini B. Anaplastic large cell lymphoma: pathological, molecular and clinical features. Br J Haematol. 2001; 114: 741–760.
20.   Jacobsen E. Anaplastic large-cell lymphoma, T-/null-cell type. Oncologist. 2006; 11: 831–840.

ACUTE LYMPHOBLASTIC LEUKEMIA AND LYMPHOMA

INTRODUCTION

Acute lymphoblastic leukemia (ALL) is a highly aggressive neoplasm of hematopoietic cells of the lymphoid lineage. Clonal expansion of aberrant T- or B-lymphoblasts manifests in the bone marrow, peripheral blood, and extramedullary sites. ALL is predominantly a childhood cancer, with two thirds of new cases diagnosed in children under 15. Uniformly fatal until the 1960s, ALL is now cured in over 80% of children due to advances in chemotherapy. Adults diagnosed with ALL, however, continue to have a poor overall prognosis. Important factors in assessing prognosis are the type of lymphoid cell involved (T-cell versus B-cell) and the presence of high-risk cytogenetic markers, such as the t(9;22) (BCR–ABL) translocation.

- Disease of childhood
- Childhood ALL has an improved overall survival relative to adult ALL
- Characterized as a highly aggressive lymphoid malignancy by World Health Organization (WHO) criteria
- Immunophenotypes: B-cell (80%) and T-cell (20%)
- Cytogenetic alterations such as t(9;22) are associated with inferior prognosis

EPIDEMIOLOGY AND ETIOLOGY

Leukemia comprises 32% of malignancies in children under 15. Of these, the majority are ALL. Each year approximately 2,400 children in the United States are diagnosed with ALL, with peak incidence in children ages 2–5. Leukemia rates are significantly higher in Caucasian children, with a nearly threefold higher incidence over African-American children. ALL is almost 30% more common in males than females. Overall, the incidence of childhood ALL has increased in the past 20 years at a rate of 0.9% per year.

Adult ALL is less common. The incidence decreases from age 15 until 50, when there is a second, minor increase in new cases. A third peak appears at age 80.

The etiology of ALL is unknown. In children, the following characteristics are associated with ALL:

- Male gender
- Age 2–5
- Caucasian race
- Higher socioeconomic status (SES)
- Hereditary factors (Down syndrome, Bloom syndrome, ataxia telangectasia, neurofibromatosis, Klinefelter syndrome, Schwachman syndrome, and Langerhans cell histiocytosis).

Various models have suggested that inadvertent exposure to radiation in utero and postnatal radiation treatment for such conditions as tinea capitus and thymic enlargement increase risk of ALL (1). A common cytogenetic translocation involving ETV-6 was retrospectively detected in neonatal blood spots of children who were diagnosed with ALL between ages 2 and 5, suggesting that ALL can be initiated by somatic translocation in utero but requires additional molecular events to fully develop (2). Limited and/or inconsistent evidence links ALL to parental smoking, infection, diet, electromagnetic fields, and hydrocarbons.

ALL CLASSIFICATION

Proper characterization of the specific hematopoietic lineage involved in ALL is crucial for assessing risk and developing a treatment plan. ALL may be classified according to the presence or absence of various cell surface and intracellular markers.

Approximately 80% of ALL patients have lymphoblasts with phenotypes corresponding to precursor B-cells (B-cell progenitors). Within the category of precursor B-ALL are the pre-B and early pre-B-cell types. Precursor B-ALL cells express CD19 and at least one other B-lineage marker such as CD20, CD24, CD22, CD21, or CD79. More than 90% also express CD10 (CALLA, common ALL antigen). Lymphoblasts typically express terminal deoxytransferase (TdT) and/or the primitive marker CD34. In addition, 25% of patients have cytoplasmic Ig staining.

Leukemias of T-cell origin are characterized according to the sequence of expression of T-cell associated surface markers during thymocyte ontogeny. Precursor T-cells leukemias express CD7, TdT, and cytoplasmic CD3 antigen. Expression of CD1a is also characteristic. More highly differentiated thymocytes acquire CD2 and CD5 and, later, CD4 and 8. Mature thymocytes express functional T-cell receptor (TCR) and surface CD3. TCR rearrangement studies may be conducted to establish clonality.

Mature B-cell ALL represents a disseminated form of Burkitt's lymphoma and accounts for 2–3% of ALL. This rare subtype is characterized by expression of surface Ig and a distinctive cellular morphology consisting of deeply basophilic cytoplasm with prominent vacuoles. Expression of cell surface markers CD19 and CD20 and absence of CD10 are characteristic. Typically, rearrangements of chromosome 8, involving the c-myc proto-oncogene, are present.

Identifying expression of cell surface and cytoplasmic proteins is accomplished using fluorescence activated cell sorting (FACS, flow cytometry) and immunohistochemistry. Using these techniques, panels of lineage-specific antibodies directed against B-lymphoid, T-lymphoid, and myeloid antigens are used to stain bone marrow and lymph node samples from patients. Common immunophenotypes are presented in Table 29-1.

Figure 29-1 provides an example of flow cytometric analysis using CD10 and CD19 to characterize precursor B-cell ALL.

In children, approximately 80% of ALL are precursor B-cell (encompassing early pre-B and pre-B-cell ALL), 2% are mature B-cell (Burkitt leukemia/lymphoma), and 15% are precursor T-cell ALL. In adults, 70% are precursor B-cell ALL, while 5% are mature B-cell ALL, and the remaining 25% are precursor T-cell ALL.

DIAGNOSIS OF ALL

Clinical Presentation

Children with ALL can have an insidious or explosive course before diagnosis, whereas adults present more uniformly with rapid-onset disease. Physical signs and symptoms are the sequelae of marrow failure and clonal proliferation. Patients commonly present with anemia, leading to pallor, fatigue, lethargy, and, in adults, cardiac angina. In particular, patients with a mediastinal mass, seen

Table 29-1

Common Immunophenotype Profiles of Lymphoid and Myeloid Malignancies

		Primitive			B-lymphoid			T-lymphoid		Myeloid		
		TdT	CD34	CD1a	CD10 (cALLa)	CD20	sIg	CD4	CD8	CD13	CD33	MPO
B-Cell	Precursor B-cell ALL	+	+	−	+	−	−	−	−	−	−	−
	Mature B-cell	−	−	−	−	+	+	−	−	−	−	−
T-Cell	Precursor T-cell ALL	+	−	+	±	−	−	+	+	−	−	−
	Mature T-cell	−	−	−	−	−	−	+	−	−	−	−
Myeloid		−	+	−	−	−	−	−	−	+	+	+

+ denotes >50% positive.

− denotes <50% positive.

NOTE. This is a general schema, exceptions exist. For example, biphenotypic and multilineage leukemias may coexpress multiple lineage markers.

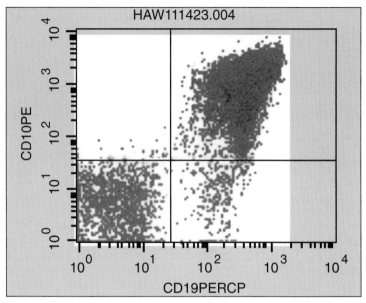

FIGURE 29-1 Flow cytometric analysis of CD10 versus CD19. (Courtesy Rob Hasserjian, MGH Cancer Center).

more often with T-cell ALL, may complain of chest discomfort, shortness of breath, and dyspnea on exertion. Large mediastinal masses have been associated with superior vena cava syndrome.

Thrombocytopenia manifests as easy bruising, bleeding, and petechiae. Underproduction of normal neutrophils predisposes patients to infection. Marrow expansion leads to bony pain, and young children may present with resistance to walking. Extramedullary deposition, resulting in lymphadenopathy, hepatosplenomegaly, and tenderness to palpation, is more commonly seen in mature B-cell ALL, as is frequent involvement of the CNS and hyperuricemia with renal failure. When present, CNS involvement may manifest in headaches, nausea/vomiting, and cranial nerve palsies.

Many patients present with fever absent infectious etiology. A summary of clinical features is presented in Table 29-2.

Diagnostic Studies

When ALL is suspected, diagnostic workup consists of a full battery of blood tests, imaging, bone marrow aspiration and biopsy, and lumbar puncture (LP) (Table 29-3). CBC and peripheral blood smear will show leukocytosis with lymphoblasts (Figure 29-2). Insidious disease can present with profound anemia and thrombocytopenia, reflective of the lag between early marrow failure and clinical presentation. Serum chemistries reflect the degree of tumor burden and cell lysis: patients may present with hyperuricemia, hypocalcemia, hyperphosphatemia, and elevated LDH. Bone marrow aspiration reveals a homogeneous lymphoblast field with hypercellular marrow. By convention, lymphoblasts must comprise 25% of cells, but most patients with ALL far exceed this minimum standard. Myeloid and erythroid precursors and megakaryocytes are normal in appearance and function, but total counts

Table 29-2

Clinical Manifestations of ALL

Marrow failure
- Anemia: pallor, fatigue, lethargy, angina
- Thrombocytopenia: bruising, petechiae
- Neutropenia: infection

Clonal expansion
- Bone pain, resistance to walking in children
- Tender lymphadenopathy
- Hepatosplenomegaly
- Fever

CNS infiltration
- Headache
- Nausea, vomiting
- Cranial nerve palsies

Table 29-3

Workup of Suspected ALL

CBC and peripheral smear
- Leukocytosis with lymphoblasts
- Anemia
- Thrombocytopenia

Serum chemistries
- Hyperuricemia
- Hypocalcemia
- Hyperphosphatemia
- Elevated LDH reflective of high-tumor burden and cell lysis

Bone marrow
- Homogenous lymphoblast field with hypercellular marrow (>25% blasts)
- Residual myeloid and erythroid precursors are morphologically normal
- A few/absent megakaryocytes

LP
- CNS blasts
- Elevated opening pressure
- Elevated protein
- Decreased glucose

Radiology
- Anterior mediastinal mass (more often associated with T-cell ALL)
- PET/CT scanning of the neck, chest, abdomen, and pelvis

are reduced. CNS involvement is present in 5–15% of adults and children, and is associated with the precursor T-cell immunophenotype. LP and subsequent CNS analysis show blasts, elevated opening pressure, elevated protein, and decreased glucose. Evidence exists that a traumatic LP may seed the CNS in unaffected children, and traumatic tap is an indication for intensification of CNS therapy (3). PA and lateral chest X-ray will show an anterior mediastinal mass in 5–10% of children and 15% of adults, a finding much more commonly associated with T-cell ALL.

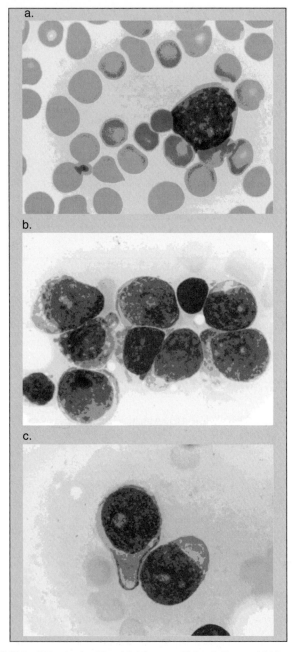

FIGURE 29-2   Slides showing (a) peripheral smear with lymphoblasts and (b) bone marrow aspirate. Leukemic lymphoblasts are large cells with a high nuclear to cytoplasmic ratio and prominent nucleoli. Cells with "hand mirror" contours may be seen in the peripheral blood in ALL. (Courtesy Rob Hasserjian, MGH Cancer Center).

RISK STRATIFICATION

Clinical Factors

Treatment of ALL is based on assignment of risk derived from immunopheno-type, cytogenetics, and clinical prognostic factors. In children, the Rome/NCI criteria have traditionally assigned children to standard versus high-risk categories for treatment based on age and WBC count at diagnosis. Children of ages 1–9 with B-cell ALL who present with WBC count <50,000/μl at diagnosis are considered standard risk, while all others are high risk. Recent trials have employed Children's Oncology Group (COG) criteria for risk assessment, in which age and WBC count determine initial risk; cytogenetics and subsequent response to therapy substratify during treatment into a four-category algorithm that maximizes cure rate and minimizes exposure to toxic chemotherapies in low-risk patients.

Factors that influence prognosis in children are summarized in Table 29-4. Overall, mature B-cell and precursor T-cell ALL immunophenotypes have poorer prognosis, and children are assigned to the high-risk treatment group regardless of blast count at presentation. Age at presentation is crucial, with the age group 1–9 being most favorable. Children less than 1 year old have an exceptionally poor prognosis, with aggressive disease (higher WBC at presentation, often accompanied by massive hepatosplenomegaly) attributed to a high frequency of the t(4;11) MLL-AF4 locus, which occurs in 50% of infants. Adolescents (10–20 years) have a poorer prognosis than younger children, presenting with more T-cell disease and poorer outcomes with Philadelphia-positive B-cell disease. When treated with pediatric protocols, however, outcomes are improved—the reason for this is not clear (4). Patient ethnicity has historically been a factor: African-Americans and Native Americans have generally experienced poorer outcomes, with higher WBC count, lymphadenopathy, and mediastinal mass on

Table 29-4

Prognostic Factors in Childhood ALL

	Favorable	Unfavorable
Age	1–9 Years at diagnosis	<1, >10 Years at diagnosis
WBC at presentation	<50,000/μl	>50,000/μl
Immunophenotype	Precursor B-cell type	Mature B-cell type Precursor T-cell type and sequelae: mediastinal mass and CNS involvement.
Race	Caucasian	Other (though normalizes with equal access to care)
Organ involvement (lymph nodes, spleen, liver,testes)	Absent	Present
CBC	Anemia and thrombocytopenia (implies indolent onset)	Absence of anemia or thrombocytopenia (implies explosive onset)
CNS involvement	Absent	Present
Response to therapy	Clearance of blasts by day 7	Nonclearance of blasts
Cytogenetics	t(12; 21) ETV-6 Hyperdiploidy >50 Trisomies 4, 10, 17	t(9; 22) BCR–ABL t(4; 11) AF4/MLL t(1; 19) E2A/PBX Hypodiploidy

presentation. However, this difference is reduced when patients are provided equal access to care (5). Important clinical factors include organ involvement (lymph nodes, spleen, liver, testes), which portends poor prognosis, as does the absence of anemia and thrombocytopenia, which correlates with explosive disease. Likewise, CNS involvement is associated with a lower rate of remission and higher rate of relapse. Finally, clearance of blasts is routinely measured at days 7 and 14 of induction chemotherapy; nonclearance of blasts is associated with a 2.7-fold relative risk of relapse in children (6).

Risk assignment in adults is less succinctly defined. In the absence of consensus guidelines, individual consortia have developed parameters to govern their trials. The Cancer and Leukemia Group B (CALGB) criteria for high-risk patients include (1) age greater than 30, which is inversely correlated with achievement of complete remission (CR), duration of CR, and overall survival. The linear worsening of prognosis with age in adult ALL makes it difficult to define a threshold of low versus high risk. (2) WBC at presentation: greater than 30,000/μl is associated with poor prognosis. (3) Presence of a mediastinal mass (which correlates with the precursor T-cell phenotype.)

Cytogenetics

Genetic lesions in ALL are common and correlated with immunophenotype, response to treatment, and disease recurrence (Figure 29-3). The WHO identifies six cytogenetic subcategories associated with prognosis in precursor B-cell ALL, summarized in Table 29-5. In children, classical cytogenetic lesions associated with favorable prognosis in precursor B-cell disease are the t(12;21) (ETV-6) translocation, found in 15–25% of children with ALL, and hyperdiploidy, with chromosome counts >50 per cell, found in 30% of children (versus 2% of adults). Trisomies of chromosomes 4, 10, 17, while not a WHO subcategory, also correlate with favorable prognosis in children (7).

Treatment failure in precursor B-cell ALL is associated with the t(4;11) (MLL-AF4) translocation, commonly found in infantile ALL with high blast counts (8). In both adults and children, the Philadelphia chromosome t(9;22) (BCR–ABL) portends negative prognosis. Prevalence of t(9;22) is striking in older adults, with 50% of patients over 50 exhibiting this mutation. Both the 210-kD gene product, identical to the one found in CML, and a smaller, 190 kD

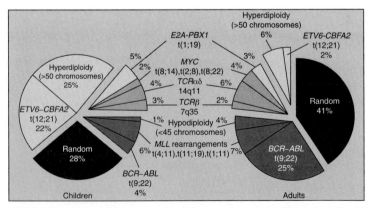

FIGURE 29-3 Estimated frequencies of specific genotypes among children and adults with ALL. (From Pui E. Drug therapy: acute lymphoblastic leukemia. New Engl J Med. 1998; 339: 605–615. Copyright © 1998 Massachusetts Medical Society. All rights reserved.)

Table 29-5

World Health Organization (WHO) Prognostic Implications of Genetic Alterations in Precursor B Lymphoblastic Leukemia

Cytogenetic finding	Genetic alteration	Function	Frequency (children)	Frequency (adults)	Prognosis
t(9;22)(q34;q11.2)	BCR/ABL	Fusion product with constitutive protein tyrosine kinase activity; enhances clone proliferation and survival.	3–4%	25%	Unfavorable
t(4;11)(q21;q23)	AF4/MLL	Disrupts homeobox genes, which regulate normal transcription of hematopoetic stem cells.	2–3%, but 50% of infants	5–6%	Unfavorable
t(1;19)(q23;p13.3)	E2A/PBX	Disrupts the activity of HOX-PBX dimers, which normally regulate hematopoetic differentiation.	6% (25% of pre-B ALL)		Unfavorable
t(12;21)(p13;q22)	ETV-6	Fusion product of two transcription factors, TEL and AML1. Inhibits normal AML1 activity, resulting in altered stem cell differentiation.	20–25%		Favorable
Hyperdiploid >50			30%	2%	Favorable
Hypodiploidy			2%	2%	Unfavorable

Adapted and expanded from Brunning RD, Borowitz M, Matutes E, et al. Precursor B lymphoblastic leuukaemia/lymphoblastic lymphoma (precursor B-cell acute lymphoblastic leukaemia). In E Jaffe, N Harris, H Stein, J Vardiman (eds.), "World Health Organization Classification of Tumors, Pathology and Genetics, Tumors of Haematopoietic and Lymphoid Tissues," IARC Press, Lyon, 2001 p. 113.

255

protein are found in Ph+ ALL, with equal prognostic implications (9). Finally, the t(1;19) (E2A-PBX1) translocation is associated with early treatment failure in pre-B-cell ALL (10).

Prognosis in T-cell ALL is less well correlated with specific cytogenetic mutations. The T-cell immunophenotype more often presents with aggressive features, including mediastinal mass and CNS infiltration, but no single karyotype confers this risk. Approximately 50% of precursor T-cell clones have activating mutations of the NOTCH1 gene, but the prognostic significance of this mutation is not yet defined (11). Translocations involving the T-cell receptor genes chromosomes 7 and 14 are common.

Application of genomic techniques to the study of ALL (expression profiling of lymphoblasts using cDNA microarrays) corroborates the clinical experience with cytogenetics playing a key role in prognosis. Expression arrays show clustering of gene expression influenced by major cytogenetic alterations. Microarray techniques may prove most useful in patients with normal cytogenetics for whom distinct molecular lesions are not identified by karyotype. Similarly, new techniques such as comparative genomic hybridization (CGH) may identify new chromosomal alterations and genetic mutations important in disease pathogenesis.

TREATMENT

Chemotherapy is the mainstay of treatment in ALL. The treatment regimen chosen is dependent upon immunophenotype and risk category. Table 29-6 provides a global approach to the treatment of patients with acute lymphoblastic malignancies.

With standard protocols, children with ALL attain remission in 98% of cases, with 80% surviving at least 5 years from diagnosis (12). In contrast, 85% of adults achieve CR, with a median duration of remission of 15 months and ultimate cure rate of only 25–40% of individuals.

Mature B-cell ALL does not respond well to chemotherapy traditionally used for precursor ALL. However, event-free survival (EFS) rates exceeding 90% have been obtained with treatments designed for Burkitt's lymphoma, which emphasize cyclophosphamide and the rapid rotation of antimetabolites in high dosages (Table 29-7). This strategy differs from therapies for precursor ALL, which involve sequential modules of remission induction, intensification, CNS prophylaxis, and maintenance. Patients with large sites of disease, as in precursor T-cell ALL with a mediastinal mass, often require involved field radiation therapy in addition to systemic chemotherapy. Typical regimens for precursor and mature B-cell ALL are provided in Table 29-8.

Remission induction aims to restore normal blood counts and marrow appearance, reduce the percentage of blasts to <5%, and eliminate extramedullary disease. Standard treatment regimens consist of vincristine, a glucocorticoid (usually prednisone), and L-asparaginase. Often an anthracycline (doxorubicin/daunorubicin) is added. Three to four drugs are used for standard-risk patients, while up to seven drugs may be used in high-risk cases. For adult patients, a five-drug regimen incorporating an alkylating agent, such as cyclophosphamide, an anthracycline, such as daunorubicin, vincristine, prednisone, and L-asparaginase, is commonly used for induction (13).

Intensification aims to eliminate residual leukemia, prevent relapse, and reduce the possible emergence of drug-resistant cells. In children, high-dose methotrexate with mercaptopurine is commonly used. Reinduction with the initial drug combination often follows after several months. In adults, current protocols use cyclophosphamide, Ara-C, mercaptopurine, vincristine, and L-asparaginase.

Table 29-6

Risk-Apdapted Stratification for Treatment of Adult ALL

Risk		Low-risk ALL	High-risk ALL	Very high risk ALL	Mature B-cell ALL
	B-lineage	WBC <30 K	WBC >30 K	Ph1/ bcr–abl* +	
	T-lineage	WBC <100 K	WBC >100 K		
	Time to CR	< 4 weeks	> 4 weeks Pro-B ALL, Pro T ALL		
Pretreatment			Consider Vinc/Pred if pretreatment for bulky disease		Cyclophos- phamide /prednisone for bulky disease
Multiple agent chemotherapy			Yes		Short, intensive cycles (4–6 depending upon regimen)
CNS prophylaxis			Yes		Yes
Consolidation / intensification			Yes		
BMT in CRI		Consider allo if MRD available	Allo if MRD available	Allo if MRD available, MUD for younger patients if MRD not available; Auto SCT for all others	No
Maintenance 6-MP/MTX intensification for 2 years		In patients not transplanted	In patients not transplanted	Yes	No

* Patients with t(9;22) should receive a bcr/abl tyrosine kinase inhibitor continuously throughout every phase of treatment.

Table 29-7

Common Adult ALL Treatment Regimens

Precursor acute B-cell lymphoblastic leukemia/lymphoma
- CALGB 19802 (Stock, et al. Blood. 2003; 102: 1375a)
- CALGB 9111 (Larson, et al. Blood. 1998; 92: 1556)

Precursor acute T-cell lymphoblastic leukemia/lymphoma
- GMALL/MSCMCC (Hoelzer, et al. Blood. 2002; 99: 4379)

Mature B-cell leukemia/Burkitt's lymphoma
- GMALL (German multicenter study group for treatment of adult ALL) (Hoelzer, Ludwig, et al. Blood. 1996; 87: 495.)
- BFM GMALL/NHL 2002(Hoelzer D, et al. Blood. 2003; 102: 236a)
- BFM 86(Reiter, et al. Blood. 1994; 84(9): 3122-3133)
- Modified Magrath Regimen (Lacasce, et al. Leuk Lymphoma. 2004; 45: 761-767.)
- (R)-HyperCVAD (Thomas et al. J Clin Oncol. 1999; 17: 2461-2470, Thomas et al. Cancer. 2006; 106: 1569-1580.)

Maintenance therapy preserves remission. In children, ALL requires 2–3 years of maintenance, significantly longer than other chemoresponsive cancers. The standard maintenance regimen in children is daily mercaptopurine and weekly methotrexate. In adults, monthly pulses of vincristine and prednisone are commonly added, though data on the benefit of maintenance in adults are inconclusive.

CNS prophylaxis While the incidence of CNS involvement is relatively rare (5–15%), the CNS can harbor ALL and be the nidus for recurrence if not treated at the outset. In CNS-negative disease, patients receive intrathecal (IT) methotrexate ±IT-Ara-C. Cranial irradiation is a standard component of therapy.

Salvage chemotherapy Relapsing patients (the majority of adults and the minority of children) will undergo reinduction with repeated use of induction agents or salvage regimens based on high-dose cytarabine in combination with other agents. Allogeneic transplantation, when possible, frequently follows for such high-risk patients if remission is attained.

Supportive care includes administration of G-CSF to maintain adequate neutrophil counts, infection prophylaxis, and treatment of the electrolyte disturbances associated with tumor lysis (alkalinization of urine, IV hydration, allopurinol, or rasburicase administration).

The efficacy of chemotherapy is evaluated by repeated analysis of peripheral blood and bone marrow samples at regular intervals. Response to therapy is measured in several ways: (1) Time interval to achieve CR with induction chemotherapy. Adults who do not achieve CR by 4 weeks are twice as likely to relapse, and have a negligible 5 year disease-free survival rate. (2) Detection of minimal residual disease. Molecular techniques (flow cytometry, quantitative PCR) can detect one lymphoblast in 10^4 and 10^6 normal cells, respectively. Current research is underway to correlate molecularly persistent disease with clinical recurrence.

Advances in survival have outpaced significant alterations in chemotherapy for ALL; survival is attributed to improvements in risk stratification such that patients receive sufficient chemotherapy while toxicities are minimized. Current investigation in pharmacogenomics may result in personalized approaches to chemotherapy types and dosages. For example, discovery of an autosomal recessive polymorphism in the thiopurine methyltransferase (TPMT) gene, responsible for inactivation of 6-mercaptopurine, has altered how chemotherapy is dosed. TPMT-deficient patients achieve toxic levels when standard doses of 6-MP are administered, but their EFS has been historically better—a finding with implications for optimal dosing in wild-type patients as well (14). In the future, pharmacogenomics will help to identify polymorphisms and permit dosing to maximal effect in patients.

Allogeneic hematopoietic cell transplantation has been shown to improve outcomes in high-risk groups such as t(9;22)-positive adults. Following remission induction, patients undergo conditioning with chemotherapy (and

Table 29-8

Common ALL Treatment Regimen

Acute lymphoblastic leukemia/lymphoma
CALGB 9111[1] (Larson, et al. Blood. 1998; 92: 1556-64)
Course I: Induction (4 weeks)

Cyclophosphamide*	IV	1,200 mg/m^2	Day 1
Daunorubicin*	IV	45 mg/m^2	Days 1, 2, 3
Vincristine	IV	2 mg	Days 1, 8, 15, 22
Prednisone*	PO/IV	60 mg/m^2/day	Days 1–21
L-asparaginase (*E coli*)	SC/IM	6,000 IU/m^2	Days 5, 8, 11, 15, 18, 22

* For patients ≥60 year old

Cyclophosphamide		800 mg/m^2	Day 1
Daunorubicin		30 mg/m^2	Days 1, 2, 3
Prednisone		60 mg/m^2/ day	Days 1–7

Course IIA: Early Intensification (4 weeks; repeat once for Course IIB)

Intrathecal methotrexate		15 mg	Day 1
Cyclophosphamide	IV	1,000 mg/m^2	Day 1
6-Mercaptopurine	PO	60 mg/m^2/ day	Days 1–14
Cytarabine	SC	75 mg/m^2/ day	Days 1–4, 8–11
Vincristine	IV	2 mg	Days 15, 22
L-asparaginase (*E coli*)	SC/IM	6,000 IU/m^2	Days 15, 18, 22, 25

Course III: CNS prophylaxis and interim maintenance (12 weeks)

Cranial irradiation		2,400 cGy	Days 1–12
Intrathecal methotrexate		15 mg	Days 1, 8, 15, 22, 29
6-Mercaptopurine	PO	60 mg/m^2/ day	Days 1–70
Methotrexate	PO	20 mg/m^2	Days 36, 43, 50, 57, 64

Course IV: Late intensification (8 weeks)

Doxorubicin	IV	30 mg/m^2	Days 1, 8, 15
Vincristine	IV	2 mg	Days 1, 8, 15
Dexamethasone	PO	10 mg/m^2/ day	Days 1–14
Cyclophosphamide	IV	1,000 mg/m^2	Day 29
6-Thioguanine	PO	60 mg/m^2/ day	Days 29–42
Cytarabine	SC	75 mg/m^2/ day	Days 29–32, 36–39

Course V: Prolonged maintenance (until 24 mo from diagnosis)

Vincristine	IV	2 mg	Day 1 of every 4 weeks
Prednisone	PO	60 mg/m^2/ day	Days 1–5 of every 4 weeks
6-Mercaptopurine	PO	60 mg/m^2/ day	Days 1–28
Methotrexate	PO	20 mg/m^2	Days 1, 8, 15, 22

(*Continued*)

Table 29-8 (*Continued*)

Common ALL Treatment Regimen

Mature B-cell lymphoma/Burkitt's lymphoma

1. BFM-86 for childhood ALL[2] (Reiter, et al., *Blood*, 80: 2471-8;1992).

ALL - BFM 86

AA

	VM-26	100	mg/m^2	1h INF.
	ARA-C	150	mg/m^2 every 12h	1h INF.
	VCR	1.5	mg/m^2	i.v.
	*MTX/ARA-C/PRED-S			i.th.
	MTX	5	g/m^2	24 h INF.
	IFO	800	mg/m^2	1h INF.
	DEXA	10	mg/m^2/day	p.o.

1 2 3 4 5   Days

BB

	DOX	25	mg/m^2	i.v.
	VCR	1.5	mg/m^2	i.v.
	*MTX/ARA-C/PRED-S			i.th.
	HD-MTX	5	g/m^2	24 h INF.
	CP	200	mg/m^2	1h INF.
	DEXA	10	mg/m^2/day	p.o.

1 2 3 4 5   Days

* i.th. Doses :	MTX	ARA-C	PRED-S
<1 Y.:	3	8	2 mg
>-1 and <2 Y.:	4	10	3 mg
>=2 and <3 Y.:	5	13	4 mg
>=3 Y.:	6:	15	5 mg

2. B-NHL 86 for mature ALL in adults[3] (German multicenter study group for treatment of adult ALL, Hoelzer, Ludwig, et al., *Blood* 87:495; 1996).

B-NHL 86

Prephase

	CP	200 mg/m^2 i.v. (1h)
	PRED	3 X 20 mg/m^2 p.o.

1 2 3 4 5 days

(*Continued*)

Table 29-8 *(Continued)*

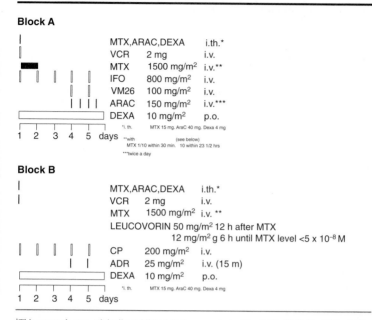

Block A

	MTX,ARAC,DEXA	i.th.*
	VCR	2 mg	i.v.
	MTX	1500 mg/m²	i.v.**
	IFO	800 mg/m²	i.v.
	VM26	100 mg/m²	i.v.
	ARAC	150 mg/m²	i.v.***
	DEXA	10 mg/m²	p.o.

1 2 3 4 5 days

*i. th.   MTX 15 mg. AraC 40 mg. Dexa 4 mg
**with   (see below)   MTX 1/10 within 30 min.   10 within 23 1/2 hrs
***twice a day

Block B

	MTX,ARAC,DEXA	i.th.*
	VCR	2 mg	i.v.
	MTX	1500 mg/m²	i.v. **
	LEUCOVORIN 50 mg/m² 12 h after MTX
	12 mg/m² g 6 h until MTX level <5 x 10⁻⁸ M
	CP	200 mg/m²	i.v.
	ADR	25 mg/m²	i.v. (15 m)
	DEXA	10 mg/m²	p.o.

1 2 3 4 5 days

*i. th.   MTX 15 mg. AraC 40 mg. Dexa 4 mg

[1]This research was originally published in Larson, et al., Blood 92: 1556-64; 1998. © The American Society of Hematology.

[2]This research was originally published in Reiter, et al., Blood, 80: 2471-8; 1992. © The American Society of Hematology.

[3]This research was originally published in German multicenter study group for treatment of adult ALL, Hoelzer, Ludwig, et al., Blood 87: 495; 1996. © The American Society of Hematology.

sometimes radiation) and transplantation with allogeneic hematopoietic cells. Transplantation not only provides hematopoietic rescue but also donor lympho- cytes, which may mediate a graft versus leukemia/lymphoma effect (15). Recent evidence suggests that even patients with normal cytogenetics benefit from allo- geneic transplantation over standard consolidation and maintenance chemotherapy if a matched related donor can be identified. Nonmyeloablative strategies are cur- rently under investigation for older patients or those unable to receive myeloabla- tive conditioning due to other medical conditions. Current research is evaluating the benefit of purged autologous hematopoietic stem cells, reduced-intensity con- ditioning regimens, and use of alternative stem cells sources such as cord blood.

Molecular agents The targeted ABL kinase inhibitor imatinib mesylate (Gleevec, Glivec) has shown activity against t(9;22)-positive disease, mainly when administered with standard chemotherapies (16). Current trials are evaluat- ing the benefit of monoclonal antibodies, such as the anti-CD20 agent rituximab (Rituxan), and inhibitors of molecular targets perturbed in ALL, such as NOTCH.

REFERENCES

1. National Cancer Institute. Adult ALL Treatment, Childhood ALL Treatment, SEER Pediatric Monograph. Available at http://www.cancer.gov/cancertopics/pdq/treat- ment/adultALL/HealthProfessional ttp://www.cancer.gov/cancertopics/pdq/treat- ment/childhoodALL/HealthProfessional. Accessed February 17, 2006.

2. Wiemels JL, Cazzaniga G, Daniotti M, et al. Prenatal origin of acute lymphoblastic leukaemia in children. The Lancet. 1999; 354: 1499–1503.
3. Gajjar A, Harrison PL, Sandlund JT, et al. Traumatic lumbar puncture at diagnosis adversely affects outcome in childhood acute lymphoblastic leukemia. Blood. 2000; 96(10): 3381–3384.
4. Boissel N, Auclerc M-F, Lheritier V, et al. Should adolescents with acute lymphoblastic leukemia be treated as old children or young adults? Comparison of the French FRALLE-93 and LALA-94 trials. J Clin Oncol. 2003; 21(5): 774–780.
5. Pui CH, Sandlund JT, Pei D, et al. Results of therapy for acute lymphoblastic leukemia in black and white children. J Am Med Assoc. 2003; 290(15): 2001–2007.
6. Steinherz PG, Gaynon PS, Breneman JC, et al. Cytoreduction and prognosis in acute lymphoblastic leukemia—the importance of early marrow response: report from the Children's Cancer Group. J Clin Oncol. 1996; 14: 389–398.
7. Brunning RD, Borowitz M, Matutes E, et al. Precursor B lymphoblastic leuukaemia/lymphoblastic lymphoma (precursor B-cell acute lymphoblastic leukaemia). In E Jaffe, N Harris, H Stein, J Vardiman (eds.), "World Health Organization Classification of Tumors, Pathology and Genetics, Tumors of Haematopoietic and Lymphoid Tissues," IARC Press, Lyon, 2001 pp. 111–117.
8. Heerema NA, Sather HN, Ge J, Arthur DC, Hilden JM, Trigg ME, Reaman GH. Cytogenetic studies of infant acute lymphoblastic leukemia: poor prognosis of infants with t(4;11)—a report of the Children's Cancer Group. Leukemia. 1999; 13(5): 679–686.
9. Secker-Walker L, Craig JM. Prognostic implications of breakpoint and lineage heterogeneity in Philadelphia-positive acute lymphoblastic leukemia: a review. Leukemia. 1993; 7: 147–1451.
10. Foa R, Vitale A, Mancini M, et al. E2A-PBX1 fusion in adult acute lymphoblastic leukemia: biological and clinical features. Br J Haematol. 2003; 120: 484–487.
11. Weng AP, Ferrando AA, Lee W, et al. Activating mutations of NOTCH1 in human T cell acute lymphoblastic leukemia. Science. 2004; 306: 269–271.
12. Maloney KW, Schuster JJ, Murphy S, Pullen J, Camitta BA. Long-term results of treatment studies for childhood acute lymphoblastic leukemia: Pediatric Oncology Group studies from 1986–1994. Leukemia. 2000; 14(12): 2276–2285.
13. Larson RA, Dodge RK, Burns CP, et al. A five-drug remission induction regimen with intensive consolidation for adults with acute lymphoblastic leukemia: cancer and leukemia group B study 8811. Blood. 1995; 85: 2025–2037.
14. Stanulla M, Schaeffeler E, Flohr T, et al. Thiopurine methyltransferase (TPMT) genotype and early treatment response to mercaptopurine in childhood acute lymphoblastic leukemia. J Am Med Assoc. 2005; 293(12): 1485–1489.
15. Dhedin N, Dombret H, Thomas X, et al. Autologous stem cell transplantation in adults with acute lymphoblastic leukemia in first complete remission: analysis of the LALA-85, -87 and -94 trials. Leukemia. 2006 Feb; 20(2): 336–344.
16. Thomas DA, Faderl S, Cortes J, et al. Treatment of Philadelphia chromosome-positive acute lymphocytic leukemia with hyper-CVAD and imatinib mesylate. Blood. 2004; 103: 4396–4407.

CHRONIC LYMPHOCYTIC LEUKEMIA

INTRODUCTION

Chronic lymphocytic leukemia (CLL) is a neoplastic disease characterized by the accumulation of monoclonal lymphocytes in blood, bone marrow, and lymphoid tissues. These lymphocytes are small, mature-appearing B cells typically expressing CD19, CD5, and CD23. It is generally a disease of older people and prognosis ranges widely from a few years to many years, but it is not considered curable outside of the bone marrow transplant setting.

EPIDEMIOLOGY

CLL is the most common form of leukemia among adults of Western societies and accounts for 30% of all leukemias. In the United States, 10,020 new cases or 2.7 per 100,000 persons and 4,660 deaths are projected for 2006 (1). The male to female ratio is approximately 2:1. CLL accounts for 0.8% of all cancers, and is a disease of older adults with a median age of 65 years; only 10% of patients are <50 year old. The disease tends to run in families. When multiple members of a family have CLL, a detectable clone of CLL cells can be found by flow cytometry in 13.5% of apparently healthy first-degree relatives of patients. Also, among normal individuals >40 years of age, a clone of B cells consistent with CLL can be found by multiparameter flow cytometry in 3.5% of subjects (2). It is uncertain whether these individuals will progress to clinically significant disease. CLL is uncommon in Asia.

BIOLOGY

Cause

The cause is unknown. Environmental factors such as exposure to radiation, sunlight, chemical toxins, or viruses are not associated with an increased incidence of the disease. HLA haplotype is not associated with disease susceptibility.

Molecular Defect

CLL cells are characterized by a defective B-cell receptor (CD79a and CD79b) that does not respond properly to antigen engagement but is associated with constitutive signaling intracellularly through ITAM's (immuno-receptor tyrosine based activation motifs) to activate a cascade of kinases including Lyn and Syk leading to proliferation, inhibition of apoptosis, or, on occasion, promotion of apoptosis. These changes lead to an accumulation of CLL cells in G0. CLL cells derive from antigen-experienced B lymphocytes and have the phenotype of activated cells. Activation status is based on the cell's overexpression of activation markers CD23, CD25, CD69, and CD71 as well as reduced expression of CD22, Fc receptor IIb, CD79b, and immunoglobulin D.

During an immune response, normal B cells encountering antigen will travel to a germinal center and undergo a series of point mutations in the immunoglobulin genes, which result in a more snug fit for the antigen in its binding site. These somatic mutations can be detected by sequencing the immunoglobulin heavy-chain variable-region (IgV_H) genes, a labor-intensive procedure not routinely available. Patients with CLL cells that contain somatic mutations in their Ig genes (a little over 50%) will have a much better prognosis than patients with CLL cells containing germline Ig sequences. Two surrogate markers for mutational status are more easily obtainable: CD38, a cell-surface enzyme involved in regulating B-cell activation, and ZAP-70, the 70 kD zeta-associated protein normally found in T cells and NK cells (3). CD38 levels tend to be high in CLL cells bearing unmutated Ig genes and can be easily assayed by routine flow cytometry. The intracellular protein ZAP-70 can also be assayed by flow cytometry, but it is technically more difficult. Elevated levels of ZAP-70 are also associated with CLL expressing unmutated Ig genes.

CLL cells can develop other cytogenetic abnormalities. Commonly detected clonal evolutions involve DNA deletions at chromosomes 13q14, 11q22-23, 17p13, and 6q21.

Immune Dysregulation

Patients with CLL frequently demonstrate immune dysregulation ranging from hyperreactivity to external stimuli such as insect bites to frank immunodeficiency with frequent infections. CLL cells elaborate immune suppressive cytokines such as CD27 or transforming growth factor-β, which impede immune activation. CLL cells can also down-modulate CD40 ligand on CD4 T cells, which results in defective function of T cells as well as the initial steps in immunoglobulin production. Paradoxically autoimmunity may develop leading to autoimmune hemolytic anemia, idiopathic thrombocytopenic purpura (ITP), pure red cell aplasia, or autoimmune neutropenia. Usually the pathogenic autoantibodies are not produced by the CLL cells but are produced by normal lymphocytes and plasma cells in response to factors produced by the CLL cells.

CLINICAL PRESENTATION

Most patients with CLL present with mild symptoms of fatigue or malaise. Over 25% will present asymptomatically with incidental lymphocytosis in blood and nearly 80% of patients have nontender lymphadenopathy. Occasionally, patients will present with advanced disease with fever, sweats, weight loss, anemia, thrombocytopenia, or recurrent infections. Although computerized axial tomography (CT) scans are not part of the routine evaluation of CLL, they can on occasion demonstrate massive lymphadenopathy not otherwise appreciated. Rarely, lymphadenopathy in CLL will be responsible for organ dysfunction such as ureteral obstruction with hydronephrosis or biliary obstruction. Splenomegaly is present initially in approximately 50% of patients and may cause discomfort or early satiety. Patients may have anemia or thrombocytopenia. It is of critical importance to assess whether the cause is bone marrow infiltration or destruction by autoantibodies as the treatment approach may vary according to the mechanism. The examination of the peripheral blood smear will generally show a lymphocytosis of mature-appearing lymphocytes with occasional larger lymphocytes and smudge cells. The smudge cells, which are broken lymphocytes resulting from the technique to prepare the blood smear, are virtually pathognomonic for CLL. Despite very high lymphocyte counts in some patients with CLL, hyperleukocytosis with pulmonary or cerebral symptoms requiring emergency intervention is rare; patients have generally tolerated lymphocyte counts as high as 800,000/μl without problems of hyperviscosity. Bone marrow biopsies performed at the time of presentation will show infiltrating CLL cells. The pattern of infiltration is said to be prognostic, and four patterns are recognized: interstitial, nodular, mixed, and diffuse (prognosis going from better to worse). A Coombs test is recommended at the time of presentation because approximately 20% of patients will test positive; however, only 8% will have autoimmune hemolytic anemia. Approximately 15% of patients will present with normochromic normocytic anemia that is not associated with anti-RBC antibodies.

DIAGNOSIS

Specific Criteria

The diagnostic criteria for CLL have evolved over time. In 1988 the National Cancer Institute-sponsored Working Group on Chronic lymphocytic leukemia (NCI-WG) published guidelines for the diagnosis and treatment of the disease, and these guidelines were updated in 1996 (4). According to the NCI-WG the diagnosis of CLL required a lymphocytosis of >5,000/μl with cells that are B cells (positive for CD19, CD20, and CD23) and carry the marker CD5. The lymphocytosis must also consist of <55% prolymphocytes, and >30% of the bone marrow needed to be infiltrated by lymphocytes. In 1997 a clinical advisory committee met to develop a classification of hematologic malignancies for the World Health Organization (WHO) and published their work in 1999 (5). Small lymphocytic lymphoma (SLL) was noted to be a tumor involving the same type of tumor cells as CLL but without blood involvement. According to the WHO criteria, the diagnosis of CLL relies almost completely on the immunophenotype of cells in tissue or blood without any requirement for certain numbers of lymphocytes in blood or bone marrow. The neoplastic B-cell population is positive for CD19 or CD20 and usually expresses CD5 and CD23. A variant, CLL with increased prolymphocytes, was defined for patients with typical CLL but with >10% but <55% prolymphocytes in blood. Additional features that help to define CLL are weak or dim expression of monoclonal surface immunoglobulin, and the absence of CD10 and cyclin D1. Rare cases of CLL can be negative for CD5 or CD23 when other features strongly support the diagnosis. Although approximately 80% of cases will have an abnormal karyotype by FISH analysis, no specific cytogenetic abnormality defines the disease.

Differential Diagnosis (see Table 30-1)

BENIGN LYMPHOCYTOSIS   Patients may present with a high lymphocyte count when infected with various organisms such as: viruses, *Bordetella pertussis*, or *Toxoplasma gondii*. Usually, the lymphocytosis is not sustained, however, and flow cytometry will not show monoclonal surface Ig or expression of CD5 on B cells.

DISTINGUISHING CLL FROM OTHER B CELL LEUKEMIAS   CLL is generally easily distinguished from other monoclonal B cell malignancies that can be associated with lymphocytosis. CLL is surface Ig weak (all others are strong), CD5 positive (all others are negative), CD23 positive (all others are negative), and CD79b/CD22 weak (all others are strong). In addition, an antibody called FMC7 does not react with CLL cells but does react with other B-cell leukemias.

PROLYMPHOCYTIC LEUKEMIA   When the percentage of prolymphocytes in blood exceeds 55% in a patient who otherwise makes criteria for CLL, a diagnosis of prolymphocytic leukemia is made. It accounts for 1% of lymphoid leukemias. The prolymphocytes are larger cells being 10–15 μm in diameter (versus 7–10 μm for CLL cells), and they have more cytoplasm, frequently have nucleoli, and stain brightly for surface immunoglobulin. Prognosis is worse for prolymphocytic leukemia.

Table 30-1

Immunophenotype of CLL and Similar Neoplasms

Neoplasm	Surface Ig	CD3	CD4	CD5	CD8	CD10	CD11c	CD19	CD20	CD23	CD103	Cyclin D1	Bcl-2	TCR
CLL/SLL[1]	dim	-	-	+	-	-	dim	+	dim	+		-		-
PLL[2]	++		-	+/-				+	+	-				
LGL[3]	-	+			+									+
HCL[4]	+			-		-	++	+	+	-	++	+/-		
MCL[5]	++			+		-		++	+	-	-	+	+	
SMZL[6]	+			-		-			+	-	-	-		
FL[7]	+			-		+		+	+	+			+	

[1]Chronic lymphocytic leukemia/small lymphocytic lymphoma.

[2]Prolymphocytic leukemia.

[3]Large granular lymphocyte leukemia.

[4]Hairy cell leukemia.

[5]Mantle cell leukemia.

[6]Splenic marginal zone lymphoma.

[7]Follicular lymphoma.

T-CLL OR T-PROLYMPHOCYTIC LEUKEMIA (T-PLL) In about 2% of cases of small lymphocytic leukemia, the blood contains small to medium sized lymphoid cells with nongranular basophilic cytoplasm and round or oval nuclei with a nucleolus. Patients often have hepatosplenomegaly and lymphadenopathy and 20% have skin infiltration. The tumor cells are CD2, CD3, and CD7 positive and TdT and CD1a negative. In 60%, the cells express CD4 but not CD8; in 15% they express CD8 but not CD4; and in 25% they express both CD4 and CD8. The course of disease is rapid with median survival of 1 year.

T-CELL LARGE GRANULAR LYMPHOCYTIC LEUKEMIA In 2–3% of cases of small lymphocytic leukemia, the cells in the peripheral blood have abundant cytoplasm that contains azurophilic granules. These patients usually present with neutropenia and minimal lymphocytosis. Flow cytometry shows these cells to be T cells being positive for CD3, CD8, CD57, and the T-cell receptor (TCR). The cells are usually negative for CD4. The course of disease is often indolent.

HAIRY CELL LEUKEMIA In about 2% of cases of small lymphocytic leukemia, the blood smear will show a minimal lymphocytosis with lymphocytes demonstrating villous projections. Flow cytometry is diagnostic with cells positive for CD19, CD20, CD22, CD25, CD103, and CD11c. Flow cytometry will be negative for CD5, CD10, CD21, and CD23. Note that some cells may be positive for cyclin D1. Soluble CD25 levels are elevated. Patients present with splenomegaly and pancytopenia; monocytopenia is often noted. Long remissions have been obtained using cladribine or other nucleosides.

MANTLE CELL LYMPHOMA WITH BLOOD INVOLVEMENT These cells in blood and lymph nodes may look very much like CLL cells, and flow cytometry is required for a secure diagnosis. The cells are positive for CD5, surface immunoglobulin, and cyclin D1, while being negative for CD10 and CD23. Prognosis for mantle cell lymphoma is generally much worse than that for CLL.

FOLLICULAR LYMPHOMA WITH BLOOD INVOLVEMENT Examination of the blood smear usually shows these cells to have cleaved nuclei, while CLL cells do not. The flow cytometry pattern shows cells positive for CD10, CD19, CD20, CD22, and surface immunoglobulin with a bright pattern. The cells are negative for CD5.

EVALUATION OF THE PATIENT

The following evaluation is commonly performed on patients with CLL:

> History and physical exam
> Complete blood count with differential
> Reticulocyte count, Coombs test, and LDH
> Routine chemistries, uric acid, liver function tests including albumin and globulin
> Serum protein electrophoresis
> Beta-2-microglobulin
> Flow cytometry of blood including a CD38 determination
> CT scans of the neck, chest, and abdomen (optional)
> Bone marrow biopsy with cytogenetics by FISH analysis (optional)

Clinical trials may require CT scans to assess response. Bone marrow biopsy is usually delayed until it is indicated to assess the pathophysiologic basis of anemia or thrombocytopenia. Peripheral blood examination and physical examination are usually adequate for initial evaluation of asymptomatic patients.

PROGNOSTIC FACTORS

Staging

Using clinical data from the physical exam and the complete blood count with differential, an estimate of prognosis can be obtained. The critical features used to assign clinical stage of disease are the presence of lymphadenopathy, splenomegaly, or hepatomegaly, and the presence of anemia and/or thrombocytopenia. The Rai (6) and Binet (7) staging classifications for CLL are shown in Table 30-2. Prognosis varies from 2 years with advanced stage disease to over 10 years with lymphocytosis.

Mutational Status

In about half of cases of CLL, immunoglobulin V_H genes have undergone somatic mutation, and this event is associated with an improved prognosis compared to patients whose cells express unmutated Ig genes. Determining mutational status of Ig genes is highly specialized and not widely available. The presence of ZAP-70 in the cytoplasm and CD38 on the surface of CLL cells has been found to correlate with the presence of unmutated Ig genes and a poorer prognosis. In one study (Figure 30-1), at approximately 10 years the mutated group and the CD38 negative group both showed 80% survival, while the unmutated group and the CD38 positive group both showed approximately 40% survival (8). Similar results have been seen when CLL patients have been analyzed based on ZAP-70 expression (9).

Table 30-2

Staging Systems for Chronic Lymphocytic Leukemia (7,8)

	Criteria	Median survival (y)
RAI STAGING SYSTEM Stage*		
O (low-risk)	Lymphocytes > 15 × 10⁹/l Bone marrow >40% Lymphocytes	>10
I and II (intermediate-risk)	Blood and bone marrow lymphocytosis, lymphadenopathy, liver or spleen enlargement	6
III and IV (high-rish)	Blood and bone marrow lymphocytosis plus anemia (hemoglobin <11 g/dl) or thrombocytopenia (platelets <100 × 10⁹/l)	2
BINET STAGING SYSTEM Group*		
A	No anemia or thrombocytopenia, less than three of the following five areas involved: axillary,inguinal, cervical (unilateral or bilateral), lymphadenopathy, liver, spleen	9
B	No anemia or thrombocytopenia; three or more involved areas	5
C	Anemia (hemoglobin <10g/dl) or thrombocytopenia (platelets <100 × 10⁹/l)	2

*Autoimmune hemolytic anemia and thrombocytopenia are independent of stage or group.

(Reproduced with permission from Handin R, Lux S, Stossel T (eds). Blood: Principles and Practice of Hematology. Philadelphia, JB Lippincott, 1995, p. 789.)

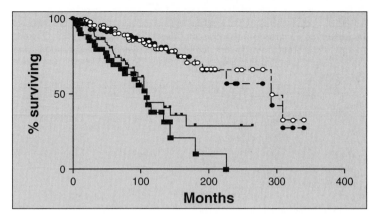

FIGURE 30-1 Survival curves of 145 patients with B-CLL. Comparisons were made of patients whose cells are CD38+ (⊥. N = 60) or CD 38-(•. N = 85) and have mutated (○. N = 95) or unmutated (■. N = 50) IgV$_H$ genes from date of diagnosis of CLL. (From Hamblin TJ, et al. CD38 expression and immunoglobulin variable region mutations are independent prognostic variables in chronic lymphocytic leukemia, but CD38 expression may vary during the course of the disease. Blood. 2002; 99: 1023-1029.)

Karyotype

Cytogenetic analysis can also identify patients with distinct prognosis (10). Surprisingly, 82% of the cases contained a chromosomal aberration by FISH techniques. The most frequent changes were a deletion in 13q, a deletion in 11q, trisomy 12, a deletion in 17p, and a deletion in 6q (Table 30-3). Prognosis varied widely with a median survival of 2.5 years for patients with the 17p deletion compared to 10 years or more for patients with a normal karyotype, trisomy 12, or a 13q deletion (Figure 30-2).

Other Factors

Short doubling time of the lymphocyte count is associated with a poor prognosis; median survival for patients with a doubling time <12 months is about 5 years compared to a survival of 12 years for a longer doubling time. Bone marrow histology for patients with CLL (as noted above) has been studied; those with a diffuse pattern of involvement have a poor prognosis and complications with cytopenias. Elevated beta-2-microglobulin is associated with poorer prognosis. Elevated LDH may indicate the presence of Richter transformation, which occurs at some point in 5–10% of patients with CLL. The transformation marks the conversion to a diffuse large B-cell lymphoma generally resistant to treatment and associated with survival of 3–6 months. Telomerase activity when high has been linked to the presence of short telomeres and aggressive histology. The patients with unmutated CLL tend to have high telomerase activity and short survival.

Most of these prognostic factors are not employed in clinical decision-making.

TREATMENT

Indications

The indications to treat CLL are the emergence of symptoms caused by the tumor mass (pain, organ compromise, or constitutional symptoms) or the development of anemia and/or thrombocytopenia. It is important to investigate the mechanism of the cytopenia. The development of autoimmune cytopenias does not influence

Table 30-3

Incidence of Chromosomal Abnormalities in 325 Patients with Chronic Lymphocytic Leukemia. (From Dohner et al. Genomic Aberrations and Survival in Chronic Lymphocytic Leukemia. N Engl J Med. 2000; 343: 1910-1916.)

Aberration	No. of patients (%)*
13q deletion	178 (55)
11q deletion	58 (18)
12q trisomy	53 (16)
17p deletion	23 (7)
6q deletion	21 (6)
8q trisomy	16 (5)
t(14q32)	12 (4)
Clonal abnormalities	268 (82)
Normal karyotype	57 (18)

*One hundred seventy five patients had one aberration, 67 had two aberrations, and 26 had more then two aberrations.

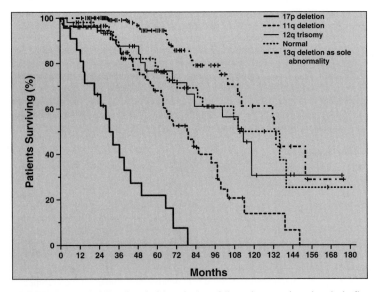

FIGURE 30-2   Probability of survival from the date of diagnosis among the patients in the five genetic categories. The median survival times for the groups with 17p deletion, 11q deletion, 12q trisomy, normal karyotype, and 13q deletion as the sole abnormality were 32, 79, 114, 111, and 133 months, respectively. Twenty-five patients with various other chromosomal abnormalities are not included in the analysis. (From Dohner H, et al. Genomic aberrations and survival in chronic lymphocytic leukemia. N Engl J Med. 2000; 343: 1910-1916.)

overall survival. These autoimmune cytopenias can be controlled by immuno-suppressive therapy with glucocorticoids or rituximab or, in some instances, by splenectomy. If marrow expansion of CLL cells is the basis for the cytopenia, aggressive therapy aimed at the tumor is indicated because the disease is in advanced stage and represents a threat to survival.

Intensity of Treatment

Once a decision is made to treat a patient, one must consider whether a mild treatment is best or a more intense approach is indicated. The clinical features used to make this decision generally are: age of the patient, performance status, comorbid conditions, ability to monitor the patient closely, and the specific wishes of the patient.

Specific Drugs or Regimens

Most patients with CLL are treated with one or a combination of the following drugs: chlorambucil, fludarabine, cyclophosphamide, rituximab, and alemtuzumab. Single-agent fludarabine is more active than chlorambucil (Figure 30-3), but patients in both groups had a median survival of approximately 5 years (11). While glucocorticoids are important for treating complicating conditions such as hemolytic anemia and ITP, they do not improve the response rate of treatment with alkylating agents. Likewise, alkylating agent based combinations such as CVP (cyclophosphamide, vincristine, and prednisone), CHOP (cyclophosphamide, doxorubicin, vincristine, and prednisone), and CAP (cyclophosphamide, doxorubicin, and prednisone) have not been proven to be better than an alkylating agent alone, and they have been inferior to single-agent fludarabine treatment, when tested head-to-head. Clinical trials have shown that responses improve, however, when cyclophosphamide or rituximab (anti-CD20) is added to fludarabine (Table 30-4). Using the three drugs together as a combination has resulted in further improvement (12). Doses and schedules of commonly used regimens are provided in Table 30-5. The role of alemtuzumab (anti-CD52) is unclear, but as a single agent in 41 patients without prior treatment, an overall response rate of 87% was observed with 19% complete responses (13). It is generally reserved for second-line therapy in patients who no longer respond to fludarabine-based therapy because of its potent immunosuppressive effects that may lead to opportunistic infection.

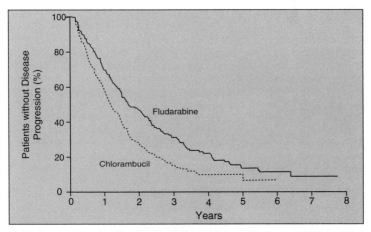

FIGURE 30-3 Proportion of CLL patients without disease progression, according to treatment group. The median time to progression was significantly longer in the fludarabine group than in the chlorambucil group (20 versus 14 months, $P < 0.001$). (From Rai KR, et al. Fludarabine compared with chlorambucil as primary therapy for chronic lymphocytic leukemia. N Engl J Med. 2000; 343: 1750-1757.)

Table 30-4

Reported Complete and Overall Response Rates (CR and OR) in Various Clinical Trials for Previously Untreated Chronic Lymphocytic Leukemia (CLL)

Regimen	Patients	CR (%)	OR (%)	Reference
Chlorambucil	181	4	37	(11)
Fludarabine	170	20	63	(11)
Fludarabine + Cyclophosphamide	34	35	88	(17)
Fludarabine + Rituximab	51	47	90	(18)
Fludarabine, Cyclophosphamide, Rituximab	224	70	95	(12)

Table 30-5

Regimens Useful in the Treatment of CLL

Regimen	Dose and schedule
Chlorambucil	10 mg/day PO or 40 mg/m^2 PO day 1 q28d
Fludarabine	25 mg/m^2 IV days 1–5 q28d
Fludarabine plus Cyclophosphamide	30 mg/m^2 IV days 1–3 q28d 300 mg/m^2 IV days 1–3 q28d
Fludarabine plus Rituximab	25 mg/m^2 IV days 1–5 q28d 375 mg/m^2 IV d1 q28d, with an extra dose on day 4 of cycle 1
Fludarabine plus Cyclophosphamide plus Rituximab	25 mg/m^2 IV on days 2–4 of cycle 1, days 1–3 of cycles 2–6 250 mg/m^2 IV for 3 days with fludarabine 375 mg/m^2 IV day 1 of cycle 1, 500 mg/m^2 IV day 1 of cycles 2–6

Bone Marrow Transplantation

There is no consensus about which patients with CLL are likely to benefit most from high-dose therapy with hematopoietic stem cell support. Since most patients with CLL are over age 60, many are too old to be eligible for allogeneic transplants. The use of autologous stem cell transplantation raises the concern about contaminating CLL cells being harvested with the marrow or peripheral blood to be reinfused. For both autologous and allogeneic transplants, the median survival is 4–8 years without a clear plateau of survival, although there have been fewer late failures among the patients undergoing allogeneic bone marrow transplantation (14). Mini-transplants are being evaluated. Younger patients with aggressive disease may be considered for an experimental approach.

FUTURE DIRECTIONS

Consolidation with Alemtuzumab

Patients with CLL characterized by deletions of 17p13 have a particularly resistant form of disease, possibly due to alterations in p53. Alemtuzumab is particularly effective in this population of patients leading to the concept of consolidating patients with alemtuzumab treatment after more conventional treatment to eradicate any resistant cells that may be left behind. Results of such studies are already being reported (15).

Minimal Residual Disease

As treatment becomes more effective, there is a need to evaluate patients with lower tumor burden than can be detected by clinical measures. Studies using PCR (polymerase chain reaction) techniques for the IgV_H gene can detect 1 CLL cell in 10,000 on a reliable basis, but the procedure is labor intensive. Multiparameter flow cytometry is also capable of detecting 1 CLL cell in 10,000 when certain antibodies are used. One set of antibodies shown to be effective for this is CD5, CD19, CD20, CD79b. Detection of minimal residual disease (MRD) is clinically useful, as trials now show a survival advantage for those patients that are rendered MRD negative (16). Most future clinical trials will include MRD monitoring. Additional data are needed to assess whether clinical decisions can be made based on the MRD results.

New Drugs

Several new drugs undergoing evaluation in clinical trials are already showing activity in CLL. Although it is unclear at this time how useful they will become, they have stirred the interest of many investigators. A short list of active new agents includes flavopiridol (a caspase 3 activator), lenalidomide (a thalidomide analog), denileukin diftitox (an IL-2 directed toxin), and oblimersan (an anti-sense compound to BCL-2).

Supportive Care

The underlying hypogammaglobulinemia along with certain agents used in treatment (fludorabine, rituxumab, alemtuzumab) can lead to an increased risk of serious infection. When a patient experiences his or her second serious infection, monthly intravenous immunoglobulin can reduce the infectious risk, but is expensive.

CONCLUSIONS

Considerable progress has been made in understanding the biology of CLL and developing new and more effective treatments. Long-term remissions are now possible in a subset of patient. Therapies are sufficiently potent that questions can now be raised about the clinical meaning of MRD. The outlook for CLL patients has improved and ongoing research promises even more progress.

REFERENCES

1. Jemal A, Slegel R, Ward E, et al. Cancer statistics. CA Cancer J Clin. 2006; 56: 106–130.
2. Rawstron AC, Green MJ, Kuzmicki A, et al. Monoclonal B lymphocytes with the characteristics of "indolent" chronic lymphocytic leukemia are present in 3.5% of adults with normal blood counts. Blood. 2002; 100: 635–9.
3. Chiorazzi N, Rai KR, Ferrarini M. Chronic lymphocytic leukemia. N Engl J Med. 2005; 352: 804–15.
4. Cheson BD, Bennett JM, Grever M, et al. National Cancer Institute-sponsored Working Group guidelines for chronic lymphocytic leukemia: revised guidelines for diagnosis and treatment. Blood. 1996; 87: 4990–7.
5. Harris NL, Jaffe ES, Diebold J, et al. World Health Organization classification of neoplastic diseases of the hematopoietic and lymphoid tissues: report of the Clinical Advisory Committee meeting-Airlie House, Virginia, November 1997. J Clin Oncol. 1999; 7: 3835–49.
6. Rai KR, Sawitsky A, Cronkite EP, et al. Clinical staging of chronic lymphocytic leukemia. Blood. 1975; 46: 219–34.

7. Binet JL, Auquier A, Dighiero G, et al. A new prognostic classification of chronic lymphocytic leukemia derived from a multivariate survival analysis. Cancer. 1981; 48: 198–206.

8. Hamblin TJ, Orchard JA, Ibbotson RE, et al. CD38 expression and immunoglobulin variable region mutations are independent prognostic variables in chronic lymphocytic leukemia, but CD38 expression may vary during the course of the disease. Blood. 2002; 99: 1023–9.

9. Rassenti LZ, Huynh L, Toy TL, et al. ZAP-70 compared with immunoglobulin heavy-chain gene mutation status as a predictor of disease progression in chronic lymphocytic leukemia. N Engl J Med. 2004; 351: 893–901.

10. Dohner H, Stilgenbauer S, Benner A, et al. Genomic aberrations and survival in chronic lymphocytic leukemia. N Engl J Med. 2000; 343: 1910–6.

11. Rai KR, Peterson BL, Appelbaum FR, et al. Fludarabine compared with chlorambucil as primary therapy for chronic lymphocytic leukemia. N Engl J Med. 2000; 343: 1750–7.

12. Keating MJ, O'Brien S, Albitar M, et al. Early results of a chemoimmunotherapy regimen of fludarabine, cyclophosphamide, and rituximab as initial therapy for chronic lymphocytic leukemia. J Clin Oncol. 2005; 23: 4079–88.

13. Lundin J, Kimby E, Bjorkholm M, et al. Phase II trial of subcutaneous anti-CD52 monoclonal antibody alemtuzumab (Campath-1H) as first-line treatment for patients with B-cell chronic lymphocytic leukemia (B-CLL). Blood. 2002; 100: 768–73.

14. Gribben JG, Zahrieh D, Stephans K, et al. Autologous and allogeneic stem cell transplantations for poor-risk chronic lymphocytic leukemia. Blood. 2005; 106: 4389–96.

15. Moreton P, Kennedy B, Lucas G, et al. Eradication of minimal residual disease in B cell chronic lymphocytic leukemia after alemtuzumab therapy is associated with prolonged survival. J Clin Oncol. 2005; 23: 2971–9.

16. Rawstron AC, Kennedy B, Evaas PA, et al. Quantitation of minimal disease levels in chronic lymphocytic leukemia using a sensitive flow cytometric assay improves the prediction of outcome and can be used to optimize therapy. Blood. 2001; 98: 29–35.

17. O'Brien SM, Kantarjian HM, Cortes J, et al. Results of the fludarabine and cyclophosphamide combination regimen in chronic lymphocytic leukemia. J Clin Oncol. 2001; 19: 1414–20.

18. Byrd JC, Peterson BL, Morrison VA, et al. Randomized phase 2 study of fludarabine with concurrent versus sequential treatment with rituximab in symptomatic, untreated patients with B-cell chronic lymphocytic leukemia: results from Cancer and Leukemia Group B 9712 (CALGB 9712). Blood. 2003; 101: 6–14.

PLASMA CELL DISORDERS

INTRODUCTION

Plasma cell disorders are a group of related diseases arising from a common progenitor belonging to the B cell lineage. They are characterized by the expansion of plasma cells in the bone marrow (BM) and nearly always accompanied by the presence of a monoclonal immunoglobulin (Ig) or Ig fragment in the serum and/or urine of patients (1). Monoclonal gammopathy of undetermined significance (MGUS), multiple myeloma (MM), Waldenstrom's macroglobulinemia (WM), primary amyloidosis, and heavy chain diseases (HCD) all belong to this group of disorders. Dysproteinemias or plasma cell dyscrasias are some of the other terms used to refer to this unique group of disorders.

Normal B cell differentiation is characterized by a process of Ig VDJ rearrangement, somatic mutation, and Ig class switching resulting in maturation of antibody-producing plasma cells. Ig variable (VH) gene sequence analysis indicates that myeloma tumor cells are postfollicular, and originate from a memory cell undergoing isotype switch events. Translocations involving switch regions indicate that the final oncogenic molecular event in myeloma occurs late in B cell ontogeny. Five heavy chain isotypes (M, G, A, D, E) and two light chain isotypes (κ and λ) are present and are typically identified by serum or urine protein electrophoresis as a sharp spike in the gamma region. The isotype is further identified and quantitated by immunofixation and is referred to as the monoclonal component, that is, arising from the neoplastic clone. This is a useful biomarker and helps determine responses in patients with plasma cell disorders. More recently an ELISA-based assay is being used to detect light chains in the serum. This is particularly useful in patients with amyloidosis, light chain MM, and nonsecretory MM.

MONOCLONAL GAMMOPATHY OF UNDETERMINED SIGNIFICANCE

Monoclonal gammopathy of undetermined significance (MGUS) is seen in 1% of patients over age 50 and 3% of people over age 70 and is associated with the presence of a monoclonal Ig which is less than 3.5 g/l (2). It is differentiated from MM by the lack of proteinuria, fewer than 5% monoclonal BM plasma cells, and lack of end organ damage like bone lesions, anemia, hypercalcemia, or renal dysfunction. In a large series of 1,384 patients followed longitudinally at the Mayo Clinic, 115 patients progressed to MM (relative risk (RR) 25), IgM lymphoma (RR 2.4), primary amyloidosis (RR 8.4), macroglobulinemia (RR 46), chronic lymphocytic leukemia (RR 0.9), or plasmacytoma (RR 8.5). The risk of progression of MGUS to MM or related disorders is about 1% per year; the initial concentration of serum monoclonal protein is a significant predictor of progression at 20 years. (2)

MULTIPLE MYELOMA

Epidemiology

MM is a plasma cell dyscrasia characterized by a clonal proliferation of lymphoid B cells and infiltration of the BM by plasma cells (1, 3). It is the second most common hematologic malignancy, and is responsible for at least 2% of cancer-related deaths. It is estimated that 19,900 new cases of MM were diagnosed in the United States and 10,790 deaths from MM occurred in 2007 (4). African-Americans and Pacific Islanders have a reported high incidence of MM followed by Europeans and North American Caucasians. Low incidence rates have been reported for Asians living in Asia and the United States (5). In addition to MGUS, potential risk factors for the development of MM include exposure to irradiation or petroleum products. Familial cases have also been reported, suggesting a possible genetic predisposition. Myeloma has also been found to occur with somewhat greater frequency in farmers, paper producers, furniture manufacturers, and wood workers.

Biology

Cytokines like interleukin-6 (IL-6) and insulin-like growth factor-1 (IGF-1) confer a growth and survival advantage to MM cells. Regulation of the mitogen activated protein kinase (MAPK) and phosphatidylinositol 3′-kinase/Akt kinase (P13 kinase/AKT) pathways by these and other cytokines and activation of the survival Janus Kinase/signal transducer and activator of transcription (JAK/STAT) pathway may be involved in the pathogenesis. The role of adhesion molecules and the BM microenvironment is also critical to tumor cell growth and survival. Adhesion molecules mediate both homotypic and heterotypic adhesion of tumor cells to either extracellular matrix (ECM) proteins or bone marrow stromal cells (BMSCs). After class switching in the LN, adhesion molecules, including CD44, VLA-4, VLA-5, LFA-1, CD56, Syndecan-1, and MPC-1, mediate homing of myeloma cells to the BM, and adhesion to BMSCs and ECM. Such binding not only localizes tumor cells to the BM microenvironment, but also stimulates IL-6 transcription and secretion from BMSCs with related paracrine growth of myeloma cells. In addition to homing to the BM, loss of some of these adhesion molecules results in migration at the time of disease progression. The binding of MM cells to BMSCs also regulates cell cycle progression and plays a role in the development of adhesion-mediated drug resistance (3).

A variety of chromosomal abnormalities are found in MM. Based on conventional cytogenetic analysis, chromosome 13 deletions were predominant and associated with a poor prognosis. Techniques like spectral karyotyping have identified chromosomal abnormalities in the majority of MM patients and are broadly classified into hyperdiploid (HRD) or nonhyperdiploid (NHRD) tumors. Five recurrent IgH translocations have been seen in MM including MMSET and FGFR3 (15%), cyclin D3 (3%), cyclin D1 (15%), c-maf (5%) genes, and MAFB (2%) accounting for a prevalence of 40%. All MM tumor cells have high levels of cyclin D1, D2, and D3 including MGUS suggesting a unifying early oncogenic event (6, 7). Dysregulation of cyclin genes renders MM cells more susceptible to proliferative stimuli resulting in selective expansion in response to BMSCs and/or cytokines like IL-6 and IGF-1. On the basis of gene expression profiles, a new molecular classification has been proposed that categorizes patients based on the five major translocations and cyclin D overexpression in MM.

Diagnostic Criteria

The diagnosis of MM is based on the presence of well defined major and minor criteria (Table 31-1) (8). These criteria help distinguish MM from other plasma cell dyscrasias and B cell malignancies associated with a paraprotein. They also help differentiate MM from solitary plasmacytoma. Solitary plasmacytomas are collections of monoclonal plasma cells originating in either bone (solitary osseous

Table 31-1

Durie-Salmon Criteria for Diagnosis of Myeloma

Major criteria
1. Plasmacytomas on tissue biopsy
2. BM plasmacytosis (>30% plasma cells)
3. Monoclonal immunoglobulin spike on serum or urine electrophoresis: IgG >3.5 g/dl or IgA >2.0 g/dl; κ or λ light chain urinary excretion > 1.0g/day

Minor criteria
a. BM plasmacytosis (10–30% plasma cells)
b. Monoclonal immunoglobulin spike present but at a lower magnitude than above
c. Lytic bone lesions
d. Normal IgM< 500 mg/l, IgA < I g/l, or IgG < 6 g/l

The diagnosis of myeloma requires a minimum of one major and one minor criterion, although (1) + (a) is not sufficient or three minor criteria that must include (a) and (b).

Patients with the above criteria associated with
- absent or limited bone lesions (≥3 lytic lesions), no compression fractures
- stable paraprotein levels IgG < 70 g/l, IgA <50 g/l
- no symptoms and associated disease features including Karnofsky performance status > 70%, hemoglobin > 10 g/l, normal serum calcium, serum creatinine <2 mg/dl, and no infections
- plasma cell labelling index ≤ 0.5%

are categorized as those with indolent myeloma and do not require immediate therapy.

Adapted from Durie, BG. Semin Oncol. 1986; 13: 300–309.

plasmacytoma, SOP) or soft tissue (extramedullary plasmacytoma, EMP) and are very responsive to local radiation treatment. The mean age of diagnosis of solitary plasmacytomas is usually younger than MM and approximately 70% of EMPs can be cured with local treatment alone. EMPs typically involve the lymphoid tissues of the upper aerodigestive tract. SOPs have a higher rate of progression to MM and therefore patients with plasmacytomas require prolonged follow-up (9).

Clinical and Laboratory Features

The mean age at diagnosis for MM is 62 years for men and 61 years for women. A slight male preponderance has been described. BM infiltration with plasma cells is commonly seen (Figure 31-1). Most of the symptoms associated with MM are a result of the end organ damage caused by either MM tumor cell infiltration and/or the associated paraprotein. Symptoms of bone pain and anemia remain the most common presenting features affecting 80% of the patients. Other features include renal insufficiency, hypercalcemia, and symptoms associated with infection and hyperviscosity (10) (Table 31-2).

Bone disease and hypercalcemia MM typically presents with osteolytic bone lesions (Figure 31-2). These may be associated with pathologic and compression fractures of the vertebral bodies. Bone scans and serum alkaline phosphatase are usually normal because of the absence of osteoblastic activity. Increased tumor burden results in production of osteoclast-activating factors like lymphotoxin (LT), TNF-α, hepatocyte growth factor (HGF), IL-6, IL-1, metalloproteinases, RANKL, and insulin-like growth factor binding protein 4 (IGFIV) resulting in increased osteoclastogenesis and increased bone resorption. Bone resorption leads to increased calcium in extracellular fluid.

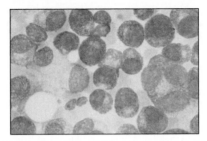

FIGURE 31-1 Multiple myeloma (marrow). The cells bear characteristic morphologic features of plasma cells, round or oval cells with an eccentric nucleus composed of coarsely clumped chromatin, a densely basophilic cytoplasm, and a perinuclear clear zone (hof) containing the Golgi apparatus. Binucleate and multinucleate malignant plasma cells can be seen. *(From Kasper DL, Braunwald, E, Fauci AS, et al. "Harrison's Principles of Internal Medicine," 16th edition. McGraw-Hill, New York, p. 657.)*

A skeletal survey is routinely performed on patients with MM to evaluate for bone disease. MRI is more sensitive and is being increasingly used in patients. In addition to defining bone disease, it can highlight BM infiltration.

Anemia Anemia in MM can be due to a number of factors, including tumor infiltration of the BM, renal impairment, the myelosuppressive effects of tumor products and chemotherapy, and a deficient production of erythropoietin (EPO) relative to the degree of anemia.

Table 31-2

Clinical Features of Multiple Myeloma

Organ involvement	Pathogenesis	Signs and symptoms
Skeletal system	↑osteoclastogenesis ↑OAFs by tumor cells Tumor cell infiltration	Bone pains Osteoporosis Lytic disease Pathologic fractures Hypercalcemia Cord compression
Hematopoietic system	Tumor cell infiltration Inhibitory cytokines ↓Erythropoietin ↑Antibodies Hyperviscosity	Anemia Neutropenia Thrombocytopenia Bleeding
Renal	Light chain disease Myeloma kidney Dehydration Amyloid Urate nephropathy	Renal failure Hypercalcemia
Immune system	Hypogammaglobulinemia ↓ neutrophil migration	Infections
Neurologic	↑Antibodies Hyperviscosity Tumor infiltration	Neuropathies Strokes Cord compression

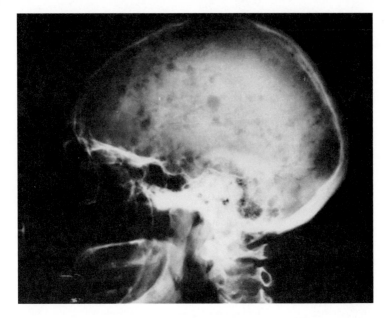

FIGURE 31-2 Bony lesions in multiple myeloma. The skull demonstrates the typical "punched out" lesions characteristic of multiple myeloma. The lesion represents a purely osteolytic lesion with little or no osteoblastic activity. (*From Kasper DL, Braunwald E, Fauci AS, et al. "Harrison's Principles of Internal Medicine," 16th edition, McGraw-Hill, New York, p. 658. Courtesy of Dr. Geraldine Schechter.*)

Renal failure Renal failure in MM predicts for an adverse outcome. The causes of renal failure in MM are often multifactorial and include hypercalcemia, MM kidney, hyperuricemia, toxicity from intravenous urography, dehydration, plasma cell infiltration, pyelonephritis, medications like nonsteroidal antiinflammatory drugs, and amyloidosis.

Hyperviscosity Hyperviscosity is characterized clinically by spontaneous bleeding with headache and neurologic and visual disorders. Hyperviscosity is commonly seen with IgM paraproteins, although the IgG3 subclass has also been associated with this syndrome.

Recurrent infections Patients with MM are at an increased risk of infections because of the underlying hypogammaglobulinemia. *Streptococcus pneumoniae* and Hemophilus infections usually occur early and typically during response to chemotherapy. Gram-negative infections occur in refractory, advancing disease; in the setting of previous antibiotic therapy; instrumentation; immobilization; colonization with hospital flora; and azotemia. Fatal infections may be hospital acquired, emphasizing the need to minimize indwelling foreign bodies such as catheters in patients with MM.

Cardiac failure The median age of patients with MM is more than 60 years; such patients are at an increased risk of cardiovascular disease. Patients are uniquely susceptible to cardiac ischemia and/or congestive heart failure (CHF) due to myocardial infiltration with amyloid, causing dilated or restricted cardiomyopathy, hyperviscosity syndrome, and/or anemia. MM patients are also susceptible to high output CHF of unclear etiology.

Neuropathies   In MM, a symmetric, distal sensory or sensorimotor neuropathy is most common and is associated with axonal degeneration, with or without amyloid deposition. In some cases, neuropathy is associated with monoclonal antibodies directed against peripheral nerve myelin.

Laboratory evaluation identifies a monoclonal Ig in serum and/or urine in the majority of cases. In most series, 50–60% of patients with myeloma have both serum and urinary monoclonal protein; 20–30% of patients have serum without urinary protein; 15–20% patients have monoclonal protein in urine only, and only 1–2% patients do not secrete monoclonal protein in blood and/or urine but have evidence of BM infiltration with plasma cells. IgG or IgA monoclonal proteins are most common, and IgD or IgE proteins are rare. The natural history of myeloma is a progressive increase in tumor growth. The M protein doubling time, which is reflective of the myeloma growth rate, shortens with each relapse. Eventually marrow failure develops, with sideroblastic anemia, leukopenia, and thrombocytopenia. The median interval from marrow failure to death is 3 (range 1–9) months. Infection (52%) and renal failure (21%) account for the majority of deaths in patients with myeloma.

Prognostic Factors

Multiple attempts have been made to define clinical and laboratory parameters which have prognostic significance. The Durie–Salmon staging system has been most commonly utilized (11). Staging in this system correlated with tumor cell mass and was further subdivided into A and B based on renal function. Based on this system, survival duration is 61.2 months for patients with Stage IA disease, 54.5 for Stages IB + IIA + IIB, 30.1 months for Stage IIIA, and 14.7 months for Stage IIIB disease. A newer staging system has been has been validated in over 10,000 MM patients based on presenting serum albumin and β2microglobulin levels (12). This system classifies patients into three stages with median survivals of 62 months for Stage I, 44 months for Stage II, and 29 months for stage III disease (Table 31-3).

Treatment

Between 5–10% of MM patients have an indolent course (see Table 31-1) and do not require immediate therapy. For the majority of patients, MM treatment is indicated at the time of diagnosis. Treatment is subdivided into specific antitumor therapy and supportive care measures.

SUPPORTIVE CARE MEASURES

Bone disease and hypercalcemia   The use of bisphosphonates for the treatment of MM-related bone disease has greatly improved the quality of life of MM

Table 31-3

New International Staging System for Multiple Myeloma

Stage	Serum β2 microglobulin	Serum albumin	Median survival
I	<3.5 mg/l	≥3.5 g/dl	62 months
II	<3.5 mg/l or 3.5–5.5 mg/l	<3.5 g/dl any level	44 months
III	≥5.5 mg/l	any level	29 months

Adapted from Greipp PR, et al. J Clin Oncol. 2005; 23: 3412-3420. Reprinted with permission from the American Society of Clinical Oncology.

patients. Clodronate, an oral bisphosphonate is commonly used in Europe. Pamidronate has demonstrated efficacy in a prospective randomized trial by reducing skeletal-related events, including pathologic fractures, radiation therapy to bone, and spinal cord compression in patients with Durie–Salmon stage III MM and ≥ one lytic bone lesion (13). More potent bisphosphonates, such as zoledronate, have undergone clinical evaluation and offer the advantage of shorter infusion times compared to pamidronate. Osteonecrosis of the jaw is a new entity increasingly reported and associated with the use of intravenous bisphosphonates (14). Ongoing work is elucidating its pathogenesis and evaluating alternate dosing strategies for bisphosphonates. Palmidronate is given at a dose of 90 mg IV given over at least 2 h every 3–4 weeks. Zoledronate is given at a dose of 4 mg IV over 15 min every 3–4 weeks.

The treatment of hypercalcemia consists of maintaining hydration, treatment of the underlying MM, as well as inhibition of osteoclastic bone resorption with glucocorticoids, calcitonin, mithramycin, and/or bisphosphonates.

Anemia   EPO administration is beneficial in managing the anemia of MM if baseline serum EPO levels are not elevated above 50 U/ml. Many physicians begin the use of EPO in patients whose hgb levels fall below 10–11 g/dl. The starting dose is 150 U/kg subcutaneously three times a week. Make sure the patient is not iron deficient before initiating EPO treatment. The dose may be doubled if no response is seen after 8 weeks of treatment.

Renal dysfunction   Aggressive hydration and treatment of the underlying MM are the usual measures taken. Decisions about dialysis are affected by the status of the underlying disease.

Hyperviscosity   Clinical findings improve with vigorous plasmapheresis, which reduces both MM protein concentration and serum viscosity. Plasmapheresis is more effective when the paraprotein is IgM, because 80% of the IgM remains intravascular. IgG hyperviscosity requires more frequent and complete plasmapheresis.

Infections   Patients should be taught to take the onset of fever seriously and seek immediate medical attention. Patients who have survived a serious infection may benefit from monthly infusions of intravenous immunoglobulin, although they are expensive.

INITIAL ANTITUMOR TREATMENT   The status of MM therapy is in a period of dynamic change. Oral administration of melphalan and prednisone (MP) has been the standard of care for over 5 decades in elderly MM patients (Table 31-4). This form of therapy produces objective response in 50–60% of patients. The shortcomings of MP have stimulated investigators to use many combinations of chemotherapeutic agents. Several different combinations have been tested and two large overviews of over 10,000 patients have demonstrated that MP had equivalent efficacy and survival to combination chemotherapy (15, 16). MP therefore still remains a very reasonable treatment strategy for elderly MM patients. A number of developments promise to be improvements over MP. Palumbo and colleagues have incorporated the use of thalidomide in combination with MP in newly diagnosed patients with MM over the age of 65 years (17). The addition of thalidomide resulted in a 76% complete or partial response rate compared to 47% in the MP arm. This translated into a doubling of the 2 year event-free survival (EFS) to 54% versus 27%. Ongoing randomized trials with the use of other novel agents like bortezomib (a proteasome inhibitor) and lenalinamide (a thalidomide analogue) with MP are currently underway.

Patients under the age of 65 years are potential autologous transplant candidates. To avoid the stem-cell-toxic melphalan, combination chemotherapy with

Table 31-4

Treatment of Myeloma

MP [15,16]	Melphalan: 10 mgs/m^2 Days 1–4 Prednisone: 100 mgs PO qd Days 1–4	Repeat every 28 days to maximum response	50–60% (newly diagnosed)
MPT [17]	Melphalan: 4 mgs/m^2 Days 1–7 Prednisone 40 mgs PO qd Days 1–7 Thalidomide: 100 mgs qhs continuous	Every 28 days × 6 cycles followed by maintenance thalidomide	75% (newly diagnosed)
Thal/Dex [19]	Thalidomide 200 mgs qhs Dexamethasone 40 mgs PO days 1–4, 9–12, 17–20 alternating with Dexamethasone 40 mgs PO days 1–4	Every 28 days × 4 cycles or maximal response	63% (newly diagnosed)
Bortezomib [30]	Bortezomib 1.3 mgs/m^2 on days 1,4,8, and 11	Every 21 days × 8 cycles	38% (relapsed/ refractory)
Lenalidomide/ Dex [29]	Lenalidomide 25 mgs days 1–21		
	Dexamethasone 40 mgs PO days 1–4, 9–12, 17–20	Every 28 days × 4 cycles or maximal response	61% (relapsed/ refractory)

vincristine, doxorubicin, and dexamethasone (VAD) was typically used in younger patients. Although VAD produces a high response rate (84%), with 28% of all patients achieving a complete response, the duration of response was only 18 months with increased toxicity and associated indwelling catheters (18). VAD-like regimens are currently being replaced by use of novel agents like thalidomide, bortezomib, and lenalinamide as upfront treatments for MM. Regimens containing pegylated liposomal doxorubicin are also replacing the use of conventional VAD. In a large randomized phase III ECOG study, thalidomide with dexamethasone (Thal/Dex) was compared with dexamethasone alone as initial therapy for MM. The response rate favored the Thal/Dex arm but was also associated with increased toxicity, specifically deep vein thrombosis and peripheral neuropathy (19). Cavo *et al* have compared VAD with Thal/Dex in a case-controlled analysis and have seen significantly higher response rates with Thal/Dex (76%) compared to VAD (52%) (20). Importantly, patients were successfully consolidated with an autologous transplant following Thal/Dex. Ongoing studies are accruing patients on initial treatment protocols containing bortezomib and lenalinamide.

High-dose therapy The rationale for the administration of high doses of alkylating agents (melphalan) with or without total body irradiation, followed by transplantation of syngeneic, allogeneic, and autologous BM or peripheral blood progenitor cells (PBPCs), is based on the fact that MM is uniformally fatal and MM cells have demonstrated a dose–response curve to chemotherapy with a high proportion of patients achieving complete responses when higher doses of therapy are given.

Allogeneic stem cell transplantation Experience with allografting has been disappointing in MM largely because of the high transplant related mortality (TRM). Syngeneic BMT has been done infrequently, but some patients reported from Seattle and the European BM Transplant Group (EBMT) have remained progression-free at long intervals post-BMT. The EBMT and Seattle groups have reported on allografting in MM with similar results demonstrating an overall survival (OS) of 20–28% associated with a high TRM of 41–44% (21, 22). Nonetheless, molecular remissions, due in part to a graft-versus-myeloma (GVM) effect, have been noted in allogeneic BMT, and the emphasis now is to develop strategies to achieve and maintain high remission rates while avoiding TRM. The use of nonmyeloablative transplantation is one such alternative strategy which preserves GVM allogeneic immunity while avoiding the toxicity of allografting and is currently under investigation. Early data demonstrate reduced TRM (10–20%) with improved OS but follow-up remains short (23).

Autologous stem cell transplantation High-dose chemoradiotherapy followed by transplantation of either autologous BM or PBPCs has achieved high (40%) CR rates, but the median duration of these responses has been only 2–3 years. The Intergroupe Francais du Myelome (IFM 90), a national French study, first demonstrated the efficacy of autologous BMT over conventional chemotherapy in 200 MM patients (24). Several randomized trials and case-controlled studies have been performed and the results have been variable. For example, the MRC randomized study confirmed a 12 month survival benefit for the transplanted arm (25). In contrast, the US Intergroup randomized trial was unable to confirm the benefits of transplantation (26). Despite the use of aggressive approaches like transplantation, few, if any, patients are cured. To improve upon the results of high-dose chemotherapy, the French group have compared single versus double autografts and their data suggest that two sequential transplants may benefit a subset of patients with MM who did not achieve a complete remission after the first transplant (27). Other strategies including use of maintenance therapy with thalidomide, and lenalinamide are under evaluation and appear promising.

Refractory Disease

Almost all patients who initially respond to treatment will eventually relapse. A major advance in the treatment of resistant MM has been the emergence of Thal as an effective therapy. The University of Arkansas Cancer Center has reported overall response rates of 37% with 2 year EFS of 20% and OS of 48% (28). Based on the impressive results of single-agent Thal in refractory relapsed MM, Thal has been coupled with Dex to treat patients with disease refractory to either agent alone; even in this setting, half of patients treated respond. Lenalinamide, an analog of Thal has completed phase I, II, and III testing in relapsed MM and is FDA approved in combination with Dex for the treatment of MM (29).

Proteosome inhibitors like bortezomib are another significant advance in the therapy of relapsed MM. Laboratory studies coupled with phase I and phase II studies of bortezomib demonstrating clinical promise led to a phase III international randomized trial, APEX. The study compared bortezomib versus Dex in relapsed MM and demonstrated an improvement in median time to progression in the bortezomib arm (6.2 versus 3.5 months) (30).

Future Directions

Despite the use of aggressive approaches like transplantation and the use of novel agents like bortezomib, thalidomide, and lenalinamide, MM remains incurable. In order to overcome resistance to current therapies and improve patient outcome, novel biologically based treatment approaches that target mechanisms whereby MM cells grow and survive in the BM are needed. Our understanding of the biology of MM has allowed the development of several promising targeted therapies that can attack the MM cell in its BM microenvironment and, it is hoped, overcome classic drug resistance. A host of other novel biologics including histone deacetylase inhibitors, heat shock protein inhibitors, and mTOR inhibitors are undergoing preclinical and clinical evaluation (31). These therapies may produce longer remissions for MM patients and assist in making MM a chronic disease, if a not-yet-curable one.

WALDENSTROM'S MACROGLOBULINEMIA (WM)

The diagnosis of WM requires an IgM serum level of at least 3.0 g/dl in association with an increase in lymphocytes or plasmacytoid lymphocytes in the marrow. WM corresponds most closely to the lymphoplasmacytic lymphoma (LPA) under the World Health Organization (WHO) classification of lymphoid tumors (LPL/immunocytoma of the Revised European–American (REAL) classification of lymphoma). Like MM, BM involvement is common; however, no lytic bone disease is noted with WM (32).

The median age of onset of WM is 61 years. Symptoms are characteristically vague and nonspecific, with the most common being weakness, anorexia, and weight loss. Symptoms due to peripheral neuropathy and Raynaud phenomenon can precede more serious manifestations. Lymphadenopathy, splenomegaly, and/or hepatomegaly are present in 30–40% of cases, and at least 20–25% lymphoplasmacytoid cells are usually present in the marrow. Visceral involvement of small bowel and peripheral nerves can cause the clinical sequelae of malabsorption and neuropathy, respectively. Hemorrhagic complications are common, attributable to abnormal bleeding times, decreased platelet adhesiveness, or direct interference by the IgM protein with the release of platelet factor 3 and with coagulation factors. An important part of the differential diagnosis is to exclude the less common entity of IgM MM, which is characterized by lytic bone disease and an absence of organomegaly and/or lymphocytic involvement; rarely, WM can progress to IgM MM. Amyloidosis occurs rarely in WM. Hyperviscosity syndrome, described earlier as a rare complication in MM, occurs more commonly in the setting of excess IgM and is characterized by mucosal bleeding and neurologic, ocular, and cardiovascular abnormalities. Plasmapheresis is more useful to remove excess IgM than it is in the setting of excess IgG monoclonal proteins and related hyperviscosity in MM.

The median survival of patients with WM is approximately 50 months. In contrast to persons with MM, many individuals with WM have indolent disease requiring no therapy for long periods of time, with survivals in excess of 20 years. A high IgM level is not in itself an indication to initiate therapy. A prognostic model has been developed for WM based on an analysis of 585 patients seen at the Mayo Clinic (33). Age greater than 65 years and organomegaly were the major risk factors; absence of both was associated with a median survival of nearly 11 years, while the presence of one or both factors predicted a median survival of 4.2 years.

A consensus panel on WM has developed recommendations for initiation of therapy in WM. Hematocrit of <30, platelet count <100,000, symptoms attributable to WM, hyperviscosity, moderate to severe neuropathies, symptomatic cryoglobulinemia, and cold agglutinin disease are some indicators to start therapy. Low-dose therapy with alkylating agents like chlorambucil has resulted in overall response rates of 50%. However, this is a stem cell toxic agent and acute leukemia has developed in patients with WM. Nucleoside analogs, fludarabine and 2-chlorodeoxyadenosine, have demonstrated efficacy with overall response rates of 30–70% with more rapid cytoreduction. Monoclonal antibody therapy with rituximab, a chimeric anti-CD20 monoclonal antibody, produces responses in both treated and untreated patients with low-grade lymphoma. Given that the CD20 antigen is typically present in WM, rituximab has been given to WM patients and a clinical response is seen in about one-third of previously treated patients. Ongoing studies are looking at combining rituximab with fludarabine in the treatment of WM. Salvage strategies for treatment of WM have included reuse of the first-line agent, combination chemotherapy like CHOP and CVP, and stem cell transplantation. Novel agents like thalidomide, lenolinamide, and bortezomib used in MM are also being studied for the treatment of WM.

HEAVY CHAIN DISEASES (HCD)

The HCD are rare lymphoplasmacytic maliganancies. They are classified based on the heavy chain isotype (34).

Gamma HCD was originally described by Franklin and coworkers in a patient with malignant lymphoma whose serum and urine contained large amounts of the Fc fragment of IgG. It is characterized by the presence of a portion of the Ig heavy chain in the serum or urine or both. The median age at diagnosis is similar to MM, about 60 years. Most common presenting symptoms are weakness, fatigue, and fever, associated with lymphadenopathy and hepatosplenomegaly. In addition to Ig heavy chain in serum or urine, a lymphoplasmacytic marrow infiltrate is noted in most cases. The clinical course can be fulminant and rapidly progressive; alternatively, the monoclonal heavy chain can persist for years in otherwise asymptomatic patients. Thus, survival is variable, but the median is only 12 months. Treatment options for patients with active disease are similar to those used for lymphoma or MM, whereas patients with indolent disease should be followed expectantly without therapy.

Cases of αHCD, μHCD, and δHCD have also been described. αHCD is typically associated with Mediterranean lymphoma affecting the gastrointestinal tract, beginning with plasma cells that produce a heavy chain and aggregate in the intestinal tract and subsequent transformation into a malignant non-Hodgkin lymphoma of the immunoblastic type. μHCD is extremely rare and may be associated with chronic lymphocytic leukemia. The ideal therapy for HCD is not known because of its rarity, but intensive chemotherapy including intravenous cyclophosphamide, doxorubicin, vincristine, and oral prednisone appears to offer some patients long-term remissions.

AMYLOIDOSIS

Amyloidosis is relatively rare as a clinically significant disease. The amyloid found in most cases of amyloidosis can be assigned to one of two types, according to whether the fibrils consist mainly of the variable region of Ig light chains (AL, or primary amyloidosis) or protein A (AA, or secondary amyloidosis). Protein A is not related to any known immunoglobulin. In AL, amyloid primarily involves the heart, tongue, gastrointestinal tract, and skin, whereas AA primarily results in fibril deposition in liver, kidney, and spleen. A review of 229 patients with AL documented MM in 47 (21%) patients. Initial presenting symptoms were fatigue and weight loss, with pain more common in those who also had MM. Hepatomegaly and macroglossia were present in up to one-third of patients with AL; renal insufficiency was present in half of patients, and proteinuria (defined as albuminuria with immune globulin, seen only in MM) was documented in 82% of patients. Nephrotic syndrome, CHF, orthostatic hypotension, carpal tunnel syndrome, and peripheral neuropathy were all more common in those without MM (30–70% of patients studied) than in persons with (< 20%) MM. Overall median survival was 12 months, 5 months for those with MM in contrast to 13 months for individuals without MM (35).

Treatment for AL is unsatisfactory. Only 18% patients responded to MP, although median survival for responders was prolonged at 89.4 months; only 5% of patients with primary AL survive ≥10 years. Early reports suggest that dose-intensive melphalan with blood stem cell support can achieve CR, with improvement in performance status and clinical remission of organ-specific disease. Attempts to improve outcomes for patients with symptomatic and advanced multisystem disease may require both solid and stem cell transplantation, as well as the use of less intensive conditioning regimens. Novel drugs with promise in the treatment of MM, are also being tested in patients with amyloidosis.

REFERENCES

1. Rajkumar SV, Kyle RA. Multiple myeloma: diagnosis and treatment. Mayo Clin Proc. 2005; 80: 1371–1382.
2. Kyle RA, Rajkumar SV. Monoclonal gammopathy of undetermined significance. Clin Lymphoma Myeloma. 2005; 6: 102–114.
3. Hideshima T., Bergsagel P. L., Kuehl W. M., Anderson K. C. Advances in biology of multiple myeloma: clinical applications. Blood. 2004; 104: 607–618.
4. Jemal, A., Siegel, R., Ward, E., et al. Cancer statistics, 2007. CA Cancer J Clin. 2007; 57: 43–66.
5. Herrinton, L. J., Weiss, N. S., Olshan, A. F. Eipidemiology of myeloma. In JS Malpas, DE, Bergsagel, R, Kyle, K Anderson (eds.), "Myeloma: Biology and Management," Oxford Medical Publications, Oxford, 1997, pp. 150.
6. Bergsagel, P. L., Kuehl, W. M. Molecular pathogenesis and a consequent classification of multiple myeloma. J Clin Oncol. 2005; 23: 6333–6338.
7. Shaughnessy, J. D., Jr. and Barlogie, B. Using genomics to identify high-risk myeloma after autologous stem cell transplantation. Biol Blood Marrow Transplant. 2006; 12: 77–80.
8. Durie, B. G. Staging and kinetics of multiple myeloma. Semin Oncol. 1986; 13: 300–309.
9. Dimopoulos, M. A., Moulopoulos, L. A., Maniatis, A., Alexanian, R. Solitary plasmacytoma of bone and asymptomatic multiple myeloma. Blood. 2000; 96: 2037–2044.
10. Kyle, R. A. Multiple myeloma: review of 869 cases. Mayo Clin Proc. 1975; 50: 29–40.
11. Durie, B. G. M. Salmon S. E. A clinical staging system for multiple myeloma. Correlation of measured cell mass with presenting clinical features, response to treatment and survival. Cancer. 1975; 36: 842–854.
12. Greipp, P. R., San Miguel, J., Durie, B. G., et al. International staging system for multiple myeloma. J Clin Oncol. 2005; 23: 3412–3420.
13. Berenson, J. R., Lichtenstein, A., Porter, L., et al. Efficacy of pamidronate in reducing skeletal events in patients with advanced multiple myeloma. Myeloma Aredia Study Group. N Engl J Med. 1996; 334: 488–493.
14. Ruggiero, S. L., Mehrotra, B., Rosenberg, T. J., and Engroff, S. L. Osteonecrosis of the jaws associated with the use of bisphosphonates: a review of 63 cases. J Oral Maxillofac Surg. 2004; 62: 527–534.
15. Gregory, W. M., Richards, M. A., Malpas, J. S. Combination chemotherapy versus melphalan and prednisolone in the treatment of multiple myeloma: an overview of published trials. J Clin Oncol. 1992; 10: 334–342.
16. Combination chemotherapy versus melphalan plus prednisone as treatment for multiple myeloma: an overview of 6,633 patients from 27 randomized trials. Myeloma Trialists' Collaborative Group. J Clin Oncol. 1998; 16: 3832–3842.
17. Palumbo, A., Bringhen, S., Caravita, T., et al. Oral melphalan and prednisone chemotherapy plus thalidomide compared with melphalan and prednisone alone in elderly patients with multiple myeloma: randomised controlled trial. Lancet. 2006; 367: 825–831.

18   Alexanian, R., Barlogie, B., Tucker, S. VAD-based regimens as primary treatment for multiple myeloma. Am. J. Hematol. 33: 86–89, 1990.

19. Rajkumar, S. V., Blood, E., Vesole, D.,et al. Phase III clinical trial of thalidomide plus dexamethasone compared with dexamethasone alone in newly diagnosed multiple myeloma: a clinical trial coordinated by the Eastern Cooperative Oncology Group. J Clin Oncol. 24: 431–436, 2006.

20. Cavo, M., Zamagni, E., Tosi, P., et al. Superiority of thalidomide and dexamethasone over vincristine-doxorubicindexamethasone (VAD) as primary therapy in preparation for autologous transplantation for multiple myeloma. Blood. 106: 35–39, 2005.

21. Gahrton, G., Svensson, H., Cavo, M., et al. Progress in allogeneic bone marrow and peripheral blood stem cell transplantation for multiple myeloma: a comparison between transplants performed 1983–93 and 1994–8 at European Group for Blood and Marrow centers. Br J Haematol. 113: 209–216, 2001.

22. Bensinger, W. I., Maloney, D., Storb, R. Allogeneic hematopoietic cell transplantation for multiple myeloma. Semin Hematol. 38: 243–249, 2001.

23. Badros, A., Barlogie, B., Siegel, E., et al. G. Improved outcome of allogeneic transplantation in high-risk multiple myeloma patients after nonmyeloablative conditioning. J Clin Oncol. 20: 1295–1303, 2002.

24. Attal, M., Harousseau, J. L., Stoppa, A. M., et al. A prospective, randomized trial of autologous bone marrow transplantation and chemotherapy in multiple myeloma. Intergroupe Francais du Myelome. N Engl J Med. 335: 91–97, 1996.

25. Child, J. A., Morgan, G. J., Davies, F. E., et al. High-dose chemotherapy with hematopoietic stem-cell rescue for multiple myeloma. N Engl J Med. 348: 1875–1883, 2003.

26. Barlogie, B., Kyle, R. A., Anderson, K. C., et al. Standard chemotherapy compared with high-dose chemoradiotherapy for multiple myeloma: final results of phase III US Intergroup Trial S9321. J Clin Oncol. 24: 929–936, 2006.

27. Attal, M., Harousseau, J. L., Facon, T., et al. Single versus double autologous stem-cell transplantation for multiple myeloma. N Engl J Med. 349: 2495–2502, 2003.

28. Singhal, S., Mehta, J., Desikan, R., et al. Antitumor activity of thalidomide in refractory multiple myeloma. N Engl J Med. 341: 1565–1571, 1999.

29. Richardson, P. G., Schlossman, R. L., Weller, E., et al. Immunomodulatory drug CC–5013 overcomes drug resistance and is well tolerated in patients with relapsed multiple myeloma. Blood. 100: 3063–3067, 2002.

30. Richardson, P. G., Sonneveld, P., Schuster, M. W., et al. Bortezomib or high-dose dexamethasone for relapsed multiple myeloma. N Engl J Med. 352: 2487–2498, 2005.

31. Hideshima, T., Chauhan, D., Richardson, P., Anderson, K. C. Identification and validation of novel therapeutic targets for multiple myeloma. J Clin Oncol. 23: 6345–6350, 2005.

32. Dimopoulos, M. A. Anagnostopoulos, A. Waldenstrom's macroglobulinemia. Best Pract Res Clin Haematol. 18: 747–765, 2005.

33. Ghobrial I.M, Fonseca, R., Gertz, M.A., et al. Prognostic model for disease-specific and overall mortality in newly diagnosed symptomatic patients with Waldenstrom macroglobulinemia. Br J Haematol. 133: 158–164, 2006.

34. Witzig, T. E., Wahner-Roedler, D. L. Heavy chain disease. Curr Treat Options Oncol. 3: 247–254, 2002.

35. Rajkumar SV, Gertz MA. advances in the treatment of amyloidosis. N Engl J Med. 356: 2413–2415, 2007.

| 32 | Eyal C. Attar |

MYELODYSPLASTIC SYNDROMES

INTRODUCTION

Myelodysplastic syndrome (MDS) represents a premalignant entity that shares many characteristics with acute myeloid leukemia (AML). This clonal hematopoietic stem cell (HSC) disorder is characterized by pancytopenia resulting from failure of normal hematopoiesis. The bone marrow shows hypercellularity, arrested maturation in one or more cellular lineages, and an increase in bone marrow myeloid precursors. Clinical symptoms result from cytopenias. Approximately 1/3 of patients ultimately progress to AML. Treatment involves supportive care and the use of agents capable of ameliorating cytopenias and delaying development of AML. However, HSC transplantation represents the only potentially curative treatment for MDS.

KEY FEATURES

- One or more peripheral blood cytopenias.
- Hematopoietic cell dysplasia.
- Bone marrow hypercellularity.
- Ringed sideroblasts (occasionally).
- Less than 20% bone marrow and peripheral blood myeloblasts.
- Abnormal cytogenetics in approximately 50% of patients. A small portion of patients have characteristic, interstitial deletions within the long arm of chromosome 5 associated with clinical response to immunomodulatory drugs (IMIDs).
- MDS may be related to prior chemotherapy and/or radiation for another medical condition (therapy-related MDS or t-MDS).
- Approximately 30% of patients with MDS develop AML.

EPIDEMIOLOGY

Approximately 15,000–30,000 new cases of MDS are diagnosed in the United States each year. MDS is 3–4 times more prevalent than AML and follows a more indolent course. MDS is underdiagnosed; the true prevalence is likely much higher. MDS is one cause of anemia in the elderly, though it is rare.

ETIOLOGY

The exact cause of MDS is unknown in most patients. However, intrinsic defects in hematopoietic cells and extrinsic defects associated with the bone marrow microenvironment are involved in the pathogenesis of this disorder.

While most patients with MDS have spontaneously arising, de novo, disease, a portion of patients have therapy-related MDS (T-MDS). Such patients have received chemotherapy and/or radiation in the past, possibly for another malignancy or autoimmune disorder. T-MDS develops within a period of 3–10 years following chemotherapy and is associated with complex chromosomal abnormalities, often involving alterations of chromosomes 5 and/or 7. In addition,

T-MDS is associated with a more aggressive clinical course and poorer prognosis in comparison to de novo MDS.

CLINICAL CHARACTERISTICS

- Median age is approximately 70 years.
- Slightly more common in males than in females.
- Prevalence is 50,000–100,000 cases in the United States.
- May be associated with prior chemotherapy, radiation, or environmental exposures to genotoxic agents.

CLASSIFICATION OF MDS

The World Health Organization (WHO) classification system (1) (Table 32-1) includes refractory anemia (RA), refractory cytopenias with multilineage dysplasia (RCMD), and MDS with isolated deletion of 5q for patients harboring a

Table 32-1

WHO Classification of Myelodysplastic Syndromes

Category	Peripheral blood	Bone marrow
RA	Anemia No or rare blasts	Erythroid dysplasia only Blasts <5% Ringed sideroblasts <15%
RARS	Anemia No blasts	Erythroid dysplasia only Blasts <5% Ringed sideroblasts ≥15%
RCMD	Cytopenias in two or more lineages No or rare blasts Monocytes <1000/μl No Auer rods	Dysplasia in ≥10% of cells in 2 or more lineages Blasts <5% Ring sideroblasts <15% No Auer rods
RCMD-RS	Bi- or pancytopenia No or rare blasts Monocytes <1000/μl No Auer rods	Multilineage dysplasia Blasts <5% Ring sideroblasts ≥15% No Auer rods
RAEB-1	Cytopenias Blasts <5% Monocytes <1000/μl No Auer rods	Uni- or multilineage dysplasia Blasts 5–9% No Auer rods
RAEB-II	Cytopenias Blasts 5–19% Monocytes <1000/μl Auer rods ±	Uni- or multilineage dysplasia Blasts 10–19% Auer rods ±
MDS-U	Cytopenias No or rare blasts No Auer rods	Unilineage dysplasia in granulocyte or megakaryocyte lineage Blasts <5% No Auer rods
MDS, isolated del(5q)	Blasts <5% Platelets normal or increased Anemia	Isolated del (5q) Blasts <5% Megakaryocytes normal or increased

RA: refractory anemia; RAEB: refractory anemia with excess blasts; RARS: RA with ringed sideroblasts; RCMD: refractory cytopenia with multilineage dysplasia; RCMD-RS: RCMD with ringed sideroblasts; MDS-U: myelodysplastic syndrome, unclassified.

distinct interstitial deletion within the long arm of chromosome 5. RA with excess blasts I and II (RAEB-I, II) indicates patients with 5–9% and 10–19% bone marrow myeloblasts, respectively. Patients with 20% or greater myeloblasts in the marrow have AML.

PROGNOSIS

The most commonly used system to assess a patient's prognosis is the International Prognostic Scoring System (IPSS) (2). This system assigns a score within each of three categories: the percentage of bone marrow blasts, cytogenetics, and the number and degrees of cytopenias (Table 32-2). The scores are added to yield the IPSS category (Low, Int-1, Int-2, and High). The median survival for patients with Low, Int-1, Int-2, and High-risk disease is 5.7, 3.5, 1.2, and 0.4 years, respectively. Importantly, this system applies only to patients with de novo MDS and was not developed using information from patients with t-MDS, who uniformly have a worse prognosis.

Other factors affect prognosis. The presence of abnormally localized immature progenitors (ALIPS) within the bone marrow worsens prognosis. These collections of immature, CD34 positive cells are displaced from their customary paratrabecular location to the central marrow space and are associated with decreased survival and increased risk of transformation to AML, even within IPSS subgroups. Dependence upon blood transfusions is associated with a 13 month median inferior survival compared to patients who are transfusion independent.

Table 32-2

The International Prognostic Scoring System (IPSS). (a) Components of the IPSS. (b) Relationship of the IPSS to Median Overall Survival and Time to 25% of Patients Transforming to AML

(a)

	Score				
	0	0.5	1.0	1.5	2.0
Percentage of BM blasts	<5	5–10	–	11–20	21–30
Karyotype	Good (NL, Y-, 5q-, 20q-)	Intermediate (all others)	Poor (complex, Chr 7)	–	–
Cytopenias	0/1	2/3	–	–	–

RBC ≡ HgB < 10
WBC ≡ ANC <1800
Plt ≡ <100 K

(b)

	Score	Overall median survival (year)	Time to 25% of patients transforming to AML (year)
Low	0	5.7	9.4
Int-1	0.5–1.0	3.5	3.3
Int-2	1.5–2.0	1.2	1.1
High	2.5–3.5	0.4	0.2

LEMENTS OF PROGNOSIS

- IPSS scoring system (Table 32-2):
  - Percentage of bone marrow blasts.
  - Cytogenetics.
  - Number and degrees of cytopenias.
- ALIPS.
- Requirement for blood product transfusions.
- Therapy-related MDS.

PATHOPHYSIOLOGY

MDS involvement of multiple hematopoietic lineages suggests the disease arises in a primitive hematopoietic cell, or HSC. However, the microenvironment, too, contributes significantly to disease pathogenesis.

MDS Is a Clonal Stem Cell Disorder

The hypercellular bone marrow in MDS is clonal in origin and the clonal genetic lesion resides within a primitive HSC. Transplantation of bone marrow from patients with MDS successfully engrafts in immunocompromised mice, with resulting blood features consistent with MDS (3). Furthermore, once engrafted, the blood cells bear the same cytogenetic lesions seen in the patients. Thus, MDS arises from a primitive, multipotent HSC capable of homing and engraftment (8).

Genomic Instability

Genomic instability within hematopoietic cells further indicates the presence of a cell-intrinsic defect. Clonal genetic abnormalities are observed in the bone marrow of 50% of patients with de novo MDS and 80% of patients with secondary MDS. The majority of abnormalities are nonrandom. The presence of genetic alterations, in most cases, is associated with inferior prognosis. However, one particular genetic alteration, interstitial deletion within the long arm of chromosome 5, paradoxically confers a favorable prognosis.

T-MDS is an example of the contribution of genomic instability to MDS pathogenesis. T-MDS occurs in younger patients than de novo MDS and is more often associated with chromosomal abnormalities. Karyotypic abnormalities include deletion of large portions of, or entire, chromosomes (-5, -7, 7q-, 13q-, 17p-, and -18) (4).

Clinically, T-MDS follows exposure to agents that cause DNA damage and accounts for approximately 10–20% of MDS/AML. Affected individuals have been previously treated for lung cancer, breast cancer, childhood acute lymphoblastic leukemia, rheumatoid arthritis, and other oncologic and autoimmune disorders requiring chemotherapy and/or irradiation. T-MDS is associated with a poorer prognosis than de novo MDS, with a median survival of approximately 9 months. Injury associated with topoisomerase inhibitor chemotherapy, such as etoposide, has the earliest onset, often within 2–3 years of exposure. Typical mutations involve core binding factor on chromosomes 16 or 21 and the mixed-lineage leukemia (MLL) gene on 11q. In contrast, alkylating agents such as chlorambucil and cyclophosphamide result in a more latent T-MDS, arising 4–7 years following exposure. Alkylator-associated T-MDS is often associated with abnormalities of chromosomes 5 and/or 7. Exposure to radiation results in the most latent form of T-MDS, peaking at approximately 10 years following exposure. This category of injury is associated with mutations in the AML1 gene.

Genotoxic insult from occupational solvents, such as benzene, is clearly associated with development of MDS/AML, and the incidence of these myeloproliferative disorders is increased in healthcare professionals, painters, machine operators, coal miners, textile workers, hairdressers, and cosmetologists.

Bone marrow disorders associated with stem cell defects, such as paroxysmal nocturnal hemoglobinuria (PNH) and aplastic anemia (AA), may evolve into MDS.

5q-Interstitial Deletion

Approximately 5–20% of patients with MDS harbor an interstitial deletion within the long arm of chromosome 5, with or without additional cytogenetic abnormalities. This represents the most common single cytogenetic abnormality in MDS (5). These patients differ from those with t-MDS, who have losses of large regions of 5q or the entire chromosome 5 and have a distinctly inferior prognosis. Instead, interstitial deletion of genomic DNA between bands q13 and q34 is prognostically favorable compared to other types of MDS. Most importantly, patients with 5q- are exquisitely responsive to the class of agents known as immunomodulators (IMIDs). Patients harboring the 5q- interstitial deletion but carrying additional cytogenetic abnormalities are also responsive to IMIDs, although they have a worse prognosis when compared to patients with isolated interstitial deletion of 5q.

Approximately half of patients with 5q- have isolated deletion of 5q- and clinical features comprising the "5q- syndrome": RA, mild leukopenia, atypical megakaryocytes, normal or increased platelets, transfusion dependence, and extended survival with low risk of transformation to AML. 5q- syndrome is twice as common in women as men and has a median age of 68 years.

Abnormal Differentiation

A major clinicopathologic feature of MDS is altered differentiation on cytologic examination of the bone marrow aspirate and biopsy, which displays arrested differentiation and dysplasias affecting one or more lineages. Altered differentiation likely results from a combination of intrinsic and extrinsic features.

In vitro differentiation of MDS bone marrow is diverted toward nonerythroid lineages, explaining the clinical anemia observed in these patients. MDS marrow contains lower levels of erythroid progenitors and requires several-fold higher concentrations of erythropoietin (Epo) to support in vitro erythroid colony growth. This is clinically relevant, as patients with MDS are often resistant to exogenous Epo or require higher doses to support erythropoiesis than required for other diseases.

Increased Proliferation and Apoptosis

Cell cycle analyses have demonstrated increased cellular proliferation in MDS marrow, particularly in the myeloid lineage. However, this is accompanied by an increase in cellular apoptosis. The net balance is a hypercellular bone marrow but ineffective hematopoiesis.

Proliferation and apoptosis have been specifically studied in primitive CD34+ cells from MDS. In early stages of disease such as RA and RARS, apoptosis is greatest and exceeds proliferation. This is associated with an increased ratio of pro-apoptotic (Bax/Bad) to antiapoptotic (Bcl-2/Bcl-X_L) Bcl-2-related protein levels. In progressive stages of disease such as RAEB, the ratio of apoptosis to proliferation equalizes. Progression to RAEB-t is associated with reductions in both proliferation and apoptosis. Compared to de novo AML, the apoptotic index is higher in RAEB and RAEB-t (6). As MDS progresses, upregulation of antiapoptotic proteins such as Bcl-2 and Bcl-X_L is associated with reduction in apoptosis and may contribute to leukemogenesis.

Microenvironment

Several abnormalities related to the environment in which hematologic progenitors proliferate may contribute to the increased apoptosis seen in MDS. In addition, there is evidence that MDS bone marrow has increased microvessel density.

T-lymphocytes are hypothesized to provide immune surveillance in MDS and undergo activation and proliferation in an attempt to eradicate the malignant clone. However, such T-cell expansions may paradoxically result in suppression of normal hematopoiesis. Indeed, use of immunosuppressive medications such as cyclosporine and eliminating activated T-cells using antithymocyte globulin (ATG) can improve cytopenias (7).

Another potential cause of increased apoptosis is increased secretion of pro-apoptotic cytokines by bone marrow fibroblasts and macrophages. Cells and stroma from MDS patients secrete increased levels of TNF-α, interleukin-6, and IFN-γ relative to normal controls. Agents such as IMIDs inhibit TNF-α and IL-6 secretion and reduce bone marrow angiogenesis.

CLINICAL PRESENTATION

The clinical presentation of MDS relates to the degree and type of cytopenias. Anemia, the most common cytopenia in MDS, may manifest as light headedness, fatigue, chest pain, dyspnea, palpitations, and depression. Leukopenia is the second most common cytopenia in MDS, present in 50% of affected individuals. Manifestations include recurrent lung, sinus, and skin infections. Thrombocytopenia is present in 25% of patients. Its manifestations include easy bruising, epistaxis, petechiae, hematochezia, and hematuria.

In addition, qualitative defects in hematopoietic cell function may result in clinical signs and symptoms, even in the presence of adequate blood counts. For example, neutrophil dysfunction may contribute to infection, while platelet dysfunction may result in hemorrhage even if the blood counts are within the normal range.

1. *Anemia.* Light headedness, fatigue, chest pain, dyspnea, palpitations, and depression.
2. *Leukopenia.* Lung, sinus, and skin infections.
3. *Thrombocytopenia.* Easy bruising, epistaxis, petechiae, hematochezia, and hematuria.

DIAGNOSTIC STUDIES

The initial evaluation of uni- or multilineage cytopenias begins with careful history taking. Medications, such as antibiotics and chemotherapeutic agents, are common causes. Also, infections caused by parvovirus, HBV, HCV, EBV, CMV, and HIV suppress hematopoiesis, and their presence may be discerned by history, physical examination, and laboratory studies.

When MDS is suspected, a complete blood count with differential is necessary to identify the number and severity of cytopenias. Examples of peripheral blood features present in MDS are provided in Figure 32-1. An elevated erythroid mean corpuscular volume (MCV) is often, though not always, present in MDS. Evaluation of iron levels by assessing the iron (Fe), total iron binding capacity (TIBC), and ferritin levels is necessary to assess baseline iron stores, to determine whether iron supplementation is required to enhance hematopoiesis, or identify situations of Fe overload. The B$_{12}$ and folate levels should also be assessed to ensure adequate substrates for hematopoiesis. An Epo level is helpful in deciding whether exogenous erythroid growth factor administration will be likely to help patients with anemia.

A B

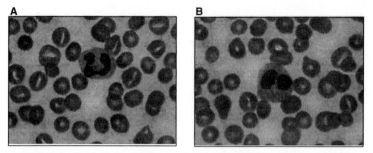

FIGURE 32-1 Peripheral blood features of MDS. (a) Neutrophil hypogranulation. The cytoplasm appears to blend with the slide background due to the absence of granules. (b) This bilobed neutrophil demonstrates the pseudo-Pelger–Huët abnormality. (Photos courtesy of Dr. Robert Hasserjian, Massachusetts General Hospital Department of Pathology.)

A bone marrow aspiration and core biopsy is essential for the diagnosis of MDS. The percentage of bone marrow cellularity is assessed on the core biopsy, while the myeloblast percentage is calculated using the aspirate. Examples of bone marrow features present in MDS are provided in Figure 32-2. Morphologic assessment of myeloid and erythroid dysplasia is made using the aspirate, while megakaryocyte dysplasia is most easily assessed on the core. Flow cytometry is utilized to identify monotypic populations of lymphoid and myeloid cells. Cytogenetic analysis is performed on the aspirate. If no aspirate can be extracted, FISH may be used to disclose critical genetic deletions.

Bone marrow studies may reveal alternative causes for cytopenias, such as other hematologic malignancies including AML and non-Hodgkin's lymphomas, and solid tumors metastatic to the bone. Hypoplastic and AA may be determined on the bone marrow core. PNH may be detected by flow cytometric assessment of the glycosylphosphatidylinositol (GPI) linked proteins CD55 and CD59.

Laboratory studies used to diagnose MDS

- Peripheral blood
  - CBC with differential, MCV
  - Fe, TIBC, ferritin
  - B12, folate
  - Epo level
- Bone marrow aspiration and biopsy
  - Morphologic analysis of dysplasia using the aspirate and core biopsy
  - Quantitation of myeloblasts using the bone marrow aspirate
  - Flow cytometry to identify monoclonal populations of lymphoid and myeloid cells
  - Cytogenetics to identify chromosomal alterations (FISH is sometimes used in patients when no aspirate may be extracted)

THERAPIES FOR MDS

The management of patients with MDS is distinct from other hematologic malignancies. A personalized approach should take into consideration the specific hematologic presentation, age, comorbidities, and prognosis. No single treatment is uniformly effective or best addresses the clinical scenario of all patients. A broad range of management options exists including amelioration of hematologic deficits with blood product support, antiinfectives, and administration of growth factors, the use of novel agents aimed at restoring normal hematopoiesis and

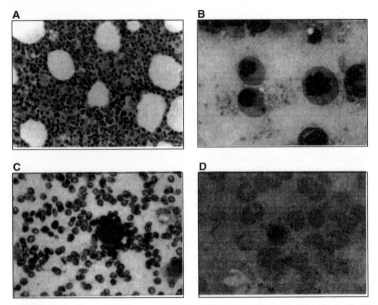

FIGURE 32-2 Bone marrow features of MDS. (a) Bone marrow hypercellularity. (b) Erythroid dysplasia is demonstrated by the convoluted nuclei within erythroid precursors. (c) Megakaryocytic dysplasia. A characteristic tri-lobed "pawn ball" megakaryocyte is demonstrated. (d) Prussian blue staining reveals iron-laden mitochondria in a perinuclear orientation in this erythroid precursor. A ringed sideroblast is characterized as having at least five positively staining granules that encircle at least 1/3 the perimeter of the nucleus. (Photos (a), (b), and (c) courtesy of Dr. Robert Hasserjian and photo (d) courtesy of Dr. Aliyah Rahemtullah, Massachusetts General Hospital Department of Pathology.)

reducing the malignant clone (Table 32-3), and stem cell transplantation (SCT) for younger patients with aggressive disease characteristics.

Supportive Care

The goal of supportive care is to reduce morbidity and improve quality of life (QoL). Supportive care for MDS consists of cytokine growth factors capable of stimulating myelo- and erythropoiesis, transfusion of red blood cells and platelets, and antibiotics. Anemia, the most common cytopenia in MDS, has been clearly linked to diminished QoL that can be improved by increasing the hemoglobin (HgB). Age, comorbidities, and lifestyle determine the optimal target HgB level for each patient. However, most patients derive clinical benefit by maintaining a HgB of at least 9 g/dl and HCT of at least 27%, though lower transfusion thresholds are required for patients with symptoms of anemia and with other comorbidities, such as cardiopulmonary disease.

Initial treatment of anemia may be achieved by periodic administration of exogenous CSFs (epoetin alfa, Procrit; darbepoetin alfa, Aranesp). Responses to epoetin alfa and darbepoetin alfa are 20–70% depending on the patient population. Epoetin alfa may be initiated at 40,000–60,000 units weekly, while darbepoetin at 200–300 mcg every 1–2 weeks. However, dose adjustment will be required to achieve the desired laboratory and clinical benefit. HgB rises of 1–4 g/dl may be achieved. Both agents appear to have similar efficacy in MDS (8). There may be potential synergy achieved by adding G-CSF (filgrastim, Neupogen), which should be considered if

Table 32-3

FDA-Approved Therapeutic Agents for MDS

Name	Class	FDA indication
5-Azacitidine (Vidaza)	Cytidine analog, DNA methyltransferase inhibitor	All FAB subtypes of MDS: • RA and RARS (if accompanied by neutropenia or thrombocytopenia or requiring transfusions) • RAEB • RAEB-T • CMMoL
Decitabine (Dacogen)	Cytidine analog, DNA methyltransferase inhibitor	• All FAB subtypes • All IPSS subtypes of MDS excluding Low-risk patients
Lenalidomide (Revlimid)	Immunomodulatory drug (IMID)	Patients with transfusion-dependent anemia due to Low and Int-1 IPSS MDS associated with deletion 5q cytogenetic abnormality, with or without additional cytogenetic abnormalities

there is no response to epoetin or darbepoetin alone after a period of 6 weeks (9). Patients with elevated endogenous Epo levels (>500 mU/ml) and those requiring RBC transfusions are unlikely to respond to erythroid growth factors alone.

Patients who fail to respond to growth factors require red blood cell supplementation via periodic transfusions. Individuals with advanced MDS by IPSS score are more likely to require RBC transfusions than those with lower risk disease. Leukodepleted products are recommended to decrease alloimmunization, prevent nonhemolytic febrile transfusion reactions, and reduce the transmission of cytomegalovirus (CMV). Other complications include iron and volume overload, infections, and graft-versus-host disease. Blood products should be irradiated to prevent potentially fatal graft-versus-host disease.

The goal of red cell transfusion support is to improve tissue oxygenation, physical and intellectual activity, and QoL. The target HgB will depend on the specific circumstances of the patient related to age, functional activity, and comorbidities. Most individuals will have improved energy with Hgb levels of 10 g/dl. A higher target may be required for persons with coexistent cardiac or pulmonary disease.

Infections are treated with antibiotics. Myeloid growth factors are not routinely used for prophylaxis of uninfected individuals, even if neutropenic. However, they may be added for resistant or recurrent infections, particularly in patients with an ANC <500/μL. Platelet transfusions are used to treat patients with thrombocytopenia. Prophylactic transfusions are used when the platelet count is <10,000/μL. However, transfusions may be required at higher levels such as 20,000 or 30,000 if accompanied by signs of bleeding or petechiae. Repeated platelet transfusions may result in alloimmunization to HLA-antigens and development of panel reactive antibodies (PRA), with resulting resistance to transfusions. In such patients, or those at high risk of bleeding or with hemorrhage, aminocaproic acid or other antifibrinolytic agents should be considered. HLA-matched platelets may also be required.

Iron-Chelation Therapy

Iron overload in MDS occurs by two mechanisms. The first is transfusional iron overload in patients receiving regular transfusions of pRBCs. Each transfusion provides 200–250 mg of iron. The second mechanism of iron overload is by dysregulation of hepcidin, a small, cysteine-rich cationic peptide produced by hepatocytes, secreted into plasma, and excreted in the urine. Hepcidin reduces iron absorption in the gut, promotes release of iron from macrophages, and regulates iron metabolism. Most patients with iron overload have elevated urinary hepcidin levels, but some patients with MDS have inappropriately suppressed levels. Thus, both increased intestinal absorption and transfusional overload account for elevated iron in MDS.

While total body iron stores are normally between 3 and 5 g, tissue overload with subsequent dysfunction occurs when the total body iron load is 15–20 g. A serum ferritin of 1000 ng/ml corresponds with a total body iron load of approximately 5 g. Current guidelines are to consider iron-chelation therapy in patients who have received more than 20–25 units of packed RBCs, or who have a serum ferritin exceeding approximately 2500 ng/ml. Chelation may be achieved by use of the parenteral agent deferoxamine (Desferal), or one of the two oral chelators, deferiprone and deferasirox (ICL-670, Exjade). Consideration must be given toward balancing the cost and convenience of chelation therapy with the potential benefit. A patient with MDS may have a very brief lifespan depending on their presentation and IPSS score. End-organ damage due to iron overload typically develops over a period of many months to years. Thus, chelation therapy should be most strongly considered in young patients with Low/Int-1 IPSS scores who have low levels of bone marrow myeloblasts and anemia requiring RBC transfusions.

Though the relationship of iron-chelation therapy to overall survival has not been prospectively assessed, one retrospective study found that transfusional iron overload, defined as a ferritin level exceeding 1000 ng/ml, was associated with inferior survival in patients with RA and RARS receiving pRBC transfusions compared to patients whose ferritin levels remained below <1000 ng/ml (10). Apart from reducing end-organ damage, iron chelation may improve hematopoiesis in MDS by reducing reactive oxygen species damaging to HSCs.

Hypomethylating Agents

Epigenetic DNA hypermethylation is common in MDS. Hypermethylation results in transcriptional silencing and may contribute to the pathogenesis of MDS by decreasing expression of tumor suppressor genes, genes involved in differentiation, and cyclin-dependent kinase inhibitors (CDKIs). DNA methyltransferase inhibitors (DMTIs) promote hypomethylation via their incorporation into DNA and inhibition of DNA methyltransferases. Like histone deacetylase inhibitors (HDACs), DMTIs have the capacity to promote cellular differentiation in vitro. Such approaches are of obvious relevance to patients with MDS, in which the bone marrow often shows hypercellularity and a block in differentiation.

The DMTI 5-azacitidine (Vidaza), a cytidine analog, was the first agent to receive approval by the FDA for the treatment of MDS. Azacitidine is approved for all FAB subtypes of MDS, including RA and RARS with neutropenia or thrombocytopenia or requiring transfusional support. Azacitidine's activity was established in a study of 191 patients with MDS randomized to receive azacitidine versus best supportive care (11). Complete and partial responses were observed in 7 and 10% of patients, respectively, treated with azacitidine compared to none in the control arm. Overall improvement was observed in 37% of patients with azacitidine versus 5% with best supportive care. Time to leukemia or death was significantly increased from 13 to 21 months in the azacitidine group. In addition, QoL in the categories of fatigue, dyspnea, physical functioning, positive affect, and psychologic distress was improved in the treatment arm.

Decitabine (5-deoxyazacitidine, Dacogen) is a deoxycytidine analog that inhibits DNA methylation. Decitabine's activity was established in a study of 170 patients with MDS randomized to receive either decitabine at a dose of 15 mg/m^2 given intravenously over 3 h every 8 h for 3 days (at a dose of 135 mg/m^2 per course) and repeated every 6 weeks, versus best supportive care (12). Responses were classified according to the International Working Group (IWG) and required that response be maintained for at least 8 weeks. Patients treated with decitabine achieved an overall response rate of 17%, including 9% complete responses. In comparison, no responses were seen in the supportive care group. In addition, patients treated with decitabine had a trend toward a longer median time to progression to AML or death compared with patients who received supportive care alone (all patients, 12.1 months versus 7.8 months ($P = 0.16$)). Improvement was statistically significant in patients with IPSS Int-2 and High-risk disease (12.0 months versus 6.8 months ($P = 0.03$)) and those with de novo disease (12.6 months versus 9.4 months ($P = 0.04$)). Further studies will help define the optimal dose, administration, and duration of treatment with decitabine. Decitabine is approved for all FAB subtypes and IPSS risk groups excluding Low-risk patients.

Immunomodulators (IMIDs)

IMIDs are oral agents that suppress secretion of inflammatory cytokines but also modulate the immune response and inhibit angiogenesis. Thalidomide (Thalomid), the first member of this family to show activity in MDS, is highly teratogenic and is associated with significant side effects including neuropathies, constipation, drowsiness and fatigue, and has been superseded by lenalidomide (Revlimid), the second agent to gain FDA approval for the treatment of MDS. Lenalidomide is approved for the subset of MDS patients who are transfusion dependent with Low or Int-1 risk and harbor the 5q- interstitial deletion. Lenalidomide is a 4-amino glutarimide derivative of thalidomide. Lenalidomide is a more potent inhibitor of TNF-α than thalidomide and more potent stimulator of T-lymphocyte proliferation and IL-2 and IFN-γ production. It also has fewer side effects than thalidomide. A specific receptor has not been identified and its therapeutic mechanism of action in MDS is unclear.

The efficacy of lenalidomide in MDS was initially observed in a phase II study of 43 patients. Erythroid and cytogenetic responses were most prominent in patients with the 5q- interstitial deletion. Therefore, two multicenter, phase II studies were conducted to further define the relationship between lenalidomide activity and cytogenetics. Both studies were identical in design. One study, MDS-003, enrolled only patients with the 5q- interstitial deletion with or without additional cytogenetic abnormalities, while the other study, MDS-002, enrolled non-5q-MDS patients. Both studies involved low and Int-I risk patients who were transfusion-dependent.

In MDS-003, 148 patients with median age 71 were enrolled (13). Isolated deletion of 5q- was observed in 73% of patients, while 18% had one additional abnormality and 8% had complex cytogenetics. Transfusion independence was achieved in 67% of patients, while an additional 9% had minor erythroid responses. The median duration of response exceeded 104 weeks. Also, 45% of patients had complete cytogenetic remissions, while another 28% had minor cytogenetic responses.

In MDS-002, 214 patients with median age 72 were enrolled. The majority of patients (78%) had a normal karyotype. Transfusion independence was achieved in 26% of patients, while an additional 17% had minor erythroid responses. Of the 47 (22%) patients with abnormal cytogenetics, 9 (19%) achieved a cytogenetic response of which four were complete. The median duration of transfusion independence was 41 weeks.

The most common toxicities of lenalidomide include neutropenia and thrombocytopenia, which appear to be more common in patients with the 5q-interstitial deletion than in other patients. Additional toxicities include diarrhea and rash. Deep venous thromboses (DVTs) are increased in patients who receive IMIDs in combination with glucocorticoids, such as those used in the treatment of multiple myeloma. However, use of these agents in the absence glucocorticoids, as in MDS, is not associated with an increased risk of DVTs.

Immune Suppression

Some patients with MDS demonstrate elevated levels of inflammatory cytokines within the blood and/or abnormal lymphoid collections within the bone marrow. These findings suggest that immune dysregulation is operative in MDS pathogenesis and raises the possibility that immune suppression may result in clinical benefit. In a study of 61 patients with primarily low-risk MDS by FAB treated with equine ATG, responses were seen in all three hematopoietic lineages (7). Of these, 21 of 61 patients became transfusion independent, with a median duration of 36 months, 10 of 21 with severe thrombocytopenia achieved sustained responses, and 6 of 11 patients with severe neutropenia had significant improvements. Other studies have shown activity of ATG in MDS, particularly in patients with RA and RARS. Variables noted to predict response to therapy include young age (<60), expression of the HLA-DR15 antigen, and shorter duration of RBC transfusion dependence.

Additional Agents under Investigation

Like DNA methyltranferases, histone deacetylases suppress gene transcription and are active in patients with MDS. Thus, the role of histone deacetylase inhibitors (HDACs) is under investigation in MDS. A trial of the orally bioavailable HDAC, vorinostat (suberoylanilide hydroxamic acid, SAHA), has shown activity. Valproic acid (VPA) is a HDAC with differentiation properties that has been studied both alone and in combination with all-trans retinoic acid (ATRA).

The Ras/Raf kinase signaling pathway is activated in a variety of malignancies including MDS and AML. Agents capable of inhibiting this pathway include arsenic trioxide (AsO_3, Trisenox), farnesyl-transferase inhibitors (FTIs), which block necessary steps required for Ras activation, and direct pathway inhibitors, such as the Raf kinase inhibitor Bay 43-9006 (Sorafenib).

The proteasome, a catalytic, multisubunit protease involved in protein degradation, is an antineoplastic target inhibited by bortezomib (PS-341, Velcade). This agent, capable of suppressing levels of the master transcription factor, nuclear factor-kappa B (NF-κB), is approved for use in multiple myeloma. Elevated levels of nuclear NF-κB have been identified in primitive leukemia cells from patients with leukemia in addition to CD34+ bone marrow cells from patients with high-risk MDS, suggesting a role for the inhibitor in myeloid malignancies.

Chemotherapy and Stem Cell Transplantation

Care of younger patients and those with advanced disease presents a considerable clinical challenge. The role of intensive chemotherapy and SCT is an important consideration.

A variety of therapies useful to treat AML have been studied in MDS. Given the important clinical role of cytarabine in AML, low-dose chemotherapy strategies have focused on cytarabine, alone or in combination with etoposide or 6-thioguanine. Other agents include gemcitabine, fludarabine, troxacitabine, melphalan, and homoharringtonine. Complete response rates vary from 16% to 64%. While these therapies reduce the blast count and improve cytopenias, overall survival rates are not significantly altered. In addition, the impaired bone marrow reserve of MDS patients and their older age compromise the ability to administer cytotoxic therapies. Intensive induction chemotherapy with an anthracycline and cytarabine at doses similar to those used in AML has been attempted (see for example (14)). Complete responses may be achieved in 50–60% of patients treated with such regimens (15). However, treatment-related mortality is approximately 20%, and less than 10% of patients are alive at 5 years.

Allogeneic stem cell transplantation remains the only potential cure for MDS, though long-term survival is only approximately 30%. An estimated 10–15% of patients are eligible for SCT, which is generally performed in younger patients with adequate performance status and for whom a suitable donor can be identified. SCT is poorly tolerated in older adults as the treatment-related morbidity and mortality increases with age. However, nonmyeloablative approaches appear better tolerated, though their efficacy remains to be defined. A retrospective study of 836 MDS patients transplanted with stem cells from HLA-identical sibling donors was conducted (16). In this study, 621 patients received standard myeloablative conditioning (SMC) and the remaining 215 received reduced-intensity conditioning (RIC). At 3 years, the probabilities of progression-free and overall survivals were similar in both groups (39% after SMC versus 33% in RIC; multivariate $P = 0.9$; and 45% versus 41%, respectively; $P = 0.8$). However, in multivariate analysis, the 3 year relapse rate was significantly increased after RIC (HR, 1.64; 95% $P = 0.001$) and the 3 year non-relapse mortality was significantly decreased in the RIC group (HR, 0.61; 95% CI, 0.41–0.91; $P = 0.015$). Thus, SMC transplants are generally conducted on younger individuals able to withstand ablative conditioning regimens, and RIC transplants are reserved for older individuals or those with comorbidities. Additional clinical studies are required to determine the optimal settings for RIC transplants. Autologous transplantation remains an option for individuals without suitable allogeneic candidates, though the majority of patients relapse within 2 years (17).

Optimal timing of allogeneic SCT represents a balance between maximizing chances of long-term survival while decreasing transplant-related morbidity and mortality. A decision-model analysis was conducted to determine the relationship between IPSS score and timing of SCT (18). This model concluded that for patients with Int-2 or High-risk disease, early SCT increased overall survival. In contrast, SCT could be delayed for a brief period of time for patients with Low or Int-1 risk disease, provided the SCT is done before leukemic transformation. This strategy maximizes overall survival for low-risk patients while decreasing the early morbidity and mortality of transplantation.

PRINCIPLES OF THERAPY

Treatment of MDS requires consideration of patient age, treatment preference, IPSS score, performance status, presence of antecedent hematologic disorder (AHD), and availability of an HLA-matched stem cell donor. A treatment schema is provided in Figure 32-3.

Patients with secondary MDS have a worse prognosis relative to those with de novo MDS. Therefore, assessing for the presence of an AHD or T-MDS is a critical initial step. If the patient is a candidate for intensive therapy, an allogeneic donor must be sought and preparations made for allogeneic SCT. If the patient is deemed unsuitable or an appropriate donor cannot be identified, therapies consisting of supportive care, azacitidine, decitabine, and/or clinical trial should be considered.

For patients with Low or Int-1 risk MDS and anemia, cytogenetic status influences the starting therapy. Initial treatment for patients with the

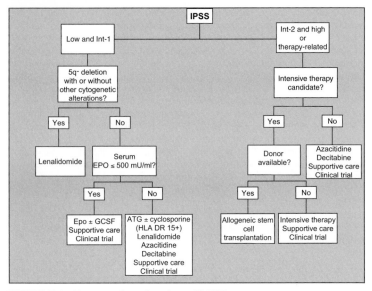

FIGURE 32-3 Treatment schema for patients with MDS.

5q-interstitial deletion, with or without additional cytogenetic abnormalities, is with lenalidomide. If an adequate response is not achieved after a period of approximately 3 months, attention is turned toward azacitidine, decitabine, or clinical trials in addition to supportive care. For Low/Int-1 risk patients lacking the 5q- cytogenetic deletion, initial treatment is based upon the serum Epo level and transfusion status. Patients with elevated serum Epo levels and/or those dependent upon RBC transfusions are unlikely to respond to exogenous erythropoietic growth factors and, therefore, treatment commences with supportive care, azacitidine, decitabine, and/or clinical trials. Lenalidomide may be effective in improving anemia, even in patients lacking the 5q- interstitial deletion.

Erythroid growth factors are used in the initial treatment of patients with serum Epo levels ≤500 mU/ml. Myeloid growth factors may be added if an inadequate response is achieved after an initial trial of Epo therapy. Patients with ringed sideroblasts demonstrate intrinsic resistance to Epo, and initial therapy with both myeloid and erythroid growth factors is often utilized. For Low/Int-1 risk patients who are suitable SCT candidates and have HLA-matched donors, delaying transplantation for a brief period of time, typically 1–2 years, maximizes overall survival.

Antilymphocyte therapy consisting of ATG may be effective in patients who are HLA-DR15 positive, who harbor trisomy 8, or who have a hypocellular MDS.

Patients with neutropenia and infections require myeloid growth factors and antibiotics. Patients with clinically significant thrombocytopenia should receive platelet transfusions and/or antifibrinolytic agents (aminocaproic acid). Azacitidine, decitabine, or clinical trials may be beneficial for individuals with thrombocytopenia and/or neutropenia.

For Int-2 and High-risk patients, SCT represents the best initial therapy for young patients with HLA-matched donors. If a donor cannot be identified, or if the patient is not a candidate for SCT, azacitidine, decitabine, chemotherapy agents, and/or supportive care are reasonable choices.

REFERENCES

1. Vardiman JW, Harris NL, Brunning RD. The World Health Organization (WHO) classification of myeloid neoplasms. Blood. 2002; 100: 2292–2307.

2. Greenberg P, Cox C, LeBeau MM, et al. International scoring system for evaluating prognosis in myelodysplastic syndromes. Blood. 1997; 89: 2079–2088.

3. Thanopoulou E, Cashman J, Kakagianne T, Eaves A, Zoumbos N, Eaves C. Engraftment of NOD/SCID-beta2 microglobulin null mice with multilineage neoplastic cells from patients with myelodysplastic syndrome. Blood. 2004; 103: 4285–4293.

4. Mauritzson N, Albin M, Rylander L, et al. Pooled analysis of clinical and cytogenetic features in treatment-related and de novo adult acute myeloid leukemia and myelodysplastic syndromes based on a consecutive series of 761 patients analyzed 1976–1993 and on 5098 unselected cases reported in the literature 1974–2001. Leukemia. 2002; 16: 2366–2378.

5. Nimer SD. Clinical management of myelodysplastic syndromes with interstitial deletion of chromosome 5q. J Clin Oncol. 2006; 24: 2576–2582.

6. Parker JE, Mufti GJ, Rasool F, Mijovic A, Devereux S, Pagliuca A. The role of apoptosis, proliferation, and the Bcl-2-related proteins in the myelodysplastic syndromes and acute myeloid leukemia secondary to MDS. Blood. 2000; 96: 3932–3938.

7. Molldrem JJ, Leifer E, Bahceci E, Saunthararajah Y, Rivera M, Dunbar C, Liu J, Nakamura R, Young NS, Barrett AJ. Antithymocyte globulin for treatment of the bone marrow failure associated with myelodysplastic syndromes. Ann Intern Med. 2002; 137: 156–163.

8. Mannone L, Gardin C, Quarre MC, et al. High dose darbopoetin alfa the treatment of lower risk MDS: results of a Phase II study. Br J Haematol. 2006; 133: 513–519.

9. Hellstrom-Lindberg E, Gulbrandsen N, Lindberg G, et al. A validated decision model for treating the anaemia of myelodysplastic syndromes with erythropoietin + granulocyte colony-stimulating factor: significant effects on quality of life. Br J Haematol. 2003; 120: 1037–1046.

10. Malcovati L, Porta MG, Pascutto C, et al. Prognostic factors and life expectancy in myelodysplastic syndromes classified according to WHO criteria: a basis for clinical decision making. J Clin Oncol. 2005; 23: 7594–7603.

11. Silverman LR, Demakos EP, Peterson BL, et al. Randomized controlled trial of azacitidine in patients with the myelodysplastic syndrome: a study of the cancer and leukemia group B. J Clin Oncol. 2002; 20: 2429–2440.

12. Kantarjian H, Issa JP, Rosenfeld CS, et al. Decitabine improves patient outcomes in myelodysplastic syndromes: results of a phase III randomized study. Cancer. 2006; 106: 1794–1803.

13. List A, Dewald G, Bennett J, et al. Lenalidomide in the myelodysplastic syndrome with chromosome 5q deletion. N Engl J Med. 2006; 355: 1456–1465.

14. de Witte T, Suciu S, Peetermans M, et al. Intensive chemotherapy for poor prognosis myelodysplasia (MDS) and secondary acute myeloid leukemia (sAML) following MDS of more than 6 months duration. A pilot study by the Leukemia Cooperative Group of the European Organisation for Research and Treatment in Cancer (EORTC-LCG). Leukemia. 1995; 9: 1805–1811.

15. Kantarjian H, Beran M, Cortes J, O'Brien S, Giles F, Pierce S, Shan J, Plunkett W, Keating M, Estey E. Long-term follow-up results of the combination of topotecan and cytarabine and other intensive chemotherapy regimens in myelodysplastic syndrome. Cancer. 2006; 106: 1099–1109.

16. Martino R, Iacobelli S, Brand R, et al. Retrospective comparison of reduced intensity conditioning and conventional high dose conditioning for allogeneic hematopoietic stem cell transplantation using HLA identical sibling donors in myelodysplastic syndromes. Blood. 2006; 108: 836–846.

17. Ducastelle S, Ades L, Gardin C, et al. Long-term follow-up of autologous stem cell transplantation after intensive chemotherapy in patients with myelodysplastic syndrome or secondary acute myeloid leukemia. Haematologica. 2006; 91: 373–376.

18. Cutler CS, Lee SJ, Greenberg P, et al. A decision analysis of allogeneic bone marrow transplantation for the myelodysplastic syndromes: delayed transplantation for low-risk myelodysplasia is associated with improved outcome. Blood. 2004; 104: 579–585.

33	Jerry L. Spivak

POLYCYTHEMIA VERA

INTRODUCTION

Polycythemia vera is a clonal disorder of a multipotent hematopoietic stem cell in which overproduction of morphologically normal red cells, white cells, and platelets occurs in the absence of an apparent cause. Polycythemia vera is an uncommon but not rare disorder, occurring at an average frequency of 2/100,000 but with increasing age, rates as high as 18/100,000 have been observed. Although there is a slight overall male predominance, below age 40, women predominate. Familial expression of the disease is well documented but uncommon.

PATHOGENESIS

The etiology of polycythemia vera is unknown and unlike certain leukemias, it has not been associated with radiation exposure. Abnormalities of chromosomes 1, 8, 9,13, and 20 have been identified in up to 30% of polycythemia vera patients, but they are neither specific for the disorder nor necessary for its pathogenesis; in many instances they appear to occur as secondary events and their expression can be enhanced by exposure to chemotherapeutic agents (1). Growth factor independent in vitro erythroid colony formation is a characteristic feature of polycythemia vera, although not specific for it, since this behavior has also been observed in idiopathic myelofibrosis and essential thrombocytosis. The molecular basis for this behavior has been identified to be constitutive activation of JAK2, (2) which is the cognate tyrosine kinase for type 1 hematopoietic growth factor receptors such as the erythropoietin, thrombopoietin, and granulocyte colony stimulating factor receptors.

In polycythemia vera and to a lesser extent in its companion myeloproliferative disorders, idiopathic myelofibrosis, and essential thrombocytosis, an acquired point mutation has been identified in the autoinhibitory JH2 domain of the JAK2 gene, causing valine to be replaced by phenylalanine (V617F) and leading to constitutive activation of this tyrosine kinase in CD34+ stem cells as well as their progeny. JAK2 is located on the short arm of chromosome 9 and loss of heterozygosity for 9p is a common cytogenetic lesion in polycythemia vera, leading to homozygosity for the JAK2 V617F mutation; in some patients, there is also reduplication of chromosome 9. In polycythemia vera, approximately 90% of patients express the JAK2 V617F mutation, of which approximately 35% are homozygous for it. Approximately 5% have an activating mutation in exon 12 of JAK2 to date, no clinical differences have been identified between heterozygotes and those homozygous for the mutation, nor are there any clinical differences between polycythemia vera patients expressing JAK2 V617F and those who do not. Thus, although the JAK2 V617F mutation provides an explanation for the hematopoietic growth factor independence of polycythemia vera hematopoietic cells in vitro, their apoptosis resistance and their uncontrolled growth in vivo, the absence of the mutation in some patients with classical polycythemia vera, and its expression in idiopathic myelofibrosis and essential thrombocytosis patients suggest that other as yet unidentified molecular lesions are involved in the pathogenesis of these disorders.

CLINICAL FEATURES

Polycythemia vera is extremely variable in its presenting manifestations as well as its clinical features, which also change over the course of the disorder. Because its onset can be insidious, an abnormal blood count is often the first sign of the disease. In approximately 40% of patients, there will be an increase in red cells, white cells, and platelets. In approximately 15% of patients, erythrocytosis will be the sole presenting manifestation. In approximately 5–10% of patients, an elevated platelet count may be the first manifestation of the disease, while in the rest, erythrocytosis and thrombocytosis or leukocytosis are the presenting blood abnormalities. Extramedullary hematopoiesis as manifested by palpable splenomegaly occurs in approximately 40% of patients at the time of diagnosis; rarely, myelofibrosis will be the initial manifestation of polycythemia vera with erythrocytosis becoming evident later on. Since polycythemia vera is a hypercoagulable state, arterial or venous thrombosis may also be the first manifestation of the disease. Classically, in young women, the thrombosis most commonly involves the hepatic veins. Pruritus, usually aquagenic, is not uncommon as a presenting manifestation, but polycythemia vera is often not initially recognized as its cause. Erythromelalgia, in which the extremities become warm, red, and painful, migraine headaches or other neurologic disturbances such as vertigo or visual disturbances are also characteristic symptoms that indicate the presence of an elevated red cell mass or thrombocytosis.

LABORATORY ABNORMALITIES

In addition to increases in the red cell, granulocyte, and platelet counts, the MCV can be low if red cell mass expansion or gastrointestinal blood loss depletes body iron stores. Hypocholesterolemia may be a consequence of blood cell expansion. An elevated leukocyte alkaline phosphatase, and serum vitamin B12 and vitamin B12 binding capacity due to increased release of granulocyte transcobalamin III reflect neutrophil activation, presumably due to JAK2 V617F, which is also responsible for the increase in expression of granulocyte PRV-1 mRNA (CD177). Serum histamine and uric acid may be increased as may homocysteine. When the platelet or leukocyte counts are elevated, spurious hyperkalemia may be observed, as can hypoglycemia and a low pO_2 if blood samples are not collected on ice and in the presence of sodium azide. Elevation of serum alkaline phosphatase occurs with extramedullary hematopoiesis and becomes more marked after splenectomy.

Abnormalities of coagulation in polycythemia vera are largely limited to platelet function. These include defective platelet aggregation to ADP, epinephrine or collagen alone or in combination and loss of alpha granules and dense bodies. However, increased thromboxane synthesis and expression of thrombospondin and P selectin indicate that platelet activation also occurs. This is in part a consequence of leukocyte activation and in part due to the erythrocytosis. When the platelet count exceeds 1,000,000/ml, higher molecular weight von Willebrand multimers will be absorbed by the platelets and degraded, leading to a reduction in ristocetin cofactor activity and an acquired form of von Willebrand's disease.

DIAGNOSIS

Elevation of the red cell mass is the sine qua non of polycythemia vera, the only feature that distinguishes it from its companion myeloproliferative disorders, idiopathic myelofibrosis and essential thrombocytosis, and the feature of the disease that is responsible for its most frequent serious consequences. Unfortunately, erythrocytosis is not unique to polycythemia vera and in recent years the very means for identifying the presence of erythrocytosis, direct determination of the red cell mass by isotope dilution, has become unavailable in many areas. Attempts to resolve this issue by the use of surrogate markers for the red cell mass determination have not proved to be useful (3). For example, specific hematocrit or hemoglobin levels are woefully inadequate as indicators of the red cell mass unless the hematocrit is 60% (hemoglobin 20 g%) in a man or 50% in a woman (hemoglobin 17 g%). The reasons for this are a consequence of blood rheology and the unique pathophysiology of polycythemia vera with respect to blood volume regulation.

For example, when erythrocytosis occurs as a consequence of hypoxia, there is a simultaneous reduction in the plasma volume as the body attempts to maintain a normal total blood volume. This contributes to the observed increase in hematocrit. In polycythemia vera, however, particularly in women, as the red cell mass rises, the plasma volume either rises or fails to decrease. Furthermore, with splenomegaly and splenic red cell sequestration, there is a compensatory increase in plasma volume. Both of these situations lead to hematocrit values that are spuriously low with respect to the actual red cell mass (4). As a corollary, a decrease in the plasma volume alone can lead to a falsely elevated hematocrit, when in fact the red cell mass is normal.

Thus, with the exception of the extreme values described above, the only method for determining whether a high hematocrit (or hemoglobin) is due to a diminished plasma volume or an absolute increase in red cell mass or both is to measure these values directly by isotope dilution. Because the plasma volume and red cell mass vary independently, it is not possible to measure one and extrapolate the value of the other with any accuracy. More importantly, because of plasma volume expansion in polycythemia vera, a normal hematocrit in this disease provides no assurance that the red cell mass is actually normal, particularly in women. Finally, given the phenotypic mimicry that characterizes the chronic myeloproliferative disorders, erythrocytosis is the only laboratory feature that can distinguish polycythemia vera from idiopathic myelofibrosis and essential thrombosis.

The recent discovery of the JAK2 V617F mutation has greatly simplified the evaluation of a high hematocrit and the diagnosis of polycythemia vera. This is because first, benign disorders causing erythrocytosis are more common than polycythemia vera (Table 33-1) and second, because surrogate markers for the latter lack sensitivity and specificity. For example, while serum erythropoietin levels are lower in polycythemia vera than in other disorders causing erythrocytosis, the serum erythropoietin level can also be normal in polycythemia vera as well as in secondary forms of erythrocytosis. Similarly, the bone marrow examination can be normal in polycythemia vera or even mimic that of idiopathic myelofibrosis. Cytogenetic abnormalities are present in only 30% of polycythemia vera patients and are not pathognomonic for the disease, while other markers such as elevation of the leukocyte alkaline phosphatase and endogenous erythroid colony formation are consequences of the constitutively active JAK2.

Figure 33-1 illustrates an algorithm for the evaluation of the patient with a high hematocrit. When red cell mass and plasma volume determinations are not available, it is reasonable to start with an assay for JAK2 V617F with the knowledge that a positive assay only indicates the presence of a myeloproliferative disorder, while a negative assay does not exclude such a disorder. In the absence of a red cell mass determination, a positive JAK2 V617F assay in a patient with a high hematocrit obligates the physician to phlebotomize the patient to the normal hematocrit for gender as discussed below.

Table 33-1

Causes of Erythrocytosis

Relative erythrocytosis
  Hemoconcentration secondary to dehydration, androgens, or tobacco abuse
Absolute erythrocytosis
  Hypoxia
    Carbon monoxide intoxication
    High affinity hemoglobin
    High altitude
    Pulmonary disease
    Right to left shunts
    Sleep apnea syndrome
    Neurologic disease
  Renal disease
    Renal artery stenosis
    Focal sclerosing or membranous glomerulonephritis
    Renal transplantation
  Tumors
    Hypernephroma
    Hepatoma
    Cerebellar hemangioblastoma
    Uterine fibronyoma
    Adrenal tumors
    Meningioma
    Pheochromcytoma
  Drugs
    Androgens
    Recombinant erythropoietin
  Familial (with normal hemoglobin function erythropoietin receptor mutations,
    chuvash polycythemia)
  Polycythemia vera

NATURAL HISTORY

Most classical textbooks of hematology suggest that the natural history of poly-cythemia vera follows an inevitable course from erythrocytosis through myelofi-brosis and myeloid metaplasia to acute leukemia if the patient does not die first from some other complication or comorbidity. This depiction, which was based on an hypothesis derived retrospectively from an analysis of a small number of patients, many of whom had been treated with chemotherapy or radiotherapy and to a standard of care unacceptable today, ignores the clinical heterogeneity of the disease and its modification by improved therapies and the earlier stages at which polycythemia vera is now usually recognized. In this regard, prognosis does not appear to be influenced by the presence or the absence of JAK2 V617F or whether this mutation is expressed homozygously or heterozygously.

The complications of polycythemia vera are listed in Table 33-2. Erythrocytosis, not thrombocytosis, is responsible for the major thrombotic complications of polycythemia vera; minor transient thrombotic or ischemic complications such as erythromelalgia, ocular migraine, or digital infarction do involve the platelets but are exacerbated by erythrocytosis, which promotes platelet activation, platelet–leukocyte interactions, and endothelial cell activa-tion and damage that enhanced thrombogenesis. Erythrocytosis can also cause hypertension and splenomegaly and exacerbate aquagenic pruritus. Acid-peptic disease leading to gastrointestinal hemorrhage and iron deficiency occur at a

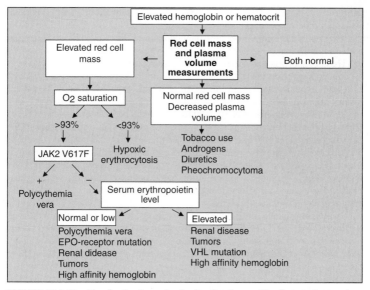

FIGURE 33-1 Algorithm for the diagnosis of polycythemia vera. The first requirement is to establish the basis for an elevated hemoglobin or hematocrit. If it is determined that there is an elevated red cell mass, an assay for JAK2 V617F will establish the diagnosis in over 90% of patients with polycythemia vera. A negative JAK2 V617F assay does not, however, exclude a myeloproliferative etiology and in the absence of splenomegaly, leukocytosis, or thrombocytosis, further studies will be required.

higher frequency in polycythemia vera patients than in the general population; the roles of vascular stasis, excess histamine, or other cytokine production or Helicobacter infection in this are unknown.

With time there will be an increase in the leukocyte and platelet counts but unless extreme, leukocytosis per se has no clinical significance and asymptomatic thrombocytosis requires no therapy either. The development of excessive extramedullary hematopoiesis with massive splenomegaly and hepatomegaly is a

Table 33-2

The Consequences of Polycythemia Vera

Consequence	Cause
• Thrombosis, hemorrhage, hypertension	• Elevated red cell mass, decreased vWF multimers
• Organomegaly	• Extramedullary hematopoiesis or elevated red cell mass
• Pruritis, acid-peptic disease	• Inflammatory mediators
• Erythromelalgia	• Thrombocytosis
• Hyperuricemia, gout, renal stones	• Increased cell turnover
• Myelofibrosis	• Reaction to the neoplastic clone
• Acute leukemia	• Therapy-induced or clonal evolution

serious complication of polycythemia vera but not one that afflicts every patient. Although this complication is frequently characterized as the spent phase of the disease, this is a misnomer because such patients are often capable of generating extremely high leukocyte and platelet counts post splenectomy and the actual red cell mass may be masked by an expanded plasma volume.

Splenomegaly can lead to mechanical discomfort, easy satiety, portal hypertension, and cachexia. Marrow myelofibrosis is another expected event in the natural history of polycythemia vera but one that has also been mischaracterized as a harbinger of marrow failure. It is essential to distinguish between the development of increased marrow reticulin as a consequence of marrow cell hyperplasia and the hematopoietic stem cell disorder, idiopathic myelofibrosis. There is no evidence that myelofibrosis in polycythemia vera represents a bad prognostic sign or that it impairs marrow function in the absence of exposure to agents that damage the bone marrow. Rarely, pulmonary hypertension has developed with long-standing disease; in some patients this may be due to extramedullary hematopoiesis, while others there may be pulmonary fibrosis.

Spontaneous acute leukemia develops in polycythemia vera at an incidence of approximately 1.5–2.5%; this usually occurs within the first 8 years of the disease and most commonly in patients older than 60 years (5). Chemotherapy or radiation-induced acute leukemia occurs at rates as high as 10% when these patients are exposed to ^{32}P or alkylating agents. The role of hydroxyurea as a leukemogen has been a matter of debate but in one randomized prospective clinical trial (6), hydroxyurea was associated with a 10% incidence of acute leukemia after 10 years; hydroxyurea is also a proven tumor promoter when used in conjunction with ^{32}P or an alkylating agent or with UV light exposure.

TREATMENT

Polycythemia is generally an indolent disease in which survival is measured in decades in the majority of patients. Most estimates of disease survival have failed to take into account the toxic forms of therapy that have been generally employed, the inadequate use of phlebotomy, and the later stages at which the disease was previously recognized clinically. Furthermore, it is now apparent that polycythemia vera is a heterogenous disorder with both indolent and aggressive forms and that aggressive chemotherapy has not improved survival (7). There is currently no curative therapy for polycythemia vera with the possible exception of allogeneic bone marrow transplantation, a therapy not suitable for the older patients who most commonly develop this disorder, and of questionable benefit in younger patients when the clinical course is measured in decades without compromise of functional capacity. Thus, treatment should be tailored to disease manifestations. Unfortunately, in contrast to idiopathic myelofibrosis, risk stratification according to laboratory features has not been possible with the exception that a prior history of thrombosis is an adverse risk factor for recurrent thrombotic events.

Erythrocytosis is the greatest initial threat because of the adverse effects of hyperviscosity (thrombosis, hemorrhage, hypertension, headache, and impaired cognitive function). Therefore, the red cell mass should be lowered by phlebotomy to achieve an hematocrit of ≤42% (hemoglobin ≤12 g%) in women and ≤45% (hemoglobin ≤14 g%) in men (8). This can done expediously in all but the most frail because phlebotomy rapidly stimulates plasma volume expansion. Repeated phlebotomies will be necessary to maintain the hematocrit and to induce iron deficiency but once this is achieved, the need for phlebotomy will diminish. Phlebotomy therapy actually improves platelet function, does not contribute significantly to thrombocytosis, and does not lead to myelofibrosis, and it must be remembered that the higher the hematocrit, the greater the extent of tissue damage with a thrombosis. Pruritus, usually aquagenic, is a distressing symptom in approximately 30% of patients. There is no single effective remedy. Phlebotomy, antihistamines, ataractics, PUVA light therapy, interferon alpha, and hydroxyurea have all been effective but none uniformly. Hyperuricemia (uric acid >10 mg%) responds to allopurinol.

Platelet-related microvascular complications include migraine, visual auras, transient ischemic attacks, erythromelalgia, and digital infarction. Aspirin is a specific remedy for erythromelalgia but with migraine, it may be necessary to lower the platelet count as well to achieve relief using conventional remedies. Symptomatic thrombocytosis causing acquired von Willebrand disease will also require platelet count reduction. Asymptomatic thrombocytosis without a significant reduction in ristocetin cofactor activity (<30%) requires no treatment in the absence of a thrombotic risk factor. In this regard, it is important to emphasize that there is no correlation between the platelet count and thrombosis, and no study to date has demonstrated that in the absence of hematocrit control, platelet count reduction prevents arterial or venous thrombosis. Hydroxyurea does appear to be more effective than anagrelide in the prevention of transient ischemic attacks but not other forms of vascular thrombosis. Because hydroxyurea is a potential tumor promoter, anagrelide is the initial drug of choice for platelet count reduction, followed by interferon alpha. The use of prophylactic aspirin therapy is no substitute for adequate, gender-specific control of the red cell mass.

Control of extramedullary hematopoiesis involving the spleen and liver is the most challenging therapeutic problem in polycythemia vera but fortunately not one that involves every patient and which is usually evident early in the course of the disease. Interferon alpha is the drug of choice for this because it lacks a potential for mutagenicity (9). Since interferon's side effects can be significant with chronic use, and it does not eradicate the malignant clone, intermittent use is a prudent strategy. In some patients, splenomegaly may be refractory to interferon and hydroxyurea, and mechanical discomfort, cachexia, and portal hypertension may dictate splenectomy. Low-dose thalidomide is another option worth considering in this situation. Splenic irradiation is only a temporary solution and not advisable unless surgery is not an option (10). Postoperative complications include wound dehiscence, bleeding, portal or mesenteric vein thrombosis, exuberant hepatic extramedullary hematopoiesis, and extreme leukocytosis and thrombocytosis, both of which can be very difficult to control.

PREGNANCY

The opportunity of pregnancy should not be denied to women with polycythemia vera who have no medical contraindications and a prior thrombosis is not one of these. The major threat to a successful outcome is failure to maintain the red cell mass at a safe level. Since there is an expansion of the plasma volume with pregnancy normally, there will be masking of the expanded red cell mass. A normal hematocrit in a pregnant woman is never normal and this is doubly true in polycythemia vera. It is essential to phlebotomize these patients to a hematocrit of <33% and avoid iron supplements; folic acid supplementation is mandatory. Thrombocytosis and splenomegaly may mandate the use of interferon alpha. Given, the elevation of von Willebrand factor that occurs during pregnancy, aspirin therapy may be prudent but this is unproved.

REFERENCES

1. Swolin B, Weinfeld A, Westin J. A prospective long–term cytogenetic study in polycythemia vera in relation to treatment and clinical course. Blood. 1988; 72: 386–395.

2. Baxter EJ, Scott LM, Campbell PJ, et al. Acquired mutation of the tyrosine kinase Jak2 in human myeloproliferative disorders. Lancet. 2005; 365: 1054–1061.

3. Johansson PL, Safai-Kutti S, Kutti J. An elevated venous haemoglobin concentration cannot be used as a surrogate marker for absolute erythrocytosis: a study of patients with polycythaemia vera and apparent polycythaemia. Br J Haematol. 2005; 129: 701–705.

4. Lamy T, Devillers A, Bernard M, et al. Inapparent polycythemia vera: an unrecognized diagnosis. Am J Med. 1997; 102: 14–20.

5. Finazzi G, Caruso V, Marchioli R, et al. Acute leukemia in polycythemia vera: an analysis of 1638 patients enrolled in a prospective observational study. Blood. 2005; 105: 2664–2670.

6. Najean Y, Rain J. Treatment of polycythemia vera: the use of hydroxyurea and pipobroman in 292 patients under the age of 65 years. Blood. 1997; 90: 3370–3377.

7. Gruppo Italiano Studio Policitemia. Polycythemia vera: the natural history of 1213 patients followed for 20 years. Ann Intern Med. 1995; 123: 656–664.

8. Spivak JL. Polycythemia vera myths, mechanisms, and management. Blood. 2002; 100: 4272–4290.

9. Silver RT. Treatment of polycythemia vera with recombinant interferon alpha (rifnalpha) or imatinib mesylate. Curr Hematol Rep. 2005; 4: 235–237.

10. Elliott MA, Chen MG, Silverstein MN, Tefferi A. Splenic irradiation for symptomatic splenomegaly associated with myelofibrosis with myeloid metaplasia. Br J Haematol. 1998; 103: 505–511.

IDIOPATHIC MYELOFIBROSIS

INTRODUCTION

Idiopathic myelofibrosis is the least common and most enigmatic of the chronic myeloproliferative disorders. Most frequent after age 60, idiopathic myelofibrosis has an incidence of approximately 1/100,000 with no significant gender predominance. Previously known as agnogenic myeloid metaplasia, primary myelofibrosis, primary osteomyelofibrosis, or myelofibrosis with myeloid metaplasia, it is important to note that both the first and last appellations actually describe a pathologic process that is not restricted to the disease idiopathic myelofibrosis but can be caused by a variety of benign and malignant processes (Table 34-1). Like its companion myeloproliferative disorders, polycythemia vera and essential thrombocytosis, idiopathic myelofibrosis is a clonal hematopoietic stem cell disorder, but in contrast to them, it is associated not only with overproduction of blood cells without an obvious cause but also, in many patients, with anemia, leucopenia, or thrombocytopenia.

PATHOGENESIS

The etiology of idiopathic myelofibrosis is unknown. Although irradiation and exposure to organic chemicals such as toluene and benzene can cause marrow fibrosis, no consistent environmental risk factors have been identified for

Table 34-1

Disorders Causing Myelofibrosis

Malignant

Acute leukemia (lymphocytic, myelogenous, megakaryocytic)
Chronic myelogenous leukemia
Hairy cell leukemia
Hodgkin disease
Idiopathic myelofibrosis
Lymphoma
Multiple myeloma
Myelodysplasia
Metastatic carcinoma
Polycythemia vera
Systemic mastocytosis

Nonmalignant

HIV infection
Hyperparathyroidism
Renal osteodystrophy
Systemic lupus erythematosus
Tuberculosis
Vitamin D deficiency
Thorium dioxide exposure
Gray platelet syndrome

idiopathic myelofibrosis and familial transmission is rare. Cytogenetic abnormalities occur in more than 50% of patients but generally involve the same chromosomes as in polycythemia vera and essential thrombocytosis and none appear to be involved in its pathogenesis. Myelofibrosis is the hallmark of the disorder but there is good retrospective histologic evidence that a premyelofibrotic phase of the disease exists (1), supporting other evidence that the fibrosis is a consequence of the disease, not its cause.

Normally, hematopoiesis is extravascular and hematopoietic progenitor cell proliferation and differentiation in the marrow are supported by accessory cells such as macrophages, adipocytes, reticulum cells, fibroblasts, and endothelial cells, all of which are embedded in an extracellular matrix of collagens (Types 1, 3 and 4), laminin and adhesive proteins such as fibronectin and vitronectin and glycosaminoglycans. Myelofibrosis represents the deposition of additional collagen fibrils that are thicker and contiguous. The earliest phase of marrow fibrosis is the deposition of reticulin, which represents collagen fibrils coated with matrix substances such as hyaluronic acid that are argyrophilic and stain with silver. As the quantity of collagen increases relative to matrix substances, the fibrils eventually become reactive with the classical histological collagen stains.

Osteosclerosis in idiopathic myelofibrosis represents the deposition of minerals on the marrow trabeculae as opposed to the combined osteoblastic and osteoclastic activity that characterizes metabolic bone disease, and is thought to be due to overproduction of osteoprotegerin, which is an osteoclast inhibitor. With advancing myelofibrosis, there is also a reduction in the number of hematopoietic cells in the marrow with the exception of the megakaryocytes. Disease duration, spleen size, and prognosis did not correlate with the degree of myelofibrosis.

The stimulus for the marrow fibrosis and osteosclerosis that are central features of idiopathic myelofibrosis and a prerequisite for its diagnosis are not entirely understood but both megakaryocytes and monocytes appear to be involved through the elaboration of the fibrogenic cytokines TGF-β, connective tissue growth factor, and bFGF. Animal models of myelofibrosis and osteosclerosis have also been created by overexpression of thrombopoietin, impaired expression of the hematopoietic transcription factor GATA-1, or transplantation of hematopoietic cells overexpressing JAK2 V617F, further implicating megakaryocytes and other hematopoietic progenitor cells in these processes.

Importantly, a variety of techniques have been employed to definitively demonstrate that the fibroblastic component of idiopathic myelofibrosis is not monoclonal and is reactive in contrast to the hematopoietic cells in this disorder, which are clonal and primary. The latter exhibit the hematopoietic growth factor hypersensitivity and growth factor independent in vitro colony forming activity that is characteristic of all three chronic myeloproliferative disorders. An increase in circulating endothelial cell progenitor cells followed by an increase in circulating CD34+ cells and their progeny are interesting and unique features of idiopathic myelofibrosis, which are thought to be a consequence of dysregulation of bone marrow neutrophil elastase, matrix metalloproteinases, and their inhibitors (2).

Bone marrow neoangiogenesis is another characteristic feature of idiopathic myelofibrosis that is thought to be a consequence of increased VEGF production. This increase in microvascularity correlates with the degree of marrow cellularity but not the degree of myelofibrosis. There is also marrow sinusoidal dilation and intravascular hematopoiesis in these sinusoids. The latter is not a consequence of reduced marrow cellularity or peculiar to idiopathic myelofibrosis, since it can be seen in other disorders causing myelofibrosis and, in these disorders as well as idiopathic myelofibrosis, results in extramedullary hematopoiesis. With the increase in marrow vascularity and metabolic activity, there is a corresponding increase in marrow blood flow, which may account for the bone pain experienced by some patients with advanced myelofibrosis.

CLINICAL FEATURES

As with the other chronic myeloproliferative disorders, idiopathic myelofibrosis may first be recognized during a routine health maintenance evaluation due to abnormal blood counts or a palpable spleen. However, in contrast to the other chronic myeloproliferative disorders, idiopathic myelofibrosis can present with significant constitutional symptoms such as fever, night sweats, weakness, fatigue, and weight loss. In some patients, thrombocytosis alone may be the first manifestation of the disease and less commonly, isolated leukocytosis. In general, such cases of so-called essential thrombocytosis take approximately 4–7 years to develop myelofibrosis but in these patients, bone marrow examination may initially reveal changes inconsistent with the diagnosis of essential thrombocytosis. This situation has been designated as the cellular or premyelofibrotic phase of idiopathic myelofibrosis (1).

Palpable splenomegaly, which can be modest or extreme, is the most common abnormality, but occasionally patients are encountered before palpable splenomegaly has developed, putting them in a diagnostic limbo. Hepatomegaly is less common and not seen in the absence of splenomegaly. Lymphadenopathy is very uncommon and when localized should suggest another diagnosis.

LABORATORY ABNORMALITIES

Any combination of blood count abnormalities can be encountered in idiopathic myelofibrosis. Anemia is the most common abnormality and a normal hematocrit in a patient with splenomegaly should suggest the presence of polycythemia vera; indeed, retrospectively approximately 10% of patients in most published series of idiopathic myelofibrosis were found to have polycythemia vera. The anemia is usually normochromic and normocytic and a hemolytic component is rare. Folic acid deficiency, however, can complicate the disorder due to an increased turnover of marrow cells. Leukocytosis is common but not usually to the degree found in chronic myelogenous leukemia. The platelet count is usually normal or elevated but modest thrombocytopenia can be seen in approximately 25% of patients. Nucleated red blood cells, myelocytes, promyelocytes, and even blast cells may be present in the blood, creating the classical leukoerythroblastic blood picture (Figure 34-1). Tear drop shaped red cells reflect the presence of splenomegaly. The

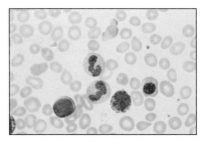

FIGURE 34-1   The peripheral blood smear in patients with myelofibrosis is described as "leuko-erythroblastic." Some RBCs are tear drop shaped based on membrane damage in the spleen. Nucleated red blood cells and immature myeloid cells may be noted. (From Spivak JL. Polycythemia vera and other myeloproliferative diseases. In DL Kasper, E Braunwald, AS Fauci, et al (eds.), "Harrison's Principles of Internal Medicine," sixteenth edition, McGraw-Hill, New York, p. 629.)

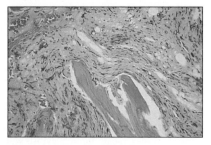

FIGURE 34-2 The bone marrow in myelofibrosis shows the marrow cavity replaced by fibrous tissue composed of collagen and reticulin fibrils. (From Spivak JL. Polycythemia vera and other myeloproliferative diseases. In DL Kasper, E Braunwald, AS Fauci, et al (eds.), "Harrison's Principles of Internal Medicine," sixteenth edition, McGraw-Hill, New York, p. 629.)

leukocyte alkaline phosphatase can be low, normal, or elevated. With hepatic extramedullary hematopoiesis, the serum alkaline phosphatase will be increased. The constitutively active JAK2 V617F mutant occurs in approximately 50% of patients and is often homozygous in its expression but this abnormality does not correlate with disease activity. Platelet function abnormalities in idiopathic myelofibrosis parallel those in the other chronic myeloproliferative disorders but idiopathic myelofibrosis patients are particularly prone to bleeding (3). In a few patients, a mutation has been identified in the thrombopoietin receptor, MPL (4).

Bone marrow is inaspirable when there is myelofibrosis. Bone marrow biopsy may reveal a hypercellular marrow with myeloid hyperplasia, an increase in large dysplastic megakaryocytes occurring in clusters and, in some patients, widening of the bony trabecula (Figure 34-2). An increase in collagen, sinusoidal dilatation, neoangiogenesis with extramedullary hematopoiesis, and a reduction in cellularity with erythroid islands and megakaryocyte sparing may also be encountered. The reticulin stain will show a dense pattern of argyrophilic fibers in a contiguous pattern with sinusoidal accentuation. If collagen deposition is extensive, the trichrome stain will be positive. It is important to remember, however, that marrow histology is not uniform with respect to biopsy sampling, and specific marrow histology cannot be relied on to stage this disorder.

RADIOLOGIC ABNORMALITIES

Osteosclerosis but not myelofibrosis can be detected radiologically, most commonly as an increase in medullary bone density in the proximal long bones. Rib and vertebral involvement are also common and even the skull can be affected. The presence of radiologically evident osteosclerosis suggests involvement of at least 40% of the marrow cavity and is related to the extent of the myelofibrosis and splenomegaly but not disease duration or prognosis. Hypertrophic osteoarthropathy with painful periostitis and onion skinning of the tibiae is an uncommon complication of idiopathic myelofibrosis and could be another consequence of the neoangiogenesis that characterizes this disorder.

CYTOGENETIC ABNORMALITIES

As mentioned above, cytogenetic abnormalities are more common in idiopathic myelofibrosis than in its companion myeloproliferative disorders, but they are mostly nonspecific. They include 20q-, 13q-, trisomy 8, trisomy 9, partial trisomy 1q, and reduplication of 9p. In contrast to its companion myeloproliferative disorders, however, trisomy 8 and 12p- as well as certain complex chromosomal abnormalities appear to confer a poor prognosis in idiopathic myelofibrosis (5).

IMMUNOLOGIC ABNORMALITIES

Autoimmune abnormalities are an unexplained feature of idiopathic myelofibrosis and include circulating immune complexes—usually IgG-antiIgG, cryoglobulinemia, antinuclear and antismooth muscle antibodies, rheumatoid factor, low C3, Coombs' positivity, and polyclonal hypergammaglobulinemia. Since myelofibrosis can complicate collagen vascular disorders such as systemic lupus erythematosus, either or both processes are probably a reaction to the underlying disease. The presence of immune abnormalities correlates with constitutional symptoms and with an increased incidence of infection.

DIAGNOSIS

Given the inability to aspirate bone marrow when myelofibrosis is present, distinguishing idiopathic myelofibrosis from the many other disorders that cause myelofibrosis (Table 34-1) is a difficult task. Clinical criteria have been formulated to facilitate this (Table 34-2), but they are either inadequate or uncritical. For example, the presence of extramedullary hematopoiesis as defined by circulating nucleated red cells, and myelocytes is a feature of many disorders other than idiopathic myelofibrosis (Table 34-3). Although splenomegaly was considered an optional diagnostic criterion, splenomegaly was present in over 90% of patients at the time of diagnosis. Thus, at a minimum, in the absence of splenomegaly, it is probably not possible to distinguish idiopathic myelofibrosis clinically from the many disorders which mimic it.

The most important disorders with respect to differential diagnosis are chronic myelogenous leukemia, polycythemia vera, acute myelofibrosis, myelodysplasia, hairy cell leukemia, primary bone marrow lymphomas, multiple myeloma, metastatic carcinoma, and systemic mastocytosis. The most difficult of this group to identify are acute myelofibrosis and myelodysplasia with myelofibrosis. The former is a rapidly progressive form of leukemia, which can have extramedullary hematopoiesis without palpable splenomegaly; the latter is somewhat more indolent but carries an equally poor prognosis. In either

Table 34-2

Diagnostic criteria for Myelofibrosis with Myeloid Metaplasia[*]

Necessary criteria
A)   Diffuse bone marrow fibrosis
B)   Absence of the Philadelphia chromosome or BCR-ABL rearrangement in peripheral blood cells

Optional criteria
1)   Splenomegaly of any grade
2)   Anisopoikilocytosis with teardrop erythrocytes
3)   Presence of circulating immature myeloid cells
4)   Presence of circulating erythroblasts
5)   Presence of clusters of megakaryocytes and anomalous megakaryocytes in bone marrow biopsy sections
6)   Myeloid metaplasia

A diagnosis of MMM is acceptable if the following combinations are present: the two necessary criteria plus any other two optional criteria when splenomegaly is present; the two necessary criteria plus any four optional criteria when splenomegaly is absent

---

*(Italian Consensus Conference on Diagnostic Criteria for Myelofibrosis with Myeloid Metaplasia. Br J Haematol 1999; 104: 730)

Table 34-3

Causes of Extramedullary Hematopoiesis and a Leukoerythroblastic Reaction

Carcinoma metastatic to the bone marrow
Lymphoma involving the bone marrow
Idiopathic myelofibrosis
Polycythemia vera
Chronic myelogenous leukemia
Myelodysplasia
Acute hepatic injury
Hemolytic anemia

instance, an increase in marrow blast cells, micromegakaryocytes, specific chromosome abnormalities, and an increase in marrow CD34+ cells favor an acute myeloid malignancy or myelodysplasia rather than idiopathic myelofibrosis.

The JAK2 V617F mutation can be used to distinguish idiopathic myelofibrosis from chronic myelogenous leukemia and the other hematopoietic malignancies in approximately 50% of cases; absence of the mutation, however, is not helpful. Furthermore, the presence of JAK2 V617F does not remove the obligation of excluding polycythemia vera masquerading as idiopathic myelofibrosis, a task that requires a red cell mass and plasma volume determination. From a diagnostic perspective, bone marrow aspiration and biopsy with cytogenetics, flow cytometry using peripheral blood, marrow immunohistochemistry with respect to CD34+ cells, and a JAK2 analysis should suffice to differentiate idiopathic myelofibrosis from the other disorders that mimic it.

NATURAL HISTORY

The natural history of idiopathic myelofibrosis is highly variable. In its most aggressive form, there is progressive bone marrow failure with expanding extramedullary hematopoiesis. The consequences of this include splenic and hepatic enlargement, portal hypertension, anemia, thrombocytopenia, leukocytosis, hyperuricemia, cachexia, and in some patients, transformation to acute leukemia. The actuarial frequency of transformation in one series was 21% at 8 years, a frequency much higher than in polycythemia vera or essential thrombocytosis (6). No organ or body space is immune to the development of extramedullary hematopoiesis, which can invade the lymph nodes, kidneys, adrenals, ovaries, dura, spinal canal, skin, mediastinum, mesentery, pulmonary parenchyma, and the pleural, peritoneal, and retroperitoneal spaces. In some patients, dense fibrous tumors develop; in others, pulmonary hypertension (7). Solitary lesions may not be recognized as such and diffuse peritoneal involvement has been mistaken for disseminated carcinoma. Progressive extramedullary hematopoiesis can also be a harbinger of leukemic transformation. Fortunately, however, this scenario is not the fate of every patient.

Although previous estimates of survival indicated that life expectancy in this disorder was distinctly inferior to its companion myeloproliferative disorders, subsequent studies have indicated that idiopathic myelofibrosis is not a monolithic illness and, with risk stratification, it has been possible to identify patients whose disease is indolent rather than progressive. Several useful risk stratification schemes have been proposed (Table 34–4). Age, anemia, leukocyte count, circulating blast cell count and cytogenetic abnormalities have been the common denominators of risk stratification. Recently, it was claimed by one group that JAK2 V617F expression conferred a poor prognosis in idiopathic myelofibrosis,

Table 34-4

Risk Stratification for Idiopathic Myelofibrosis

A. Prognostic factors*
   Hemoglobin <10 gm%
   White cell count <4,000/μl or >30,000/μl

Number of prognostic factors	Risk group	Median survival (months)
0	Low	93
1–2	High	17

B. Prognostic factors+
   Hemoglobin <10 g%
   Constitutional symptoms
   Blast cells >1%

Number of prognostic factors	Risk group	Median survival (months)
0–1	Low	99
2–3	High	21

C. Prognostic factors ++

	Median survival (months)
Age <65 years Hemoglobin ≤10 g%	
Karyotype Normal	54
Abnormal	22
Age <65 years Hemoglobin >10 g%	
Karyotype Normal	180
Abnormal	72
Age >65 years Hemoglobin >10 g%	
Karyotype Normal	44
Abnormal	16
Age >65 years Hemoglobin >10 g%	
Karyotype Normal	70
Abnormal	78

*From Dupriez, et al. Blood. 1996; 88: 1013.

+From Cervantes et al. Br J Haematol. 1998; 102: 684.

++From Reilly et al. Br J Haematol. 1997; 98: 96.

but another study indicated that the mutation correlated only with older age at diagnosis and a history of thrombosis or pruritus (8). Since both studies were retrospective and the red cell mass was not measured in either, the actual correlations between JAK2 V617F expression and the clinical features of idiopathic myelofibrosis must await comprehensive prospective studies.

TREATMENT

There is no specific therapy for idiopathic myelofibrosis and allogeneic bone marrow transplantation is the only potentially curative therapy. Unfortunately, this approach has been most effective in patients under age 45 with good prognosis disease. Transplant-related mortality was high at 27–32% and while survival was greater than 60% at 5 years for patients less than 45 years of age, it was only 14% for older patients (9). Recently, reduced intensity conditioning was found to decrease transplant-related mortality and achieve remission rates of greater than 70% (10). However, prospective studies will be required to establish the most effective conditioning regimen, whether there is a role for T-cell depletion, the optimal timing for transplantation, and which patients will benefit the most from this procedure.

Bone marrow failure and progressive splenomegaly are the two most pressing problems in the management of idiopathic myelofibrosis. Anemia is the most common problem and can be multifarious with respect to etiology, which can include hemodilution, blood loss, and folic acid deficiency. In patients with constitutional symptoms, prednisone therapy may be effective in alleviating anemia as well as the constitutional symptoms. If the serum erythropoietin level is less than 125 mU/mL, a trial of recombinant erythropoietin is worthwhile with the caveat that it could increase spleen or liver size (9). Impeded androgens such as danazol have been tried in this situation with modest success, but these agents have side effects that make their long-term use unattractive.

Progressive splenomegaly with or without hepatomegaly is the most difficult therapeutic problem in idiopathic myelofibrosis since it gives rise to mechanical problems such as easy satiety, diarrhea, abdominal discomfort, sequestration of leukocytes and platelets, splenic infarction, portal hypertension, and esophageal varices. Cachexia is an inevitable complication. A number of therapies have been tried in this situation including low dose alkylating agents, hydroxyurea, interferon alpha, imatinib mesylate, and thalidomide. Alkylating agents such as busulfan and melphalan at doses of 2–4 mg per day have proved effective but have the potential for substantial hematologic and nonhematologic toxicity and are also leukemogenic; their use should be reserved for specific situations where other remedies have not been effective. Hydroxyurea is effective in controlling leukocytosis and thrombocytosis but can exacerbate anemia. Neither interferon nor imatinib has proved effective in idiopathic myelofibrosis and both appear to have substantial toxicity in this group of patients. Thalidomide at low doses in combination with prednisone has proved to be effective in ameliorating anemia as well as thrombocytopenia in idiopathic myelofibrosis patients and reducing spleen size in approximately 20% (11).

In some patients, splenectomy may be necessary for massive splenomegaly because of the failure of other treatment options (9). This is a major undertaking with significant postoperative complications including hemorrhage, splanchnic vein thrombosis, infection, hepatomegaly, exuberant leukocytosis or thrombocytosis, and abdominal hernias. Neither anemia nor thrombocytopenia is significantly improved in most patients. In one series, the incidence of acute leukemia increased postsplenectomy. Splenic irradiation has been employed in patients thought to be unfit for surgery. This is often effective in reducing spleen size and ameliorating symptoms temporarily and can be repeated. However, myelosuppression is frequent and the mortality rate as a consequence can be as high as 50%. By contrast, irradiation can be useful in controlling localized soft tissue sites of extramedullary hematopoiesis or periostitis. In summary, lacking specific therapy for idiopathic myelofibrosis, treatment in this disorder must be tailored to the individual patient.

REFERENCES

1. Thiele J, Kvasnicka HM. Hematopathologic findings in chronic idiopathic myelofibrosis. Semin Oncol. 2005; 32: 380–394.
2. Barosi G, Hoffman R. Idiopathic myelofibrosis. Semin Hematol. 2005; 42: 248–258.

3. Murphy S, Davis JL, Walsh PN, Gardner FH. Template bleeding time and clinical hemorrhage in myeloproliferative disease. Arch Intern Med. 1978; 138: 1251–1253.
4. Guglielmelli P, Pancrazzi A, Bergamaschi G, et al. Anaemia characterizes patients with myelofibrosis harbouring Mpl mutation. Br J Haematol. 2007; 137: 244.
5. Tefferi A, Mesa RA, Schroeder G, et al. Cytogenetic findings and their clinical relevance in myelofibrosis with myeloid metaplasia. Br J Haematol. 2001; 113: 763–771.
6. Cervantes F, Tassies D, Salgado C, et al. Acute transformation in nonleukemic chronic myeloproliferative disorders: actuarial probability and main characteristics in a series of 218 patients. Acta Haematol. 1991; 85: 124–127.
7. Rumi E, Passamonti F, Boveri E, et al. Dyspnea secondary to pulmonary hematopoiesis as presenting symptom of myelofibrosis with myeloid metaplasia. Am J Hematol. 2006; 81: 124–127.
8. Tefferi A, Lasho TL, Schwager SM, et al. The JAK2(V617F) tyrosine kinase mutation in myelofibrosis with myeloid metaplasia: lineage specificity and clinical correlates. Br J Haematol. 2005; 131: 320–328.
9. Cervantes F. Modern management of myelofibrosis. Br J Haematol. 2005; 128: 583–592.
10. Rondelli D, Barosi G, Bacigalupo A, et al. Allogeneic hematopoietic stem-cell transplantation with reduced-intensity conditioning in intermediate- or high-risk patients with myelofibrosis with myeloid metaplasia. Blood. 2005; 105: 4115–4119.
11. Mesa RA, Steensma DP, Pardanani A, et al. A phase 2 trial of combination low-dose thalidomide and prednisone for the treatment of myelofibrosis with myeloid metaplasia Blood. 2003; 101: 2534–2541.

ESSENTIAL THROMBOCYTOSIS

INTRODUCTION

Essential thrombocytosis is the most nebulous of the chronic myeloproliferative disorders, since its only identifying marker, thrombocytosis, is not specific for it. Like idiopathic myelofibrosis and polycythemia vera, essential thrombocytosis is a clonal disorder involving a multipotent hematopoietic stem cell. Clinically, however, unlike its companion myeloproliferative disorders, hematopoiesis is not globally disturbed, women predominate, and overall life span is superior. The frequency of essential thrombocytosis is approximately 2/100,000. The frequency of the disorder increases with age with a mean age at diagnosis of 51 years. In women, the incidence appears to be biphasic with a peak at age 50 and a second at age 70.

PATHOGENESIS

The etiology of essential thrombocytosis is unknown. Furthermore, why a disorder involving a multipotent hematopoietic progenitor cell should be expressed primarily by overproduction of one cell line remains a conundrum, particularly since hematopoietic progenitor cells in essential thrombocytosis exhibit the same growth factor independence and hypersensitivity that are seen in polycythemia vera and idiopathic myelofibrosis. Although thrombopoietin is essential for the survival of primitive hematopoietic stem cells, overproduction of thrombopoietin does not recapitulate essential thrombocytosis in animal models nor in familial thrombocytosis due to a mutation in the 5′ UTR of the thrombopoietin gene. In contrast to polycythemia vera, where the plasma level of erythropoietin is severely reduced due to the expansion of the red cell mass, in essential thrombocytosis, the thrombopoietin level is normal or elevated despite expansion of the megakaryocyte mass, preventing its distinction from secondary forms of thrombocytosis on this basis.

A number of epigenetic abnormalities found in polycythemia vera and idiopathic myelofibrosis, such as increased expression of granulocyte PRV-1 mRNA and reduced expression of the thrombopoietin receptor, Mpl, in megakaryocytes and platelets, are also found in essential thrombocytosis. Cytogenetic abnormalities similar to those found in polycythemia vera and idiopathic myelofibrosis are present in essential thrombocytosis as well but at a much lower frequency. The frequency of the JAK2 V617F mutation is also lower in this disorder than the other chronic myeloproliferative disorders and homozygosity for the mutation is rarely found. Some investigators have claimed that essential thrombocytosis patients expressing JAK2 V617F have a "polycythemia vera-like" phenotype. However, a consistent failure on the part of these investigators to exclude polycythemia vera by performing a red cell mass determination renders these claims dubious (Table 35-1).

Table 35-1

Polycythemia Vera Masquerading as Essential Thrombocytosis

An asymptomatic 61 year old woman was referred for evaluation of thrombocytosis

2003	The platelet count = 480,000/μl
2004	The platelet count = 600,000/μl
2005	The platelet count = 799,000/μl
	Hemoglobin = 14.9 g%; white cell count =12,700/μl
	MCV = 93 fl; reticulocyte count = 1.9 %

Bone marrow: cellular with increased megakaryocytes
and stainable iron
(serum ferritin = 33 ng/ml)

Bcr-Abl FISH is negative
Jak2 V617F + (heterozygote)
Red cell mass: 38.5 ml/kg   (20–30 ml/kg)
Plasma volume: 47.1 ml/kg   (30–45 ml/kg)

CLINICAL FEATURES

Since it was first recognized in 1920, essential thrombocytosis has been known by a variety of names, including hemorrhagic thrombocythemia, idiopathic thrombocytosis, and primary thrombocytosis. This ambivalence reflects the lack of a specific diagnostic marker for essential thrombocytosis and the fact that the thrombocytosis can be associated with either thrombosis or hemorrhage. Furthermore, with the advent of electronic particle counters, thrombocytosis is now being recognized in individuals who are asymptomatic. This was most often true in women and did not vary with age. Microvascular occlusive syndromes such as migraine, transient ischemic attacks, visual disturbances, dizziness, or erythromelalgia are the most common presenting complaints but are, of course, not specific for the disease. Hemorrhage, usually involving the mucous membranes and generally mild has been more common in some series than thrombotic episodes, which could be arterial or less frequently venous. Interestingly, hemorrhage was more common with platelet counts greater than 1,000,000/μl, and thrombosis when the platelet count was lower. The actual frequency of either thrombosis or hemorrhage in essential thrombocytosis is, of course, currently obscured by ascertainment bias in most published reports.

The physical examination in essential thrombocytosis is usually normal. Splenomegaly was present in less than 30% of reported patients at diagnosis and even then was minimal in extent. Significant splenomegaly, isolated hepatomegaly, or lymphadenopathy should suggest another cause for the thrombocytosis.

LABORATORY ABNORMALITIES

Thrombocytosis is the major laboratory abnormality in essential thrombocytosis with the platelet count averaging 1,000,000/μl or greater in most large studies. It is not possible, however, to distinguish reactive thrombocytosis from essential thrombocytosis simply on the basis of platelet number. Anemia is uncommon and usually mild and an elevated hemoglobin or hematocrit level should suggest the presence of polycythemia vera. A mild neutrophilic leukocytosis is common but when the leukocyte count is greater than 15,000/μl or there is a leukoery-throblastic reaction, another diagnosis should be considered. Many patients are iron deficient but paradoxically correction of the deficit usually does not influence the platelet count. Pseudohyperkalemia occurs as a consequence of platelet potassium release during blood clotting when the platelet count is elevated. A very high-platelet count can also cause pseudohypoglycemia and hypoxemia if blood for glucose and oxygen tension measurements is not collected on ice and in the presence of a metabolic inhibitor. It is of interest that the serum erythropoietin level can be low in essential thrombocytosis, making this test not useful for distinguishing between polycythemia vera and essential thrombocytosis.

Coagulation abnormalities in essential thrombocytosis are a consequence of intrinsic platelet abnormalities or the platelet count (1). Abnormalities of platelet structure include an increase in mean platelet volume and distribution width, loss of alpha granules and dense bodies, and disorganization of the platelet microtubular and canalicular systems. Surface expression of CD41 and the thrombopoietin receptor, Mpl, are decreased, while the expression of P-selectin and thrombospondin are increased; intracellularly, ADP, PF4, and 5-HT content is reduced. The majority of patients have increased platelet aggregation in response to epinephrine, ristocetin, ADP, and collagen. Paradoxically, however, the bleeding time is increased in less than 20 % of patients. Thromboxane excretion is frequently increased and suppressible by salicylate therapy, suggesting continuous intravascular platelet activation. However, there is no correlation between the platelet abnormalities and thrombosis in this disorder.

Acquired von Willebrand's disease is an interesting feature of essential thrombocytosis as well as the other chronic myeloproliferative disorders (2). As the platelet count increases, generally above 1,000,000/μl, the platelets adsorb and destroy the largest molecular weight plasma von Willebrand multimers, leading to a reduction in ristocetin cofactor activity. Patients with this abnormality are at risk of bleeding, particularly if exposed to salicylates.

CYTOGENETIC ABNORMALITIES

Cytogenetic abnormalities are uncommon in essential thrombocytosis and none is pathognomonic for the disorder. The common cytogenetic abnormalities include trisomy 1, 8, 9, and 21, 1q-, 13q-, and 20q- (3). Since chronic myelogenous leukemia and the 5q- syndrome can present with thrombocytosis, cytogenetic analysis constitutes an important part of the diagnostic evaluation.

DIAGNOSIS

Establishing a diagnosis of essential thrombocytosis is more difficult than for the other chronic myeloproliferative disorders because so-called essential thrombocytosis lacks any unique identifying characteristics or a specific diagnostic marker and because thrombocytosis can be the initial manifestation of polycythemia vera or idiopathic myelofibrosis, either of which may not become clinically apparent for many years after the onset of the thrombocytosis (4, 5). Furthermore, there is as yet no agreement as to what platelet count threshold should be used for the diagnosis of essential thrombocytosis. A number of diagnostic criteria have been developed, but they rely on the exclusion of other disorders and their complexity emphasizes the difficulties inherent in the diagnostic process for this disease. The extent of the problem can be simply visualized from the number of benign and malignant disorders that can cause thrombocytosis (Table 35-2). Furthermore, it is apparent from epidemiologic studies of JAK2 V617F expression, platelet Mpl expression, and clonality that there is substantial heterogeneity among essential thrombocytosis patients with respect to these abnormalities and, except for lack of JAK2 V617F homozygosity, no specificity.

Table 35-2

Causes of Thrombocytosis

Tissue inflammation
  Collagen vascular disease, inflammatory bowel disease
Malignancy
Infection
Myeloproliferative disorders
  Polycythemia vera, idiopathic myelofibrosis, essential
  thrombocytosis, chronic myelogenous leukemia
Myelodysplastic disorders
  5q- syndrome, idiopathic refractory sideroblastic anemia
Postsplenectomy, or hyposplenism
Hemorrhage
Iron deficiency anemia
Surgery
Rebound
  Correction of vitamin B12 or folate deficiency, post ethanol abuse
Hemolysis
Familial
  Thrombopoietin overproduction, constitutive Mpl activation

From a prognostic prospective, the most serious illnesses associated with thrombocytosis that need to be excluded are chronic myelogenous leukemia, myelodysplasia (5q- syndrome), sideroblastic anemia, idiopathic myelofibrosis, and polycythemia vera. It also needs to be emphasized that chronic myelogenous leukemia can present with isolated thrombocytosis alone in the absence of leukocytosis or basophilia. From this perspective, a bone marrow aspirate and biopsy for morphology, flow cytometry, cytogenetics, and peripheral blood FISH for bcr-abl, since this can be present in the absence of the Philadelphia chromosome, are the essential diagnostic tests. The leukocyte alkaline phosphatase can be normal or high. A negative assay for JAK2 V617F does not exclude the diagnosis of essential thrombocytosis nor does its presence have any implications with respect to the clinical course.

NATURAL HISTORY

Most but not all studies of essential thrombocytosis have found that life span was not significantly different from the general population. Differences with respect to longevity reflect in part lack of a uniform means for diagnosis, lack of clinically validated forms of therapy, the use of myelotoxic drugs, and biologic heterogeneity in the patient populations studied. Risk factors for thrombosis in essential thrombocytosis include age $\geq$ 60 years, prior thrombosis, presence of other causes for thrombophilia, and leukocytosis (15,000/μl), while risk factors for survival included age $\geq$ 60 years, leukocytosis, tobacco use, and diabetes.

The major risk factor for hemorrhage was a platelet count of 1,500,000/μl or greater. Transformation to myelofibrosis or polycythemia vera occurs in approximately 10% of patients over the first decade after diagnosis (4, 5). Spontaneous leukemic transformation occurs but is uncommon and the vast majority are a consequence of exposure to myelotoxic drugs.

TREATMENT

The first rule of therapy for essential thrombocytosis is accuracy in diagnosis, particularly because life span is generally not reduced in this disease and its treatment differs from the other chronic myeloproliferative diseases that it mimics.

The second rule of therapy is to do no harm. Stated differently, the treatment cannot be worse than the disease. Unfortunately, most prior studies of essential thrombocytosis have violated these rules, making it difficult to use an evidence-based approach to formulate therapeutic options. Thrombosis, either macrovascular or microvascular, is the major impediment to health in essential thrombocytosis but there is no correlation between the height of the platelet count and thrombosis, rendering problematic the formulation of a treatment endpoint on that basis. In general, patients with essential thrombocytosis who have had a prior major vessel thrombosis should be treated no differently with respect to anticoagulation and risk factor reduction than their counterparts with a normal platelet count. The most difficult decision then becomes how to manage the platelet count (6).

Patients with essential thrombocytosis under age 60 years, who have no cardiovascular risk factors or a prior thrombosis, are not at a greater risk of thrombosis than their age-matched counterparts with a normal platelet count (7). Treatment in these patients should be directed at the alleviation of microvascular symptoms such as ocular migraine or erythromelalgia. Aspirin is a specific remedy for these and can be given daily or on as needed basis. Ibuprofen can be substituted if a shorter acting agent is required. When the platelet count is greater than 1,000,000/μl, ristocetin cofactor activity should be measured before using either agent in a symptomatic patient and, if reduced, platelet count reduction rather than platelet inactivation is a safer approach. In some patients, particularly those with migraine, platelet inactivation may not be sufficient to control symptoms. The safest method to lower the platelet count then becomes the major issue.

Current therapy for controlling the platelet count includes hydroxyurea, anagrelide, interferon alpha, alkylating agents, and ^{32}P. All of these agents are usually effective but each has distinct disadvantages. The most serious of these is myelotoxicity leading to acute leukemia, which has been demonstrated unequivocally for the alkylating agents and ^{32}P. Whether hydroxyurea is leukemogenic has been a matter of debate. Hydroxyurea is unequivocally a tumor promoter. It also enhances the leukemogenic effect of the alkylating agents and ^{32}P whether given before or after them. Since the use of chemotherapeutic agents has not been shown to improve longevity in the chronic myeloproliferative disorders, their use should be restricted to situations where other forms of therapy have been ineffective.

Two randomized clinical trials provide some guidance to this end. In a study of essential thrombocytosis patients older than 60 years, hydroxyurea was not more effective than aspirin in preventing arterial thrombosis (8). In a much larger study of high-risk patients with thrombocytosis taking aspirin, in whom the platelet count was normalized, hydroxyurea was not more effective than anagrelide in preventing arterial thrombosis and was actually less effective in preventing venous thrombosis. Hydroxyurea was, however, more effective in preventing transient ischemic attacks (9). Therefore, in patients over age 60 years who have risk factors for thrombosis and who are experiencing transient ischemic attacks, hydroxyurea is the drug of choice. Otherwise, a safer alternative such as interferon alpha or anagrelide should be used when there is a clinical indication to lower the platelet count. In the case of interferon, given the side effects associated with long-term use, its use should be intermittent if possible. The recent claim that anagrelide causes myelofibrosis was not supported by any data but the drug does have inotropic effects and can cause anemia and fluid retention (10). If long-term use is planned, periodic cardiac monitoring is also indicated. Finally, the combination of aspirin and anagrelide has been associated with an increased incidence of gastrointestinal hemorrhage (9).

Acquired von Willebrand syndrome caused by thrombocytosis requires no treatment unless there is a need for surgery or the patient experiences spontaneous bleeding (2). In this instance, platelet count reduction will be required. In an emergent situation, plateletpheresis can be employed but this is not a particularly efficient approach when there is extreme thrombocytosis. Administration of epsilon aminocaproic acid is an effective remedy for bleeding in this situation.

PREGNANCY

Special mention needs to be made about pregnancy since essential thrombosis is so common in young women. Pregnancy has an ameliorating effect on the thrombocytosis in this disorder and, while first trimester abortions were increased, there was no correlation between platelet count and obstetrical complications. No specific therapeutic intervention has been proved to be uniformly effective but low-dose aspirin has been recommended as prophylactic therapy and, when there has been prior thrombosis, low molecular weight heparin. Interferon alpha can also be given safely during pregnancy if platelet count reduction is desired. Perhaps the most important recommendation is to be sure that patient does not actually have polycythemia vera. Stated differently, a normal hematocrit in a pregnant woman with essential thrombocytosis should suggest the presence of polycythemia vera.

REFERENCES

1. Wehmeier A, Sudhoff T, Meierkord F. Relation of platelet abnormalities to thrombosis and hemorrhage in chronic myeloproliferative disorders. Semin Thromb Hemost. 1997; 23: 391–402.
2. Michiels JJ, Budde U, van der PM, et al. Acquired von Willebrand syndromes: clinical features, aetiology, pathophysiology, classification and management. Best Pract Res Clin Haematol. 2001; 14: 401–436.
3. Steensma DP, Tefferi A. Cytogenetic and molecular genetic aspects of essential thrombocythemia. Acta Haematol. 2002; 108: 55–65.
4. Jantunen R, Juvonen E, Ikkala E, et al. Development of erythrocytosis in the course of essential thrombocythemia. Ann Hematol. 1999; 78: 219–222.
5. Cervantes F, Alvarez-Larran A, Talarn C, Gomez M, Montserrat E. Myelofibrosis with myeloid metaplasia following essential thrombocythaemia: actuarial probability, presenting characteristics and evolution in a series of 195 patients. Br J Haematol. 2002; 118: 786–790.
6. Schafer AI. Thrombocytosis. N Engl J Med. 2004; 350: 1211–1219.
7. Ruggeri M, Finazzi G, Tosetto A, et al. No treatment for low-risk thrombocythaemia: results from a prospective study. Br J Haematol. 1998; 103: 772–777.
8. Cortelazzo S, Finazzi G, Ruggeri M, et al. Hydroxyurea for patients with essential thrombocythemia and a high risk of thrombosis. N Engl J Med. 1995; 332: 1132–1136.
9. Harrison CN, Campbell PJ, Buck G, et al. Hydroxyurea compared with anagrelide in high-risk essential thrombocythemia. N Engl J Med. 2005; 33: 353: 33–45.
10. Wagstaff AJ, Keating GM. Anagrelide: a review of its use in the management of essential thrombocythaemia. Drugs. 2006; 66: 111–131.
11. Steurer M, Gastl G, Jedrzejczak W-W, et al. Anagrelide for thrombcytosis in myeloprliferative disorders. A prospective study to assess efficacy and adverse event profile. Cancer 2004; 101: 2239–2246.

36	Yi-Bin Chen

HIGH-DOSE CHEMOTHERAPY

HIGH-DOSE CHEMOTHERAPY

High-dose chemotherapy (HDC) followed by either autologous or allogeneic hematopoietic stem cell transplant has become an important modality of treatment for many malignancies. It is used both in the realm of consolidation therapy when disease is minimal and as a strategy of salvage therapy for refractory or relapsed disease. While initially thought of as an emerging therapy for both hematological and solid tumors, results of large clinical trials have shown HDC to be of no overall long-term benefit for the vast majority of solid tumors, most likely due to their inherent relatively low sensitivity to chemotherapy. Thus, the current use of HDC is mainly restricted to hematological malignancies and life-threatening benign bone marrow disorders with the exceptions of relapsed or refractory germ cell tumors and childhood neuroblastoma.

The rationale for HDC derives from the experimental observation that there is a linear relationship between drug dose and cell kill for alkylating agents in experimental therapy of murine leukemias. Several traditional chemotherapeutic regimens have been used in various high-dose combinations with or without total body irradiation (TBI). Examples are shown in Table 36-1. Each agent at

Table 36-1

Common High-Dose Chemotherapy (HDC) Regimens

Busulfan / cytoxan (BuCy2)
- Busulfan 0.8 mg/kg IV q6h on days –7, –6, –5, –4
- Cyclophosphamide 1,800 mg/m^2 IVB on days –3, –2

Cytoxan / TBI
- Cyclophosphamide 1,800 mg/m^2 IVB on days –5, –4
- TBI on days –3, –2, –1, –0

CBV
- Cyclophosphamide 750 mg/m^2 q12h on days –6, –5, –4, –3
- BCNU 112.5 mg/m^2 QD on days –6, –5, –4, –3
- Etoposide 200 mg/m^2 IV BID on days –6, –5, –4, –3
- MESNA 750 mg/m^2 IVCI Q24H on days –6, –5, –4, –3, –2

BEAM
- BCNU 300 mg/m^2 IV on day –8
- Etoposide 200 mg/m^2 IV on days –7, –6, –5, –4
- Cytarabine 200 mg/m^2 IV q12h on days –7, –6, –5, –4
- Melphalan 140 mg/m^2 on day –3

Melphalan
- Melphalan 140–240 mg/m^2 × 1 or divided over 2–5 days

such high doses brings its own pharmacokinetic and pharmacodymanic profile along with specific toxicities. Therapy based on pharmacokinetic targets such as AUC (area under the curve), C_{max}, or other parameters has been difficult to apply to the majority of antineoplastic therapies including HDC due to several obstacles, including the lack of reproducible assays with rapid turnaround times, undefined target concentrations for most agents, and very little knowledge about the activity and potential contribution of metabolites (1). However, treatment may eventually shift toward such an approach given the narrow therapeutic window for most chemotherapeutic agents, the high potential for various drug–drug interactions, the known interpatient variability, and the potential to improve patient outcomes while decreasing overall morbidity. For now, the majority of drugs are still dosed based on the crude index of body surface area (BSA) without corrections for individual pharmacokinetic differences.

The rationale for HDC differs depending on the specific indication and on whether autologous or allogeneic stem cells are used for hematological rescue. In the autologous setting, the sole goal is to effect as much tumor cytoreduction as possible, and, thus, the agents used are commonly the ones most effective against the specific malignancy being treated. In the allogeneic setting, the goals include delivering maximal antitumor activity, but also achieving myeloablation and immunosuppression to allow donor cells to engraft. The benefits of allogeneic therapy extend beyond the intrinsic cytotoxic activity of the conditioning regimen and include an immunological graft-versus-tumor effect mounted by the allogeneic immune cells. Recently, in efforts to extend allogeneic therapy to more patients, conditioning regimens have been scaled down to reduce the toxicity and maximize the graft-versus-tumor effect. These so-called reduced intensity or nonmyeloablative conditioning regimens remain experimental and will not be discussed further here (2). The morbidity and mortality of HDC are not trivial with commonly quoted early transplant-related mortality rates of 1–3% for autologous protocols and up to 20% for allogeneic transplants.

Several classes of chemotherapeutic drugs are commonly used in HDC combination regimens, and this chapter focuses on the specific characteristics and toxicities of these agents in HDC regimens (see Table 36-2). The general mechanisms, pharmacokinetics, and toxicities of conventional doses of these agents are discussed in other chapters. Traditionally, HDC combinations were designed to consist of agents with nonoverlapping toxicities to allow the use of each of the individual agents in full doses. There have been very few prospective randomized trials comparing different regimens in a head-to-head manner, and,

Table 36-2

Common Agents in HDC Regimens with Pharmacokinetics, Mechanism of Clearance, and Toxicities

Drug	Clearance	PKs: elimination Half-life*	Specific toxicities
Cyclophosphamide	Hepatic	Nonlinear 4–8 h	GU, cardiac, VOD
Ifosfamide	Hepatic	Nonlinear 11–15 h	CNS, GU, VOD
Busulfan	Hepatic	Linear 1–7 h	VOD, CNS, lung
Melphalan	Hydrolysis	Linear 1–2 h	Mucositis
BCNU	Hepatic	Linear 30–45 min	VOD, pulmonary, renal
Carboplatin	Renal	Linear 1–4 h	Renal, ototoxicity, neuropathy
Etoposide	Hepatic / renal	Linear 4–15 h	Mucositis, diarrhea

* Linear: drug concentration in plasma is linearly correlated with dose.

thus, standard regimens differ from center to center. The most commonly used agents include alkylating agents (cyclophosphamide, ifosfamide, busulfan, melphalan, carmustine (BCNU)), carboplatin, and etoposide. Other agents used previously such as taxanes or thiotepa will not be discussed here as they were reserved mainly for patients with solid tumors, for which HDC is no longer thought to be of significant benefit. In addition, cytarabine is used in some regimens (i.e., BEAM), but the doses are similar to standard doses used in leukemia therapy.

ALKLYLATING AGENTS

Cyclophosphamide is a classic alklyating agent which is widely used in combination regimens of HDC. Non-HDC conventional doses are less than 1,000 mg/m^2, while doses in HDC regimens range from 4,000 to 7,200 mg/m^2. Cyclophosphamide is a pro-drug which undergoes bioactivation via hepatic P450 enzymatic processes to a variety of active and inactive metabolites. At HDC doses, clearance of both parent drug and the active intermediates, aldophosphamide and phosphoramide mustard, depends not only on renal clearance, but also on hepatic microsomal metabolism and other enzymatic and chemical detoxifying interactions. Elimination at such doses is nonlinear with a half-life ranging anywhere from 3 to 9 h. Strategies based on pharmacokinetic targets have been difficult to develop partly because it is unclear whether PK parameters of parent cyclophosphamide correlate with the PK of the active metabolites responsible for the actual cytotoxic and toxic effects. Assays for these metabolites, which include 4-hydroxycyclophosphamide (4-HC) and aldophosphamide, have been limited in the past by the instability of these intermediates (1).

While noted for its relative sparing of oral or GI mucosa, cyclophosphamide at doses used in HDC regimens has major organ toxicities including hemorrhagic cystitis, acute cardiotoxicity, and, in combination with other alklyating agents or TBI, hepatic veno-occlusive disease (VOD). Hemorrhagic cystitis is mediated by a toxic metabolite, acrolein, and can be prevented by vigorous IV hydration and coadministration of equimolar doses of 2-mercaptoethanesulfonate (MESNA) which conjugates acrolein in the urine. Acute cardiotoxicity, while rare and usually reversible, can be life threatening, and occurs in the form of a hemorrhagic myopericarditis that develops within the first 7–10 days after administration. Monitoring of symptoms, auscultatory findings (diminished hearts sounds, new friction rub), and electrocardiograms (diffuse loss of voltage) is essential. Hepatic VOD is seen when combining cyclophosphamide with busulfan or TBI, and separate pharmacokinetic measurements of certain cyclophosphamide metabolites (specifically, o-carboxyethyl-phosphoramide mustard) have actually shown a correlation with hepatic injury (3). VOD is discussed below. Ifosfamide, very similar in structure to cyclophosphamide, is also activated by hepatic metabolism, and shares many systemic toxicities. Acrolein is one of its metabolites and, thus, MESNA is administered to prevent renal injury and hemorrhagic cystitis. Unique to ifosfamide is its neurotoxicicty which is thought to be due to accumulation of the metabolite chloracetaldehyde. The primary manifestation is acute encephalopathy with altered mental status which usually resolves spontaneously within a few days. Other reported effects have included generalized seizures and cerebellar ataxia.

The primary advantage of busulfan in HDC regimens is its marked myeloablative effect and lesser GI toxicity. It is most commonly combined with cyclophosphamide, but has also been used in combination with TBI or etoposide. Busulfan is metabolized to inactive compounds in the liver, and has a linear elimination with a half-life of 2–3 h. Until relatively recently, busulfan was only available in an oral form, leading to significant inter- and intrapatient pharmacokinetic variability in high dose Therapy. With IV busulfan now available, intrapatient variability has virtually been eliminated, but interpatient variation remains. IV busulfan is cleared from plasma in a manner consistent with a single-compartment first-order elimination, and assays to allow rapid and accurate AUC determination are being developed for potential PK-directed dosing (1). Moreover, toxicity and therapeutic outcomes correlate with total drug exposure as measured by area under the curve of concentration (AUC) $\times$ time (4). Indeed, the risks of developing hepatic VOD, the most serious consequence of busulfan therapy, and mucositis, both increase with increasing AUC measurements (5). At HDC doses, busulfan can also cause generalized seizures, and, thus, routine prophylaxis with phenytoin is usually recommended during administration. In addition, busulfan can cause chronic pulmonary fibrosis. Symptoms include cough and dyspnea. Pulmonary function tests reveal a restrictive picture, and standard treatment is with corticosteroids.

Melphalan is given at doses of 180–200 mg/m^2 as part of HDC regimens (compared to approximately 30 mg/m^2 in conventional doses). Most commonly, it is used with autologous rescue as consolidation therapy for patients with multiple myeloma. It does not require metabolic activation, undergoes spontaneous hydrolysis in the plasma, and 15% of the intact drug is excreted in the urine. Melphalan PK remains linear in the dose ranges used for HDC and its distribution fits a two-compartment model with a half-life of 45–60 min (1). Caution is exercised when patients have significant renal insufficiency as the effect of decreased renal function on PK and toxicity has not been well studied. At these doses, melphalan causes significant mucositis.

The nitrosurea carmustine (BCNU) has a similar mechanism to alkylating agents, but is not thought to be cross-reactive in regard to tumor resistance. Its adduct with DNA is repaired by guanine alkyl transferase, which also repairs busulfan methylation of DNA. The DNA adducts formed by classical alkylating agents are repaired by the nucleotide excision repair process, while BCNU-induced DNA cross-links and those of other cross-linking alkylators are reversed by the more complex process of homologous recombination. It is eliminated via hydrolysis and hepatic inactivation with a clearance that is linear with dose. It has a half-life of 30–45 min. BCNU is incorporated into HDC regimens because of its predominant myelotoxicity at conventional doses and is most commonly used in the BEAM and CBV regimens (see Table 36-1) for non-Hodgkin's and Hodgkin's lymphomas. Additional toxicities of BCNU when given as HDC are idiopathic pneumonia syndrome (see below), renal failure secondary to interstitial nephritis, and hepatic VOD (see below).

PLATINUM ANALOGS

Carboplatin has been included in HDC regimens, because unlike cisplatin, dose escalation of carboplatin results in significant myelosuppression without severe nephrotoxicity and ototoxicity. The combination of carboplatin with etoposide is a common choice of HDC for relapsed or refractory germ cell tumors given their inherent sensitivity to these agents. Much like with conventional use, high-dose carboplatin illustrates the successful application of a pharmacokinetically directed therapy, as dosing is based on the calculation of the patient's creatinine clearance (CrCl). At high doses, high dose carboplatin exhibits a linear elimination with a half-life of 60–200 min. Even though less harmful than cisplatin, monitoring of renal function as well as ototoxicity and neuropathy remains essential to supportive care.

TOPOISOMERASE II INHIBITORS(CONTINUE)

Etoposide is a podophyllotoxin derivative whose primary mechanism of action is topoisomerase II inhibition. It undergoes both hepatic metabolism and urinary excretion and has a half-life of 4–15 h. Its main uses in HDC regimens at a dose range of 750–2400 mg/m^2 are for non-Hodgkin's lymphoma and germ cell tumors. Severe mucositis and diarrhea are its main toxicities at such high doses.

TOXICITIES COMMON TO DRUG CLASS

In addition to drug-specific toxicities as discussed above, there are certain general toxicities of HDC. These include immunodeficiency, infertility, oral mucositis, hepatic VOD, pulmonary complications, and secondary hematological malignancies.

Relative immunodeficiency is a sustained condition and lasts well beyond neutrophil engraftment. After HDC and autologous transplant, the length of clinically significant immunodeficiency is likely 3–6 months, and patient activities and exposures are restricted during this time for fear of infection. This period is significantly longer after allogeneic protocols given the need for immunosuppressive medications and the common occurrence of graft-versus-host disease (GVHD). Some centers will restrict patient activities for up to 1 year or more after allogeneic transplantation. Specific infectious complications are beyond the scope of this chapter, but are a significant source of morbidity and mortality especially after allogeneic transplantation.

Infertility for both male and female patients is a virtual certainty after HDC protocols with a few exceptions. Current recommendations include routine sperm banking for males and embryo preservation for females. Unfortunately, unfertilized ova cryopreservation is not possible at this time.

Oral mucositis is a significant cause of morbidity in up to 75% of patients undergoing HDC. While self-limited in course, mucositis is one of the most bothersome complaints of patients after HDC. Besides causing severe discomfort, mucositis also prolongs hospital stays and predisposes patients to systemic infection. In addition, there are rare cases of significant mucosal edema leading to airway compromise requiring intubation. Injury to the oral mucosa from HDC regimens results from two major events: direct mucosal basal cell injury leading to atrophy and ulcerations, and the effect of opportunistic local infection which is exacerbated during the prolonged period of neutropenia (6). Pretherapy periodontal disease, TBI, HDC regimens containing high-dose melphalan or etoposide, and allogeneic protocols seem to predict for worse disease.

Symptoms of oral mucositis usually begin around 3–10 days after HDC and can range from mild soreness and burning to severe erosive mucositis requiring narcotics for pain control. Total parenteral nutrition (TPN) may be necessary to sustain nutrition. Local infections, most commonly candidiasis and HSV, should be treated, and care should be taken to monitor for dissemination of secondary fungal or bacterial infections. In addition, thrombocytopenia can exacerbate oral bleeding from ulcerative lesions, oftentimes requiring higher platelet transfusion goals. Physical findings of oral mucositis progress from soft tissue erythema to focal white desquamative patches and eventually to frank ulcerations with pseudomembranes. The National Cancer Institute (NCI) has standardized a grading scale from 1 to 4 which is commonly used (see Table 36-3) to convey severity. Recommendations for reducing the severity of mucositis include a thorough oral hygiene exam prior to HDC and the use of oral nonalcohol antiseptic rinses. Recently, keratinocyte growth factor (KGF or Kepivance), which is known to stimulate growth of resting epidermal keratinocytes, was tested in a randomized placebo-controlled trial of patients undergoing HDC followed by autologous stem cell rescue. Given for 3 days prior to conditioning (HDC + TBI), KGF was shown to reduce the incidence of severe mucositis, the duration of symptoms, the use of opioid analgesics, and the use of TPN (7). Treatment of established oral mucositis is mainly supportive with good oral hygiene, pain control (with both local analgesic

Table 36-3

Mucositis Grading (NCI, 2003)

Grade	Clinical exam	Functional or symptomatic
1	Erythema of mucosa	Minimal symptoms; normal diet
2	Patchy ulcerations or pseudomembranes	Symptomatic but can eat and swallow modified diet
3	Confluent ulcerations or pseudomembranes; bleeding with minor trauma	Symptomatic and unable to adequately aliment and hydrate orally
4	Tissue necrosis; significant spontaneous bleeding; life-threatening consequences	Symptoms associated with life-threatening consequences

mouthwashes and systemic narcotics), careful monitoring for infection, and daily assessments of proper nutritional intake. Symptoms usually last for 7–10 days with resolution occurring around the time of neutrophil recovery.

Hepatic VOD contributes significantly to treatment-related morbidity and mortality associated with HDC. It is characterized by the clinical constellation of weight gain, right upper quadrant pain, hepatomegaly, jaundice, and ascites. VOD has a spectrum of severity from very mild disease to fulminant hepatic failure, and usually occurs within the first 30 days after transplantation. Its incidence is difficult to estimate (anywhere from 5 to 50%) given the range of presentations and the heterogeneity of protocols used; however, about 25–30% of cases are thought to be severe and life threatening (8). Risk factors are thought to include preexisting liver disease, a history of abdominal radiation, allogeneic transplantation, and inclusion in the conditioning regimen of certain agents such as cyclophosphamide, busulfan, and BCNU. The pathophysiology of VOD is rooted in the occlusion of hepatic venules, and, thus, has a clinical presentation quite similar to the Budd–Chiari syndrome. The initial step in VOD is thought to be injury to the hepatic venous endothelium stimulating a local hypercoagulable state followed by focal deposition of fibrinogen and factor VIII leading to progressive occlusion and further injury. The diagnosis is often made clinically, but needs to be distinguished from other processes including hepatic GVHD, viral infection, cholestasis from sepsis, and drug toxicity. Treatment of VOD is difficult. IV heparin and alteplase (tPA) have been attempted with some success but also pose significant risk of major hemorrhage. Recently, the synthetic polydexoyribonucelotide, defibrotide, which has multiple ani-thrombotic and thrombolytic actions has been used with promising success (9). Many centers have also begun to use prophylaxis with either low-dose heparin or ursodeoxycholic acid (ursodiol) as preliminary evidence has suggested a benefit (10).

Two types of pulmonary complications after HDC warrant mention: diffuse alveolar hemorrhage (DAH) and the idiopathic pneumonia syndrome (IPS). DAH tends to occur within the first 30 days after transplant. Risk factors are older age, preexisting renal insufficiency, and thoracic radiation. Different case series report the incidence anywhere between 2 and 14%. Among all HDC patients admitted to the ICU for respiratory failure, approximately 40% have DAH (11). The clinical presentation of DAH includes the acute onset of dyspnea, hypoxia, and cough. Frank hemoptysis is the exception, and occurs in only about 10–15% of patients. The pathophysiology is unclear, but DAH usually occurs around the time of engraftment, and is thought to represent a syndrome of capillary leak with hemorrhage aggravated by concomitant thrombocytopenia. Diagnosis is confirmed by ruling out infection and repeated bronchoalveolar lavage revealing increasingly hemorrhagic results. Treatment is usually with high-dose IV corticosteroids, although prospective data are lacking. If patients proceed to respiratory failure requiring mechanical ventilation, which many will need, the mortality rate is as high as 80% (11).

IPS usually develops weeks after engraftment, but within the first 100 days after transplant. It has been defined as "evidence of widespread alveolar injury in the absence of active lower respiratory tract infection after BMT" (12). Its incidence is estimated to be about 10–20% after allogeneic transplant, and lower after autologous therapies. The pathophysiology of IPS is unclear, as it is most likely a heterogeneous group of disorders which result in similar clinical manifestations and pathological findings of interstitial pneumonitis and diffuse alveolar damage. Injury from HDC is certainly thought to play a crucial role as evidenced by the much lower incidence reported for nonmyeloablative conditioning regimens (13). Treatment of IPS is usually with high-dose IV corticosteroids, but the prognosis has historically been poor. Recently, promising results have been shown with etanercept, a synthetic fusion protein designed to inhibit tumor necrosis factor, but confirmatory trials are needed (14).

Development of secondary myelodysplastic syndrome (MDS) or acute myelogenous leukemia (AML) is a feared complication of chemotherapy. There is a general consensus that HDC regimens with or without TBI significantly increase this risk, although studies have suggested, that in some situations, the abnormal clones are present even prior to receiving HDC (15). Given the differences in regimens used and the significant treatment histories of most patients prior to HDC, estimations of this risk are difficult to quantify. Alkylating agents and topoisomerase II inhibitors are thought to be the most likely culprits. Alklyating agent induced disease usually has a latency period of 5–7 years with characteristic cytogenetic changes of partial or complete loss of chromosomes 5 and/or 7. Invariably, the prognosis for these patients is poor. Topoisomerase II inhibitors, such as etoposide, cause a disease with a shorter latency period of only around 1–3 years. These patients generally have a better chance of achieving remission than alkylator-induced MDS/AML, and have characteristic rearrangments involving the MLL gene at 11q23 (16). In addition, it has also been recently reported that topoisomerase II inhibitors can lead to acute promyelocytic leukemia (APML) with the characteristic t(15;17) rearrangement, and these patients appear to have a prognosis that is similar to those with de novo disease (17).

In conclusion, HDC followed by autologous or allogeneic hematopoietic stem cell rescue continues to be an important form of therapy for many hematological malignancies with rare applications for solid tumors as well. As practitioners have recognized the interpatient variability in pharmacokinetics of each of these agents and the significant toxicity of using these cytotoxic drugs at such escalated doses, there has been a movement toward more pharmacokinetically directed dosing. Although dosing of the vast majority of drugs is still adjusted according to BSA, with better understanding and more standardized assays, this may soon change. HDC has unique toxicities, some of which are specific to the agents used, and others of which are generalized to the class of drugs. It is important for the prescribing practitioner to understand these toxicities in order to provide the optimal supportive care through the immediate transplant period and thereafter.

REFERENCES

1. Nieto Y, Vaughan WP. Pharmacokinetics of high-dose chemotherapy. Bone Marrow Transplant. 2004; 33: 259–269.
2. Satwani P, Harrison L, Morris E, et al. Reduced-intensity allogeneic stem cell transplantation in adults and children with malignant and nonmalignant diseases: end of the beginning and future challenges. Biol Blood Marrow Transplant. 2005; 11: 403–422.
3. McDonald, GB, Slattery JT, Bouvier ME. Cyclophosphamide metabolism, liver toxicity, and mortality following hematopoietic stem cell transplantation. Blood. 2003; 101: 2043–2048.
4. Andersson BS, Thail PF, Madden T. Busulfan systemic exposure relative to regimen-related toxicity and acute graft-versus-hose disease: defining a therapeutic window for IV BuCy2 in chronic myelogenous leukemia. Biol Blood Marrow Transplant. 2002; 8: 477–485.
5. Dix SP, Wingard JR, Mullins RE. Association of busulfan area under the curve with veno-occlusive disease following BMT. Bone Marrow Transplant. 1996; 17: 225–230.
6. Stiff P. Mucositis associated with stem cell transplantation: current status and innovative approaches to management. Bone Marrow Transplant. 2001; 27(S2): S3–S11.
7. Spielberger R, Stiff P, Bensinger W. Palifermin for oral mucositis after intensive therapy for hematologic cancers. N Engl J Med. 2004; 351: 2590–2598.
8. Bearman SI. Avoiding hepatic veno-occlusive disease: what do we know and where are we going? Bone Marrow Transplant. 2001; 27: 1113–1120.
9. Richardson PG, Murakami C, Jin Z. Multi-institutional use of defibrotide in 88 patients after stem cell transplantation with severe veno-occlusive disease and multisystem organ failure: response without significant toxicity in a high-risk population and factors predictive of outcome. Blood. 2002; 100: 4337–4343.
10. Essel JH, Schroeder MT, Harman GS. Ursodiol prophylaxis against hepatic complications of allogeneic bone marrow transplantation. A randomized, double blind, placebo-controlled trial. Annal Intern Med. 1998; 128: 285–291.
11. Afessa B, Tefferi A, Litzow MR. Diffuse alveolar hemorrhage in hematopoietic stem cell transplant recipients. Am J Respir Crit Care Med. 2002; 166: 641–645.
12. Yen KT, Lee AS, Krowka MJ. Pulmonary complications in bone marrow transplantation: a practical approach to diagnosis and treatment. Clin Chest Med. 2004; 25: 189–201.
13. Fukuda T, Hackman RC, Guthrie KA. Risks and outcomes of idiopathic pneumonia syndrome after nonmyeloablative and conventional conditioning regimens for allogeneic hematopoeitic stem cell transplantation. Blood. 2003; 102: 2777–2785.
14. Yanik G, Hellerstedt B, Custer J. Etanercept (Enbrel) administration for idiopathic pneumonia syndrome after allogeneic hematopoietic stem cell transplantation. Biol Blood Bone Marrow Transplant. 2002; 8: 395–400.
15. Lillington DM, Micallef IN, Carpenter E. Detection of chromosome abnormalities pre-high-dose treatment in patients developing therapy-related myelodysplasia and secondary acute myelogenous leukemia after treatment for non-Hodgkin's lymphoma. J Clin Oncol. 2001; 19: 2472–2481.
16. Libura J, Slater DJ, Felix CA. Therapy-related acute myeloid leukemia-like MLL rearrangements are induced by etoposide in primary human CD34+ cells and remain stable after clonal expansion. Blood. 2005; 105: 2124–2131.
17. Beaumont M, Sanz M, Carli PM. Therapy related acute promyelocytic leukemia. J Clin Oncol. 2003; 21: 2123–2137.

BONE MARROW TRANSPLANTATION

INTRODUCTION

Bone marrow transplantation (BMT) is a potentially curative therapy for a wide variety of life-threatening congenital and acquired hematopoietic stem cell disorders and other neoplastic diseases. With the development of human leukocyte antigen (HLA) typing to identify suitably matched donors, together with pre-clinical experience that established the requisites for conditioning therapy, GVHD prophylaxis, etc., clinical BMT became a reality. Although, much of the initial clinical BMT experience was directed toward acute leukemia and severe aplastic anemia, the demonstration of donor lymphohematopoietic reconstitution, the powerful cytoreductive effect of intensive conditioning therapy, and the observation of a potent immunologically mediated graft-versus-tumor (GVT) effect led to the application of BMT for drug resistant hematologic malignancies and many other disorders (1).

The principal functions of BMT are to provide:

1. *Rescue* (i.e., the circumvention of the myeloablative effects of the conditioning regimen by the infusion of pluripotential hematopoietic progenitor cells.)
2. *Replacement* (i.e., the replacement of a diseased hematopoietic stem cell population by healthy stem cells.)
3. *An immunological platform.* As mixed lymphohematopoietic chimerism often develops after reduced intensity preparative regimens, BMT may induce an immunological platform for adoptive cellular immunotherapy via donor lymphocyte infusions (DLI) (2).

Because of the various sources of stem cells for transplantation, hematopoietic stem cell transplantation (SCT) is now more widely used than BMT to describe the field. Diseases for which SCT, because it allows ablative, potentially curative doses of chemoradiotherapy and/or replacement of a diseased hematopoietic stem cell population with a healthy immunocompetent one, are shown in Table 37-1.

DONOR ORIGIN OF HEMATOPOIETIC STEM CELLS

- *Autologous SCT* refers to the collection and subsequent reinfusion of hematopoietic stem cells from the patient. Intensive conditioning (preparative) therapy is given in an effort to cytoreduce a malignancy or, in some cases, to provide immunoablation for a refractory autoimmune disease. Host hematopoietic stem cells are then infused to *rescue* the patient from the myeloablative effects of the preparative regimen.
- *Allogeneic SCT* refers to the transplantation of hematopoietic stem cells from an HLA matched or partially matched donor. Allogeneic SCT may occur after myeloablative or reduced intensity (nonmyeloablative) conditioning therapy. In addition to the cytoreductive effects of the preparative therapy, allogeneic SCT confers a potentially potent immunologically mediated effect of donor immune cells versus host tumor cells.
- *Syngeneic SCT* refers to transplantation of hematopoietic stem cells from an identical twin. While a GVT effect does not likely occur after syngeneic SCT, the stem cell product may have an advantage compared to an autologous stem cell product in that there are no contaminating tumor cells.

Table 37-1

Hematopoietic Stem Cell Transplantation: Selected Indications

Allogeneic: acquired	Autologous: acquired
• Hematologic malignancies	• Hematologic malignancies
AML	AML/CR
ALL	ALL/CR
CML	Multiple myeloma
Multiple myeloma	Non-Hodgkin lymphoma
Non-Hodgkin lymphoma	Hodgkin lymphoma
Hodgkin lymphoma	• Selected solid tumors
MDS	Neuroblastoma
• Nonmalignant stem cell disorders	Germ cell tumors
Aplastic anemia	• Autoimmune diseases
PNH	SLE
IMF	Scleroderma
	MS

Allogeneic: congenital

- Primary immunodeficiency diseases
- Hemoglobinopathies
  - Sickle cell anemia
  - Thalassemia major
- Metabolic diseases
  - Gaucher's disease
  - Mucopolysaccharidosis
  - X-linked adrenoleukodystrophy
  - Others
- Bone marrow failure states
  - Fanconi anemia
  - Diamond–Blackfan anemia
  - Others
- Disorders of phagocytosis
  - Osteopetrosis
  - Familial hemophagocytic lymphohistiocytosis

AML: acute myeloid leukemia; ALL: acute lymphoblastic leukemia; CML: chronic myeloid leukemia; CLL: chronic lymphocytic leukemia; MDS: myelodysplastic syndrome; PNH: paroxysmal nocturnal hemoglobinuria; IMF: idiopathic myelofibrosis; CR: complete remission; SLE: systemic lupus erythematosis; MS: multiple sclerosis.

STEM CELL SOURCES FOR ALLOGENEIC SCT

A preference is given to related donors who are HLA-identical (as determined by molecular class I and II HLA-typing) to the recipient. As each sibling inherits two haplotypes, one from each parent, there is only a 25% chance that two siblings will be genotypically identical. Therefore, alternative, HLA-nongenotypically identical donor sources have been increasingly utilized (3–5). These sources include:

- HLA phenotypically matched unrelated donors
- HLA haploidentical related donors
- Umbilical cord blood

Hematopoietic stem cells capable of restoring hematopoiesis and immune function following transplantation can be procured from:

- *Bone marrow* (following an intraoperative bone marrow harvest procedure)

- *Peripheral blood* (following "mobilization" with chemotherapy and/or recombinant hematopoietic growth factor(s)
- *Umbilical cord* (following full-term delivery)

While the exact morphologic and immunophenotypic characteristics of the pluripotential hematopoietic stem cell have not been fully defined, a number of surrogate markers for an early hematopoietic progenitor cell capable of restoring hematopoiesis following conditioning therapy have been established. CD34, a surface glycoprotein expressed on a small percentage of normal hematopoietic progenitor cells, is a useful marker of such an early progenitor population. Sustained hematologic recovery following transplantation correlates with the number of CD34+ progenitor cells infused. Following autologous SCT, for example, prompt and durable hematologic recovery occurs following the infusion of $\geq 2 \times 10^6$/kg CD34+ progenitor cells. While the transplanted umbilical cord blood CD34+ cell dose is substantially smaller (approximately one log lower) than an adult stem cell graft, similar correlates have been established between the number of infused CD34+ progenitors and the speed and durability of engraftment (6).

PREPARATIVE THERAPY FOR SCT

A strong dose–response relationship of chemoradiotherapy has been demonstrated in vitro and in preclinical animal models. A logarithmic increase in tumor cell kill has been shown after exposure of a number of tumor cell lines to alkylating agents and ionizing radiation. Based on these principles, many different preparative regimens, primarily utilizing total body irradiation (TBI) or alkylating agents, have been developed for SCT.

Reduced intensity (nonmyeloablative) preparative regimens for SCT have been increasingly utilized to avoid many of the potentially lethal complications of myeloablative conditioning. These regimens were developed after the observation that a potent GVT effect could occur after allogeneic SCT and that mixed lymphohematopoietic chimerism could be induced after highly immunosuppressive, but nonmyeloablative conditioning. These strategies have expanded the application of allogeneic SCT to older patients and patients with substantial comorbidity, who might not tolerate a fully ablative regimen.

AUTOLOGOUS SCT: INDICATIONS, RISKS, AND OUTCOMES

The principle indications for autologous SCT are chemotherapy-sensitive hematologic malignancies for which no other potentially curative therapies are available (7). Prospective randomized trials have demonstrated disease (or event) free survival and/or overall survival advantages for several hematologic malignancies including (1) recurrent chemotherapy-sensitive aggressive non-Hodgkin lymphoma, (2) recurrent chemotherapy-sensitive indolent non-Hodgkin lymphoma, (3) recurrent Hodgkin lymphoma, and (4) newly diagnosed multiple myeloma. A disease-free, but not overall, survival advantage has been demonstrated for acute myeloid leukemia (AML) in first remission. Autologous SCT may also have curative potential for patients with AML in second or subsequent remission, who are considered to be incurable with standard chemotherapy.

Autologous SCT has also been performed in patients with treatment refractory autoimmune diseases. Durable remissions have been achieved in some patients with systemic lupus erythematosus, scleroderma, multiple sclerosis, and idiopathic thrombocytopenic purpura. Prospective randomized trials are in progress to determine whether autologous SCT offers a survival benefit for patients with advanced autoimmune disease.

The risks of autologous SCT include early toxicities of chemoradiotherapy (e.g., gastrointestinal toxicities, oropharyngeal mucositis, severe pancytopenia with risk of infection, and/or hemorrhage and organ injury such as interstitial pneumonitis and hepatic veno-occlusive disease) and late toxicities (particularly secondary malignancies such as myelodysplastic syndrome or AML. Early (before day 100 post-SCT) mortality after autologous SCT is now ≤5%. Depending on the underlying disease and the conditioning regimen, late secondary hematologic malignancy risk may be as high as 5–10%. The specific patterns of toxicity and the pharmacokinetics of high-dose chemotherapy are discussed in detail in the chapter on alkylating agents.

The outcomes of autologous SCT are variable, and depend upon the underlying disease and the remission status of the disease. For example, a long-term disease-free survival probability of approximately 40% has been achieved following autologous SCT for recurrent chemotherapy-sensitive aggressive non-Hodgkin lymphoma. The primary reason for treatment failure is recurrent lymphoma (which occurs in ≥50% of transplanted patients).

ALLOGENEIC SCT: INDICATIONS, RISKS, AND OUTCOMES

Allogeneic SCT is considered for patients with diseases which can be cured by cytoreduction of the disease by the preparative regimen, replacement of a diseased hematopoietic stem cell population, and by induction of a GVT effect (8). Central to the induction of a GVT effect is graft-vs-host alloreactivity, which is induced by the exposure of donor T-cells to host minor (or major in the situation of haploidentical SCT) histocompatibility antigens. Separation of GVT from clinical GVHD is a primary goal of allogeneic SCT strategies. In some situations, the choice of either an autologous or an allogeneic SCT exists (e.g., AML in second or subsequent remission). The treatment decision is based on both patient factors (e.g., the risk for relapse of the leukemia as determined by cytogenetic status, etc., and the age and health status of the patient) and the donor availability (i.e., health status and histocompatibility).

Indications for allogeneic SCT include a variety of congenital disorders (e.g., sickle cell anemia), acquired life-threatening hematopoietic stem cell diseases (e.g., severe aplastic anemia), and a wide variety of malignant diseases involving the lymphohematopoietic compartment (e.g., acute or chronic leukemia) (see Table 37-1). In addition to cytoreduction of the disease by the preparative regimen, allogeneic SCT confers a potent immunologically mediated GVT effect, which results in a lower probability of relapse compared to an autologous SCT.

The risks of allogeneic SCT may include similar early toxicities as autologous SCT when myeloablative preparative therapy is given. In addition, there is a risk of acute GVHD, which occurs in 20–80% of patients, depending on histocompatability of the donor and recipient, and GVHD prophylaxis strategy employed, and a 50–80% risk of chronic GVHD (9). Acute GVHD is a multiorgan system disease initiated by immunocompetent T-cells in the donor graft. The primary targets of involvement of acute GVHD are the skin (rash), gastrointestinal tract (nausea, vomiting, diarrhea), and liver (jaundice, enzyme elevation). The histopathology of cutaneous and gastrointestinal GVHD, emphasizing the prominent epithelial cell injury in this disorder, are shown in Figures 37-1 and 37-2. The prognosis of GVHD is related to its stage (which is dependent upon the severity of individual organ involvement), and response to treatment. Chronic GVHD, which typically presents after day 100 post-SCT, is manifested by a wider spectrum of organ involvement. Chronic GVHD mimics many autoimmune disorders with, for

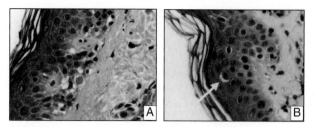

FIGURE 37-1 (a) Vacuolar epidermal changes and (b) focal epidermal keratinocytic dyskeratosis. These changes are consistent with acute graft-versus-host disease.

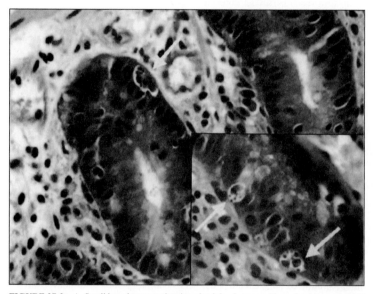

FIGURE 37-2 A. Small bowel mucosa showing glandular damage with moderate to prominent apoptotic activity consistent with grade III/IV graft-versus-host disease (inset showing another gland with prominent apoptotic bodies).

example, sclerodermatous skin changes, a Sjögren's disease-like sicca complex, esophageal dysmotility, and cholestatic hepatopathy. Patients with acute, and particularly chronic GVHD, have a lower probability of relapse of their underlying malignancy. In some hematologic malignancies, this reduction in relapse probability has translated into an overall survival advantage.

The outcomes of allogeneic SCT are also highly variable. In prospective and retrospective comparisons of autologous with allogeneic SCT for aggressive non-Hodgkin lymphoma, long-term survival probabilities are similar. Following allogeneic SCT, there is considerably higher early mortality risk (in the 20–30% range) but a substantially lower relapse probability.

Reduced intensity SCT is also associated with a potent GVT effect. For more indolent hematologic malignancies, such as chronic lymphocytic leukemia and indolent non-Hodgkin lymphoma, similar disease-free and overall survival probabilities compared to transplants in which myeloablative conditioning was used have been achieved. A GVT effect may be induced or enhanced by the

Table 37-2

Supportive Care for Stem Cell Transplantation

Issue infection	Autologous	Allogeneic
Prophylaxis	• Antibacterial (e.g., quinolone) • Antifungal (e.g., fluconazole) • Antiviral (acyclovir) • Antipneumocystis (TMP-SMX)	• Antibacterial(e.g., quinolone) • Antifungal (e.g., fluconazole) • Antiviral (acyclovir) • Antipneumocystis (TMP-SMX)
Treatment	• Broad spectrum antibiotics for febrile neutropenia • Broader antifungal coverage for persistent febrile neutropenia	• Preemptive treatment of CMV infection
GVHD		
Prophylaxis	NA	Calcineurin inhibitor: (cyclosporine or tacrolimus) + • methotrexate or • MMF or • Sirolimus versus T-cell depletion of the stem cell graft
Treatment	NA	Corticosteroids ± • polyclonal (e.g., antithymocyte globulin) or monoclonal T-cell antibodies or • TNF inhibitor • MMF or • sirolimus

TMP-SMX: trimethoprim sulfamethoxazole; GVHD: graft versus host disease; CMV: cytomegalovirus; MMF: mycophenolate mofetil; TNF: tumor necrosis factor; NA: not applicable.

administration of DLI, used to treat persistent malignancy or to convert mixed lymphohematopoietic chimerism to full donor hematopoiesis.The role of reduced intensity allogeneic SCT in most patient populations remains to be defined.

SUPPORTIVE CARE FOR SCT

Many of the advances in SCT over the past three decades have been the result of better prevention of infectious complications and prevention and treatment of GVHD. Antiinfective prophylaxis is now routinely employed. Guidelines established by the CDC/ASBMT/IDSA have included (10):

• Antifungal prophylaxis with fluconazole
• Antiviral prophylaxis with acyclovir
• Anti-Pneumocystis prophylaxis with trimethoprim sulfamethoxazole.

Newer generation broad-spectrum antibiotics and antifungal agents with reduced toxicity and a broader spectrum of coverage are available for patients with suspected or established opportunistic infections.

Cytomegalovirus (CMV), which was the chief infectious cause of mortality in the early allogeneic SCT experience, may be prevented by donor selection (CMV seronegative donors for CMV seronegative patients whenever possible), the routine monitoring for CMV infection posttransplant (by PCR or antigenemia assay), and the preemptive use of ganciclovir for patients with infection.

GVHD may be effectively prevented by ex vivo depletion of T-cells from the donor graft. T-cell depletion of a graft, however, is complicated by a higher rate of engraftment failure and a higher risk of relapse (owing to the loss of a GVT effect). An improved arsenal of immunosuppressive drugs is available for pharmacoprophylaxis of GVHD (see Table 37-2).

- Calcineurin inhibitor (cyclosporine or tacrolimus) based GVHD prophylaxis is standard
- Corticosteroid based treatment regimens are generally used for patients with established GVHD

While management of grades I–II acute GVHD is usually successful, more advanced (grades III–IV) GVHD is more difficult to manage, with mortality rates of greater than 50%.

Other important supportive care measures include red blood cell and platelet transfusional support. Blood products are irradiated to prevent transfusion associated GVHD, and third generation leukocyte reduction filters are used to prevent allosensitization, febrile nonhemolytic transfusion reactions, and CMV transmission. Total parenteral nutrition is often required because of patients' poor oral nutrition resulting from oropharyngeal mucositis and frequent nausea and vomiting.

FUTURE DIRECTION

Hematopoietic SCT has become more widely applicable in large part due to expansion of donor sources (matched unrelated donors, cord blood, etc.) which allow for transplantation of the majority of patients who do not have an HLA-identical sibling donor, and the expansion of eligibility criteria for many patients who were previously believed to be too old or too ill to have a transplant (reduced intensity conditioning, improved supportive care, etc.). Further improvement in the outcomes of SCT will depend upon (1) more effective eradication of the underlying disease (via more targeted therapies) and (2) manipulation of the cellular environment to favor a GVT effect, while avoiding the deleterious effects of GVHD. Building upon the experience in which mixed chimerism is induced as *an immunological platform* for adoptive cellular immunotherapy, the infusion of specific cell populations which mediate an antitumor effect and/or suppress GVHD alloreactivity, may improve transplant outcomes. Additional prospective, randomized trials are required to define the efficacy of autologous compared to allogeneic SCT, myeloablative compared to reduced intensity SCT, and SCT compared to a number of emerging and promising therapies for hematologic malignancies.

REFERENCES

1. Spitzer TR, McAfee SL. Bone marrow transplantation. In LC Ginns, AB Cosimi, PJ Morris (eds.), "Transplantation," Blackwell Science, Cambridge, MA, 1999 pp. 560–587.
2. Champlin R, Khouri I, Anderlini P, et al. Nonmyeloablative preparative regimens for allogeneic hematopoietic transplantation. Biology and current indications. Oncology. 2003; 17: 94–100.
3. Grewal SS, Barker JN, Davies SM, Wagner JE. Unrelated donor hematopoietic cell transplantation: marrow or umbilical cord blood? Blood. 2003; 101: 4233–4244.
4. Ballen KK. New trends in umbilical cord blood transplantation. Blood. 2005; 105: 3786–3792.

5. Spitzer TR. Haploidentical stem cell transplantation: the always present but overlooked donor. Hematology (Am Soc Hematol Educ Program). 2005; 390–395.

6. Schmitz N, Barrett J. Optimizing engraftment—source and dose of stem cells. Semin Hematol. 2002; 39: 3–14.

7. Blume KG, Tomas ED. A review of autologous hematopoietic cell transplantation. Biol Blood Marrow Transplant. 2000; 6: 1–12.

8. Craddock C. Haemopoietic stem-cell transplantation—recent progress and future promise. Lancet Oncol. 2000; 1: 227–234.

9. Ferrara JL, Vanik G. Acute graft versus host disease—pathophysiology, risk factors, and prevention strategies. Clin Adv Hematol Oncol. 2005; 3: 415–428.

10. Sullivan KM, Dykewicz CA, Longworth DL, et al. Practice guidelines and beyond. Preventing opportunistic infections after hematopoietic stem cell transplantation: the Centers for Disease Control and Prevention, Infectious Disease Society of America, and American Society for Blood and Marrow Transplantation Practice Guidelines and Beyond. Hematology (Am Soc Hematology Educ Program). 2001: 392–421.

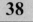

| 38 | Abraham B Schwarzberg, M. Dror Michaelson |

RENAL CELL CARCINOMA

INTRODUCTION

Renal cell carcinoma (RCC) represents approximately 3% of all adult malignancies in the United States. In 2005 there were an estimated 36,160 new cases and, despite recent advances in diagnosis and treatment, 12,660 deaths (1). RCC is the 7th most common malignancy in men and the 12th in women with a male to female ratio of 1.6:1. The median age at diagnosis is 64 years of age and more that half of patients are identified through incidental findings on imaging studies. Prognosis of early stage disease is excellent; however, 25% of patients have advanced disease at initial presentation. Median survival for patients with metastatic disease is 12–15 months with a 10% 5 year survival (2). Advances in the understanding of the pathophysiology of RCC combined with the development of novel targeted therapies have begun to redefine the standard management of this challenging disease.

ETIOLOGY AND PATHOGENESIS

Numerous environmental, lifestyle and genetic factors have been linked to the development of RCC (Table 38-1). Cigarette smoking is associated with an increased relative risk of 30–100%. Obesity is a potential risk factor, with some suggestion that the relative risk rises along with increasing body mass index.

Several hereditary syndromes predispose patients to RCC (3). Insight into the Von Hippel Lindau (VHL) disease has led to the foundation of our

Table 38-1

Risk Factors for The Development of Renal Cell Carcinoma

Environmental/lifestyle
  Smoking
  Obesity
  Hypertension
  Acquired cystic kidney disease associated with end-stage renal disease
  Asbestos
  Trichloroethylene
  Cadmium
Hereditary
  Von Hippel Lindau disease
  Familial clear cell renal cancer
  Hereditary paraganglioma
  Hereditary papillary renal carcinoma
  Birt–Hogg–Dube
  Hereditary leiomyomatosis and renal cell cancer

understanding of clear cell RCC tumor genesis. Features of VHL disease include the following:

- Autosomal dominant disease affecting 1 in 36,000 individuals
- Clinical manifestations include hemangioblastomas (cerebellum and retina), pheochromocytomas, pancreatic islet cell tumors, and clear cell renal carcinomas
- Mortality generally related to CNS tumors
- VHL tumor suppressor gene, located on chromosome 3

In the hereditary form, one allele is inherited as an abnormal gene. Development of RCC occurs when the second allele is altered by deletion, hypermethylation, or mutational inactivation. Biallelic gene alteration leads to loss of function of the tumor suppressor protein and is observed in nearly 100% of the hereditary cases as well as >75% of sporadic cases of clear cell renal carcinoma. The VHL protein normally functions to inhibit cellular growth and is involved in regulating the expression of several genes involved in angiogenesis. Under normoxic conditions, the VHL protein targets Hypoxia-inducible factor (HIF)-1α and HIF-2α for degradation via the ubiquitination pathway. Loss of the VHL protein leads to elevated levels of intracellular HIF proteins with subsequent increased expression of downstream gene targets including vascular endothelial growth factor (VEGF), platelet-derived growth factor (PDGF), and transforming growth factor (TGF-α) (Figure 38-1). The overexpression of HIF-α seems to be necessary but not sufficient for the tumorigenesis of clear cell renal carcinomas.

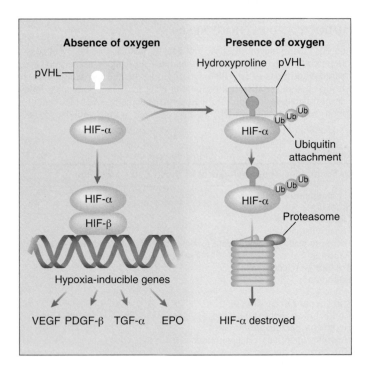

FIGURE 38-1 VHL pathway. (George DJ, Kaelin WG. The von Hippel-Lindau protein, vascular endothelial growth factor, and kidney cancer. N Engl J Med. 2003; 349:419-421.) (4).

The development of papillary renal cell cancer is seen in hereditary papillary renal carcinoma (HPRC). This syndrome is an autosomal dominant disorder involving an activating mutation of the MET proto-oncogene at 7q31.3. The MET mutation leads to autoactivation of the tyrosine kinase domain and increased duplication of chromosome 7. This syndrome results in multifocal bilateral papillary renal cell cancers. MET mutations are infrequently seen in the sporadic forms of papillary renal cell cancer.

The Birt–Hogg–Dube (BHD) syndrome is a rare autosomal dominant syndrome that arises from a mutated BHD gene on chromosome 17 that codes for an apparent tumor suppressor protein, folliculin. BHD syndrome results in hair-follicle hamartomas (fibrofolliculomas) of the face and neck, pulmonary cysts, and renal tumors. Renal tumors can be chromophobe (34%), mixed chromophobe-oncocytoma (50%), and less commonly oncocytoma, clear cell carcinoma or papillary RCC.

Hereditary leiomyomatosis and renal cell cancer (HLRCC) is an autosomal dominant syndrome associated with mutations in the fumarate hydratase (FH) gene. Patients develop cutaneous and uterine smooth-muscle tumors, and aggressive papillary renal cell cancers.

PATHOLOGIC CLASSIFICATION

The majority of kidney cancers (>85%) arise from the renal parenchyma with the remainder originating from the renal pelvis (Table 38-2). High-grade variants are described as having sarcomatoid growth patterns, and typically confer a poor prognosis.

CLINICAL PRESENTATION

A majority of patients diagnosed with RCC are asymptomatic at the time of presentation. The classic triad of hematuria, abdominal pain, and flank/abdominal mass is currently seen in only 10% or fewer of patients. Patients with RCC may present with a wide range of signs and symptoms (Table 38-3). Multiple paraneoplastic syndromes are associated with RCC including polycythemia, nonmetastatic hepatic liver abnormalities (Stauffer syndrome), and hypercalcemia secondary to the production of parathyroid-like hormone.

At presentation, a quarter of patients present with locally advanced or metastatic disease. Of those who undergo surgical resection of apparently localized disease, about 33% will eventually develop disease recurrence. RCC can metastasize

Table 38-2

Histologic Characterization

Histologic cell type	Frequency (%)	Syndrome	Gene	5 Year survival
Clear cell	60–75	VHL disease/HP FCRC	VHL/SDHB 3p del	~60%
Papillary	12	HPRC HLRCC	MET FH	~80%
Chromophobe	4	BHD syndrome	BHD	~90%
Oncocytoma	4	BHD syndrome	BHD	Benign
Collecting Duct	<1	–	–	<5%
Medullary	<1	–	Sickle trait	Rare

FCRC: familial clear cell renal cancer; HP: hereditary paraganglioma; SDHB: succinate dehydrogenase B; HPRC: hereditary papillary renal carcinoma; HLRCC: hereditary leiomyomatosis and renal cell cancer: and FH: fumarate hydratase.

Table 38-3

Clinical Presentation

Presenting signs and symptoms	% of patients
Hematuria	59
Palpable mass	45
Flank pain	41
Weight loss	28
Anemia	21
Fever	20
Hypertension	20
Abnormal liver function	15
Hypercalcemia	5
Polycythemia	3
Neuromyopathy	3
Amyloidosis	3
Acute varicocele	2

Table 38-4

Sites of Metastatic Disease

Sites of metastasis at presentation	%
Lung	61
Lymph nodes (retroperitoneal, mediastinal)	35
Bone	27
Adrenal	16
Liver	13
Brain	6
Soft tissue	4

to nearly any anatomic location, but most commonly metastasizes to lungs, mediastinum, liver, pancreas, retroperitoneum, adrenals, and bone (Table 38-4).

The diagnostic evaluation of suspected RCC has evolved over the past several years. CT and MRI have largely replaced intravenous pyelograms. Initial evaluations should include:

- Family history screening for familial syndromes, especially if <50 years of age
- Abdominal and pelvic CT Scan with contrast
- Chest x-ray
- Consider MRI evaluation of involvement of renal vein and inferior vena cava
- Note that bone scintigraphy and Positron Emission Tomography (PET) scan are relatively insensitive for RCC, and are not recommended for routine staging purposes.

STAGING

See Table 38-5 for staging classifications.

PROGNOSIS

Prognosis in RCC is closely related to T-N-M staging (Table 38-6). In the setting of metastatic disease patient prognosis can be stratified according to poor risk features. One common classification system uses Karnofsky performance status, elevated serum lactate dehydrogenase, low hemoglobin, absence of prior nephrectomy, and elevated serum calcium (Table 38-7) (5).

Table 38-5

Staging Classifications

Primary tumor (T)

TX	Primary tumor cannot be assessed
T0	No evidence of primary tumor
T1	Tumor 7 cm or less in greatest dimension limited to the kidney
T2	Tumor more than 7 cm in greatest dimension limited to the kidney
T3	Tumor extends into major veins or invades the adrenal gland or perinephric tissues, but not beyond Gerota's fascia
T3a	Tumor invades the adrenal gland or perinephric tissues but not beyond Gerota's fascia
T3b	Tumor grossly extends into the renal vein(s) or vena cava below the diaphragm
T3c	Tumor grossly extends into the renal vein(s) or vena cava above the diaphragm
T4	Tumor invades beyond Gerota's fascia

Regional lymph nodes (N)*

NX	Regional lymph nodes cannot be assessed
N0	No regional lymph node metastases
N1	Metastases in a single regional lymph node
N2	Metastases in more than one regional lymph node

*Laterality does not affect the N classification

Distant metastasis (M)

MX	Distant metastasis cannot be assessed
M0	No distant metastasis
M1	Distant metastasis

Stage grouping

Stage I	T1	N0	M0
Stage II	T2	N0	M0
Stage III	T1	N1	M0
	T2	N1	M0
	T3a	N0	M0
	T3a	N1	M0
	T3b	N0	M0
	T3b	N1	M0
	T3c	N0	M0
	T3c	N1	M0
Stage IV	T4	N0	M0
	T4	N1	M0
	Any T	N2	M0
Any T	Any N	M1	

(Used with the permission of the American Joint Committee on Cancer (AJCC), Chicago, Illinois. The original source for this material is the AJCC Cancer Staging Manual, 6th edition (2002) published by Springer-New York, www.springeronline.com.)

TREATMENT

Localized Disease

- *Radical nephrectomy*: mainstay of treatment, and consists of removal of Gerota's fascia, kidney, ureter, ipsilateral adrenal gland, and adjacent hilar lymph nodes (LNs).

Table 38-6

Five Year Survival Correlates Closely With TNM Staging

TNM stage	% 5 Year survival
T1	95
T2	88
T3	59
T4	20
M1	10–20

Table 38-7

Prognostic Factors in Metastatic RCC

Risk group	# of risk factors	Median survival (month)	% of patients
Favorable	0	20	25
Intermediate	1–2	10	53
Poor	3 or more	4	22

- *Nephron-sparing procedures* (*partial nephrectomy*): reasonable alternative in selected patients, multiple case series support safety and feasibility, but no randomized clinical trials comparing outcomes with radical nephrectomy. Consider in patients with:
  1. Preexisting renal disease in the contralateral kidney
  2. Genetic syndromes that may predispose patients to multifocal disease (VHL, HPRC)
  3. Small tumors (≤ 4 cm)
  4. Coincident medical conditions that may lead to renal insufficiency

- *Radiofrequency ablation (RFA) or cryotherapy*: may be alternatives in selected patients who cannot tolerate definitive curative surgical resection. There is only short-term follow-up to date and no controlled trials have been done comparing outcomes with surgery. Single-center case series have shown excellent outcome and good tolerability with RFA in tumors < 3 cm.

Adjuvant Therapy

Several studies have evaluated the role of adjuvant therapy for patients with RCC and all have demonstrated no benefit. Two recent studies using adjuvant immunotherapy confirmed the lack of benefit of systemic therapy following nephrectomy. In the study by Messing et al., 283 patients with T3-T4a or N1 disease were randomized to observation or interferon (IFN)-α following nephrectomy and lymphadenectomy (6). After a 10 year median follow up there was no difference in overall survival or relapse free survival. Another randomized study was terminated early due to an interim analysis after 69 patients were accrued. It was determined that the study would fail to demonstrated the 30% benefit to disease-free survival for patients randomized to HD-IL2 compared to observation (7). Despite the clear need for adjuvant therapy in high-risk patients, there is currently no role for adjuvant medical therapy except in the context of a clinical trial.

Metastatic Disease

Median survival for metastatic disease is 12–15 months with a 5 year survival of approximately 10%. The main focus of systemic therapy, until recently, has been immunotherapy, and cytotoxic chemotherapy has a little or no activity. Although spontaneous tumor regressions have been documented in patients with RCC, it is a rare event.

Nephrectomy

Two prospective phase III randomized trials evaluated the benefit of nephrectomy in patients with metastatic RCC (8, 9). Both studies demonstrated a statistically significant increase in median survival for patients treated with nephrectomy followed by IFN-α· when compared with IFN-α alone. Both studies included patients with performance status of 0 or 1 and no prior treatment. Despite the difference in median survival there was no observed difference in response to immunotherapy in the two groups (Table 38-8). The results of these studies support the role of nephrectomy in selected patients with good performance status. Furthermore, the treatment of solitary metastases, both synchronous and metachronous, should be carefully considered in selected patients.

Chemotherapy/ Biochemotherapy

Metastatic RCC is refractory to chemotherapeutic agents in multiple phase II trials. Due to the modest success of biologic therapy, there have been attempts to combine cytokine therapy with cytotoxic agents in an attempt to improve response rates and ultimately survival. To date, the addition of agents including vinblastine and 5-fluorouracil (minimally active cytotoxic agents) to IFN-α and/or IL2 have not led to cleary improved outcomes, and are rarely used outside of clinical trials.

Immunotherapy

Until recently, high-dose (HD) IL2 had been the only approved treatment for metastatic RCC in the United States. In 1992, the FDA reviewed data on 255 patients collected from 7 phase II clinical trials with HD-IL2 (10). Overall, there were 17 (7%) complete responses (CRs) and 20 (8%) partial responses (PRs) with a median survival of 16 months and a 4% treatment related mortality. HD-IL2 was typically given as either 600,000 or 720,000 IU/kg via a 5 min intravenous infusion every 8 h for up to 14 consecutive doses over 5 days as tolerated. A second identical course was given following 5–9 days of rest. Three large clinical trials compared different dosing regimens for IL2 with or without IFN (Table 38-9) (11–13). The data from the three trials indicated that bolus HD-IL2 is the most effective immunotherapy treatment when measuring response rates, but there was no consistent difference in overall survival. Studies have evaluated the addition of IFN-α to IL2 and a summary of these results demonstrates that combined therapy increases toxicity but offers no improvement in response rates or survival (Table 38-10). The major limitations to treatment with HD-IL2 are its life-threatening side effects including severe

Table 38-8

IFN-α Versus IFN-α + Nephrectomy in Patient With Metastatic RCC

		Median survival (month)		
	# of patients	IFN	IFN+ nephrectomy	*P*
SWOG 8949 (8)	241	8.1	11.1	0.05
EORTC 30947 (9)	85	7	17	0.03
Combination	331	7.8	13.6	0.002

Table 38-9

RCT of IL2 for Treatment of Metastatic RCC

	Dose IL2	# of Pts	# of CR	# of PR	RR(%)
Negrier et al. (11)	18×10^6 IU/M²/day as continuous infusion $\times$ 5 days (intermediate dose IL2)	138	2	7	6.5
	18 IU/M²/day $\times 10^6$ as above + IFN-α 6×10^6 IU SC 3 days/week	140	1	25	18.6[†]
Yang et al. (12)	720,000 IU/kg q8h (high-dose IL2)	155	11	22	21[†]
	72,000 IU/kg q8h (low-dose IL2)	149	6	13	13
McDermott et al. (13)	5 MIU/m² s.c. q8h $\times$ 3 doses then daily for 5 days/week (low-dose IL2) + INF-α 5 MIU/m² s.c. 3 days/week for 4 weeks	91	3	6	9.9
	600,000 IU/kg q8h (high-dose IL2)	95	8	14	23[†]

[†]$P < 0.05$ for RR but no survival difference.

Table 38-10

Summary of Chemotherapy and Immunotherapy in Metastatic RCC

Treatment	Infusion regimens	Overall response rate (%)
Cytotoxic chemotherapy		<10
IFN-α	5–10 MIU/m² s.c. 3–5 times/week	8–15
HD-IL2	600,000–720,000 IU/kg IV infused over 15 min q8h $\times$ 14 doses then 5–9 day rest and repeat cycle If patien responding repeat every 8–12 weeks	15–23
LD-IL2	72,000 IU/kg IV q8h $\times$ 15 doses q7–10 days for two cycles. If patient responding repeat every 8–12 weeks	13–15
IFN + IL2	LD-IL2 (5 MIU/m² s.c. q8h $\times$ 3 doses then daily 5 days/week) + INF-α (5 MIU/m² s.c. 3 days/week for 4 weeks)	15–25
IFN + others		5–25
IL2 + others		5–25

hypotension and capillary leak syndrome. Therefore, HD-IL2 should be administered in experienced centers with the necessary monitoring and supportive measures available.

Targeted Therapy

Improved understanding of tumorigenesis in clear cell RCC has led to novel therapeutic approaches aimed at inhibiting the down stream products of HIF-α, which include VEGF and PDGF (Figure 38-1). Bevacizumab, a monoclonal antibody against VEGF ligand (Figure 38-2), was evaluated in a phase II study randomizing patients to placebo, low-dose (3mg/kg) or high-dose (10 mg/kg) bevacizumab (14). There was a significant difference in time to progression: 2.5 months in the placebo arm compared with 4.8 months in the high-dose arm. There was no difference in overall survival, although the study was not powered for this endpoint. Two randomized phase III trials are comparing first-line interferon-α to interferon-α in combination with high-dose bevacizumab and are currently ongoing.

Two small molecule inhibitors of the VEGF receptor and PDGF receptor tyrosine kinases have been approved for the treatment of advanced kidney cancer. Sunitinib is a tyrosine kinase inhibitor of the VEGF receptor (Figure 38-2) and was tested in a randomized phase III trial versus interferon-α in the first-line treatment of metastatic clear cell RCC. Sunitinib demonstrated an improvement in progression-free survival (11 versus 5 mo) and in overall response rate (31% vs. 6%) in comparison to interferon-α and has become the reference standard for first-line therapy of advanced RCC (15). Sorafenib is another tyrosine kinase inhibitor of the VEGF and PDGF receptors (Figure 38-2). In a phase III randomized trial for cytokine-refractory patients, sorafenib demonstrated a significant improvement in progression-free survival of 5.5 months versus 2.8 mo in the placebo group (16). The activity of one anti-angiogenic agent after failure of another is not well studied to date. Both sunitinib and sorafenib are well tolerated, with serious toxicity only rarely seen. The most common side effects are fatigue and diarrhea with sunitinib, and hand–foot syndrome and hypertension with sorafenib.

Temsirolimus has also been recently approved for the treatment of advanced kidney cancer. Temsirolimus inhibits the mammalian target of rapamycin (mTOR) kinase, resulting in inhibition of intracellular pathways involved in the growth and proliferation of tumor cells. A first-line phase III trial in patients with multiple adverse prognostic factors demonstrated significant improvement in overall survival in those treated with temsirolimus alone versus those treated with interferon alone. Treatment with both temsirolimus and interferon did not improve survival compared with interferon alone (Table 38-11) (17). Overall survival times in the interferon group, the temsirolimus group, and the combination-therapy group were 7.3, 10.9, and 8.4 months, respectively. Rash, peripheral edema, hyperglycemia, and hyperlipidemia were the most common side effects.

FUTURE DIRECTIONS

Localized RCC is effectively treated with surgery, and increasingly now with less invasive approaches. The roles of laparoscopic surgery, percutaneous therapy of localized tumors, and adjuvant medical therapy are areas of active research. Despite recent positive developments, treatment options for advanced RCC remain limited and additional therapies are needed. Future directions will include establishing the optimal dosage and scheduling of the newly approved therapies. Additional clinical trials are evaluating sequential and combination therapy with targeted agents and immunotherapy or chemotherapy. Other targeted agents are actively being investigated, including agents that inhibit other products of the HIF pathway, the mammalian target of rapamycin (mTOR) pathway, and the epidermal growth factor (EGF) pathway. Hopefully, deeper understanding of the underlying biology of kidney cancer will continue to result in improved therapeutic options for patients suffering from this disease.

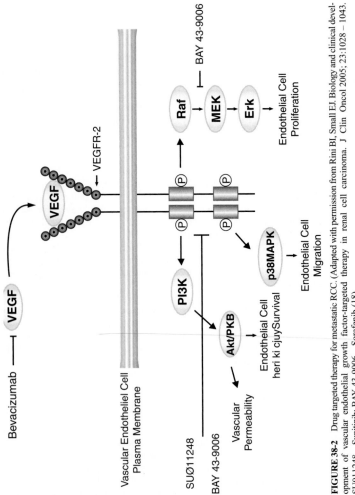

FIGURE 38-2   Drug targeted therapy for metastatic RCC. (Adapted with permission from Rini BI, Small EJ. Biology and clinical development of vascular endothelial growth factor-targeted therapy in renal cell carcinoma. J Clin Oncol 2005; 23:1028 – 1043. SU011248 – Sunitinib; BAY 43-9006 – Sorafenib (18).

Table 38-11

Randomized Trials of Antiangiogenenic Therapy for Metastatic RCC

Trial	# of patients	Treatment (Dosage)	ORR (%)	PFS (month)	Survival (month)
Motzer et al. (15)	750	IFN (3x/wk SC 9 MIU)	6	5	**
		Sunitinib (50mg PO QD 4 wks on followed by 2 wks off)	31	11	**
*Escudier et al. (16)	903	Placebo	2	2.8	**
		Sorafenib (400mg PO BID)	10	5.5	**
Hudes et al. (17)	626	IFN (3x/wk SC 3-18 MIU)	4.8	3.1	7.3
		TEMSR (25mg IV weekly)	8.6	5.5	10.9
		TEMSR (15mg IV weekly) – IFN (3x/wk SC 6 MIU)	8.1	4.7	8.4

IFN – interferon–α, TEMSR – temsirolimus, ** – data not mature
* Second-line study in cytokine-refractory patients

REFERENCES

1. Jemal A, Murray T, Ward E, et al. Cancer Statistics, 2005. CA Cancer J Clin 2005; 55: 10–30.
2. DeVita VT, Hellman S, Rosenberg SA. "Cancer Principles & Practice of Oncology," 7th edition, Lippincott Williams & Wilkins, Philadelphia, PA, 2005.
3. Iliopoulos O, Eng C. Genetic and clinical aspects of familial renal neoplasms. Semin Oncol. 2000; 27(2): 138–149.
4. George DJ, Kaelin WG. The von Hippel-Lindau protein, vascular endothelial growth factor, and kidney cancer. N Engl J Med. 2003; 349: 419–421.
5. Motzer RJ, Mazumdar M, Bacik J, et al. Survival and prognostic stratification of 670 patients with advanced renal cell carcinoma. J Clin Oncol. 1999; 17: 2530–2540.
6. Messing EM, Manola J, Wilding G, et al. Phase III study of interferon alfa-NL as adjuvant treatment for resectable renal cell carcinoma: an Eastern Cooperative Oncology Group/Intergroup trial. J Clin Oncol. 2003; 21: 1214–1222.
7. Clark JI, Atkins MB, Urba WJ, et al. Adjuvant high-dose bolus interleukin-2 in patients with high-risk renal cell carcinoma—a Cytokine Working Group Phase III trial. J Clin Oncol. 2003; 21: 3133.
8. Flanigan RC, Salmon SE, Blumenstein BA, et al. Nephrectomy followed by interferon alfa-2b compared with interferon alfa-2b alone for metastatic renal-cell cancer. N Engl J Med. 2001; 345: 1655–1659.
9. Mickisch GH, Garin A, van Poppel H, et al. Radical nephrectomy plus interferon-alfa-based immunotherapy compared with interferon alfa alone in metastatic renal-cell carcinoma: a randomized trial. Lancet. 2001; 358: 966–970.
10. Fyfe G, Fisher RI, Rosenberg SA, et al. Results of treatment of 255 patients with metastatic renal cell carcinoma who received high-dose recombinant IL-2 therapy. J Clin Oncol. 1995; 13: 688–696.

11. Negrier S, Escudier B, Lasset C, et al. Recombinate human interleukin-2, recombinate human interferon alfa-2a, or both in metastatic renal-cell carcinoma. N Engl J Med. 1998; 338: 1272–1278.

12. Yang JC, Sherry RM, Steinberg SM, et al. Randomized study of high-dose and low-dose interleukin-2 in patients with metastatic renal cancer. J Clin Oncol 2003; 21: 3127–3132.

13. McDermott DM, Regan MM, Clark JI, et al. Randomized phase III trial of high-dose interleukin-2 versus subcutaneous interleukin-2 and interferon in patients with metastatic renal cell carcinoma. J Clin Oncol 2005; 23: 133–141.

14. Yang, JC, Haworth L, Sherry, RM, et al. A randomized trial of bevacizumab, an anti-vascular endothelial growth factor antibody, for metastatic renal cancer. N Engl J Med. 2003; 349: 427–434.

15. Motzer RJ, Hutson TE, Tomczak P, et al. Sunitinib versus interferon alfa in metastatic renal-cell carcinoma, N Engl J Med 2007; 356(2): 115–124.

16. Escudier B, Eisen T, Stadler WM, et al. Sorafenib in advanced clear-cell renal-cell carcinoma. N Engl J Med 2007; 356(2): 125–134.

17. Hudes G, Carducci M, Tomczak P, et al. Temsirolimus, interferon alfa, or both for advanced renal-cell carcinoma. N Engl J Med 2007; 356(22): 2271–2281.

18. Rini BI, Small EJ. Biology and clinical development of vascular endothelial growth factor-targeted therapy in renal cell carcinoma. J Clin Oncol. 2005; 23: 1028–1043.

LOCALIZED PROSTATE CANCERS

EPIDEMIOLOGY

In the United States, an estimated 232,090 men were diagnosed with prostate cancer in 2005. There were 30,350 deaths attributed to prostate cancer (1). These statistics highlight the paradox of prostate cancer. Although it is the second leading cause of cancer death for men in the United States, only a handful of men diagnosed with prostate cancer will actually die of disease. This chapter will present guidelines for the management of localized prostate cancer. It will describe the controversies associated with PSA screening, describe the work up and staging of prostate cancer, and finally discuss treatment options for localized disease.

PSA

PSA is a serine protease secreted by normal prostate epithelium. An abundant protein in the exocrine secretions of the prostate, it functions in seminal clot lysis. Although imperfect, serum PSA has become a standard screening tool for prostate cancer. In addition to prostate cancer, PSA elevations may be the result of a variety of nonmalignant conditions including benign prostatic hypertrophy, inflammation, or urinary tract infection. Traditionally, 4.0 ng/ml has been considered the upper limit of normal for serum PSA; however, recent data demonstrate that many men with a serum PSA in the normal range have prostate cancer if biopsied (2). Conversely, many men with elevated PSA levels do not. As PSA normally rises with age, an age-specific algorithm may be a more effective screening approach. Age-specific PSA normal ranges have been shown to aid in finding important early cancer in younger men and avoiding unnecessary procedures and overdiagnosis in older men (Table 39-1).

CURRENT RECOMMENDATIONS FOR SCREENING

Prostate cancer screening is a controversial issue. Although PSA screening has led to the detection of earlier prostate cancer, it is not clear if this has led to better outcomes for the screened men. Many screen detected cancers may be incidental cancers that would have never resulted in clinical sequelae within the man's lifetime. Still, most men pursue radical treatment. The American Cancer Socity currently recommends that men with average risk of prostate cancer undergo screening only after a discussion with their primary physician regarding the questionable efficacy of PSA screening including the potential benefits

Table 39-1

Age-Specific PSA Ranges

PSA Values (ng/ml)	Age
0.0–0 2.5	40–49
0.0–3.5	50–59
0.0–4.5	60–69
0.0–6.5	70–79

and risks of an early prostate cancer diagnosis. For men who elect screening, PSA and digital rectal examination (DRE) should be offered annually starting at age 50. Continued screening is most appropriate in men with a life expectancy of at least 10 years. Factors that increase the risk of prostate cancer include sub-Saharan African decent or prostate cancer diagnosis in a first-degree relative before the age of 65. If more than one first-degree relative has been diagnosed before the age of 65, the American Cancer Society recommends screening begin at age 40.

Digital Rectal Examination

Although the majority of prostate cancer is detected by PSA screening, others are diagnosed based on an abnormal DRE even in the setting of a normal PSA. Both PSA and DRE should be incorporated into the screening process. A palpable nodule or a discrete indurated area constitutes a suspicious DRE which should prompt further evaluation.

Diagnosis

Prostate cancer is diagnosed exclusively by the use of a transrectal ultrasound guided needle biopsy (Figure 39-1). This is an outpatient office based procedure performed under local anesthetic. It has a very low-complication rate estimated at 1 serious complication per 1,000 procedures. There is no radiographic modality adequate for diagnosis without the use of the biopsy. Ultrasound may show a hypoechoic area which corresponds to localized carcinoma, but this is an unreliable finding and not sufficient for diagnosis. An abnormal PSA or DRE in an appropriate screening candidate should prompt a transrectal ultrasound and prostate biopsy. The proper technique for prostate biopsy has been well studied. The standard approach is a systematic sampling of all areas of the prostate in a grid pattern (Figure 39-2). Most urologists employ a technique of sampling 6–12 regions of the prostate. The cancer detection rate is substantially higher with a 10–12 biopsy technique. There has certainly been some concern raised about this technique uncovering a higher percentage of "clinically insignificant cancers."

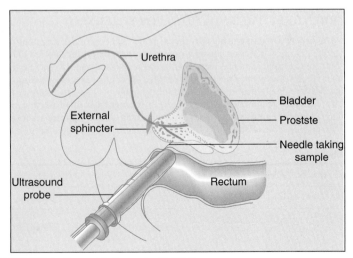

FIGURE 39-1   Transrectal ultrasound guided biopsy.

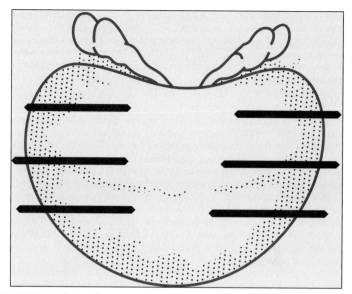

FIGURE 39-2 Sextant biopsy pattern.

Gleason Score (Table 39-2)

The histologic grading of prostate cancer is described using the Gleason scoring system. This system assigns two numeric scores to the carcinoma. As there is often heterogeneity within the cancer, the first score describes the dominant pattern and the second the secondary pattern. For example, Gleason 3 + 4 indicates the primary pattern is 3. Gleason 4 + 3 indicates that the higher grade predominates. This is clinically important because prognosis is substantially related to the primary Gleason score. In discussing prostate cancer staging, the Gleason sum, that is, the sum of the individual scores, is commonly referenced. Although the Gleason sum is one of the most important prognostic features, the primary and secondary scores should also be reported as they may refine a patient's prognosis. For instance, Gleason sum of 3 + 4 and 4 + 3 are both 7, though the latter cancer has a worse prognosis.

In the absence of prostate cancer, there are other common histologic findings that warrant consideration. Atypical small acinar proliferation (ASAP) is frequently an inadequately sampled carcinoma escaping definitive diagnosis. A repeat biopsy is indicated. High-grade prostatic intraepithelial neoplasia (HGPIN) is commonly found on prostate biopsies. The significance of this finding

Table 39-2

Gleason Score Frequency for PSA Detected Prostate Cancers (17)

Gleason Score	Percentage
2–4	<5
5–6	60–65
7	15–20
8–10	10

is controversial. Some believe it is a precursor of invasive adenocarcinoma, but definitive proof is lacking. Standard practice calls for continued close monitoring and rebiopsy of these patients. Perineural invasion (PNI) is a finding often reported in men who have prostate cancer. Some investigators believe this is associated with a higher risk of extra prostatic tumor spread, but this has been an inconsistent finding.

STAGING

The most important independent variables used in staging prostate cancer are the patient's PSA, the DRE findings, and the Gleason score. Using these clinical features, significant prognostic judgment can be made. The Partin tables assess the likelihood of pathologic stage based on these clinical variables. They are very useful in counseling patients about appropriate treatment options (3). Metastatic workup includes CT scanning of the abdomen and pelvis to assess for pelvic and retroperitoneal lymphadenopathy. A bone scan may pick up bone metastases. Because of the extremely small likelihood of positive findings, these studies are not indicated for patients with a PSA of less than 10, Gleason score 6, and normal prostate exam. In general, these studies are indicated only in patients with Gleason 4 + 3 or higher cancer, PSA greater than 10, or clinical high local stage tumor, clinical T2-B or higher.

Endorectal MRI has been extensively studied for its role in local staging of prostate cancer. Modest accuracy in the prediction of extra capsular disease limits the use of this study.

Treatment Options

Definitive local treatment is primarily a curative strategy in patients with localized disease, but it is occasionally employed to prevent symptoms from locally advanced disease even in men with evidence of distant metastasis.

Watchful Waiting/Active Surveillance

Prostate cancer frequently behaves in an indolent fashion. Watchful waiting or active surveillance is an excellent strategy for men with less than a 10 year life expectancy or with low-volume Gleason 3 + 3 disease. Population-based studies suggest only a small minority of men with Gleason 3 + 3 carcinoma will develop metastatic or life-threatening disease within 10 years if left untreated (4). Still, a randomized trial performed in Europe demonstrated that radical prostatectomy reduced the risk of death, metastatic dissemination, and local progression as opposed to watchful waiting in men with early prostate cancer (5). As the majority of these men did not have screen detected cancers, this study does not truly represent watchful waiting as practiced in the United States. It does support the efficacy of local treatment in the management of more significant prostate cancers. Active surveillance with selective delayed intervention is an approach gaining popularity in Canada for men with favorable risk disease. It relies on serial PSA follow-up and repeat biopsies allowing significant cancers to declare themselves early in follow-up. Patients with significant cancers are offered treatment in a timely fashion, while patients with indolent prostate cancer are spared radical treatment and the associated sequelae. Series have reported prostate cancer specific survival of 99% with 65% of men averting treatment at 8 years (6).

Treatment Options

Several well-proven treatment options for local prostate cancer are available. Radical prostatectomy is the standard surgical procedure comprising complete removal of the prostate and seminal vesicles. This procedure is done using several different approaches. All of them have been proven to be safe and effective. Radical retropubic prostatectomy involves a midline incision from the umbilicus to a synthesis pubis. Radical perineal prostatectomy is performed through a midline incision between the scrotum and the anus. Minimally invasive surgical approaches are now in wide use. A laparoscopic approach through the lower abdomen can be accomplished by standard laparoscopic technique or with the aid of a surgical robot. Radical prostatectomy is one of the most commonly performed major surgical operations. In skilled hands, the mortality and major morbidity rates are extremely low. Major potential complications of surgical removal of the prostate are urinary incontinence, erectile dysfunction, significant hemorrhage, and bladder neck contracture. In properly selected patients, severe incontinence occurs in less than 1% of patients. Mild stress urinary incontinence in which the patient may require pads in his underwear to catch some occasional urinary leakage is found in less than 10% of patients. Erectile dysfunction rates vary widely with patients' preoperative sexual function, the choice of surgical approach (nerve sparing or nonnerve sparing), and the patient's age. In early stage disease, bilateral nerve sparing surgery may result in preservation of erectile function in over 80% of younger men with preoperatively normal sexual function. More aggressive surgical resection which includes one of the pairs of neurovascular bundles which run posteriolaterally to the prostate result in less than 50% of patients recovering spontaneous erectile function. If both nerve bundles are sacrificed, spontaneous erectile function is unlikely to recover. Bladder neck contracture results when dense scar tissue obstructs the point of anastamosis of the urethra and bladder. This may result in acute urinary retention in the early postoperative period. Repeated urologic procedures may be necessary to restore adequate urinary function. Significant hemorrhage may be encountered during radical prostatectomy. It is common practice for surgeons to bank autolagous blood prior to radical prostatectomy. Blood loss on average is much reduced with peritoneal and laparoscopic approaches to radical prostatectomy. Regional pelvic lymph nodes are routinely sampled during radical retropubic and laparoscopic radical prostatectomy. This may give important staging information. It is not possible to sample pelvic lymph nodes through the perineal approach.

RADIATION THERAPY OPTIONS *External beam radiation therapy.* External beam radiation therapy has a well-established track record in the management of localized prostate cancer (7). It is a noninvasive form of treatment delivered in daily fractions over the course of several weeks. Modern trials have demonstrated that higher doses, on the order of 78–79 Gy, are more efficacious for cancer control when external radiation is used as monotherapy (8, 9). Conformal radiation therapy utilizing CT planning is necessary for the safe delivery of sufficient radiation dose in this setting. Daily prostate imaging using either transabdominal ultrasound or radiographic visualization of implanted fiducial markers allows more accurate targeting of the prostate. This facilitates the delivery of high-radiation doses to the prostate while minimizing dose to nontarget tissue, such as the bladder and rectum, which is the primary cause of late morbidity. A variety of external beam radiation techniques are acceptable forms of treatment including multifield 3D conformal radiation, intensity modulated radiation therapy (IMRT), and proton radiation therapy. The technique employed is less important than the quality of the radiation plan as assessed by dose volume histogram and the proper delivery of treatment at a facility which employs strict quality assurance measures over the course of treatment. Complications of external beam radiation therapy include radiation proctitis, cystitis, and urethritis. The rates of these complications are on the order of 10%. Similar to surgery, erectile dysfunction is the most common side effect of treatment. Rates of erectile dysfunction vary with patient age and the presence of medical comorbidities, particularly cardiovascular disease, obesity, diabetes, and smoking. Late sequelae are not always noted until years after treatment.

Prostate brachytherapy Prostate brachytherapy is another excellent treatment modality for early prostate cancer. When used as monotherapy, it should be restricted to patients with low-intermediate risk disease. Modern prostate brachytherapy is typically delivered under transrectal ultrasound guidance using a transperineal approach (Figure 39-3). This technique resulted in dramatic improvements in dose distribution and outcome as compared to prior efforts using an open approach and freehand seed placement. As modern series have matured, results have been comparable to surgical and external beam radiation for early stage disease. Commonly, this procedure is performed in an operating room under either general or spinal anesthesia. An ultrasound probe is placed in the rectum and needles containing radioactive seeds are guided into the prostate using a transperineal template or grid. These seeds typically contain either Iodine-125 or Palladium-103 whose half-lives are 60 and 17 days, respectively. They remain in the prostate permanently and deliver the full dose of radiation over several months. This procedure is termed transperineal permanent low-dose rate (LDR) prostate brachytherapy. It differs from high-dose rate (HDR) brachytherapy where temporary catheters are placed in the prostate using a similar placement technique. The catheters serve as avenues for a HDR radioactive wire which contains a high-activity source, typically Iridium-192. High-dose brachytherapy requires the delivery of several fractions, necessitating repeated catheter placement. This treatment is most frequently combined with external radiation, but is also used as monotherapy. Although promising, results are immature to date. The brachytherapy techniques described are those most commonly used, but there are notable and interesting variations including the use of CT or MRI as opposed to ultrasound to guide needle placement. Brachytherapy is an excellent way of delivering a high dose of radiation to the prostate. It is conformal and safe. A LDR implant is a very convenient approach as it is a one time outpatient procedure. For well-selected patients, this may be more attractive than a protracted course of external beam radiation.

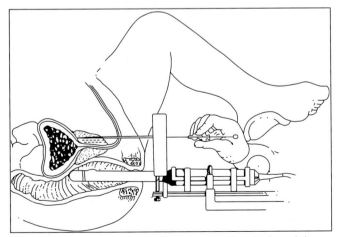

FIGURE 39-3   Ultrasound guided transperineal permanent prostate implant technique.

The most troublesome acute side effects of brachytherapy are obstructive urinary symptoms including urgency and frequency. They are most severe the first month, but occasionally persist for several months. Poorly selected patients with larger prostates or preexisting obstructive symptoms are at risk of urinary retention. Late sequelae include radiation urethritis, cystitis, and proctitis which may result in prolonged symptoms or bleeding. Erectile dysfunction is a more common side effect with rates comparable to external beam radiation. As monotherapy, prostate brachytherapy may be less effective in patients with Gleason 7 or higher, palpable cancer, or PSA greater than 10. When combined with a short course of androgen deprivation therapy or external radiation, it is comparable to surgery or high-dose external radiation (10).

Adjuvant androgen deprivation therapy The benefit of the addition of androgen deprivation therapy to external radiation for patients with locally advanced prostate cancer has been demonstrated in several large randomized studies (11-14). Some have demonstrated an overall survival benefit, while all have demonstrated a benefit in terms of biochemical and local control, decreased distant metastasis, and prostate cancer specific survival. These trials suggest a benefit to a prolonged course of ADT both prior to and after radiation (2–3 years) as opposed to a shorter course of treatment preceding and continuing to the end of radiation (4–6 months in total) (14). In clinical practice, the use of ADT has been extended to lower risk patients. A short course of ADT (4–6 months) has been demonstrated to improve outcome in intermediate risk patients in smaller trials, but larger trials are pending (15). Patients treated in all of these studies were treated to lower doses than commonly used in current practice. There is no evidence that ADT is of any benefit for low-risk patients.

Cryotherapy Liquid nitrogen delivered through probes in the perineum guided by transrectal ultrasonography has been employed to treat localized prostate cancer. This procedure is FDA approved and in common usage throughout the United States. Its efficacy and safety are far less certain than with the above mentioned surgical or radiation therapy techniques. Significantly more research efforts will be required to establish this technique as an acceptable alternative.

HI INTENSITY FOCUSED ULTRASOUND Hi intensity focused ultrasound is an investigational technology which employs a transrectal probe to deliver very intense focused pulses of ultrasound energy through the rectal wall into the prostate. Several centers have explored its use. It remains an investigational technique. Serious complications of urinary retention, rectal urethral fistula, have been reported in the early series. Its efficacy as an oncologic procedures remains unproven.

REFERENCES

1. American Cancer Society. "Cancer Facts and Figures 2003," American Cancer Society, Atlanta, GA, 2005.
2. Thompson IM, Pauler DK, Goodman PJ, et al. Prevalence of prostate cancer among men with a prostate-specific antigen level ≤4.0 ng per milliliter. N Engl J Med. 2004; 350: 2239-2246.
3. http://urology.jhu.edu/prostate/partintables.php.
4. Albertsen PC, Hanley JA, Fine J. 20-year outcomes following conservative management of clinically localized prostate cancer (see comment). J Am Med Assoc. 2005; 293: 2095-2101.
5. Bill-Axelson A, Holmberg L, Ruutu M, et al. Radical prostatectomy versus watchful waiting in early prostate cancer (see comment). N Engl J Med. 2005; 352: 1977-1984.

6. Klotz L. Active surveillance for prostate cancer: for whom? J Clin Oncol. 2005; 23: 8165-8169.

7. Kuban DA, Thames HD, Levy LB, et al. Long-term multi-institutional analysis of stage T1–T2 prostate cancer treated with radiotherapy in the PSA era (see comment). Int J Radiat Oncol, Biol, Phys. 2003; 57: 915-928.

8. Zietman AL, DeSilvio ML, Slater JD, et al. Comparison of conventional-dose vs high-dose conformal radiation therapy in clinically localized adenocarcinoma of the prostate: a randomized controlled trial (see comment0. J Am Med Assoc. 2005; 294: 1233-1239.

9. Pollack A, Zagars GK, Starkschall G, et al. Prostate cancer radiation dose response: results of the M. D. Anderson phase III randomized trial (see comment). Int J Radiat Oncol, Biol, Phys. 2003; 53: 1097-1105.

10. D'Amico AV, Whittington R, Malkowicz SB, et al. Biochemical outcome after radical prostatectomy, external beam radiation therapy, or interstitial radiation therapy for clinically localized prostate cancer (see comment). J Am Med Assoc. 1998; 280: 969-974.

11. Bolla M, Collette L, Blank L, et al. Long-term results with immediate androgen suppression and external irradiation in patients with locally advanced prostate cancer (an EORTC study): a phase III randomised trial (see comment). Lancet. 2002; 360: 103-106.

12. Lawton CA, Winter K, Murray K, et al. Updated results of the phase III Radiation Therapy Oncology Group (RTOG) trial 85-31 evaluating the potential benefit of androgen suppression following standard radiation therapy for unfavorable prognosis carcinoma of the prostate. Int J Radiat Oncol, Biol, Phys. 2001; 49: 937-946.

13. Pilepich MV, Winter K, John MJ, et al. Phase III radiation therapy oncology group (RTOG) trial 86-10 of androgen deprivation adjuvant to definitive radiotherapy in locally advanced carcinoma of the prostate. Int J Radiat Oncol, Biol, Phys. 2001; 50: 1243-1252.

14. Hanks GE, Pajak TF, Porter A, et al. Phase III trial of long-term adjuvant androgen deprivation after neoadjuvant hormonal cytoreduction and radiotherapy in locally advanced carcinoma of the prostate: the Radiation Therapy Oncology Group Protocol 92-02 (erratum appears in J Clin Oncol. 2004; 15; 22(2): 386). J Clin Oncol. 2003; 21: 3972-3978.

15. D'Amico AV, Manola J, Loffredo M, Renshaw AA, DellaCroce A, Kantoff PW. 6-month androgen suppression plus radiation therapy vs radiation therapy alone for patients with clinically localized prostate cancer: a randomized controlled trial (see comment). J Am Med Assoc. 2004; 292: 821-827.

16. Oesterling JE, Jacobsen SJ, Chute CG, et al. Serum prostate-specific antigen in a community-based population of healthy men. Establishment of age-specific reference ranges. J Am Med Assoc. 1993; 270: 860-864.

17. Schroder FH, van der Maas P, Beemsterboer P, et al. Evaluation of the digital rectal examination as a screening test for prostate cancer. Rotterdam section of the European Randomized Study of Screening for Prostate Cancer (see comment). J Natl Cancer Inst. 1998; 90: 1817-1823.

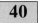

TESTICULAR CANCER

EPIDEMIOLOGY

Testicular cancer is by far the most common malignancy in men aged 15–35 years, and represents nearly 25% of all cancers diagnosed in that age range. However, due to the high cure rate of this disease, it represents fewer than 5% of cancer deaths during those ages. Compared to other cancers across the life-span, testis cancer is rare with about 8,000 new cases and 400 deaths expected in 2006 in the United States. Incidence is increasing while mortality has been in decline. The cause of the rise in incidence is unclear but the declining mortality rate is attributed to the development of curative chemotherapy for advanced disease, improved treatment algorithms, earlier stage at presentation, and a growing proportion of seminomas compared to nonseminomas. The US male lifetime risk of being diagnosed with testis cancer is between 3 and 4 in 1,000. Testis cancer is exceedingly rare in men of African ancestry: white non-Hispanic Americans are more than four times more likely to be diagnosed than black Americans and more than twice as likely to be diagnosed as Hispanic-, Asian-, and Native Americans.

The major risk factors for testis cancer include cryptorchidism, a family history of testicular cancer, and a personal history of testicular cancer. Having a brother with testis cancer raises a man's risk about 8–10-fold, whereas testis cancer in the father raises the son's risk fourfold. The risk for testis cancer in men with cryptorchidism is estimated to be 10–15 times higher than in the general population resulting in a roughly 2–3% lifetime risk of testis cancer. Prepubertal orchiopexy is strongly recommended in men with cryptorchidism to facilitate detection of testis cancer (in addition to other benefits), but whether orchiopexy reduces the risk of testis cancer remains unanswered and controversial. Men who have had testis cancer diagnosed have about a 3% risk of developing a second cancer in the contralateral testis.

PATHOLOGY

The vast majority of testicular neoplasms are germ cell tumors (GCT), which include the following subcategories:
- seminoma
- embryonal carcinoma
- teratoma
- yolk sac tumor (aka endodermal sinus tumor)
- choriocarcinoma

It is important to note that choriocarcinoma in men is a different disease than gestational choriocarcinoma in women. For management purposes, GCTs in men are divided into pure seminomas and nonseminomas. Nonseminomas most often consist of a mixture of two or more GCT subtypes, and one of these subtypes may be seminoma. Seminomas, in contrast, are pure by definition and may contain no other GCT elements.

Serum tumor markers (STMs) are elevated in over half of all testis cancer patients but a substantial minority of men with testis cancer have normal STMs. STMs are more likely to be elevated in advanced stage than localized disease.

The following STMs all play a critical role in the diagnosis, staging, and management of testicular cancer:

- alpha-fetoprotein (AFP) (half-life = 5–7 days)
- human chorionic gonadotropin (HCG) (half-life = 24–36 h)
- lactate dehydrogenase (LDH)

One critical fact is that seminomas do not produce alpha-fetoprotein, so an elevated serum AFP level precludes a diagnosis of seminoma regardless of the histopathology unless an alternative source for the AFP is clearly identified. The degree of elevation of STMs following orchiectomy but prior to other treatment carries strong staging and prognostic implications. Similarly, a slower than expected rate of decline of AFP and HCG during chemotherapy is associated with chemoresistance and a worse prognosis. Persistently elevated STMs following orchiectomy indicate the presence of metastatic disease (unless a compelling alternative explanation is identified), while rising STMs are often the earliest indication of relapse.

GCT are not the only cause of elevated AFP, HCG, and LDH. Elevations of AFP are seen in hepatocellular carcinoma, hepatitis, and cancers of the stomach, colon, rectum, and other gastrointestinal sites. AFP can be elevated due to hepatotoxicity from chemotherapy, so elevations of AFP at the conclusion of treatment cannot always be interpreted as indicative of residual disease. Elevations of HCG are seen in biliary, pancreatic, and many other cancers but in non-GCT neoplasms, the elevation is typically mild. Hypogonadism resulting in elevated serum gonadotropins can result in false elevations of HCG due to assay cross-reactivity with luteinizing hormone. Elevations of LDH are seen in a host of cancers and other diseases, including lymphoma, liver disease, myocardial infarction, and other conditions associated with cell death.

DIAGNOSIS AND STAGING

Testis cancer typically presents with a painless or painful testicular mass. Other much less common presenting symptoms include gynecomastia, gynecodynia, testicular atrophy, infertility, and, in advanced stage disease, back pain, supraclavicular adenopathy, thromboembolic events, or pulmonary symptoms. If a testicular tumor is suspected from the history and/or physical examination, a scrotal ultrasound should be ordered to evaluate both testicles. If the ultrasound indicates that a tumor is present, the usual series of steps for establishing the diagnosis and stage are:

- measure serum AFP, HCG, LDH
- radical/inguinal orchiectomy if ultrasound indicates a tumor is present
- CT scan of the abdomen and pelvis
- Chest x-ray if the CT of the abdomen/pelvis is normal
- Chest CT if the CT of the abdomen/pelvis shows nodal or visceral metastases
- if any STM was elevated before orchiectomy, recheck STMs after orchiectomy
- brain MRI or CT in patients with metastatic choriocarcinoma, postorchiectomy AFP or HCG > 5000, or signs or symptoms intracranial metastases

Staging

Testicular cancer divides into three stages:

I.   limited to the testis, spermatic cord, and scrotum
II.   metastatic disease to retroperitoneal and/or pelvic lymph nodes *and* STMs normal or mildly elevated

III. visceral or distant nodal metastases or the combination of regional nodal metastases plus moderately or highly elevated STMs

Although patients with persistently elevated STMs following orchiectomy are technically labeled stage I if there is no radiographic evidence of metastatic disease (stage IS), they are nonetheless treated as stage III patients for presumed micrometastatic disease.

Stage I is further subdivided based on tumor stage:

IA	T1	limited to testis with or without invasion of tunica albuginea
IB	T2	lymphovascular invasion or invasion of the tunica vaginalis
	T3	invasion of the spermatic cord
	T4	invasion of the scrotum
IS	any	T stage plus elevated markers

Stage II is subdivided based on the number and size of enlarged lymph nodes:

IIA	fewer than six enlarged nodes, none measuring more than 2 cm in greatest diameter
IIB	any node between 2 cm and 5 cm or more than five enlarged nodes with none greater than 5 cm
IIC	a nodal mass greater than 5 cm

Stage III is subdivided based on the level of STMs and the location of metastases. However, treatment decisions about advanced stage disease are based on the International Germ Cell Consensus Classification system that was derived from a pooled analysis of patients with disseminated GCT treated with multiagent cisplatin-based regimens (1). This system divides patients into risk categories (Table 40-1).

Stage I and II Seminomas

STAGE I SEMINOMA   Stage I seminomas carry an outstanding prognosis with fewer than 1% of patients expected to die as a result of the disease. There are three management options for these patients following surgical removal of the involved testis (2):

- surveillance
- external beam radiation therapy
- single-agent carboplatin chemotherapy

None of these options has been shown to produce better or worse long-term survival, but each has distinct risks and benefits. Historically, radiation therapy was preferred but as long-term follow-up data became available, seminoma patients receiving radiation therapy were found to have an excess risk of developing secondary malignancies and some studies found an increased risk of cardiovascular disease and death. Surveillance was then investigated and has produced survival rates indistinguishable from those associated with radiation therapy. The relapse rate for stage I patients put on surveillance following orchiectomy is about 18% compared to 4% after radiation therapy. The vast majority of these can be cured with radiation therapy at the time of relapse, while almost all of the others can be cured with chemotherapy. Risk factors for relapse during surveillance include a large tumor (e.g., >4 cm) and invasion of the rete testis (3). Risk of relapse is about 10%, 16%, and 32% for men with zero, one, or both risk factors, respectively. A common surveillance schedule is to perform a physical examination, chest x-ray, STM measurement, and an abdominopelvic CT scan at the following intervals:

- years 1–3:   every four months
- years 4–6:   every six months
- years 7–10:   annually

Table 40–1

International Germ Cell Consensus Classification System Risk Categories

Good prognosis

Nonseminoma	Seminoma
Testis/retroperitoneal primary and	Any primary site and
No nonpulmonary visceral metastases and	No nonpulmonary visceral metastases and
All of the following: AFP < 1000 ng/ml HCG < 5000 mIu/ml LDH < 1.5 × upper limit of normal (ULN)	Normal AFP, any HCG, any LDH
5 year progression-free survival = 89%	5 year progression-free survival = 82%
5 year overall survival = 92%	5 year overall survival = 86%

Intermediate prognosis

Nonseminoma	Seminoma
Testis/retroperitoneal primary and	Any primary site and
No nonpulmonary visceral metastases and	Nonpulmonary visceral metastases and
Any of the following: AFP ≥ 1,000 and ≤ 10,000 ng/ml HCG ≥ 5,000 and ≤ 50,000 mIU/ml LDH ≥ 1.5 × ULN and ≤ 10 × ULN	Normal AFP, any HCG, any LDH
5 year progression-free survival = 75%	5 year progression-free survival = 67%
5 year overall survival = 80%	5 year overall survival = 72%

Poor prognosis

Nonseminoma	Seminoma
Mediastinal primary and/or	
Nonpulmonary visceral metastases and/or	No seminoma patients classified as poor prognosis
Any of the following: AFP > 10,000 ng/ml HCG > 50,000 mIu/ml LDH > 10 × ULN	
5 year progression-free survival = 41%	
5 year overall survival = 48%	

An alternative strategy for avoiding the late toxicity of radiation therapy is carboplatin chemotherapy given as either one or two cycles at a dose of either 400 mg/m^2 or an AUC of 7. A randomized trial comparing a single cycle of carboplatin to external beam radiation reported no difference in relapse rate. Studies of two cycles of carboplatin have reported lower relapse rates of about 2% (4). Very limited long-term follow-up for patients treated with carboplatin is available but disease-specific survival in reported series is 100%. Little is known about the hypothetical risk of late relapse and late toxicity (Table 40-2).

STAGE II SEMINOMA   Treatment of stage II seminoma has never been investigated in well-designed, adequately powered randomized trials, largely due to the small number of patients. Historically, management has been based on disease bulk. Stage IIA patients typically receive radiation therapy, stage IIC patients are treated with cisplatin-based chemotherapy for disseminated disease,

Table 40–2

Outcomes for Stage I Seminoma in Published Series

	N	Relapses	Relapse rate (%)	5 year DSS
Surveillance	1,032	190	18.4	99.6
Carboplatin (two cycles)	650	11	1.7	100
Radiation	4,005	154	3.8	99.6

DSS: disease-specific survival.

and stage IIB patients can be treated with either approach. The cure rate for IIA/IIB disease is 90–95% and 85–90% for IIC.

Stage I and II Nonseminomatous Germ Cell Tumors

STAGE I NSGCT   Men with stage I NSGCTs who have persistently elevated STMs should be treated as stage III patients using cisplatin-based chemotherapy. Persistently elevated STMs usually indicate distant metastases. Stage I NSGCTs in men with normal postorchiectomy STMs can be managed successfully with any of the following three strategies:
- surveillance
- surgery (retroperitoneal lymph node dissection)
- two cycles of BEP chemotherapy (BEP = bleomycin, etoposide, cisplatin)

Each results in a disease-specific survival of about 99%. Men on surveillance face a 30% risk of relapse on average but the risk is higher for men with lymphovascular invasion and/or a predominance of embryonal carcinoma. Surveillance requires frequent doctor visits and medical tests:

Year 1:	monthly visits for PE*, STMs, CXR.	abdominopelvic CT every 3 months
Year 2:	Bi-monthly PE, STMs, CXR	abdominopelvic CT every 4 months
Year 3:	PE, STMs, CXR every 3 months	abdominopelvic CT every 4 months
Year 4:	PE, STMs, CXR every 4 months	abdominopelvic CT every 6 months
Year 5:	PE, STMs, CXR every 6 months	abdominopelvic CT annually
Years 6+:	PE, STMs, CXR, annually	abdominopelvic CT annually

*PE = physical examination

Retroperitoneal lymph node dissection reduces the risk of relapse, permits more precise staging, and appears to reduce the risk of late relapse, presumably by removing any metastatic teratoma (5). However, this operation should be performed by a highly experienced surgeon in order to avoid incomplete resections and/or unnecessary side effects such as infertility. If no cancer is found at surgery, the risk of relapse is 5–10% but if cancer is found, adjuvant chemotherapy is often recommended, particularly if the pathological stage is IIB or IIC. Adjuvant chemotherapy with two cycles of BEP or EP following retroperitoneal lymph node dissection reduces the relapse risk to about 1%.

Primary chemotherapy refers to chemotherapy given as primary treatment following orchiectomy. Two cycles of BEP in this setting results in a relapse risk of less than 3%. Primary chemotherapy is thus the most effective treatment at preventing relapses. However, there is some concern that these patients may be at increased risk of late relapse due to incompletely treated cancers or unresected, chemoresistant teratomatous elements and there is some concern about late toxicity from BEP. As a result, the question of which of the three treatment options for stage I NSGCT is best remains highly contentious.

STAGE II NSGCT   Stage II NSGCTs are treated either with retroperitoneal lymph node dissection or with cisplatin-based chemotherapy for disseminated disease. A significant number of men with radiographic evidence of low-volume (IIA) disease and normal STMs will turn out to have benign pathological findings at surgery and will thus be pathological stage I. Thus, one main goal of RPLND in clinical stage IIA patients is to obtain accurate staging and to avoid administering unnecessary chemotherapy. Stage II patients undergoing RPLND should be warned that they will probably be advised to undergo adjuvant chemotherapy with two cycles of BEP or EP chemotherapy.

Men with bulkier nodal disease on CT scans and/or elevated STMs are generally treated with three cycles of BEP or four cycles of EP chemotherapy. RPLND in the setting of elevated STMs is associated with a very high risk of relapse. Men undergoing chemotherapy for stage II NSGCT should be warned that they will probably be advised to undergo a postchemotherapy RPLND to resect any residual GCT.

ADVANCED STAGE TESTIS CANCER

First-Line Chemotherapy

First-line chemotherapy for testicular cancer is usually curative and optimal regimens have been well defined in randomized controlled trials. Deviations from standard care are to be avoided. The following guidelines should be followed:
- avoid treatment delays and dose reductions
- monitor for pulmonary toxicity if administering bleomycin
- recommend sperm banking prior to chemotherapy

First-line chemotherapy for good risk patients:
- three cycles of BEP chemotherapy (6), or
- four cycles of EP chemotherapy

First-line chemotherapy for intermediate risk and poor risk patients:
- four cycles of BEP chemotherapy, or
- four cycles of VIP (etoposide, Ifosfamide, cisplatin) chemotherapy (7, 8)

Salvage Chemotherapy

Salvage chemotherapy is less well defined for testicular cancer as few randomized trials have been conducted. Salvage chemotherapy produces a substantially lower cure rate (25–50%) than first-line chemotherapy. Patients with pure seminoma are more likely to be cured by second-line chemotherapy than patients with nonseminomatous GCTs. The proper role, if any, for high-dose chemotherapy in this setting remains unclear.

Salvage chemotherapy regimens:
- four cycles of VeIP (vinblastine, ifosfamide, cisplatin)
- four cycles of TIP (paclitaxel, ifosfamide, cisplatin)
- two cycles of high-dose chemotherapy with autologous peripheral stem cell rescue

Third-line chemotherapy:
- cisplatin, gemcitabine, paclitaxel
- gemcitabine, paclitaxel

MANAGEMENT OF RESIDUAL MASSES

Nonseminomas. Residual masses following chemotherapy in patients with NSGCTs may consist of fibrosis (45–50%), teratoma (40–45%), or viable cancer (10%). Radiographic imaging, including PET, cannot reliably distinguish these entities. *When surgically feasible, all residual postchemotherapy masses in patients with NSGCTs should be resected* (9). This can include excision of pulmonary, hepatic, and retroperitoneal masses. Persistent elevation of STMs following chemotherapy is not a contraindication to resection but salvage chemotherapy should be strongly considered as initial treatment if markers are rising. Teratomatous elements of NSGCTs can be highly chemotherapy resistant. If left unresected, these elements can transform into carcinomas, sarcomas, and other cancers. Thorough postchemotherapy resections in these patients can be technically difficult and risky; referral to a highly experienced surgeon is appropriate (5).

Seminomas. Residual masses following chemotherapy in men with seminomas are usually benign. The most common clinical criteria for deciding whether a residual mass is malignant are (1) size by CT scan (< versus > 3 cm) and (2) FDG–PET results. This is *the one setting* in testicular cancer in which PET appears to be useful (10). In the largest study of this issue, the specificity, sensitivity, positive predictive value, and negative predictive values of FDG–PET were 100%, 80%, 100%, and 96%, respectively. Suspected residual malignant disease should be histopathologically confirmed and treated with salvage chemotherapy.

REFERENCES

1. International Germ Cell Cancer Collaborative Group. International Germ Cell Consensus Classification: a prognostic factor–based staging system for metastatic germ cell cancers. J Clin Oncol. 1997; 15(2): 594–603.
2. Schmoll HJ, Souchon R, Krege S, et al. European consensus on diagnosis and treatment of germ cell cancer: a report of the European Germ Cell Cancer Consensus Group (EGCCCG). Ann Oncol. 2004; 15(9): 1377–1399.
3. Warde P, Specht L, Horwich A, et al. Prognostic factors for relapse in stage I seminoma managed by surveillance: a pooled analysis. J Clin Oncol. 2002; 20(22): 4448–4452.
4. Oliver RT, Mason MD, Mead GM, et al. Radiotherapy versus single-dose carboplatin in adjuvant treatment of stage I seminoma: a randomised trial. Lancet. 2005; 366(9482): 293–300.
5. Stephenson AJ, Sheinfeld J. The role of retroperitoneal lymph node dissection in the management of testicular cancer. Urol Oncol. 2004; 22(3): 225–33.
6. Saxman SB, Finch D, Gonin R, et al. Long-term follow-up of a phase III study of three versus four cycles of bleomycin, etoposide, and cisplatin in favorable-prognosis germ-cell tumors: the Indian University experience. J Clin Oncol. 1998; 16(2): 702–6.
7. de Wit R, Stoter G, Sleijfer DT, et al. Four cycles of BEP vs four cycles of VIP in patients with intermediate-prognosis metastatic testicular non-seminoma: a randomized study of the EORTC Genitourinary Tract Cancer Cooperative Group. European Organization for Research and Treatment of Cancer. Br J Cancer. 1998; 78(6): 828–32.
8. Nichols CR, Catalano PJ, Crawford ED, et al. Randomized comparison of cisplatin and etoposide and either bleomycin or ifosfamide in treatment of advanced disseminated germ cell tumors: an Eastern Cooperative Oncology Group, Southwest Oncology Group, and Cancer and Leukemia Group B Study (see comment). J Clin Oncol. 1998; 16(4): 1287–93.

9.   Oldenburg J, Alfsen GC, Lien HH, et al. Postchemotherapy retroperitoneal surgery remains necessary in patients with nonseminomatous testicular cancer and minimal residual tumor masses. J Clin Oncol. 2003; 21(17): 3310–7.

10.   De Santis M, Becherer A, Bokemeyer C, et al. 2-18fluoro-deoxy-D-glucose positron emission tomography is a reliable predictor for viable tumor in postchemotherapy seminoma: an update of the prospective multicentric SEMPET trial. J Clin Oncol. 2004; 22(6): 1034–9.

BLADDER CANCER

SCREENING AND EARLY DETECTION

Screening for microhematuria has not been particularly useful in the detection of bladder cancer. If significant microhematuria is detected, then specific diagnostic studies are performed. When individuals are screened, 4–20% are found to have microhematuria. Of those with microhematuria, only 0.1%–6.6% have bladder tumors. When urothelial cancer is suspected, noninvasive screening may be performed, including cytology and urinary biomarkers, but the definitive diagnosis can be established only by cystoscopy and biopsy. Cytology is, nevertheless, regarded as the gold standard for noninvasive screening of urine for bladder cancer. It has a sensitivity of 40–60% with a specificity of greater than 90%.

Cancers of the bladder may be grouped into three general categories by their stages at presentation: superficial cancers, muscularis propria-invasive cancers, and metastatic cancers. Each differs in clinical behavior, primary management, and outcome. When treating superficial tumors, the aim is to prevent recurrences and progression to a life-threatening stage. With muscularis propria-invasive disease, the main issue is to determine which tumors require cystectomy, and which can be successfully managed by bladder preservation, utilizing combined modality therapy. Combination chemotherapy is the standard for treating metastatic disease. Despite reports of complete responses in more than 40% of cases, however, the duration of response and overall cure rates remain low. Nonetheless, newer therapies with improved chemotherapeutic regimens, possibly including rationally targeted agents against tumor specific growth factor pathways, offer the hope that these response rates, long-term control rates, and survival may improve in the future.

CLINICAL PRESENTATION AND STAGING

The work up of suspected bladder cancer should include a cytology, a cystoscopy, and an upper tract study. The preference for the upper tract study is a spiral CT as both the ureter and the renal pelvis can be particularly well visualized by the use of that technique as well as the relevant lymph nodes and the kidney parenchyma. Careful staging is important and should include a complete blood count, full blood chemistries, an abdominal pelvic CT scan, a chest CT scan, and a bone scan, as treatment is dependent on the initial stage of the disease. The clinical stage of the primary tumor is determined by transurethral resection of the bladder tumor (TURBT).

The primary bladder cancer is staged according to the depth of invasion into the bladder wall or beyond. The urothelial basement membrane separates superficial bladder cancers into Ta (noninvasive) and T1 (invasive) tumors. The muscularis propria separates superficial disease from deeply (muscularis propria) invasive disease. Stage T2 and higher T stage tumors invade the muscularis propria–the true muscle of the bladder wall. If the tumor extends through the muscle to involve the full thickness of the bladder and into the serosa, it is classified as T3. If the tumor involves contiguous structures such as the prostate, the vagina, the uterus, or the pelvic sidewall, the tumor is classified as stage T4.

Patients who have documented muscularis propria-invasive bladder cancer require an additional set of studies: chest CT, liver function studies, creatinine clearance, and electrolytes and an evaluation of the pelvic and retroperitoneal lymph nodes by CT scan.

TREATMENT

Superficial Bladder Cancer (Ta, Tis, T1)

Seventy percent of patients with bladder cancer have superficial disease at presentation. Approximately 15–20% of these patients will progress to stage T2 disease or greater over time. Fifty to 70% of those presenting with Ta or T1 disease will have a recurrence following initial therapy. Low-grade tumors (grade I or II) and low-stage (Ta) disease tend to have a lower recurrence rate at about 50% and a 5% progression rate, whereas high-risk disease (grade III, T1 associated with CIS and multifocal disease) has a 70% recurrence rate and a 30% progression rate to stage T2 disease or greater disease. Fewer than 5% of patients with superficial bladder cancer will develop metastatic disease without developing evidence of muscularis propria invasion (stage T2 disease or greater) of the primary lesion. Patients with superficial bladder cancer (<T2) require close urologic follow-up indefinitely, consisting of cystoscopy and urine cytology every 3 months. This is generally done as an office procedure, with examination under anesthesia and biopsy reserved for patients with positive findings at cystoscopy.

Patients who are at significant risk for development of progressive disease or recurrent disease following TURBT are generally considered candidates for adjuvant intravesical drug therapy. This for practical purposes would include those with multifocal CIS, CIS associated with Ta or T1 tumors, any grade III tumor, multifocal tumors, and those whose tumors rapidly recur following TURBT of the initial bladder tumor. A number of drugs have been used intravesically, including Bacillus Calmette-Guérin (BCG), Interferon + BCG, ThioTEPA, Mitomycin C, Doxorubicin, and Gemcitabine (under study). The proposed benefit of intravesical chemotherapy is to lessen the rate of recurrences and reduce the incidence of progression. Unfortunately, it cannot be clearly stated that any of these drugs accomplish these goals over the long term. Many studies have demonstrated that over the short term there is a reduction in the recurrence rate of superficial tumors, but in many of these studies the follow up is less than 2 years.

TREATMENT OF MUSCULARIS PROPRIA-INVASIVE DISEASE

Surgical Approaches

The standard of care for squamous cell carcinoma, adenocarcinoma, transitional cell carcinoma, and spindle cell carcinoma invading the muscularis propria of the bladder is a bilateral pelvic lymph node dissection and a cystoprostatectomy with or without a urethrectomy in the male. In the female an anterior exenteration is performed, which includes removal of the bladder and urethra (the urethra may be spared if uninvolved and an orthotopic bladder reconstruction is to be performed), the ventral vaginal wall, and the uterus. A radical cystectomy may be indicated in nonmuscularis propria-invasive bladder cancers when grade III disease is multifocal and/or associated with CIS or when bladder tumors rapidly recur, particularly in multifocal areas following intravesical drug therapy. When the prostate stroma is involved with transitional cell carcinoma or when there is concomitant carcinoma in situ of the urethra, a cystoprostatourethrectomy is the treatment of choice.

Survival

The probability of survival from bladder cancer following cystectomy is determined by the pathologic stage of the disease. Survival is markedly influenced by the presence or absence of positive lymph nodes, for example, no nodes—50%; positive nodes—25%. Positive perivesical nodes have a less ominous prognosis than involvement of iliac or para-aortic nodes.

Selective Bladder-Preserving Approaches

In the United States, radical cystectomy with pelvic lymph node dissection is the standard method used to treat patients with muscle-invasive disease, but utilizing conservative management with organ preservation, radical surgery can be avoided in selected patients. There are several reports from North America and Europe of long-term results using multimodality treatment of muscularis propria-invading bladder cancer, with appropriate safeguards for early cystectomy should this treatment fail.

Successful approaches have evolved over the past two decades following the initial reports of the effectiveness of cisplatin against transitional cell carcinoma and reports of added efficacy when it is given concurrently with radiation. From 1981 to 1986 the National Bladder Cancer Group first used cisplatin as a radiation sensitizer in 68 patients with muscularis propria-invading bladder cancer who were unsuitable for cystectomy. The long-term survival rate with stage T2 tumors (64%) and for stage T3–T4 tumors (22%) was encouraging. One key to the success of such a program is the selection of patients for bladder preservation on the basis of the initial response of each individual patient's tumor to therapy. Cystectomy is recommended for those patients whose tumors respond only incompletely or who subsequently develop an invasive tumor. All of the protocols developed at the Massachusetts General Hospital (MGH) or within the RTOG since 1986 explicitly direct discontinuation of the bladder-sparing effort in favor of radical cystectomy at the earliest sign of failure of local control. The current MGH/RTOG protocol for bladder-preserving treatment of muscle-invasive bladder cancer is shown in Table 41-1. One third of the patients entering a potential bladder-preserving protocol with trimodality therapy (initial TURBT followed by concurrent chemotherapy and radiation) will require radical cystectomy.

For almost two decades, the MGH and the RTOG have evaluated concurrent radiochemotherapy plus neoadjuvant chemotherapy or adjuvant chemotherapy and two large centers in Europe (Erlangen, Germany and Paris, France) evaluated concurrent radiochemotherapy without neoadjuvant or adjuvant chemotherapy. Radiosensitizing drugs studied in these series, either singly or in various combinations, include cisplatin, carboplatin, pacilitaxel, and 5FU.

The University of Erlangen recently updated the largest bladder-sparing study to date, 415 patients treated from 1982 to 2000 (1). This report included 126 patients who received radiation without any chemotherapy and 89 patients who were not clinical stage T2–T4 but classified as "high risk T1." The complete response (CR) rate of all 415 patients was 72% and local control of the bladder tumor after the CR without a muscle-invasive relapse was maintained in 64% of the patients at 10 years. The 10 year disease-specific survival was 42% and more than 80% of these survivors preserved their bladder. The latest North American protocol for bladder-sparing treatment (RTOG 02-33) recently opened. This is a randomized phase II study comparing two combinations of radiosensitizing chemotherapy, (cisplatin plus paclitaxel versus cisplatin plus 5FU) each given concurrently with an induction course of twice daily radiation treatment. This is followed in patients whose tumors initially respond completely by consolidation chemoradiation and in those with incompletely responding

Table 41-1

RADIATION THERAPY ONCOLOGY GROUP

RTOG 0233

A PHASE II RANDOMIZED TRIAL FOR PATIENTS WITH MUSCLE-INVADING BLADDER CANCER EVALUATING TRANSURETHRAL SURGERY AND BID IRRADIATION PLUS EITHER PACLITAXEL AND CISPLATIN OR 5-FLUOROURACIL AND CISPLATIN FOLLOWED BY SELECTIVE BLADDER PRESERVATION AND GEMCITABINE/PACLITAXEL/CISPLATINADJUVANT CHEMOTHERAPY

SCHEMA

Transurethral	Stratify →	R	Induction Chemoradiotherapy →	Post-Induction
→				
Surgery (TUR)	T Stage	A	Treatment starts 4–8 weeks post	Response
	1. T2	N	TUR; Weeks 1–3	Evaluation
	2. T3/T4	D		Week 7
		O →	†**Arm 1(a)**: paclitaxel (Taxol®), cisplatin, and b.i.d. irradiation (TCI)	
		M		
		I	†**Arm 2(b):** 5FU, cisplatin,	
		Z	and b.i.d. irradiation (FCI)	
		E		

Consolidation Chemoradiotherapy

Tumor Response	→		Adjuvant Chemotherapy
		Weeks 8–9	4 cycles, Weeks 21–33
T0, Ta, Tcis* →			with paclitaxel, cisplatin
*At site distant from original tumor (Section 11.2.1)		**Arm 1(c)**: paclitaxel (Taxol®), cisplatin, and b.i.d. irradiation (TCI)	and gemcitabine
		Arm 2(d): 5FU, cisplatin, and b.i.d. irradiation (FCI)	
≥ T1** →		**Radical Cystectomy** →	**Adjuvant Chemotherapy**
**On rebiopsy, the tumor persists and invades into or beyond the lamina propia		Week 9	4 cycles, Weeks 17–29 with paclitaxel, cisplatin and gemcitabine

---

tumors by radical cystectomy. All patients then undergo a three-drug adjuvant treatment with cisplatin, gemcitabine, and paclitaxel. (2)

Predictors of Outcome

A recent update from our institution includes all 190 patients with muscularis propria-invading bladder cancer clinical stages T2–T4a treated on successive prospective selective bladder-preserving protocols from 1986 to 1997. (3) The disease-specific survival rate stratified by clinical stage is shown in Figure 41-1.

Selective bladder sparing by trimodality therapy should be one of the approaches considered in the treatment of patients with muscle-invading bladder cancer. While it is not suggested that it will replace radical cystectomy, sufficient data now exist from many national and international prospective studies to

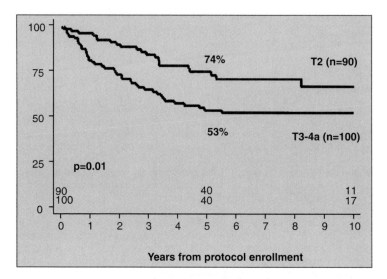

FIGURE 41-1   Disease specific survival with bladder preservation for 190 patients treated on protocol at the MGH from 1986 to 1997. (Modified from WU Shipley et al. Urology. 2002; 60: 62–67.)

demonstrate that it represents a valid alternative. This contribution to the quality of life of patients so treated represents a unique opportunity for urologic surgeons, radiation oncologists, and medical oncologists to work hand-in-hand.

EVOLVING STANDARDS FOR SYSTEMIC CHEMOTHERAPY

Neoadjuvant Chemotherapy

There is abundant evidence that muscularis propria-invasive transitional cell cancer of the bladder is associated with occult metastases, with the likelihood that micrometastases are present, in many cases, at the time of initial discovery of the bladder tumor. Although down-staging of the primary tumor has been demonstrated, randomized studies utilizing single-agent neoadjuvant chemotherapy have failed to demonstrate a survival benefit or a reduction in the development of distant metastases.

Despite more than two decades of clinical experience and investigation with neoadjuvant chemotherapy, followed either by radiochemotherapy as part of bladder-sparing or radical cystectomy, there is still uncertainty as to whether treatment, timed in this way, affects survival.

Raghavan et al. published a meta-analysis of all completed randomized trials (4) of neoadjuvant chemotherapy for invasive bladder cancer. Their analysis, comprising 2,688 patients, led the authors to the following conclusions: single-agent neoadjuvant chemotherapy is ineffective and should not be used; current combination chemotherapy regimens improve the 5 year survival by 5% which reduces the risk of death by 13% compared with the use of definitive local treatment alone (i.e., from 43% to 38%). Though each of the studies cited above were adequately designed and sufficiently powered to settle the question as to whether neoadjuvant chemotherapy should be considered the new standard of care in invasive bladder cancer, a careful review of all of the published material on this subject suggests the following conclusion: while the published data on neoadjuvant chemotherapy do not meet the required standard to declare neoadjuvant chemotherapy the new standard of care in muscularis propria bladder cancer, the data in support of benefit are sufficiently compelling that patients should be informed of the potential benefits versus the risks of neoadjuvant chemotherapy as part of the discussion leading to a decision to proceed with cystectomy.

Adjuvant Chemotherapy

The obvious advantage of adjuvant, as opposed to neoadjuvant chemotherapy, is that pathologic staging allows for a more accurate selection of patients. This approach facilitates the separation of patients in stage pT2 from those in stages pT3 or pT4 or node-positive disease, all at a high risk for progression. The major disadvantage is the delay in systemic therapy for occult metastases while the primary tumor is being treated. It is not possible to assess response to treatment, as there is no clinical endpoint except for clinically detectable disease progression. The place of adjuvant chemotherapy post cystectomy has been studied, but the results are not clear, as several of the reported studies were small phase II studies utilizing a variety of chemotherapeutic regimens. Many of the early studies utilized drug combinations now little-used as combinations of newer drugs have come to the forefront. Investigators generally agree that in the face of positive nodes and even with negative nodes and high-pathologic stage of the primary tumor, adjuvant chemotherapy is worthy of consideration.

Chemotherapy for Metastatic Disease

An estimated 12,500 deaths per year in the United States are due to metastatic bladder cancer. (5) Initial spread of bladder cancer most typically is to pelvic lymph nodes. Through lymphatic and hematogenous means, bladder cancer can then metastasize to distant organs, most commonly the lungs, bones, liver, brain, and elsewhere. The prognosis of metastatic bladder cancer, as with other metastatic solid tumors, is poor, with a median survival on the order of 12 months. Nevertheless, since the discovery that platinum-containing agents have significant antitumor effect in bladder cancer, there has been great interest in the use of chemotherapy for advanced disease.

Compared with other solid tumor malignancies, transitional cell cancer is particularly chemo-sensitive. In contemporary phase II clinical trials, overall response rates are as high as 70–80%, and even in phase III clinical trials, response rates are on the order of 50%. This compares favorably to other solid malignancies, such as lung, colon, or breast cancer, which typically have much lower response rates in phase III studies. Moreover, a small but substantial minority of responding patients manifest a CR, and among these patients some long-term, durable responses are observed. Overall, however, the duration of response in TCC is short, with a median of 4–6 months, and thus the impact of chemotherapy on survival has been disappointing. The hope is that newer cytotoxic chemotherapy and biologic agents will further increase the response rates and the percentage of patients with CRs, ultimately translating into a meaningful improvement in survival among patients with advanced TCC.

Cisplatin-Based Combination Chemotherapy

The standard chemotherapy regimen for advanced bladder cancer for over a decade was methotrexate, vinblastine, doxorubicin, and cisplatin (MVAC), developed at Memorial Sloan-Kettering Cancer Center in the 1980s. The published response rate to MVAC is 40–65%, and there is improved progression-free and overall survival compared with either single-agent cisplatin or CISCA (cisplatin, cyclophosphamide, doxorubicin). CR is seen in 15–25% of patients, but with an expected median survival of only 12 months.

Three phase II studies explored the use of gemcitabine and cisplatin together (GC) in metastatic bladder cancer. (6) This combination has attracted particular interest because of its favorable modest side effect profile.

Because of its apparently comparable efficacy and improved tolerability, GC was compared to standard MVAC in a multicenter phase III study (7). MVAC was administered as described above, and GC was administered in 28 day cycles with gemcitabine 1,000 mg/m^2 (days 1, 8, 15) and cisplatin 70 mg/m^2 (day 2). Four hundred and five patients were randomized to one of the two treatment arms, and the two groups exhibited similar characteristics, with slightly more adverse factors on the GC arm. Median survival was 13.8 months with GC and 14.8 months with MVAC, which were statistically comparable. At 6, 12 and 18 months, survival rates were 82%, 58%, and 37%, respectively, with GC, and 81%, 63%, and 38% with MVAC. The response rates were 49% for the GC arm and 46% for the MVAC arm. There was no significant difference in time to progression or time to treatment failure. (7) Thus gemcitabine and MVAC appear to have equal effectiveness as primary chemotherapy regimens.

Taxane- and Platinum-Containing Regimens

Taxanes are clearly active as single agents in patients progressing after MVAC or gemcitabine, yielding response rates of approximately 20%. The addition of taxanes to cisplatin-based regimens as primary therapy for metastatic disease has been the subject of numerous phase II trials in bladder cancer, and these regimens do not offer clear improvement over gemcitabine or MVAC.

SUMMARY

Our understanding of cancer of the urinary bladder is in a state of evolution, with important advances in our appreciation of multiple risk factors, strategies of prevention, and possibly earlier detection through screening. Superficial bladder cancer accounts for the majority of patients at presentation, and though it uncommonly progresses to muscularis propria-invasive disease, it is difficult to eradicate by local treatment. The mainstay of treatment following TURBT is intravesical therapy using either one of several chemotherapeutic agents, or BCG, with BCG the initial treatment of choice of most urologists. For muscularis propria-invasive disease, there have been improvements in surgical techniques, including continent diversions and neobladders, which have the potential of improving quality of life for patients. Bladder preservation approaches, while still under study in the interest of improving results and limiting side effects, are now moving into the mainstream of treatment with results in comparable patients equal to those achieved by radical cystectomy, and with increasing numbers of patients expressing an interest in organ-sparing treatment. Quality of life considerations have come to the forefront in the care of patients with bladder cancer, much as they have in other cancers, and there are now some important scientific data documenting the quality of life following cystectomy as well as with bladder-sparing treatment. (8)

Whether bladder sparing or cystectomy is used as local treatment, combined modality approaches are essential if treatment is to be optimal. Neoadjuvant chemotherapy has been carefully studied and appears to be of value in improving survival, though further studies will be necessary before this combined approach can be considered standard treatment. For adjuvant treatment, the data are much less convincing. The results of studies have recently begun utilizing newer drug combinations, which may help establish the role of adjuvant chemotherapy in improving survival. In advanced (metastatic) disease, several newer drug combinations have led to an improvement in overall and disease-specific response rates as compared to single-agent therapy, but thus far there has been no demonstrated improvement in survival.

REFERENCES

1. Rodel C, Grabenbauer GG, Kuhn R, et al. Combined-modality treatment and selective organ preservation in invasive bladder cancer: long-term results. J Clin Oncol. 2002; 20: 3061–3071.
2. Shipley WU, Kaufman DS, Tester WJ, et al. An overview of bladder cancer trials in the Radiation Therapy Oncology Group (RTOG). Cancer. 2003; 97(suppl): 2115–2119.
3. Shipley WU, Kaufman DS, Zehr E, et al. Selective bladder preservation by combined modality protocol treatment: long-term outcomes of 190 patients with invasive bladder cancer. Urology. 2002; 60: 62–67.
4. Raghavan D, Quinn D, Skinner DG, et al. Surgery and adjunctive chemotherapy for invasive bladder cancer. Surg Oncol. 2002; 11: 55–59.
5. Jemal A, Murray T, Samuels A, et al. Cancer statistics, 2003. CA Cancer J Clin. 2003; 53: 5–26.
6. Kaufman DS, Raghavan D, Carducci M, et al. Phase II trial of gemcitabine plus cisplatin in patients with metastatic urothelial cancer. J Clin Oncol. 2000; 18(9): 1921–1927.
7. Von der Maase H, Hansen SW, Roberts JT, et al. Gemcitabine and cisplatin versus methotrexate, vinblastine, doxorubicin and cisplatin in advanced or metastatic bladder cancer: results of a large, randomized, multinational, multicenter, phase II study. J Clin Oncol. 2000; 18(17): 3068–3077.
8. Zietman AL, Sacco D, Skowronski U, et al. Organ-conservation in invasive bladder cancer treated by transurethral resection, chemotherapy, and radiation: results of a urodynamic and quality of life study on long-term survivors. J Urol. 2003; 170: 1772–1776.

ADVANCED PROSTATE CANCER

INCIDENCE

Prostate cancer is the most commonly diagnosed cancer in men and a leading cause of cancer death. In the United States, there were approximately 234,460 new prostate cancer cases and 27,350 deaths in 2006 (1). Incidence and mortality rates for prostate cancer are highly variable worldwide.

Prostate cancer incidence in the United States increased steadily throughout the second half of the 20th century. This increase appears related to the increase in life expectancy and associated increase in number of older men at risk for prostate cancer. Other factors including widespread use of prostate specific antigen (PSA) screening also appear to have contributed to the increase in annual prostate cancer incidence. PSA screening identified a large number of prevalent cases of asymptomatic prostate cancer. The annual incidence of prostate cancer peaked at 350,000 cases in 1993. After declining in the late 1990s, the annual incidence of prostate cancer is rising again. In contrast to the striking variations in annual rates of prostate cancer diagnosis, prostate cancer mortality rates have declined steadily since 1990.

SPECTRUM OF ADVANCED DISEASE

Prostate cancer preferentially spreads to regional lymph nodes and bone. Clinically significant metastases to liver, lung, or other visceral organs are less common. Bone scans are routinely used to assess skeletal involvement. Computed tomography scans or magnetic resonance imaging scans may be used to assess regional lymph nodes.

The spectrum of advanced disease has markedly changed in recent decades. Prostate cancer screening with serum PSA has been accompanied by a dramatic stage migration and now less than 10% of men in the United States have radiographic evidence of metastases at initial diagnosis. Additionally, PSA testing is routinely used for surveillance after surgery or radiation therapy for early stage disease. As a result, advanced prostate cancer now includes men with rising serum PSA levels as the only indication of disease progression after prior treatment for early stage disease.

HORMONE THERAPY (TABLE 42-1)

The Hypothalamic–Pituitary–Gonadal Axis

Prostate cancers ubiquitously express the androgen receptor and require androgens for growth and survival. Testosterone synthesized by the Leydig cells of the testis is the primary source of androgens in men. Leydig cell synthesis of testosterone is regulated by luteinizing hormone (LH) of pituitary origin. The release of LH is regulated by gonadotropin-releasing hormone (GnRH) from the hypothalamus. Levels of circulating testosterone are maintained within normal limits by negative feedback at the level of the hypothalamus and pituitary.

Approximately 98% of plasma testosterone is present in a biologically inactive protein bound form. Free testosterone enters cells by diffusion across the cell membrane. In some tissues, including the brain, pituitary, and kidney,

Table 42-1

Hormone Therapy for Prostate Cancer

Class	Agents	Mechanism of action
GnRH agonist	Leuprolide acetate, goserelin	Down-regulation of GnRH receptors
GnRH antagonist	Abarelix	Inhibits GnRH receptors
Estrogen	Diethylstilbestrol	Suppresses pituitary LH production
Antiandrogen	Flutamide, bicalutamide	Competitively inhibits androgen receptors
Steroid synthesis inhibitor	Ketoconazole	Inhibits adrenal androgen synthesis

unmodified testosterone is bound by the androgen receptor. In other tissues, including the prostate, seminal vesicles, epididymis, adrenals, liver, and skin, testosterone is efficiently converted to dihydrotestosterone (DHT) by membrane bound 5α-reductase type II. DHT binds the androgen receptor with approximately threefold greater affinity than testosterone. In adipose tissue, testosterone is converted to estradiol by cytochrome P450-dependent aromatization.

Under the influence of pituitary adrenocorticotropin (ACTH), the adrenal glands produce androstenedione, dehydroepiandosterone (DHEA), and dehydroepiandosterone sulfate (DHEA-S). These compounds, collectively known as the adrenal androgens, have relatively weak androgenic activity. Androstenedione can be converted to testosterone in peripheral tissues and in the prostate. In normal men, the adrenal cortex is a minor source of androgen production. Residual adrenal androgens, however, may be important in promoting disease progression in men with advanced prostate cancer following medical or surgical castration.

Androgen Deprivation Therapy

The mainstay of treatment for metastatic prostate cancer is androgen deprivation therapy (Table 42-2). Permanent androgen deprivation can be accomplished by bilateral orchiectomies. Reversible methods of androgen deprivation therapy include diethylstilboestrol (DES), gonadotropin hormone releasing hormone (GnRH) agonists, and GnRH antagonists. DES suppresses pituitary LH production resulting in castrate testosterone levels. Administration of GnRH agonists causes an initial stimulation of pituitary LH production and rise in serum testosterone levels. Chronic administration of GnRH agonists causes down-regulation of pituitary GnRH receptors and prompt suppression of testicular androgen production. GnRH antagonists directly inhibit pituitary GnRH receptors.

The various forms of androgen deprivation therapy have similar efficacy. A meta-analysis of 10 randomized controlled trials, for example, concluded that bilateral orchiectomies and GnRH agonists have equivalent progression-free and overall survival (2). GnRH agonists have become the most prevalent form of androgen deprivation therapy because they are convenient, potentially reversible, and lack the psychological implications of bilateral orchiectomies. DES is not routinely used because of increased risk of thromboembolic events.

Androgen deprivation therapy achieves prompt marked decline in PSA in nearly all cases and symptomatic improvement in most men with disease-related symptoms. For men with bone metastases, the median time to disease progression is 12–18 months and median survival is 24–30 months. In men without

Table 42-2

Randomized Controlled Trials of Docetaxel for Androgen-Independent Prostate Cancer

Study	Treatment arms	Response rate	Survival
SWOG 9916 (5)	Mitoxantrone/ prednisone versus docetaxel/ estramustine	27% versus 50%	16 versus 18 months (hazard ratio 0.8, $p = 0.01$)
TAX 327 (6)	Mitoxantrone/ prednisone versus docetaxel/ prednisone	32% versus 45%	16 versus 19 months (hazard ratio 0.76, $p = 0.009$)

radiographic evidence of metastases, response duration and survival are much longer. The median survival for men with receiving adjuvant therapy for regional lymph node metastases, for example, is greater than 10 years.

For men without clinical or radiographic evidence of metastases, the optimal timing of hormone therapy is controversial (3). Three randomized controlled trials have compared immediate versus delayed androgen deprivation therapy for men with locally advanced disease or regional lymph node metastases. Early primary androgen deprivation therapy improved survival for men with locally advanced nonmetastatic prostate cancer. Adjuvant androgen deprivation therapy improves survival for men with locally advanced prostate cancer treated with radiation therapy and men with lymph node-positive prostate cancer treated with radical prostatectomy and pelvic lymphadenectomy. The effects of early androgen deprivation therapy on clinical outcomes for men with "PSA-only"disease are unknown.

Most adverse effects of androgen deprivation therapy are due to severe gonadal steroid deficiency. These include loss of lidido, hot flashes, fatigue, and osteoporosis. Androgen deprivation therapy also increases fat mass and decreases insulin sensitivity.

ANTIANDROGENS

Nonsteroidal antiandrogens including bicalutamide, flutamide, and nilutamide competitively inhibit the binding of testosterone and DHT to the androgen receptor. These nonsteroidal antiandrogens bind to the androgen receptor with <2% of the affinity of DHT. Monotherapy with nonsteroidal antiandrogens is inferior to castration for metastatic prostate cancer, likely due to their relatively low binding affinity.

Combination therapy with a GnRH agonist and a nonsteroidal antiandrogen, termed combined androgen blockade, has the potential advantage of inhibiting testicular androgen production and blocking the action of residual adrenal androgens. The concept of combined androgen blockade was first assessed in a randomized controlled trial of leuprolide versus leuprolide plus flutamide in men with metastatic prostate cancer. Compared to leuprolide alone, combined androgen blockade significantly increased median time to disease progression and survival. A subsequent larger study of orchiectomy versus orchiectomy plus flutamide found no benefit for combined androgen blockade. Three meta-analyses concluded that combined androgen blockade provides a slight but significant survival advantage compared to castration alone (4). Combined androgen blockade with flutamide is associated with increased incidence of anemia and diarrhea.

Secondary Hormone Therapy

Advanced prostate cancer almost always progresses after androgen deprivation therapy, a disease state termed andogen-independent prostate cancer. A rise in serum PSA is usually the first indication of disease progression and may predate clinical or radiographic evidence of progression by many months to several years. Secondary hormone treatment with antiandrogens, estrogens, or ketonconazole may achieve responses in as many as half of patients. Most responses to secondary hormone therapy are transient. Little is known about the effects of secondary hormonal therapy on clinical outcomes.

CHEMOTHERAPY

Chemotherapy has a recognized role in management of men with androgen-independent metastatic prostate cancer. In two randomized controlled trials, mitoxantrone plus a corticosteroid improved patient-reported pain and quality of life but not survival compared to a corticosteroid alone. These studies led to the approval of mitoxantrone in combination with corticosteroids as initial chemotherapy for the treatment of men with pain related to advanced hormone-refractory prostate cancer in 1996.

In two recent randomized controlled trials in men with androgen-independent prostate cancer, docetaxel improved overall survival compared to mitox-antrone plus prednisone (Table 42-2) (5, 6). Based on the results of these studies, docetaxel plus prednisone was approved for androgen-independent metastatic prostate cancer in 2004. Docetaxel plus prednisone is now standard first-line chemotherapy for androgen-independent metastatic prostate cancer. Additional studies are necessary to determine the optimal timing of chemotherapy for men with androgen-independent disease and to evaluate the efficacy of adjuvant chemotherapy.

There is no standard second line chemotherapy for prostate cancer. Mitoxantrone and ixabepilone have modest activity as salvage therapy after docetaxel. An ongoing phase III study is evaluating satraplatin in men with progressive disease after first-line chemotherapy.

BONE-TARGETED THERAPY

Bone metastases are a major cause of morbidity for men with prostate cancer. Complications of bone metastases include pain, fractures, and spinal cord compression. Although they appear osteoblastic by radiographic imaging, most bone metastases are characterized by excess osteoclast number and activity. Zoledronic acid, a potent inhibitor of osteoclast activity, differentiation, and survival, decreases the risk of skeletal complications in men with androgen-independent prostate cancer and bone metastases (7).

Radiation therapy has an important role in the palliative management of men of men with bone metastases. Local field external beam radiation therapy provides pain relief in approximately 80% of men with symptomatic bone metastases. Bone-seeking radiopharmaceuticals, including strontium-89 and samarium-153, decrease pain in most men with symptomatic bone metastases.

REFERENCES

1. Jemal A, Siegel R, Ward E, et al. Cancer statistics, 2006. CA Cancer J Clin. 2006; 56(2): 106–130.
2. Seidenfeld J, Samson DJ, Hasselblad V, et al. Single-therapy androgen suppression in men with advanced prostate cancer: a systematic review and meta-analysis. Ann Intern Med. 2000; 132(7): 566–577.

3. Loblaw DA, Mendelson DS, Talcott JA, et al. American Society of Clinical Oncology recommendations for the initial hormonal management of androgen-sensitive metastatic, recurrent, or progressive prostate cancer. J Clin Oncol. 2004; 22(14): 2927–2941.

4. Sharifi N, Gulley JL, Dahut WL. Androgen deprivation therapy for prostate cancer. J Am Med Assoc. 13 2005; 294(2): 238–244.

5. Petrylak DP, Tangen CM, Hussain MH, et al. Docetaxel and estramustine compared with mitoxantrone and prednisone for advanced refractory prostate cancer. N Engl J Med. 2004; 351(15): 1513–1520.

6. Tannock IF, de Wit R, Berry WR, et al. Docetaxel plus prednisone or mitoxantrone plus prednisone for advanced prostate cancer. N Engl J Med. 2004; 351(15): 1502–1512.

7. Michaelson MD, Smith MR. Bisphosphonates for treatment and prevention of bone metastases. J Clin Oncol. 2005; 23(32): 8219–8224.

43	
	Geoffrey Liu

ESOPHAGEAL CANCER

GENERAL INFORMATION

Epidemiology of Esophageal Cancer (EC)

- >14,500 cases of EC and >13,700 deaths (in year 2006).
- Incidence has increased dramatically over the past four decades.
- Median age at diagnosis is 67 years.
- Over 50% of patients are incurable/palliative at diagnosis.

Types of EC

- Two major histologic subtypes: squamous cell carcinoma and adenocarcinoma.
- Squamous cell carcinomas occur throughout the esophagus, while adenocarcinomas are usually located in the distal third of the esophagus or at the gastro-esophageal junction.
- Stable/declining squamous cell carcinoma incidence, while incidence of adenocarcinoma has grown greatly (e.g., fourfold increase in Caucasian men over a decade period).

Risk Factors

- Squamous cell carcinoma is strongly associated with heavy cigarette smoking and alcohol consumption, previous traumatic injury to the esophagus (including ionizing radiation), esophageal anatomic abnormalities (e.g., achalasia, esophageal webs, and Zenker's diverticula), and history of other diseases with similar risk factors such as head and neck cancers. Familial tylosis (nonepidermolytic palmoplantar keratoderma) is a known risk factor.
- Adenocarcinoma of the esophagus is associated with BE, chronic gastroesophageal reflux symptoms, obesity, higher socioeconomic classes, and only somewhat associated with tobacco use.

Barrett's Esophagus (BE)

- BE is the replacement of the normal stratified squamous epithelial lining of the distal esophagus with specialized columnar epithelium normally seen in the stomach or intestine.
- This intestinal metaplasia can transform into dysplastic tissue with distorted glandular architecture, hyperchromatism, and nuclei crowding that can transform further into frank cancer.
- Annual rates of cancer transformation from BE range from 0.5% to 1.0%/year, while high-grade dysplasia transforms at over 10–15%/year.

Screening

- Unclear whether screening is cost-effective and which groups to screen. Chronic gastro-esophageal reflux affects up to 10% of the US adult population and may be too broad as an eligibility criterion. Individuals with BE develop low-grade, high-grade dysplasia and cancer at a rate of approximately 4%, 1%, and 0.5% per year, respectively, and may be reasonable candidates to screen every 3–5 years (1). A diagnosis of dysplasia would lead to more frequent endoscopies.

DIAGNOSIS AND STAGING

History and Physical Exam

- Seventy five percent of EC patients have dysphagia; 50% have weight loss; 25% complain of gastroesophageal reflux; and <25% complain of odynophagia.

Endoscopy

- Usually diagnostic when combined with tissue biopsy. Common findings are ulceration and friable masses.

CT Scanning

- Contrast-enhanced computed tomography of the chest, abdomen, and pelvis is used to detect distant spread (metastases).

Endoscopic Ultrasound (EUS)

- Patients with nonmetastatic disease on CT scan may benefit from EUS and EUS-guided needle biopsies, most commonly used to detect liver and locoregional lymph nodes spread. EUS is also a reasonable tool for T-staging.

PET Scanning

- FDG-positron emission tomography is used more commonly now as a staging tool, primarily to detect occult metastatic disease. Laporascopy and laporotomy, both invasive staging techniques, are rarely necessary since the advent of both CT and PET scanning.

Staging

- See Table 43-1 for TNM staging; see Table 43-2 for AJCC staging.
- Preoperative staging of EC is often difficult. Standard noninvasive techniques are imprecise, particularly the use of CT scans for T- and N-staging (only 50–80% accuracy). EUS has an accuracy of 80–90%. This imprecision has led to treating patients with locally advanced EC across stages similarly.
- The current staging reflects registration data of mainly upper and mid-thoracic squamous cell carcinomas from Japan from over 20 years ago.
- T4NanyM0 disease (partial definition for stage III and IVA) is generally considered unresectable due to inability to achieve clean surgical margins.

Prognosis

- Table 43-2 also shows ranges of survival by stage. Overall 5 year survival rates are approximately 15%.

Table 43-1

TNM Staging for EC

TX: Primary tumor cannot be assessed
T0: No evidence of primary tumor
Tis: Carcinoma in situ
T1: Tumor invades lamina propria or submucosa
T2: Tumor invades muscularis propria
T3: Tumor invades adventitia
T4: Tumor invades adjacent structures
NX: Regional lymph nodes cannot be assessed
N0: No regional lymph node metastasis
N1: Regional (mediastinal/intrathoracic) lymph node metastasis
MX: Distant metastasis cannot be assessed
M0: No distant metastasis
M1: Distant metastasis
  For tumors of the lower thoracic esophagus:
    M1a: Metastasis in celiac lymph nodes
    M1b: Other distant structures
  For tumors of the midthoracic esophagus
    M1a: not applicable
    M1b: Nonregional lymph nodes and/or other distant metastasis
  For tumors of the upper thoracic esophagus:
    M1a: Metastasis in cervical nodes
    M1b: Other distant metastasis

Table 43-2

AJCC Staging

Stage	T	N	M	5 Year survival (%)	General category
0	Tis	N0	M0	>95	Preinvasive
I	T1	N0	M0	60–80	Early stage
IIA	T2-3	N0	M0	30–40	Node-negative locally advanced
IIB	T1-2	N1	M0	10–30	Node-positive locally advanced
III	T3	N1	M0	5–15	Node-positive locally advanced
	T4	Any	M0		Unresectable locally advanced
IVA	T1-3	Any	M1a	<5	Node-positive locally advanced or metastatic
	T4	Any	M1a		Unresectable locally advanced or metastatic
IVB	Any	Any	M1b	<1	Metastatic

- Patients with metastatic disease have a median survival of less than 1 year.
- Staging is the most important prognostic variable. In addition to higher stage, poor prognostic factors include significant weight loss (>10% of baseline), significant dysphagia, large tumors, older patients, and lymphovascular spread.

TREATMENT

Surgical and Invasive Approaches

- Several approaches to esophagectomy have been used: (a) In the transhiatal approach, the anastamosis is between the cervical esophagus and the stomach (in the neck). (b) In another approach, the stomach is mobilized through the abdomen, and then anastomosis occurs with either the cervical or upper thoracic esophagus after a transthoracic esophagectomy.
- Both approaches have similar quality-adjusted survival and median disease-free survival.

Radiation

- Conventional dose radiation (total 45–50 gray) is potentially useful in conjunction with chemotherapy for the first-line treatment of locally advanced EC. New planning strategies (3D, conformal, intensity modulated) may further reduce toxicity to adjacent anatomic structures.
- At lower doses in the palliative setting, it can relieve obstruction by tumor.
- Radiation is used rarely to cure locally advanced and early stage EC because results with radiation alone are far inferior to combined chemoradiation.

Chemotherapy

- Platinum-based chemotherapy is active in EC (Table 43-3). The platinum agent (usually cisplatin) is combined with at least another agent, usually 5-fluorouracil, irinotecan, an anthracycline or a taxane.
- Older regimens including variations of stomach cancer treatments, such as FAMTX (5FU, adriamycin, methotrexate), have been superseded by these newer regimens.

TREATMENT BY STAGE (TABLE 43-4)

High-Grade Dysplasia, Carcinoma in Situ and Early Stage ECs

- Stage 0 and I cancers are usually treated with esophagectomy with excellent prognosis.
- High-grade dysplasia is also an indication for esophagectomy, since the rate of occult frank carcinoma is frequent, and transformation rates may approach 50% in some studies. Mucosal ablation and photodynamic therapy (PDT) are being considered for the frail.
- Older patents in good health should be offered esophagectomy.

Table 43-3

Common Combination Chemotherapeutic Regimens

Regimen	Example of dose and schedule
Cisplatin (C) + 5FU (F)	C: 25 mg/m^2 days 1–4 q28 days F: 1,000 mg/m^2 days 1–4 Continuous Infusion q28 days
Cisplatin (C) + taxane	C: 75 mg/m^2 D1 q21 days paclitaxel: 200 mg/m^2 D1 q21 days
Cisplatin (C) + irinotecan (I)	C: 35 mg/m^2 D1, 8 q21 days I: 60 mg/m^2 D1, 8 q21 days

Table 43-4

General Treatment Guidelines for EC

Category	Treatment
Preinvasive	Esophagectomy
Early stage	Esophagectomy
Locally advanced	
Node-negative	Neoadjuvant chemo, neoadjuvant chemoradiation, surgery alone, or adjuvant chemoradiation[*],[**]
Node-positive	Neoadjuvant chemo, neoadjuvant chemoradiation, surgery alone, or adjuvant chemoradiation[*],[**]
Unresectable (T4)	Chemoradiation, palliative radiation, or palliative chemotherapy[**]
Metastatic	Palliative chemotherapy, palliative radiation

[*]Upper third and cervical ECs are more often treated without surgery (since occult involvement of trachea would preclude resection), while mid and lower third ECs are more often treated with surgery (with or without other modalities).

[**] Lack of consensus reflects imprecision of staging, changing histology/location of tumors, variable chemotherapeutic, and radiation regimens, all of which contributed to conflicting results from multiple randomized controlled studies.

Locally Advanced EC

SURGERY

- Surgery alone has survival rates about approximately 30–35%. Thus, the role of "adding" other therapies either adjuvantly (after surgery) or neoadjuvantly (prior to surgery) has been the focus of much research.
- Conflicting data exist as to whether platinum-based chemotherapy improves survival of locally advanced ECs when used neoadjuvantly/adjuvantly, alone or when combined with radiation.

DEFINITIVE CHEMORADIATION

- Definitive chemoradiation can result in up to 25% survival, significantly better than with radiation alone (<5–10%). However, standard treatments generally have included surgery as the backbone of therapy, relegating definitive chemoradiation to individuals with unresectable T4 lesions, or in the medically inoperable.

PREOPERATIVE CHEMOTHERAPY

- For preoperative (neoadjuvant) chemotherapy, a 440 patient Intergroup study found no benefit(2), but a 800 patient British study found benefit favoring preoperative chemotherapy (survival rate improved from 34% to 43%)(3). It is difficult to reconcile these disparate results even with the differences in study design.

TRIMODALITY THERAPY

- Preoperative chemoradiation (or trimodality therapy, since surgery is also performed) has been evaluated in at about a dozen randomized studies in the past few decades. The results are contradictory, in part, because of different radiation and chemotherapy regimens and because the majority of studies were underpowered (total $n = 60–80$). Until recently, Walsh et al. had the only positive study favoring trimodality treatment,(4) but the study was criticized because the benefit likely came from an unexpectedly poor survival from the standard surgery-only arm. Two larger studies with over 100 patients per arm had negative results, but one employed a higher toxicity radiation regimen,(5) while the other employed suboptimal doses of chemotherapy and radiation(6). A recent small ($n = 56$) but well-designed Intergroup study did find a significant benefit to trimodality therapy(7).

- Neoadjuvant therapy has become commonplace in the US despite the lack of a definitive large study.

ADJUVANT CHEMORADIATION   Macdonald et al.(8) evaluated both gastric/gastro-esophageal junction cancers and found that 5FU-based chemotherapy with a chemoradiation component given after surgery improved survival. Unfortunately, 80% of the patients had gastric cancer and only 20% had gastro-esophageal junction adenocarcinoma, so the applicability across histologic subtypes and to other tumor locations is unknown.

TREATMENT OF INVOLVED CELIAC LYMPH NODES   Another problematic group is the stage IVA patients with distal esophageal adenocarcinoma and celiac node involvement or IVB patients solely on the basis of gastrohepatic ligament node involvement. These individuals could be treated as locally advanced EC, since their involved nodes could fall within an acceptable radiation field, but their prognosis is worse than stage II/III patients. Hence, some institutions will group these patients with locally advanced patients, while others will group with the metastatic patients. As expected, individualization of therapy in the absence of good data will hinge on other factors such as patient preference or baseline health of patient.

SUMMARY

- Evidence is available arguing to treat ECs with surgery alone, with neoadjuvant platinum-based chemotherapy, with trimodality therapy, or with adjuvant 5FU-based chemotherapy (for gastro-esophageal junction cancers only). No consensus exists for how to treat these locally advanced EC.
- In practice, small T2N0 tumors may be treated with surgery alone, while node-positive individuals are strongly considered for neoadjuvant or adjuvant therapy.

Metastatic or Recurrent EC

- EC (whether adenocarcinoma or squamous cell carcinoma) may respond to chemotherapy. In the palliative setting, 15–30% partial responses have been documented for 5FU, a taxane or irinotecan, while combining one or more of these agents with cisplatin increases partial response rates to 35–50%.
- Typical responses last only several months and overall survival is under 1 year. The chance of response must be weighed against risks of side effects on an individual basis.

SPECIAL COMPLICATIONS

Obstruction (Dysphagia)

GENERAL APPROACH

- Surgery is a most effective palliation tool. Unfortunately, many patients are unresectable; under these circumstances, cisplatin-based palliative chemotherapy and/or radiation are both reasonable alternatives. Balloon

dilatation, expandable metal stents, laser ablation, and PDT are other methods to treat obstruction or dysphagia.
- For palliative purposes, partial obstructions can be treated with expandable esophageal stents, laser therapy, electrocoagulation to destroy the obstructing portion of the cancer, and PDT.

ESOPHAGEAL STENTS

- Expandable esophageal stents are placed endoscopically and brace the wall of the esophagus, keeping tumors from compressing the lumen. Potential complications include tumor bleeding (the stent makes it difficult to reach the bleeding vessels to coagulate or inject with epinephrine); stent migration (stents moving out of position) particularly if concurrent radiation or chemotherapy shrinks the tumor; and obstructing growth around and beyond the esophageal stent. Thus, stents are used practically after other local modalities of therapy have failed. Newer removable stents may be useful to patients undergoing neoadjuvant therapy to allow oral feeding; if the stent migrates, then it can be removed. Finally, stents have one added problem: if the cancer is in the distal esophagus or gastro-esophageal junction, then the stent may actually keep open the gastro-esophageal junction permanently. This can lead to debilitating acid reflux symptoms.

PHOTODYNAMIC THERAPY (PDT)   PDT treatment uses a photosensitizing drug that is activated into cell-killing free-radicals in the presence of a particular wavelength of light. After intravenous injection of this drug, the patient is shielded from light for a few weeks to keep from developing skin toxicity. In the meantime, an endoscope is inserted and a high-intensity light of the appropriate wavelength is shone directly onto the tumor. This causes tumor necrosis and can open up a lumen. PDT is not used more commonly because of the major side effect of having to keep the patients away from all sources of ultraviolet and natural light for several weeks after injection.

Airway-Esophageal Fistula

- This life-threatening complication may result from tumors of the upper thoracic and cervical esophagus. Fistulas form from the direct invasion of the airway by tumor or by tumor necrosis after radiation or chemoradiation.
- >50% involve the trachea.
- >50% have cough, 37% have aspiration symptoms, and 25% have systemic symptoms of infection (fever or pneumonia). Expandable metal stents are excellent tools to seal these fistulas.

REFERENCES

1. Shaheen N, Ransohoff DF. Gastroesophageal reflux, Barrett's esophagus, and esophageal cancer: scientific review. J Am Med Assoc. 2002; 287: 1972–81.
2. Kelsen DP, Ginsberg R, Pajak TF, et al. Chemotherapy followed by surgery compared with surgery alone for localized esophageal cancer. N Engl J Med. 1998; 339: 1979–84.
3. Medical Research Council Oesophageal Cancer Working Group. Surgical resection with or without preoperative chemotherapy in oesophageal cancer: a randomised controlled trial. Lancet. 2002; 359: 1727–33.
4. Walsh TN, Noonan N, Hollywood D, et al. A comparison of multimodal therapy and surgery for esophageal adenocarcinoma. N Engl J Med. 1996; 335: 462–7.
5. Bosset JF, Gignoux M, Triboulet JP, et al. Chemoradiotherapy followed by surgery compared with surgery alone in squamous-cell cancer of the esophagus. N Engl J Med. 1997; 337: 161–7.

6. Burmeister BH, Smithers BM, Gebski V, et al. Surgery alone versus chemora-diotherapy followed by surgery for resectable cancer of the oesophagus: a ran-domised controlled phase III trial. Lancet Oncol. 2005; 6: 659–68.

7. Krasna M, Tepper JE, Niedzwiecki D, et al. Trimodality therapy is superior to surgery alone in esophageal cancer: results of CALGB 9781. Proc Am Soc Clin Onc Gastrointest Symp. 2006; 3: (abstract)4.

8. Macdonald JS, Smalley SR, Benedetti J, et al. Chemoradiotherapy after surgery compared with surgery alone for adenocarcinoma of the stomach or gastroe-sophageal junction. N Engl J Med. 2001; 345: 725–30.

GASTRIC CANCER

Although the incidence of gastric cancer has steadily declined in the United States for over half a century, it remains the second most common cause of cancer-related mortality throughout the world. Over half of all gastric cancers occur in developing countries with the highest incidence in East Asia, South America (Andes Region), and Eastern Europe. Following migration to areas of lower risk, subsequent generations experience a risk approaching that of the surrounding population, implicating an important role for environmental factors on the development of gastric cancer. In the United States, an estimated 22,280 new cases were diagnosed and 11,430 deaths occurred due to gastric cancer in 2006 (1). Advances in prevention, early detection, aggressive surgery, the use of adjuvant therapy, and more effective antineoplastic agents will hopefully reduce the incidence and improve survival.

RISK FACTORS

- Diets rich in salty or smoked foods, nitroso compounds, low in vegetable, and antioxidants.
- Helicobacter pylori infection, which is dependent on genotype and host factors (polymorphisms).
- Smoking increases the risk by about 1.5-fold.
- Atrophic gastritis increases the risk by nearly sixfold.
- Prior gastric surgery with the highest risk at 15–20 years. The risk is greater following Billroth II than Billroth I anastomosis.
- Ionizing radiation was associated with a relative risk of 3.7 in survivors of the Japanese atomic bomb.
- Blood group A is associated with a 20% higher incidence.
- Low-socioeconomic group results in an increase in distal cancers, whereas high-socioeconomic group increases the risk of proximal cancers.
- Epstein–Barr virus associated gastric cancer is related to DNA methylation of promoter genes of various cancer-associated genes. They may have a more favorable prognosis.
- Several familial syndromes have been associated with a predisposition to gastric cancer: hereditary nonpolyposis colorectal cancer (HNPCC)/Lynch syndrome, E-cadherin mutation (diffuse type), familial adenomatous polyposis, and Peutz–Jeghers syndrome.

PATHOLOGY

Intestinal Type (Expanding)

The intestinal type of gastric cancer is characterized by the formation of distinct glands, and typically involves the cardia, corpus, or antrum. It is often associated with mutlifocal (atrophic) gastritis and intestinal metaplasia of the antrum, as well as pernicious anemia, older age, male sex, and various environmental factors, including H. pylori. There has been a dramatic decrease in the incidence of this form of gastric cancer in developing countries.

Diffuse Type (Infiltrative)

The diffuse type of gastric cancer often presents as linitus plastica. It is characterized by poorly organized clusters or signet-ring cells (mucin containing). They often arise in the corpus and affect a generally young population. There is a propensity for these tumors to develop in patients with superficial gastritis related to H. pylori without atrophy or metaplasia, as well as those who have the type A blood group. Familial clusters are common. These tumors generally tend to be more aggressive than the intestinal type.

SIGNS AND SYMPTOMS

Abdominal pain and weight loss are common presenting complaints. Nausea and vomiting are more commonly seen with distal tumors, whereas early satiety is more common with linitus plastica tumors. Gastric cancers may bleed, leading to hematemesis, melena, and anemia. Malignant ascites, resulting in increased abdominal girth, is more commonly seen in patients with linitus plastica.

DIAGNOSIS AND STAGING

- Physical examination may be remarkable for cachexia, abdominal distension, hepatomegaly in the case of liver metastases, and lymphadenopathy.
- Upper GI series may demonstrate a stricture at the GE junction in the case of GE junction cancers, a filling defect along the gastric wall, or decreased distensibility of the stomach due to a linitis plastica tumor.
- Esophagogastroduodenoscopy is the mainstay of diagnosis. Deep biopsies are often necessary if linitis plastica is suspected as the tumor tends to infiltrate the submucosa. A single biopsy of a malignant ulcer has a 70% sensitivity rate of diagnosis and seven biopsies increase the sensitivity to 98%.
- Endoscopic ultrasound aids in determining the depth of invasion, which may be important for clinical trial considerations.
- CT scan of the chest abdomen and pelvis is important for the identification of metastatic disease. CT imaging is 40–60% accurate in assessing depth of invasion and nodal involvement.
- Bone scan is typically reserved for patients with symptoms suggesting osseous metastases.
- PET scan's role has not entirely been defined, but may be most helpful in identifying occult metastatic disease.
- Laparoscopy may detect occult peritoneal or hepatic metastases too small to be appreciated by CT scan.
- Tumor markers including CEA and CA 19-9 are sometimes helpful in monitoring patients but are frequently not elevated.

STAGING (AJCC)

The American Joint Committee on Cancer is the system used for gastric cancer staging in most countries (2). The T-classification is based on depth of invasion (T1 invades the lamina propria or submucosa, T2a invades the muscularis propria, T2b invades the subserosa, T3 penetrates the serosa, and T4 invades adjacent structures), nodal status (N0 signifies no nodal involvement, N1 indicates 1–6 nodes involved by tumor, N2 indicates 7–15, and N3 indicates > 15 nodes involved by tumor), and absence or presence of metastases (M0 versus M1). The 5 year survivals for resected gastric cancer are as follows: stage Ia (T1N0M0) 78%, stage Ib (T2N0M0 or T1N1M0) 58%, stage II (T1N2M0, T2N1M0 or T3N0M0) 34%, stage IIIA (T2N2M0,

T3N1M0 or T4N0M0) 20%, stage IIIB (T3N2M0) 8%, and stage IV (T4 NanyM0, T1-3N3M0 or TanyNanyM1) 7% (3).

TREATMENT OF LOCALIZED DISEASE

Surgery

Approximately 50% of gastric cancers present with locoregional disease. The 5 year survival of patients with gastric cancer is only 15–20%, but in those with disease only involving the stomach, the 5 year survival is 50%. Survival falls to about 20% once the regional nodes are involved by tumor. Curative surgery typically consists of a subtotal or total gastrectomy. Although the incidence of gastric cancer has been decreasing, the rate of proximal gastric cancer and cancers of the gastroesophageal (GE) junction have increased dramatically. These more proximal tumors are associated with a poorer prognosis than their distal counterparts.

- Distal tumors–tumors arising in the distal two thirds of the stomach are typically amenable to subtotal gastrectomy.
- Proximal tumors are usually managed with a total gastrectomy.
- Linitus plastica tumors are diffusely infiltrative, more commonly seen in young, and typically metastatic at the time of diagnosis. If surgery is indicated, a total gastrectomy is the preferred operation.
- GE junction tumors are divided into several types:
  - Type I—esophageal carcinoma extending to the GE junction or arising in Barrett's esophagus. These typically require both a transthoracic and transabdominal approach.
  - Type II—arising within 2 cm of the squamocolumnar junction. These may be amenable to a transabdominal approach alone.
  - Type III—tumors arising in the subcardial region. These may be amenable to a transabdominal approach.
- Superficial lesions may be amenable to less invasive approaches:
  - Endoscopic mucosal resections (EMR)—may be performed in T1 tumors < 2 cm in size, without lymphatic invasion and no evidence of nodal metastases, although this is not commonly practiced in the Unites States as finding such early stage tumors is uncommon. In countries where endoscopic screening is widespread, such as Japan, early tumors are more commonly discovered and EMR employed.
  - Photodynamic therapy—a photosensitizing agent is administered and then the stomach is exposed to a laser.

Lymph Node Dissection

The magnitude of lymph node dissection has remained a contentious area of debate in the surgical management of gastric cancer. For many years, the Japanese have advocated for an extended lymph node dissection in which the lymph nodes of the perigastric (D1 dissection), in addition to the lymph nodes of the hepatic, left gastric, celiac, splenic arteries, and splenic hilum (D2 dissection) as well as the nodes in the porta hepatis and periaortic areas (D3 dissection), are removed. Proponents of the extended lymph node dissection argue that patients will be more accurately staged, leading to a better stage-related survival. Such aggressive dissections may require a distal pancreatectomy and splenectomy, leading to considerable additional morbidity. Randomized trials have failed to demonstrate an improvement in survival for the more aggressive dissections.

ROLE OF ADJUVANT THERAPY

Despite advances in staging and operative techniques, the long-term survival for patients undergoing resection for gastric cancer remains under 50%. Investigators have evaluated the role of chemotherapy and radiation in both the preoperative (neoadjuvant) and postoperative setting.

Gastric Cancer

Many randomized trials comparing surgery versus radiation or chemotherapy failed to demonstrate an improvement in survival; however, meta-analyses have suggested a benefit. The Gastrointestinal Intergroup Study (0116) randomized 556 patients with GE junction and gastric cancers postoperatively to receive bolus 5-fluorouracil (5FU) and leucovorin by the Mayo Clinic schedule for one cycle, followed by an abbreviated course of 5FU and leucovorin for two cycles with 45 Gy of radiation, and then completing with two more cycles of 5FU and leucovorin, versus no further therapy (4). The median overall, 3 year survival and disease-free survival, favored the adjuvant therapy group: 36 months, 50%, and 30 months versus 27 months, 41%, and 19 months, respectively. Although a D2 resection was recommended, only 10% had such an extensive surgery and 54% had a D0 resection, which would be considered an inadequate surgery. Since this study was conceived, more effective chemotherapy regimens have been developed. This study established a new standard of care for the management of patients with resected gastric cancer. The Cancer and Leukemia Group B is currently comparing epirubicin, cisplatin, and 5FU (ECF) to the treatment arm of INT-0116 in CALGB-80101. Both arms receive radiation therapy, but instead of administering it with bolus 5FU and leucovorin, 5FU is administered as a continuous infusion. Gastrectomy is major surgery and many patients are unable to complete the prescribed chemoradiation due to postoperative complications or impaired performance status. A major criticism of the INT-0116 study is the inadequate lymph node sampling, and it is suggested that radiation may be more beneficial in such a population. In the MAGIC (MRC Adjuvant Gastric Infusional Chemotherapy) Trial, the Medical Research Council randomized 237 patients with lower esophageal and gastric cancers to receive three cycles of ECF prior to and following surgery, versus surgery alone (5). Patients underwent endoscopic ultrasound as part of their preoperative staging. The median, 5 year and progression-free survivals, favored the treatment arm: 24 months, 36%, and 19 months, versus 20 months, 23%, and 13 months, respectively. A significant reduction in tumor size was also appreciated: 5 cm versus 3 cm. Based on these trials, adjuvant therapy is considered the standard of care, but the exact role of radiation therapy and the benefit of neoadjuvant versus postoperative adjuvant therapy are yet to be determined.

Gastroesophageal Junction Cancer

The role of adjuvant and neoadjuvant chemotherapy in the management of esophageal cancers is discussed elsewhere in this text. GE junction cancers are typically included in clinical trials of esophageal cancer and gastric cancer. Both the INT-0116 and MAGIC trial demonstrated improvements in survival for patients who received adjuvant chemotherapy with or without chemoradiation. It would therefore appear prudent to offer these patients adjuvant therapy. This group of patients is often managed differently based on the bias of the institution and whether they are cared for by thoracic or gastrointestinal multidisciplinary teams. One could argue that the more proximal GE junction tumors be treated as esophageal cancers, where the debate over adjuvant therapy is still ongoing.

MANAGEMENT OF ADVANCED AND METASTATIC DISEASE

The median survival for patients with metastatic gastric cancer is approximately 4 months. GE junction and gastric cancer most commonly metastasize to the liver, abdominal cavity, and lymph nodes (perigastric, retroperitoneal, left supraclavicular and left axillary), but also metastasize to the ovaries (Krukenberg tumor), lung, bone, and brain. Patients may experience complications related to the primary tumor that require intervention. These includes pain, early satiety, nausea, and vomiting due to obstruction, and bleeding, which may be managed conservatively with pain medications, promotility agents, stent placement, and external beam radiation. Palliative resection may improve symptom control and perhaps survival, but there is no proven benefit in performing total gastrectomy. Management of malignant ascites may be challenging in these patients, requiring frequent paracenteses if not permanent peritoneal catheter placement. Malignant ascites is more commonly seen in young patients, particularly women, and in those with poorly differentiated or signet-ring cell carcinoma. Hepatic metastases are more commonly seen in patients with well moderately differentiated tumors, and more frequently in males. Systemic chemotherapy is the cornerstone of therapy for these patients. Several randomized trials have now demonstrated an improvement in survival for those receiving chemotherapy.

Systemic Chemotherapy

Multiple chemotherapy agents have documented activity in this disease. These include 5FU (and capecitabine), mitomycin-C, cisplatin, irinotecan, epirubicin, paclitaxel, and docetaxel. Single-agent response rates are generally up to 20%. Many combinations have been tested, and most of them contain 5FU as the backbone (See Tables 44-1 and 44-2). Based on these studies, ECF and DCF should be considered standard regimens; however, the combination of irinotecan and cisplatin is considered by many to be an appropriate first line regimen due to its activity in phase II trials and acceptable toxicity profile. The TAX 325 trial reported a very high-adverse event rate, including 82% grade 3–4 neutropenia and a 30 day mortality (postlast infusion) of about 12% and a toxic death rate of 6.3%. An unfavorable feature of the ECF regimen is the need to wear the infusional 5FU continuously, without break. The REAL 2 trial demonstrated noninferiority for the substitution of capecitabine for 5FU and oxaliplatin for cisplatin.

Table 44-1.

Selected Phase II Trials

Author	Regimen	N	RR (%)	TTP (months)	Survival (months)
Ajani (6)	Irino[a]/CDDP[b]	36	58	6	9
Pozzo (7)	Irino/FU[c]/FA[d]	59	42.4	6.5	10.7
	Irino/CDDP	56	32.1	4.2	6.9
				(P < 0.0001)	(P = 0.0018)
Louvet (8)	FOLFOX[e]	53	44.9	6.2	8.6

[a]irino-irinotecan, [b]CDDP-cisplatin, [c]FU5-fluorouracil, [d]FA-folinic acid, [e]FOLFOX-5-fluorouracil, leucovorin (folinic acid), and oxaliplatin.

Table 44-2.

Selected Phase III Trials

Author	Regimen	N	RR (%)	TTP (months)	Survival (months)
Webb, et al (9)	ECF[a]	126	45	7.4	8.9
	FAMTX[b]	130	21	3.3	5.7
			(P < 0.001)	(P < 0.001)	(P < 0.001)
Cunningham, et al (10)	ECF	263	37.7	6.2	9.9
	EOF[c]	245	40.4	6.5	9.3
					(HR = 0.95)
	ECX[d]	250	40.8	6.7	9.9
					(HR = 0.92)
	EOX[e]	244	46.8	7.0	11.2
					(HR = 0.80)
Van Cutsem, et al (11)	DCF[f]	227	37	5.6	9.2
	CF[g]	230	25	3.7	8.6
			(P = 0.011)	(P < 0.001)	(P = 0.02)
Dank, et al. (12)	IFL[h]	170	31.8	5.0	9.0
	CF	63	25.8	4.2	8.7
			(P = 0.125)	(P = 0.088)	(P = 0.530)

[a]ECF-epirubicin, cisplatin, and 5-fluorouracil, [b]FAMTX-5-fluorouracil, doxorubicin, and methotrexate, [c]EOF-epirubicin, oxaliplatin, and 5-fluorouracil, [d]ECX-epirubicin, cisplatin, and capecitabine, [e]EOX-epirubicin, oxaliplatin, and capecitabine, [f]DCF-docetaxel, cisplatin, and 5-fluorouracil, [g]CF-cisplatin and 5-fluorouracil, [h]IFL-irinotecan, 5-flourouracil, and leucovorin.

REFERENCES

1. Jemal, A, Siegel, R, Ward, E, et al. Cancer statistics 2006. CA Cancer J Clin. 2006; 56: 106–130.
2. American Joint Committee on Cancer. In FL Greene, Page, DL, Fleming, ID, et al (eds.), "AJCC Cancer Staging Handbook," 6th edition. Springer, New York, 2002, p. 111.
3. Hundahl SA, Phillips JL, Mevick, HR, et al. The national cancer data base report on poor survival of US gastric carcinoma patients treated with gastrectomy. Cancer 2000; 88: 921–932.
4. MacDonald JS, Smalley SR, Benedetti J, et al. Chemoradiotherapy after surgery compared with surgery alone for adenocarcinoma of the stomach or gastroesophageal junction. N Engl J Med. 2001; 345: 725–730.
5. Cunningham D, Allum WH, Stenning SP, et al. Perioperative chemotherapy versus surgery alone for resectable gastroesophageal cancer. N Engl J Med. 2006; 355: 11–20.
6. Ajani JA, Baker J, Pisters PWT, et al. CPT-11 plus cisplatin in patients with advanced untreated gastric or gastroesophageal junction carcinoma: results of a phase II study. Cancer. 2002; 94: 641–646.
7. Pozzo C, Barone C, Szanto J, et al. Irinotecan in combination with 5-fluorouracil or with cisplatin in patients with advanced gastric or esophageal junction adenocarcinoma: results of a randomized phase II study. Ann Oncol. 2004; 15: 1773–1781.
8. Louvet C, Andre T, Tigaud JM, et al. Phase II study of oxaliplatin, fluorouracil, and folinic acid in locally advanced or metastatic gastric cancer patients. J Clin Oncol. 2002; 20: 4543–4548.
9. Webb A, Cunningham D, Scarffe JH, et al. Randomized trial comparing epirubicin, cisplatin and fluorouracil versus fluorouracil, doxorubicin and methotrexate in advanced esophagogastric cancer. J Clin Oncol. 1997; 15: 261–267.

10. Cunningham D, Rao S, Starling N, et al. Randomised multicentre phase III study comparing capecitabine with fluorouracil and oxaliplatin with cisplatin in patients with advanced oesophagogastric (OG) cancer: the REAL 2 trial. ProcASCO. 2006; 24: LBA 4017.

11. van Cutsem E, Moiseyenko VM, Tjulandin S, et al. Phase III study of docetaxel and cisplatin plus fluorouracil compared with cisplatin and fluorouracil as first-line therapy for advanced gastric cancer: a report of the V325 study group. J Clin Oncol. 2006; 24: 4991–4997.

12. Dank M, Zaluski J, Barone C, et al. Randomized phase III trial of irinotecan (CPT-11) + 5FU/folinic acid (FA) vs CDDP + 5FU in 1st-line advanced gastric cancer patients. ProcASCO 2005; 23: 308s, abstract 4003.

PANCREATIC CANCER

INTRODUCTION

For most patients, pancreatic adenocarcinoma remains highly lethal. Less than 5% survive 5 years after diagnosis. Surgical resection is the only curative treatment. However, the cure rate with surgery is only 18–25% and most patients are not surgical candidates. Patients with unresectable disease can have symptoms palliated by chemotherapy and/or radiation therapy. However, these have not significantly impacted 5 year survival. Improved understanding of pancreatic cancer biology continues to provide new therapeutic ideas. Trials are evaluating whether new approaches to earlier diagnosis or improvements in radiation therapy, chemotherapy (including targeted therapy), and/or immunotherapy (e.g., vaccines) can impact survival.

INCIDENCE AND EPIDEMIOLOGY

- Increases with age, slight male predominance, increased incidence in African Americans, variation in prevalence by world region (higher in western Europe, Scandinavia, the United States, and New Zealand) (1).
- Risk factors for pancreatic adenocarcinoma include (2, 3)

  Environmental

  - Cigarette smoking, history of diabetes mellitus, previous radiation therapy to the pancreas as treatment for other malignancies (such as Hodgkin's disease, or testicular cancer) and chronic relapsing pancreatitis (especially that due to genetic risk factors); increased body mass index may be a risk factor.

  Genetic

  - Mutations in: p16; mismatched repair genes (hMSH2 and hMLH1); BRCA1 (rare pancreatic cancers); BRCA2; STK11/LKB1 (Peutz–Jeghers syndrome); ataxia telangectasia (AT); p53 (Li–Fraumeni syndrome); APC (familial adenomatous polyposis); von Hippel-Lindau (VHL); cationic trypsinogen; and cystic fibrosis transmembrane regulator (CFTR) genes (4, 5).
  - Families with increased risk of pancreatic cancer without as get defined genetic abnormalities.
  - Overall, approximately 5–10% of patients with pancreatic cancer will have a first-degree relative who develops pancreatic cancer (2–5).

PATHOLOGY

Normal pancreatic cell types include ductal, acinar, endocrine/neuroendocrine, connective tissue support, endothelial, and lymphocytes. Malignancies can arise from each cell type. Approximately 90% are adenocarcinomas derived from duct cells with approximately two-thirds arising in the head, and one-third being in the body/tail or multicentric (4, 6, 7). Other histologic subtypes of ductal origin include pleomorphic carcinomas, giant cell carcinomas, microglandular adenocarcinomas, and cystic neoplasms. Cystic neoplasms comprise a small but increasingly identified subgroup of pancreatic tumors (6). They can be divided into serous cyst adenomas (usually benign) and mucinous cystadenocarcinomas. A higher percentage of these tumors occur in middle-aged women as compared to ductal adenocarcinomas. They appear to be divided into a group that has benign or borderline malignant cells with good prognosis and a group with carcinoma that metastasizes widely and has a prognosis similar to that of other ductal adenocarcinomas. Pancreatic papillary cystic tumors tend to occur in women of reproductive years with relatively good prognosis after surgical excision. There are also noncystic mucin producing tumors of the pancreas that tend to have a better prognosis after surgical excision. Acinar cell carcinomas make up 1–2% of pancreatic cancers. Acinar cell tumors occur most commonly in the elderly, but they also occur in younger patients and comprise a higher percentage of tumors seen in children. Overall, adult patients with acinar cell carcinomas tend to have a slightly better clinical course than those with ductal adenocarcinomas. Children have a better prognosis (7). Uncommon pancreatic tumors include pancreatic inflammatory tumors and small cell undifferentiated carcinomas. Tumors with mixed histologies including adenosquamous carcinomas and carcinosarcomas can occur and tend to have a poor prognosis. Pancreatoblastomas are rare neoplasms arising from multipotential cells that can differentiate into mesenchymal, endocrine, or acinar cells which occur primarily in children, although rare cases can occur in adults. They frequently have elevated alpha feto protein levels and are potentially curable when localized. Metastatic pancreaticoblastomas are often responsive to chemotherapy. Other pancreatic tumors found in children include solid psuedopapillary tumors, pancreatic endocrine neoplasms, PNET, and acinar cell tumors (7).

Endocrine cell cancers comprise approximately 5–10% of pancreatic tumors (8). Although associated with longer survival than pancreatic adenocarcinomas, they frequently metastasize. Lymphomas, sarcomas, and other mesenchymal tumors (e.g., teratomas, schwannomas, and neurofibromas) make up only a small proportion of pancreatic cancers (less than 2%). Their biology is similar to that of malignancies of similar histology arising in other areas of the body.

A wide variety of neoplasms can metastasize to the pancreas, including breast, lung, melanoma, renal, gastrointestinal, and other sites.

BIOLOGY OF PANCREATIC ADENOCARCINOMA

Pancreatic adenocarcinomas have frequently invaded locally and/or metastasized by the time initially detected. Local spread is directly to soft tissues and adjacent organs (9, 10). They tend to metastasize widely including lymph nodes, liver, peritoneum, lungs, adrenal glands, and, less commonly, bone and brain.

The biology of pancreatic ductal adenocarcinoma has provided targets for earlier diagnosis, potential therapy, and possible avenues for prevention in the future (4–6, 9, 10). Frequent mutations have been found in proteins involved in cell signaling pathways (especially K-ras-(70–90%)) as well as a number of tumor suppressor genes (p53, p16, and DPC4/Smad4). A number of growth factor receptor families, including insulin-like growth factor receptors, the epidermal growth factor receptors (EGFRs), and fibroblast growth factor receptors are highly expressed in a proportion of pancreatic adenocarcinomas. The life-span of cells is limited by shortening of telomeric DNA at chromosomal ends. Telomerase (the enzyme important in maintaining telomeric DNA at chromosomal ends) activity is elevated in a high percentage of pancreatic carcinomas.

The potential role of some of the mutations found in familial pancreatic cancer (e.g,. BRCA2 or mismatched repair genes) in the development of non-hereditary pancreatic cancers is unclear. The frequency of these mutations in sporadic cases is low. Tumors that have mutations in mismatched repair genes but not Ras genes are characterized by the appearance of "pushing borders" on histopathology and a better prognosis.

PRESENTING SYMPTOMS AND SIGNS

The initial symptoms produced by pancreatic cancer are insidious. Most patients have nonspecific symptoms for several months prior to diagnosis (9, 10). Tumors in the head of the pancreas sometimes produce obstruction of the bile duct and therefore jaundice at a relatively earlier stage, although most of these tumors are still unresectable. Fatigue, weight loss, anorexia, abdominal pain, back pain, jaundice/light stools/dark urine/pruritus (for head lesions), nausea, vomiting, early satiety, dyspnea, and glucose intolerance are the most common presenting symptoms. Depression is seen in a significant percentage of patients. There is a relatively high incidence of blood clot formation and some patients present with thrombophlebitis. Patients who develop verices (due to portal or splenic vein obstruction) can present with hematemesis or ascites. Ascites may also be due to metastatic disease to the peritoneum.

DIAGNOSTIC WORKUP

The diagnosis should be considered in individuals who present with the above symptoms, especially with several symptoms. A careful history should be obtained including review for the above symptoms, history of cigarette smoking or other risk factors, and a family history. Physical exam should include evaluation for evidence of weight loss, lymph node enlargement (especially in the supraclavicular or periumbilical areas), jaundice, hepatosplenomegaly, ascites, peripheral edema, and evidence of coagulopathy. For most patients, findings on physical exam are nonspecific.

Laboratory tests should include a complete blood count (CBC) and liver function tests, although, in general, laboratory studies are nonspecific and not particularly helpful in making a diagnosis. CA19-9 is the most useful tumor marker and is elevated in 70–90%. Although not useful as a screening tool due to relative nonspecificity, it is useful in helping to follow a patient's therapeutic response. Although less frequent, CEA is occasionally elevated in patients who do not have CA19-9 elevations and can be used to follow response to therapy.

Radiological evaluation plays a key role. Computerized tomographic (CT) scan currently is the most commonly used modality for assessing for a pancreatic mass, potential vascular invasion, and determining whether the tumor has metastasized. Alternatively, MRI can be utilized. Pulmonary metastases in the absence of abdominal metastases are relatively uncommon but can occur and imaging of the chest is also important.

Pathology is ultimately required to make a diagnosis. Biopsies of either the pancreas or nodal lesions can be obtained at the time of endoscopic ultrasound (EUS). These theoretically carry less potential risk of peritoneal seeding than percutaneous biopsies. Although ideally a diagnosis can be made preoperatively, for patients with a potentially resectable pancreatic mass, surgery is often necessary in any case even if the initial fine needle biopsy was not diagnostic. For patients with unresectable disease, percutaneous biopsy under radiological guidance of either the pancreas itself or of a metastatic lesion is usually obtained.

STAGING AND TREATMENT DECISIONS

The American Joint Commission on Cancer (AJC) staging system with the TNM format is utilized to group patients into stages I–IV. Although different stages by the TNM classification have prognostic significance (i.e., survival decreases with increasing stage), for purposes of treatment decisions, there are three groups of patients that need to be defined: potentially resectable, localized but unresectable, and metastatic. Once pancreatic cancer is diagnosed, the most important question is whether it is potentially resectable. Unless findings on physical exam or radiological studies indicate that the disease is already metastatic, findings from CT/MRI scans, including a careful evaluation of the question of vascular involvement by the tumor, are usually the critical factor in helping determine potential resectability. Tumors are generally considered unresectable if there is (1) metastatic disease; (2) encasement or occlusion by the tumor of the superior mesenteric vein (SMV) or SMV–portal vein confluence; or (3) direct involvement by the tumor of the aorta, celiac plexus, inferior vena cava (IVC), or the superior mesenteric artery (SMA). FDG positron emission tomography (PET) scanning has been shown to have good sensitivity in detecting potentially metastatic disease and may be helpful, but a definitive role has not yet been established. As newer approaches combining CT or MRI with PET imaging are developed and enhanced, they may allow the best features of each technique to be combined for staging patients.

EUS is increasingly being utilized as part of staging. This can be combined with endoscopic retrograde cholangiography (ERCP) for stent placement allowing both diagnostic information and a palliative approach for maintaining bile duct patency in patients who do not have potentially resectable disease.

If preliminary staging findings indicate that the tumor is potentially resectable, then the next step is either laparoscopic staging or proceeding directly to exploratory laparotomy with resection, if possible. There remains debate about the exact value of laparoscopic staging and this is an area of ongoing study.

SURGERY

There are four main surgical approaches for resecting pancreatic cancer depending on the exact nature of the disease (9, 10). These are (1) the pancreaticoduodenectomy (Whipple's procedure with various modifications that are utilized by different surgeons), (2) total pancreatectomy, (3) regional or extended pancreatectomy, and (4) distal pancreatectomy and splenectomy. Pancreaticoduodenectomies are the most commonly performed procedure for lesions in the head of the pancreas or peri-ampullary lesions. Distal pancreatectomy with splenectomy is usually used for body and tail lesions. Laparoscopic approaches are being used with increased frequency, and their exact role is being defined in ongoing studies. Morbidity and mortality after surgery for pancreatic cancer have significantly declined with most centers reporting mortality rates less than 2–5%. Median survival is approximately 18 months with approximately 20% of patients alive at 5 years. Features associated with a lower cure rate include increased tumor size, positive margins, or positive lymph nodes.

Palliative surgical approaches to delay or prevent biliary and duodenal obstruction are utilized for patients who undergo exploration but are not resectable. The major alternatives to surgical palliation of biliary and gastrointestinal obstruction are endoscopically placed stents. Stenting of the gastrointestinal tract itself remains of somewhat limited efficacy, although improvements in stents have allowed this to be used more commonly.

RADIATION ± CHEMOTHERAPY IN THE ADJUVANT OR NEO-ADJUVANT SETTING

Clinical trials have not yet established a definitive role for preoperative, intraoperative, or postoperative radiation therapy utilized alone for improving survival of patients who have resected pancreatic cancer (9, 10). Intraoperative radiotherapy (IORT) may increase local control rate but has not yet been shown to affect overall survival. Improvements in delivery of IORT make this an area of continued study. Even when local control can be achieved with radiation therapy, the primary issue remains that the majority of patients die from metastatic disease.

Most adjuvant or neo-adjuvant trials have utilized combined modality therapy integrating surgery and chemotherapy ± radiation (9–12). A randomized GI Tumor Study Group (GITSG) trial of combined postoperative treatment (external beam radiation therapy (EBRT) and chemotherapy (5FU)) and subsequent nonrandomized trials at a number of centers suggest that adjuvant or neo-adjuvant chemotherapy and radiation therapy may lead to a longer survival than surgery alone. In contrast, recent randomized trials from Europe (ESPAC1) have not shown a statistically significant improvement in survival for combined chemotherapy and radiation therapy although they have shown a survival benefit for chemotherapy.

Thus, despite trials suggesting benefit, overall evidence remains inconclusive as to whether adjuvant chemotherapy plus radiation therapy produce a long-term survival advantage for resected pancreatic cancer patients. In an attempt to better define the roles of radiation and chemotherapy in this setting, additional studies are currently ongoing. Since a number of studies have shown same survival benefit for chemotherapy, there is general consensus that adjuvant chemotherapy is of volume. In the USA, radiation therapy is also usually given.

A number of studies have evaluated the potential for neo-adjuvant chemotherapy (primarily 5FU based) alone or combined with EBRT to enhance the ability to adequately deliver adjuvant therapy to a higher percentage of patients and potentially to convert what appear to be unresectable lesions to resectable ones. Most of these studies indicate an overall ability to resect approximately 10–15% of lesions that were deemed unresectable prior to therapy. Since it is not possible to be certain what percentage of these patients would have been resectable without neo-adjuvant therapy, the magnitude of the benefit cannot be absolutely defined. However, the potential benefit of neo-adjuvant therapy utilizing current chemotherapy approaches appears to be relatively limited for this purpose. At present, the emphasis of those pursuing neo-adjuvant therapy is focused on trying to define better therapeutic approaches, especially utilizing newer agents. Eventually randomized studies will be needed to establish whether neo-adjuvant therapy would lead to enhanced survival as compared with postoperative adjuvant therapy.

PATIENTS WITH LOCALIZED BUT UNRESECTABLE DISEASE

Chemotherapy ± Radiation Therapy for Unresectable Patients

Definitive radiation therapy is not curative for the vast majority of patients whose tumors cannot be resected (9–11). However, it can palliate symptoms (especially pain) and possibly lead to slight survival prolongation. Addition of 5FU-based chemotherapy may increase survival over that seen with radiation therapy alone but this benefit is modest. A number of studies are currently addressing the question of whether other agents, such as gemcitabine, taxanes, oxaliplatin, or cisplatin, alone or in combination with each other, or in combination with 5FU and/or radiation might enhance efficacy.

Systemic chemotherapy alone can provide palliation for some patients with locally advanced disease. Since a randomized study of gemcitabine based chemotherapy versus chemoradiation in this setting has not been done, it is not possible to determine the relative merits of each of these. At present, combined therapy with both chemotherapy and radiation therapy remains the most commonly used standard approach for locally advanced disease.

CHEMOTHERAPY FOR METASTATIC DISEASE

Overall, median survival of patients with metastatic pancreatic cancer is short with ranges of 5–8 months in most large series (9, 10). The most active single agents produce response rates in the 5–20% range and there is minimal impact of treatment on 2 year survival. Clinical benefit may be seen in a slightly higher percentage of patients with approximately 25% achieving short-term clinical benefit with gemcitabine which is the standard agent based on a randomized trial that showed a slight survival advantage as compared with 5-fluorouracil (5FU). The standard schedule gives gemcitabine over 30 min once weekly. Phase II trials have suggested that giving the gemcitabine infusion over a slightly longer period (dose rate schedule) might improve its antitumor activity. This has been further evaluated in a randomized trial (results pending).

Other agents with some activity against pancreatic cancer include 5FU (including oral capecitabine), taxanes (most frequently docetaxel), oxaliplatin, cisplatin, camptothecins, and erlotinib (small molecule EGFR inhibitor). A number of combinations of agents with gemcitabine have been evaluated in phase III studies compared to gemcitabine alone, but the only two that have shown a survival advantage are gemcitabine and erlotinib, and gemcitabine and capecitabine. However, even for these the evidence for additional benefit is either modest (increase of approximately 2 weeks in median survival with erlotinib) or there are other phase III studies that have not shown a survival benefit (gemcitabine plus 5FU). Information from additional studies evaluating these and other combinations should help guide the next steps in improving therapy.

HORMONAL AND IMMUNOTHERAPY

There is no evidence for significant antitumor benefit for either hormonal or immunotherapy. The utilization of vaccine therapy for patients with resected pancreatic cancer is currently being studied, although there is not yet clear evidence for benefit.

FUTURE THERAPEUTIC DIRECTIONS

Given the limited effectiveness of current approaches against pancreatic cancer, continued studies of disease biology and clinical trials are vital in making progress (9, 10). Perhaps most promising for the future are therapies based on increased understanding of the biological processes important for proliferation, survival, or metastasis of neoplastic pancreatic cells. Compounds developed using biochemical and molecular biological approaches to target these are already providing new agents for testing in the treatment of this disease.

MANAGEMENT OF SYMPTOMS

Supportive care and management of symptoms are vitally important (9, 10). The majority of patients will develop significant pain at some point. Management includes opioid analgesics, nonsteroidals, acetaminophen, and other analgesic agents. Celiac plexus blocks can be utilized if the pain cannot be controlled by medication. Malnutrition is a significant problem. Pancreatic enzymes can sometimes help ameliorate malabsorption. Antacids may be useful in both enhancing the benefit of pancreatic enzymes and decreasing reflux symptoms. Megestrol acetate, dronabinol, or steroids can help stimulate appetite in some patients. There is a relatively high incidence of depression. This is often in the setting of increased anxiety, fatigue, and loss of any ambition making it more difficult to treat. A multidisciplinary approach to palliate symptoms is often helpful, including pain and palliative care teams.

ENDOCRINE PANCREATIC TUMORS

Islet cell tumors make up less than 10% of pancreatic cancers (8). Different functional tumors (producing symptoms related to hormone(s) that are produced) can occur or they may be nonfunctional. Types of tumors include insulinomas, glucagonomas, somatostatinomas, gastrinomas, Vipomas, PPomas, GRFomas, ACTHomas, carcinoids, tumors that produce hypercalcemia, and nonfunctioning tumors. Tumors can produce more than one peptide hormone. Except for insulinomas (which have a lower risk of metastasizing), they have similar clinical features and are malignant in the majority of cases. They tend to metastasize to lymph nodes and liver. Certain of these tumors can occur as part of multiple endocrine neoplasia syndrome I (MEN-I). MEN-I is an autosomal dominant trait that is associated with tumors or hyperplasia of multiple endocrine organs, often including pancreatic endocrine tumors (most frequently gastrinomas or insulinomas).

General treatment principles are similar for most of these tumors, although there are specific aspects of each that need to be addressed as well. Treatment includes surgical resection when that can be done especially for cure. Even when curative surgery may not be feasible, palliative cytoreduction may be of value in controlling symptoms. Symptoms can be ameliorated utilizing agents that block the effects of produced hormones. Many of these tumors can have symptoms somewhat palliated by somatostatin analogs. Although somatostatin analogs do not significantly increase long-term survival, they can markedly improve quality of life. A number of chemotherapeutic agents have some activity against these tumors. However, they are not curative, and overall activity of any one agent or combination is limited. Recent evidence suggests that dacarbazine (or its oral equivalent temozolamide) has moderate activity, and this continues to be explored both alone and in combination. Interferon a has also been utilized either alone or in combination with octreotide and/or chemotherapy to control disease for variable periods of time although a recent study did not show additional benefit over that with octreotide alone. Hepatic arterial embolization or chemoembolization can palliate symptoms in patients with functional tumors and a significant tumor burden in the liver. Radiolabeled octreotide is being pursued as a potential means of relatively specifically targeting those tumors that are positive on octreotide scan, although the exact clinical value has not yet been established.

LYMPHOMAS AND SARCOMAS

Lymphomas and sarcomas arising within the pancreas are both uncommon neoplasms. The most important issue is establishing the diagnosis histologically, so that appropriate staging and therapeutic decisions can be made. For the most part these malignancies behave with a similar clinical course to tumors of the same histology arising in other organs.

SUMMARY

Pancreatic adenocarcinoma remains a disease with poor long-term survival. Curative surgery is only achievable in a relatively small percentage of patients. Clearly, improvements in earlier diagnosis and continued development and evaluation of novel treatment approaches are needed. Clinical trials are evaluating the efficacy of approaches combining new antitumor agents, radiation therapy, and surgery. Chemotherapeutic agents are being studied alone or in combinations with each other or newer agents (e.g. targeted agents, vaccines) for treatment of patients with metastatic disease.

Despite limited clinical progress, significant advances in information about cellular and molecular biology of pancreatic cancers have been made. The nature of biological mechanisms (such as angiogenesis) important for growth and metastasis of cancers within the host are being elucidated. Increased knowledge about the molecular origins and progression of pancreatic cancer has led to evaluation of novel approaches specifically targeting proteins important for cancer cell proliferation or survival. These include vaccines, gene therapy, monoclonal antibodies, and small-targeted molecules. Improved understanding of how the immune system functions and therefore how it might be utilized for control of malignant cells has led to renewed efforts to try to develop effective vaccine therapy. Continued development of these exciting new approaches is needed to improve treatment of this usually fatal disease. Enhanced understanding of the biology of pancreatic cancer should also provide avenues to pursue for prevention and earlier detection with prospects for decreasing deaths from pancreatic cancer.

REFERENCES

1. Chang KJ, Parasher G, Christie C, et al. Risk of pancreatic adenocarcinoma: disparity between African Americans and other race/ethnic groups. Cancer. 2005; 103: 349–357.
2. Lowenfels AB, Maisonneuve P. Risk factors for pancreatic cancer. J Cell Biochem. 2005; 95: 649–656.
3. Michaud DS. Epidemiology of pancreatic cancer. Minerva Chir. 2004; 59: 99–111.
4. Sakorafas GH, Tsiotos GG. Molecular biology of pancreatic cancer: potential clinical implications. BioDrugs. 2001; 15: 439–452.
5. Hahn SA, Bartsch DK. Genetics of hereditary pancreatic carcinoma. Clin Lab Med. 2005; 25: 117–133.
6. Brugge WR, Lauwers GY, Sahani D, et al. Cystic neoplasms of the pancreas. N Engl J Med. 2004; 351: 1218–1226.
7. Shorter NA, Glick RD, Klimstra DS, et al. Malignant pancreatic tumors in childhood and adolescence: The Memorial Sloan–Kettering experience, 1967 to present. J Pediatr Surg. 2002; 37: 887–892.
8. Clark OH, Ajani J, Benson AR, et al. Neuroendocrine tumors. J Natl Compr Cancer Netw. 2006; 4: 102–138.
9. Tempero MA, Behrman S, Ben-Josef E, et al. Pancreatic adenocarcinoma: clinical practice guidelines in oncology. J Natl Compr Canc Netw. 2005; 3: 598–626.
10. Lockhart AC, Rothenberg ML, Berlin JD. Treatment for pancreatic cancer: current therapy and continued progress. Gastroenterology. 2005; 128: 1642–1654.
11. Eckel F, Schneider G, Schmid RM. Pancreatic cancer: a review of recent advances. Expert Opin Investig Drugs 2006; 15: 1395–1410.
12. Regine WF, Abrams RA. adjuvant Therapy for pancreatic cancer: current status, future directions. Semin oncol 2006; 33: 510–513.

Andrew X. Zhu

HEPATOCELLULAR CARCINOMA

INTRODUCTION

Hepatocellular carcinoma (HCC) is the most common primary cancer of the liver, accounting for more than 90% of primary liver cancer. Worldwide, HCC is the fifth most common cancer and the third most common cause of cancer-related death (1). In the United States, 18,510 new cancers of the liver and intra-hepatic bile duct are expected in 2006, with an estimated 16,200 deaths (2). The incidence rates for HCC in the United States continue to rise steadily through 1998 and have doubled during the period 1975–1995 (3, 4). Treatment outcomes are dependent on the clinical stage at diagnosis. While patients with early stage HCC can be cured by surgical resection or liver transplantation, unresectable or metastatic HCC carries a poor prognosis with a median survival of 6–8 months.

EPIDEMIOLOGY AND RISK FACTORS (TABLE 46-1)

HCC is a heterogeneous disease in terms of etiology and underlying associations with significant geographic variation in distribution worldwide. It occurs most frequently in Southeast Asia and sub-Saharan Africa. The prevalence of HCC in these areas is more than 100/100,000 population, whereas in Europe and North America it is estimated as 2–4/100,000 population.

HCC develops commonly, but not exclusively, in a setting of liver cell injury, which leads to inflammation, hepatocyte regeneration, liver matrix remodeling, fibrosis, and ultimately cirrhosis. The major etiologies of liver cirrhosis are diverse and include chronic hepatitis B (HBV) and C (HCV), alcohol consumption, certain medications or toxic exposures, and genetic metabolic diseases. More than 80% of HCC occurs in HBV-infected populations worldwide. The geographic distribution of HCC correlates with the prevalence of HBV. HCC incidence is greatest in Eastern Asia and sub-Saharan Africa, which correlates with the highest rates of chronic HBV infection in these areas. It is estimated that HBV infection may increase the risk of developing HCC more than 100-fold. The incidence of cirrhosis is approximately 25–50% in HBV infection.

Table 46-1

Risk Factors for HCC

HBV
HCV
Alcohol
Aflatoxin B
Hemochromatosis
α1-antitrypsin deficiency
Hereditary tyrosinemia
Porphyria cutanea tarda
Wilson's disease
Primary biliary cirrhosis
Oral contraceptives
Nonalcoholic steatohepatitis (NASH)

HCV infection has been increasingly recognized as another serious risk factor for HCC. It is estimated that approximately 3.9 million people in the United States and 100 million people worldwide are infected with HCV. Approximately 70–80% HCV-infected patients will develop chronic HCV infection and 15–20% will eventually develop cirrhosis. Once cirrhosis develops, HCC will develop at a rate of 1–4 % per year with 5–10 % of all patients with chronic HCV infection developing HCC eventually.

Aflatoxin B1 (AFB1), produced by the fungi *aspergillus flavus* and *aspergillus parasiticus*, is also a significant risk factor for HCC in endemic areas. Humans are exposed to AFB1 by eating contaminated rice, corn, peanuts, or products of animals that have ingested contaminated food. The highest exposure to AFB1 occurs in southern China and southern Africa. Interestingly, p53 mutations are common in HCC in these areas and a specific mutation in the p53 gene has been identified. AFB1 appears to be synergistic with HBV exposure for the development of HCC.

PATHOLOGY

HCCs range from well-differentiated to highly anaplastic undifferentiated lesions. Macroscopically they can be nodular, massive, or diffuse types. The fibrolamellar variant of HCC usually occurs in young patients and is more common in women. It is usually not associated with HBV or HCV and cirrhosis and tends to have a better prognosis. Rarely, a mixed HCC–cholangiocarcinoma variant can be seen. The two cellular components may be separate, adjacent to each other, or intimately mixed.

CLINICAL FEATURES

Presentation varies according to the size and location of the HCC lesions and the presence and severity of underlying cirrhosis. Small tumors are often detected on ultrasound performed for other reasons or during screening. Some patients may have mild to moderate upper abdominal pain, weight loss, early satiety, or a palpable mass in the upper abdomen. These symptoms often indicate a large lesion. Obstructive jaundice may develop due to the invasion of the biliary tree, compression of the intrahepatic duct, or, rarely, as a result of hemobilia. Ascites can be seen due to underlying cirrhosis, portal hypertension, or peritoneal disease. Patients may have diarrhea. Bony pain, dyspnea on exertion, chest pain, or cough may occur due to the presence of metastatic disease. Intraperitoneal bleeding as a result of tumor rupture is a serious complication, which is associated with sudden onset of severe abdominal pain with distension, an acute drop in the hematocrit and hypotension. This is usually seen in patients with underlying HBV infection without cirrhosis. Fever may develop in HCC, which could be related to the presence of central tumor necrosis.

Paraneoplastic syndromes include hypercalcemia, hypoglycemia, erythrocytosis, hypercholesterolemia, dysfibrinogenaemia, carcinoid syndrome, and sexual changes due to hormonal imbalance (gynecomastia, testicular atrophy, precocious puberty) can develop. Several cutaneous changes including porphyria cutanea tarda, dermatomyositis, and pemphigus foliaceus can occur in HCC.

DIAGNOSIS

The diagnosis of HCC can be difficult, and often requires the use of serum markers, one or more imaging modalities, and histologic confirmation. If the diagnosis of HCC is considered, a careful history should be taken to inquire potential risk factors for HCC and family history for hereditary liver disease.

A careful physical examination should focus on findings of hepatomegaly, liver mass, and other signs of cirrhosis. Complete blood counts, liver function tests, HBV/HCV serology, prothrombin time, and serum alfa-fetoprotein (AFP) are usually performed. Due to the absence of pathognomonic symptoms and the liver's large functional reserve, HCC is frequently diagnosed late in its course. For patients with underlying cirrhosis or chronic HBV or HCV infection, the diagnosis of HCC is often suspected with a rising serum AFP level or the appearance of a new hepatic lesion on ultrasound. A CT scan of the liver and/or magnetic resonance imaging (MRI) study should be pursued to better characterize the lesion(s). In cirrhotic patients, any dominant solid nodule that is hypervascular with increased T2 signal intensity, presence of venous invasion, or associated elevated AFP should be considered a HCC unless proven otherwise. If surgical resection will be performed, a preoperative biopsy may not be necessary to confirm the diagnosis if the lesion is characteristic of and highly suspicious for HCC. Biopsy carries a small risk of tumor seeding of the needle tract and increased complications in cirrhotic patients.

For noncirrhotic patients, the diagnosis of HCC should be considered for any hepatic lesion that is not clearly a hemangioma or focal nodular hyperplasia. In the absence of specific clues to the diagnosis, biopsy would be appropriate.

AFP is a glycoprotein that is normally produced during gestation by the fetal liver and yolk sac with a half-life of approximately 6 days. AFP is the most commonly used marker in HCC and is elevated in approximately 80% of patients with HCC. Elevated serum AFP can also be seen in pregnancy, with tumors of gonadal origin, and in patients with chronic HBV or HCV hepatitis without HCC. Not all HCCs secrete AFP, and serum AFP concentrations are normal in up to 20% of HCCs. For patients with HCC, those with underlying viral hepatitis are more likely to have elevated AFP than those with alcoholic disease. The sensitivity, specificity, and predictive value for the serum AFP in the diagnosis of HCC depends upon the characteristics of the population under study, the cutoff value chosen for establishing the diagnosis, and the gold standard used to confirm the diagnosis. Using a cutoff value of >20 ng/ml, it has a sensitivity of approximately 60% and a specificity of 90%. Unfortunately, serum AFP has a low positive predictive value, particularly in a population with low HCC prevalence.

STAGING AND PROGNOSTIC SCORING SYSTEMS

The AJCC TNM staging system (identical to that of the Union Internationale Contre le Cancer (UICC)) is the most widely used staging system, which was last revised and simplified in 2002. This system recognizes the importance of vascular invasion by the tumor and underlying liver fibrosis as most important predictors of prognosis. The presence and degree of severe cirrhosis or fibrosis can be used to stratify outcome for every tumor (T) classification.

A number of prognostic scoring systems, including the Okuda system, the Cancer of the Liver Italian Program (CLIP) score, the Barcelona Clinic Liver Cancer (BCLC) staging classification, and the Chinese University Prognostic Index (CUPI), have been proposed to predict the prognosis for HCC. These systems incorporate some of the other important factors for prognosis including the severity of underlying liver disease, the extent of the tumor, extension of the tumor into portal vein, the presence of metastases, and performance status.

SURGICAL TREATMENTS

Surgical resection or orthotopic liver transplantation (OLT) represents the only potential curative treatments for HCC, associated with significant prolongation of survival.

Surgical Resection

The aim of surgical resection is to remove the entire portal territory of the neoplastic segment(s) with clear margins, while preserving maximum liver parenchyma to avoid hepatic failure. Due to the presence of extrahepatic disease, severe underlying cirrhosis, anatomical location of tumor, and vascular invasion, less than 20% of HCC are suitable for surgical resection. Patients ideally suited for partial hepatectomy include a solitary HCC confined to the liver with no radiographic evidence of invasion of the hepatic vasculature, no evidence of portal hypertension, and well-preserved hepatic function. The surgical outcome is dependent on the institutional experience and patient selection. Estimated 5 year survival rates are in the range of 26–50%, and disease-free survival is 13–29%.

Liver Transplantation

OLT is a curative option for HCC. Selection for appropriateness for liver transplant often uses the "Milan" criteria which is based on data indicating that the long-term survival of HCC patients who undergo liver transplantation is highest in patients with either a single lesion ≤ 5 cm or 3 lesions ≤ 3 cm each and no evidence of gross vascular invasion (5). Based on a retrospective review of liver transplantations performed in the United States during three time intervals between 1987 and 2001, a significant improvement in survival over time was found to be associated, in part, with changes in the patient selection criteria. The current 1 and 5 year survival rates for HCC patients undergoing OLT are 77.0% and 61.1%, respectively (6). However, a major challenge with OLT is the long waiting time for donor organs. In the United States, liver allocation for adults is based upon the "model for end stage liver disease" or MELD score (7). Nevertheless, even with higher priority MELD scores, waiting times for a donor organ may be as long as 1 year. Bridging therapy with transarterial chemoembolization (TACE), radiofrequency ablation (RFA), or partial hepatectomy may be considered, while a patient with HCC is on the waiting list for an OLT.

LIVER DIRECTED LOCALIZED TREATMENTS

Table 46-2 lists some of the liver directed localized treatment options for HCC. The limitations of these approaches include the size, number, and location of the lesion(s), portal vein involvement, and the presence of micrometastatic disease. In general, these approaches are operator/institution dependent. Of all the liver directed treatment modalities, TACE and RFA are the most commonly used.

The observation that the majority of the blood supply to HCCs is derived from the hepatic artery has led to the development of techniques designed to decrease the blood supply to the tumor or to administer cytotoxic chemotherapy directly to the tumor. TACE, a technique combining intrahepatic arterial chemotherapy and selected ischemia using embolic particles, has been studied extensively. Despite several earlier negative studies, a modest survival advantage has been demonstrated in two randomized controlled trials and a meta-analysis in highly selected patients (8, 9). In the study by Lo and colleagues, only 80 of 279 Asian patients presenting with unresectable HCC fulfilled the strict entry criteria. The actuarial survival was significantly higher in the treated group at 1, 2, and 3 years (57%, 31%, and 26%, respectively) compared to controls (32%, 11%, and 3%, respectively) (9). In the second study by Llovet et al., only 112 of 903 assessed HCC patients were eligible. The 1 and 2 year survival probabilities were significantly greater with chemoembolization (82% and 63%) but not arterial embolization (75% and 50%) when compared to control (63% and 27%) (8). Several chemotherapeutic agents including cisplatin and doxorubicin have been commonly used in transarterial chemotherapy.

Table 46-2

Localized Treatment Options for HCC

Hepatic artery transcatheter treatment
   Transarterial embolization
   Transarterial chemotherapy
   Transarterial chemoembolization
   Transarterial radioembolization
Local ablative therapy
   Ethanol
   Acetic acid
   Radiation
   Radiofrequency
Debulking surgery
   Palliative resection
   Cryosurgery
   Microwave surgery

Contraindications to TACE include portal vein thrombosis, encephalopathy, biliary obstruction, and severe underlying cirrhosis (Child–Pugh C). TACE should be limited to the minimum number of procedures necessary to control the tumor to minimize the risk of hepatic decompensation.

For patients with small HCC who are poor surgical candidates due to impaired liver function or serious comorbid medical conditions, local ablative therapy represents another treatment option. Percutaneous ethanol injection (PEI) and RFA are commonly used. The outcomes are better with small lesions for both PEI and RFA, in particular, lesions less than 4 cm in size. Several studies have demonstrated improved outcomes for RFA over PEI with respect to local recurrence-free survival.

SYSTEMIC TREATMENT

Despite extensive efforts by many investigators, systemic chemotherapy for HCC has been quite ineffective, as evidenced by low response rates and no demonstrated survival benefit. HCCs are heterogeneous due to the multiple etiologies and risk factors and may have different pathways in hepatocarcinogenesis. The underlying cirrhosis in most patients may lead to portal hypertension with hypersplenism, platelet sequestration, varices and gastrointestinal bleeding, hepatic encephalopathy, hypoalbuminemia, differential drug binding and distribution, and altered pharmacokinetics, limiting the selection and adequate dosing of most cytotoxic agents. HCCs are inherently chemotherapy-resistant tumors and are known to express the multidrug resistant gene MDR-1.

The finding that various hormone receptors including estrogen receptors are present on HCC has led many investigators to examine the role of hormonal manipulation in this disease. Despite earlier reports showing significantly improved survival in patients treated with tamoxifen, several subsequent larger randomized studies failed to demonstrate improved survival with tamoxifen.

Although a large number of controlled and uncontrolled studies have been performed with most classes of chemotherapeutic agents, no single or combination chemotherapy regimen is particularly effective in HCC. The response rate tends to be low and the response duration is short. More importantly, the survival benefit of systemic chemotherapy for HCC has not been demonstrated. Agents with limited activity include doxorubicin, 5FU, interferon, and cisplatin, with doxorubicin being the most widely used agent. Several combination chemotherapy regimens have been tested in HCC including gemcitabine combined with oxaliplatin (GEMOX), and the combination of cisplatin, alpha-interferon, doxorubicin, and 5FU (PIAF). Despite the initial encouraging results with PIAF with a 26% response rate in a phase II study, a subsequent large phase III study comparing PIAF with doxorubicin failed to demonstrate overall survival benefits with PIAF regimen (10).

Improved understanding of the mechanisms of hepatocarcinogenesis coupled with the arrival of many newly developed molecularly targeted agents with better safety profiles has provided the opportunity to study some of these targeted agents in advanced HCC. Agents currently being tested at different phases of clinical trials include bevacizumab (avastin), BAY43-9006 (sorafenib), and erlotinib (tarceva).

In the absence of standard systemic therapy, patients with advanced HCC should be encouraged to participate in clinical trials. Patients with poor performance status and severe underlying cirrhosis should be offered best supportive care.

REFERENCES

1. Parkin DM, Bray F, Ferlay J, et al. Estimating the world cancer burden: Globocan 2000. Int J Cancer. 2001; 94(2): 153–156.
2. Jemel A, Siegel R, Ward E, et al. Cancer statistics, 2006. CA Cancer J Clin. 2006. 56(2): p. 106–30.
3. El-serag HB, Mason AC. Rising incidence of hepatocellular carcinoma in the United States. N Engl J Med. 1999; 340(10): 745–750.
4. El-serag HB, Davila JA, Petersen NJ, et al. The continuing increase in the incidence of hepatocellular carcinoma in the United States: an update. Ann Intern Med. 2003; 139(10): 817–823.
5. Mazzaferro V, Regalia E, Doci R, et al. Liver transplantation for the treatment of small hepatocellular carcinomas in patients with cirrhosis. N Engl J Med. 1996; 334(11): 693–699.
6. Yoo HF, Patt CH, Geschwind JF, et al. The outcome of liver transplantation in patients with hepatocellular carcinoma in the United States between 1988 and 2001: 5-year survival has improved significantly with time. J Clin Oncol. 2003; 21(23): 4329–4335.
7. Kamath PS, Wiesner RH, Malinchoc M, et al. A model to predict survival in patients with end-stage liver disease. Hepatology. 2001; 33(2): 464–470.
8. Llovet JM, Real MI, Montana X, et al. Arterial embolisation or chemoembolisation versus symptomatic treatment in patients with unresectable hepatocellular carcinoma: a randomised controlled trial. Lancet. 2002; 359(9319): 1734–1739.
9. Lo CM, Ngan H, Tso WK, et al. Randomized controlled trial of transarterial lipiodol chemoembolization for unresectable hepatocellular carcinoma. Hepatology. 2002; 35(5): 1164–1171.
10. Yeo W, Mok TS, Zee B, et al. A randomized phase III study of doxorubicin versus cisplatin/interferon alpha-2b/doxorubicin/fluorouracil (PIAF) combination chemotherapy for unresectable hepatocellular carcinoma. J Natl Cancer Inst. 2005; 97(20): 1532–1538.

CHOLANGIOCARCINOMA AND
GALLBLADDER CANCERS

INTRODUCTION

Biliary tract cancers (BTC) are invasive carcinomas that arise from the epithelial lining of the gallbladder and bile ducts. The term cholangiocarcinoma has been used to refer to bile duct cancers arising in the intrahepatic, perihilar, or distal biliary tree, exclusive of gallbladder or ampulla of Vater (Figure 47-1). Tumors involving the proper hepatic duct bifurcation are collectively referred to as Klatskin tumors. The vast majority of cholangiocarcinomas and gallbladder cancers are adenocarcinoma. While anatomically these malignancies are related and have similar metastatic patterns, each has a distinct clinical presentation, molecular pathology, and prognosis. This group of tumors is characterized by local invasion, extensive regional lymph node metastasis, vascular encasement, and distant metastases. Complete surgical resection offers the only chance for cure; however, only 10% of patients present with early-stage disease and are considered surgical candidates. Among those patients who do undergo "curative"

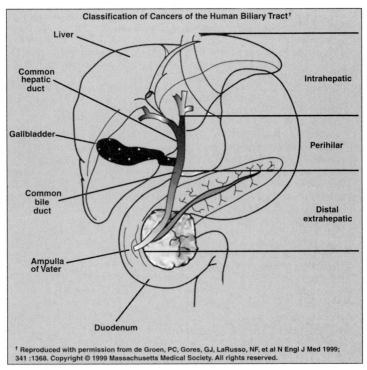

Classification of Cancers of the Human Biliary Tract[†]

Liver

Common hepatic duct

Intrahepatic

Gallbladder

Perihilar

Common bile duct

Distal extrahepatic

Ampulla of Vater

Duodenum

FIGURE 47-1 Classification of biliary tract cancers. (From deGroen PC, Gores GJ, LaRusso NF, et al. N Engl J Med. 1999; 341. Copyright © 1999 Massachusetts Medical Society. All rights reserved.)

resection, recurrence rates are high. Patients with unresectable or metastatic BTC have a poor prognosis with median overall survival of less than a year.

EPIDEMIOLOGY AND RISK FACTORS

It is estimated that there are 8,570 new cases of BTC and 3,260 deaths in the United States, in 2006 (1) Since intrahepatic bile duct cancers are included with primary livers cancers in the national databases, the total number of BTC is unknown.

Cholangiocarcinomas account for approximately 3% of all gastrointestinal (GI) malignancies, with an incidence in the United States being one or two cases per 100,000 people.

For unclear reasons, the incidence of intrahepatic cholangiocarcinoma has been rising over the past two decades in Europe and North America, Asia, Japan, and Australia, while rates of extrahepatic cholangiocarcinoma are declining internationally.

In the United States, GBC is the fifth most common GI cancer, and the most common involving the biliary tract. In contrast to the general population, GBC is the most common GI malignancy in both Southwestern Native Americans and in Mexican-Americans. Worldwide, there is a prominent geographic variability in GBC incidence that correlates with the prevalence of cholelithiasis. High rates of GBC are seen in Chile, Bolivia, Japan, and Southeast Asia. Incidence steadily increases with age, women are affected two to six times more often than men, and GBC is more common in Caucasians than in blacks.

The risk factors for cholangiocarcinoma and GBC are shown in Table 47-1. For cholangiocarcinoma, these include primary sclerosing cholangitis (PSC), congenital abnormalities of the biliary tree (Caroli's syndrome, congenital hepatic fibrosis, choledochal cysts), parasitic infection of the liver flukes of the genera Clonorchis and Opisthorchis, hepatolithiasis, toxic exposures including radiologic contrast agent thorotrast (a radiologic contrast agent banned in the 1960s for its carcinogenic properties), Lynch syndrome II and multiple biliary papillomatosis, and possibly hepatitis C infection (2).

PSC is strongly associated with ulcerative colitis (UC) with the incidence of colitis around 90% in patients with PSC. Nearly 30% of cholangiocarcinomas are diagnosed in patients with UC and PSC. The annual incidence of cholangiocarcinoma in

Table 47-1

Risk Factors for Biliary Tract Cancers

Cholangiocarcinoma
      Primary sclerosing cholangitis (PSC)
      Congenital abnormalities of the biliary tree (Caroli's syndrome, congenital hepatic fibrosis, choledochal cysts)
      Parasitic infection of the liver flukes
      Hepatolithiasis
      Toxic exposures including thorotrast
      Lynch syndrome II and multiple biliary papillomatosis
      ?Hepatitis C infection
Gallbladder cancer
      Gallstones
      Porcelain gallbladder
      Gallbladder polyps
      Chronic salmonella infection
      Congenital biliary cysts
      Abnormal pancreaticobiliary duct junction

---

patients with PSC has been estimated to be between 0.6 and 1.5% per year, with a lifetime risk of 10–15%. Cholangiocarcinoma develops at a significantly younger age (between the ages of 30 and 50) in patients with PSC than in patients without PSC.

For GBC, several conditions associated with chronic inflammation are considered risk factors, which include gallstone disease, porcelain gallbladder, gallbladder polyps, chronic salmonella infection, congenital biliary cysts, and abnormal pancreaticobiliary duct junction.

Gallstones are present in 70–90% of patients with GBC, and there appears to be a relationship between gallstones and the development of GBC. Those with symptomatic gallbladder disease, larger gallstones, and longer duration of cholelithiasis have higher risks for the development of GBC. It should be noted that despite the increased risk of GBC in patients with gallstones, the overall incidence of GBC in patients with cholelithiasis is only 0.5–3%.

An increased risk of GBC has been described in workers in the oil, paper, chemical, shoe, textile, and cellulose acetate fiber manufacturing industries, and in miners exposed to radon. The association between certain medications and GBC remains to be determined.

PATHOLOGY

The majority of bile duct and gallbladder cancers are adenocarcinoma, although other histologic types are occasionally found, including small cell cancer, squamous cell carcinoma, lymphoma, and sarcoma.

CLINICAL FEATURES

The clinical presentations may vary depending on the location of the disease. Extrahepatic cholangiocarcinomas usually become symptomatic when the tumor obstructs the biliary drainage system, causing painless jaundice. Common symptoms include pruritus, abdominal pain, weight loss, and fever. The pain is generally described as a constant dull ache in the right upper quadrant. Patients with underlying PSC and cholangiocarcinoma tend to present with a declining performances status and increasing cholestasis. Other symptoms related to biliary obstruction include clay-colored stools and dark urine. Patients with intrahepatic cholangiocarcinomas usually present with a history of dull right upper quadrant pain and weight loss, an elevated serum alkaline phosphatase, and normal or only slightly elevated serum bilirubin levels.

Patients with early invasive GBC are most often asymptomatic, or have nonspecific symptoms that mimic or are due to cholelithiasis or cholecystitis. The diagnosis of GBC should be considered if a compression of the common hepatic duct by an impacted stone in the gallbladder neck is identified (the Mirizzi syndrome). Patients with more advanced GBC may present with abdominal pain, anorexia, nausea, or vomiting, malaise, and weight loss.

DIAGNOSIS

Ultrasound (US) is often used as the initial imaging test due to its easy availability. Intrahepatic cholangiocarcinomas would appear as a mass lesion on US. Perihilar and extrahepatic cancers may not be detected, especially if small, but indirect signs (ductal dilatation throughout the obstructed liver segments) may point toward the diagnosis. Computed tomography (CT) is useful for detecting intrahepatic tumors, assessing the level of biliary obstruction, and the presence of liver atrophy and distant metastases. Ductal dilatation in both hepatic lobes with a contracted gallbladder suggests a Klatskin tumor, while a distended gallbladder without dilated intrahepatic or extrahepatic ducts suggests cystic duct stones or tumor. A distended gallbladder with dilated intrahepatic and extrahepatic ducts is more typical of tumors involving the common bile duct. Dilatation of the ducts within an atrophied hepatic lobe, in conjunction with a hypertrophic contralateral lobe (the atrophy–hypertrophy complex) suggests invasion of the portal vein. Magnetic resonance cholangiopancreatography (MRCP) is a noninvasive technique for evaluating the intrahepatic and extrahepatic bile ducts (Figure 47-2). Unlike conventional ERCP, MRCP does not require contrast material to be administered into the ductal system, thus avoiding the morbidity associated with endoscopic procedures and contrast administration. MRCP has advantages over CT because it not only can image the liver parenchyma and intrahepatic lesions but also create a three-dimensional image of the biliary tree (allowing assessment of the bile ducts both above and below a stricture), and vascular structures. MRCP provides information about disease extent and potential resectability that is comparable to the combined information obtained from CT, cholangiography, and angiography. Cholangiography involves an injection of radiographic contrast material to opacify the bile ducts; it can be performed by endoscopic retrograde pancreatography (ERCP) or via a percutaneous approach (percutaneous transhepatic cholangiogram (PTC)) (Figure 47-3). However, MRCP and dynamic CT have largely replaced invasive cholangiography in patients thought to have a hilar cholangiocarcinoma. Cholangiography may still be indicated if the suspected level of obstruction is distal, or if preoperative drainage of the biliary tree is needed. Endoscopic ultrasound (EUS) can be helpful in the diagnosis of distal bile duct cancer. It can visualize the extent of the primary tumor and the status of regional lymph nodes, and guide the fine needle aspiration and biopsy of primary tumors and enlarged nodes. EUS is

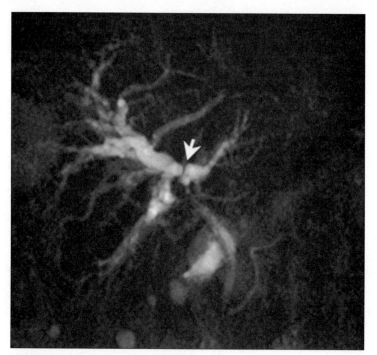

FIGURE 47-2   Klatskin tumor shown on MRCP.

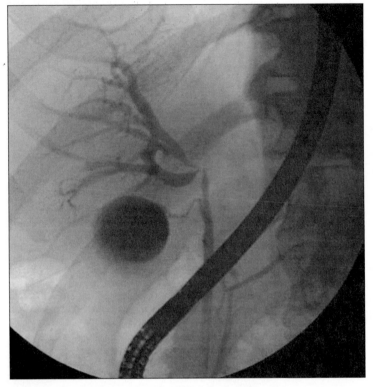

FIGURE 47-3 Klatskin tumor shown by ERCP cholangiography.

more accurate for imaging the gallbladder than is extracorporeal US. The role of positron emission tomography (PET) scan in bile duct cancers is being investigated.

Establishing a tissue diagnosis in bile duct cancers can be challenging. Sampling of bile by PTC or ERCP alone will only have a 30% positive rate in detecting malignant cells by cytology for cholangiocarcinoma. For GBC, EUS guided sampling of bile for cytologic analysis will have a sensitivity of 73% for the diagnosis of GBC. The diagnostic yield can be increased if the suspected lesion is biopsied or brushings taken from the duct for cytologic examination. The necessity of establishing a tissue diagnosis prior to surgery depends upon the clinical situation. For patients with characteristic findings of malignant biliary obstruction or mass lesion, a preoperative biopsy may not be necessary. Cholecystectomy should be strongly considered for patients with gallbladder polyps >1 cm as they are likely to contain an invasive cancer. A biopsy should be obtained for patients who would undergo chemotherapy, radiation therapy, or participation in a therapeutic clinical trial. It should be considered for patients with biliary strictures of clinically indeterminate origin, for example, in patients with a history of biliary tract surgery, bile duct stones, or PSC.

Although not specific for cholangiocarcinoma, the presence of certain tumor markers in the serum or bile of patients with cholangiocarcinoma may be of diagnostic value. Serum levels of carcinoembryonic antigen (CEA) are neither sufficiently sensitive nor specific to diagnose cholangiocarcinoma. Serum levels of cancer antigen (CA) 19-9 are widely used, particularly for detecting cholangiocarcinoma in patients with PSC. However, the accuracy of serum CA 19-9 as a tumor marker for cholangiocarcinoma is variable in different studies depending on the cut-off values used with a sensitivity of 53–79% and specificity of 98–100%. The presence of cholangitis and cholestasis may influence the optimal cut-off value for serum CA 19-9 that best discriminates between benign or malignant biliary tract diseases. CEA or CA 19-9 levels are not diagnostically useful for GBC because of lack of specificity and sensitivity.

STAGING AND PROGNOSTIC SCORING SYSTEMS

The tumor staging systems for intrahepatic and extrahepatic cholangiocarcinoma are slightly different, and they are both based upon the TNM system devised by the American Joint Committee on Cancer (AJCC). The current TNM classification schemes for both hilar and distal cholangiocarcinoma were refined and simplified with the 2002 revision of the AJCC staging criteria. Several staging systems have been used for GBC and the TNM staging system of AJCC is the preferred classification scheme in the United States. This current 2002 staging system differs from the 1997 version in that regional lymph node metastases (cystic duct or periportal lymph nodes) are now classified as stage IIB rather than stage III, stage III indicates locally unresectable disease, stage IV indicates distant metastatic disease, and peripancreatic lymph nodes are now considered to represent metastatic (M1) disease.

TREATMENT

Surgery represents the only potentially curative treatment modality. Less than 30% of patients have surgically resectable disease. The resectability rates are higher for distal cholangiocarcinomas and lower for proximal (particularly perihilar) tumors. Absolute contraindications to surgery include liver or peritoneal metastases, ascites, encasement or occlusion of major vessels including portal vein and hepatic arteries, and extensive involvement of the regional lymph nodes. The surgical procedure required for definitive resection varies depending on the sites and extent of disease. For distal cholangiocarcinoma, a pancreatico-duodenectomy (Whipple procedure) is required. For perihilar cholangiocarcinomas, bile duct resection alone leads to high local recurrence rates due to early involvement of the confluence of the hepatic ducts and the caudate lobe branches. For intrahepatic cholangiocarcinoma, hepatic resection is indicated with intent to achieve negative margins.

For patients known to have gallbladder cancer preoperatively, a simple cholecystectomy is usually not recommended. Rather, many surgical oncologists recommend a radical or extended cholecystectomy which includes removal of the gallbladder plus at least 2 cm of the gallbladder bed. In addition, dissection of the regional lymph nodes from the hepatoduodenal ligament behind the second portion of the duodenum, head of the pancreas, and the celiac axis is recommended if a gallbladder cancer is known or suspected. If a gallbladder cancer is known to invade the liver, resection of the involved liver (segmental or lobar) is often performed.

For patients who are diagnosed incidentally at the time of cholecystectomy, reexploration and radical resection is warranted if disease extent is T2. This benefit is based on the fact that more than 50% of patients with ≥T2 or greater disease will have node positive disease upon reexploration. The benefit of reexploration for patients with incidentally diagnosed T1 disease is more controversial as the incidence of liver invasion and nodal metastases is less. While simple cholecystectomy may be sufficient for many patients with T1 lesions, reexploration should be considered for patients with T1b disease (tumor invading the muscularis layer).

The outcome for patients undergoing resection of a primary bile duct or gall bladder cancer depends upon the stage of disease. The 5 year survival rate for patients with completely resected bile duct and gall bladder cancers is in the range of 20–50%. Due to the rarity of bile duct and gallbladder cancer, the role of adjuvant radiation therapy has not been definitively evaluated in randomized trials. Most studies consist of small, heterogeneous groups of patients seen in single institutions. Several retrospective series and small phase II studies suggest superior outcomes for patients who receive postoperative chemoradiotherapy. The most common chemotherapeutic agent used is 5-fluorouracil (5FU) given concurrently with radiation.

For patients with locally advanced unresectable biliary tract and gallbladder cancer, radiation, usually given in combination with concurrent 5FU-based chemotherapy, can offer palliation and may improve local control. However, the overall impact of chemoradiation on survival is unknown.

Systemic chemotherapy for BTC occasionally improves symptoms and may improve survival when compared to a historical series of supportive care alone. In one earlier study, patients with advanced biliary and pancreatic cancer were randomized to best supportive care alone or best supportive care plus chemotherapy with 5FU, etoposide, and leucovorin (FELV) (3). The median survival for the chemotherapy arm was significantly higher compared to best supportive care alone for all patients (6.5 versus 2.5 months, $P < 0.01$). Since response rates to chemotherapy for biliary tract and gallbladder adenocarcinoma are similar, most recent studies have combined patients from either site of origin. Several single agents have been tested with response rate of less than 20% and these include 5FU, gemcitabine, capecitabine, irinotecan, and docetaxel. Several combination regimens have also been studied with improved response rates of 30–45% and these regimens include ECF (epirubicine, cisplatin, 5FU), gemcitabine with cisplatin, gemcitabine with oxaliplatin, and gemcitabine with capecitabine. Future randomized studies are needed to better define the most active and tolerable systemic chemotherapy regimens.

REFERENCES

1. Jemal, A, Siegel R, Ward E, et al. Cancer statistics, 2006. CA Cancer J Clin. 2006; 56(2): 106–130.
2. Shaib YH, El-Serag HB, Davila JA, et al, Risk factors of intrahepatic cholangiocarcinoma in the United States: a case-control study. Gastroenterology. 2005; 128(3): 620–626.
3. Glimelius B, Hoffman K, Sjoden PO, et al. Chemotherapy improves survival and quality of life in advanced pancreatic and biliary cancer. Ann Oncol. 1996; 7(6): 593–600.

COLON CANCER

EPIDEMIOLOGY

Statistics

In the United States, 106,680 new cases of colon cancer were expected in 2006 (men 49,220; women 57,460) (1), and 41,930 new cases of rectal cancer were expected in 2006 (men 23,580; women 18,350). Colorectal cancer is the second leading cause of cancer related death in the United States with 68,000 deaths annually representing 10% of all cancer deaths. Age is a major risk factor in developing colon cancer. The lifetime risk of developing colorectal cancer is approximately 5% with the vast majority of cancers occurring after age 50. The overall incidence has been falling perhaps due to screening.

Epidemiologic Associations

The vast majority of colorectal cancers are sporadic and not familial. Epidemiologic studies demonstrate an increased risk of colorectal cancer with the following conditions/characteristics:

- Family history of colorectal cancer is associated with an increased risk of developing colorectal cancer. If one first-degree family member had colorectal cancer, the risk increases 1.7-fold
- Western/urbanized societies
- Diet high in red or processed meat
- Increased bowel anaerobic flora
- Diabetes mellitus/insulin resistance: the risk of colon cancer may be 30% higher in diabetics compared with nondiabetics
- Inflammatory bowel disease. Increased incidence is seen with both Crohn's disease and ulcerative colitis and is associated with the severity, extent, and duration of disease affecting the colon. The risk of colon cancer in ulcerative colitis is approximately 10% at 10 year duration, 20% at 20 year duration, and >35% at 30 year duration. Total colectomy eliminates the risk of colon cancer
- Cigarette smoking
- Alcohol consumption
- Ureterosigmoidostomy
- Streptococcus bovis bacteremia
- Prior pelvic radiation

Inherited Syndromes

Fewer than 10% of colon cancers are due to an inherited predisposition to colon cancer. The most common inherited syndromes are FAP and HNPCC. The MYH gene mutations are associated with an inherited predisposition to colon cancer as well (2).

FAMILIAL ADENOMATOUS POLYPOSIS (FAP)   Most cases of FAP are due to mutations in the APC gene on chromosome 5q21. These mutations are inherited in an autosomal dominant fashion.

APC is a tumor suppressor gene whose product interacts with critical cell proliferation genes in part by its interaction with transcription factor, beta catenin.

FAP is associated with hundreds to thousands of polyps throughout the colon. Fewer polyps and a later onset of colorectal cancer characterize an attenuated form of FAP. The use of COX-2 inhibitors can result in regression of some polyps.

By age 10, 15% of carriers will have adenomas; by age 20, 75% will have adenomas; and by age 30 more than 90% will have adenomas. Screening of first-degree relatives should be done by age 10. Treatment is a total proctocolectomy.

FAP accounts for <1% of colon cancers and is associated with congenital hypertrophy of the retinal pigment, desmoid tumors (Gardner's syndrome), and brain tumors (Turcot's syndrome).

HEREDITARY NONPOLYPOSIS COLON CANCER (HNPCC) HNPCC is due to mutation in mismatch repair genes (e.g., MLH1, MSH2) which leads to microsatellite instability and errors in DNA replication. Inherited in an autosomal dominant fashion, HNPCC may account for up to 6% of all colon cancers. The median age for development of colon cancer is less than 50. Right-sided tumors are much more common than left-sided tumors. HNPCC is associated with endometrial cancer, ovarian cancer, upper gastrointestinal cancers, and transitional cell cancers of the renal pelvis/ureter.

An individual is likely to belong to a family with HNPCC and require genetic testing if (1) three or more relatives have had colon cancer (or another cancer associated with HNPCC such as uterine, small bowel, urethral, or renal pelvic cancer) and at least one of the relatives is a first-degree relative; (2) two or more generations of the family have colon cancer; or (3) one or more relatives were diagnosed with colon cancer before age 50. Screening should begin by age 21 in affected patients and be done at least every 5 years thereafter.

These criteria for identifying HNPCC are referred to as the Amsterdam II Criteria. The Bethesda criteria modify the Amsterdam II Criteria to include in the evaluation those patients who have had family members with adenomatous colonic polyps in addition to colon cancers.

MYH MYH is a base excision repair gene located on the short arm of chromosome (1). Homozygous mutations in MYH have been associated with a syndrome manifesting itself as multiple colonic polyps and colorectal cancer. It is inherited in an autosomal recessive fashion. MYH mutations are thought to account for less than 1% of colorectal cancers.

PRIMARY PREVENTION AND SCREENING

Prevention Strategies

Nonsteroidal antiinflammatory drugs (NSAIDS), calcium, folate, and estrogens prevent the development of polyps, but there is no clear prevention of cancer. Their role is unknown in the patient who is getting adequately screened (3).

Antioxidants do not prevent colon cancer and conflicting data exist for the preventive ability of calcium, vitamin D, and statins. Diets high in fiber do not prevent colon cancer and diets high in red/processed meat and low in fish have been associated with an increased risk of colon cancer. However, physical activity may have a protective effect.

Screening

Most colorectal cancers arise from adenomatous polyps. The progression of adenomatous polyps from small polyps, to larger polyps, to dyspastic polyps, and finally to cancer occurs over at least a 10 year period. Villous adenomas have a higher rate of progression to colon cancer than tubular or hyperplastic polyps. It is generally felt that only 1% of polyps will progress through this sequence to

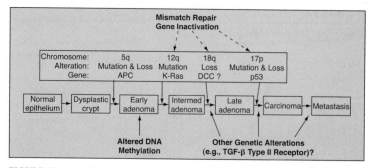

FIGURE 48-1   Vogelgram model of colon carcinogenesis.

form a cancer. This progression is due to a series of acquired mutations and is often referred to as the Vogelgram model after Bert Vogelstein who initially described these events (Figure 48-1). The purpose of screening is to detect polyps before they turn into cancer. Guidelines for screening take into account the effectiveness, sensitivity, specificity, cost, and morbidity of the test (4).

Approximately 3–6% of Americans undergoing colonoscopic screening in their 50s will have a colon cancer, dysplastic polyp, or villous adenoma. Over the last 20 years, there has been a movement away from barium enema as the screening tool of choice toward endoscopic screening. The preferred method (i.e. flexible sigmoidoscopy versus colonoscopy) is controversial, but it is clear that colonoscopy is a more effective means of detecting any polyps in the colon. Any diagnosis of a polyp on sigmoidoscopy should prompt a full colonoscopy examination.

For patients without a family history of colon cancer, the United States Multisociety Task Force recommends screening patients beginning at age 50 with annual fecal occult blood test as well as sigmoidoscopy every 5 years.

Alternatively, the task force recommended screening colonoscopy beginning at age 50 and repeated every 10 years in those patients without any colonic pathology.

For patients with two or more affected first-degree relatives or any first-degree relative with colon cancer under the age of 60, screening should begin by age 40 or at least 10 years younger than the age at which the affected family member was diagnosed.

Some experts recommend colonoscopy rather than FOBT and sigmoidoscopy on the basis of the following facts: (1) the combination of FOBT and sigmoidoscopy has a sensitivity of 75%, that is, it will miss 25% of lesions; (2) approximately 2% of asymptomatic adults at age 50 will have a precancerous or cancerous proximal colonic lesion and have a totally normal sigmoidoscopy (5, 6).

PRESENTATION AND STAGING

Signs and Symptoms

Nearly 50% of colon cancers are found in the right side of the colon that is different than 50 years ago when the majority of tumors were found on the left side of the colon. The reason for this change is not known. The presenting symptoms depend on the location of the tumor. Obstruction, perforation, change in stool character, and hematochezia are more common with left-sided tumors. Fe-deficiency anemia is more common with right-sided tumors.

Table 48-1

Categories for Colorectal Cancer

Stage	TNM	5 year survival (%)
Stage I	T1-2, N0, M0	>90
Stage IIa	T3, N0, M0	~85
Stage IIb	T4, N0, M0	~75
Stage IIIa	T1-2, N1, M0	~80
Stage IIIb	T3-4, N1, M0	~65
Stage IIIc	T any, N2, M0	~45
Stage IV	T any, N any, M1	~10

Staging of Colon Cancer

The process of staging a colon cancer is based on the American Joint Committee on Cancer (AJCC) TNM system and replaces the previous Duke's and Astler–Collier's systems (Table 48-1).

T CATEGORIES FOR COLORECTAL CANCER The T stage describes the extent through the bowel wall that the cancer spread. The N stage describes the presence of regional nodal metastases

Tx. No description of the tumor's extent is possible because of incomplete information.

Tis. The cancer is in the earliest stage. It involves only the mucosa. It has not grown beyond the muscularis mucosa (inner muscle layer) of the colon or rectum. This stage is also known as carcinoma in situ or intramucosal carcinoma.

T1. The cancer has grown through the muscularis mucosa and extends into the submucosa.
T2. The cancer has grown through the submucosa, and extends into the muscularis propria.
T3. The cancer has grown completely through the muscularis propria into the subserosa but not to any neighboring organs or tissues.
T4. The cancer has spread completely through the wall of the colon or rectum into nearby tissues or organs.

N CATEGORIES FOR COLORECTAL CANCER N categories indicate whether or not the cancer has spread to nearby lymph nodes and, if so, how many lymph nodes are involved.

Nx. No description of lymph node involvement is possible because of incomplete information.
N0. No lymph node involvement is found.
N1. Cancer cells found in one to three regional nodes. Regional nodes depend upon the location of the colon cancer and are located along the course of major vessels supplying the colon, along the vascular arcades of the marginal artery, and along the mesocolic border of the colon.
N2. Cancer cells found in four or more regional lymph nodes.

M CATEGORIES FOR COLORECTAL CANCER M categories indicate whether or not the cancer has spread to distant organs, such as the liver, lungs, or distant lymph nodes.

Mx. No description of distant spread is possible because of incomplete information.
M0. No distant spread is seen.
M1. Distant spread is present.

TREATMENT

Surgical Management

At presentation, the initial evaluation should consist of routine chemistries and a complete blood count. An elevated carcinoembryonic antigen (CEA) preoperatively is associated with a poor prognosis. The routine use of imaging is controversial. It is reasonable to obtain CT scans of the chest, abdomen, and pelvis to evaluate for the presence of metastatic disease.

For patients with stage I, II, or III colon cancer, surgical resection of the colon cancer is the mainstay of therapy. Open colectomy or laparoscopic colectomy is equally effective. For patients with stage IV colon cancer who are not considered candidates for cure, resection of the primary lesion can be based upon the symptoms of the patient. In the asymptomatic patient, surgical resection of the primary tumor is not necessary and can be deferred until the patient experiences local symptoms. Some patients will die of metastatic disease without ever experiencing symptoms from the primary tumor.

Stage 1

Surgical resection cures >90% of patients with stage 1 colon cancer. Adjuvant therapy is not recommended. Patients should undergo surveillance colonoscopy within 3–5 years of diagnosis. Patients with more than two first-degree relatives with colon cancer, a first-degree relative with colon cancer under the age of 50, or who are under 50 themselves, should undergo evaluation in a genetic/high-risk clinic.

Stage 2

Surgical resection cures approximately 80% of patients with stage 2 colon cancer. The use of adjuvant chemotherapy is controversial and is currently not recommended by the American Society of Clinical Oncology. Randomized studies have not shown a statistically significant benefit for the use of adjuvant chemotherapy in patients with stage 2 colon cancer. However, many experts advocate for the use of adjuvant chemotherapy in high-risk patients, because these patients carry a greater than 20% risk of dying from recurrent disease. Patients with stage 2 colon cancer who are considered high risk carry the following features

- T4 disease
- Presentation with perforation or obstruction
- Inadequate nodal evaluation; the American College of Pathology recommends that at least 12 regional lymph nodes be examined for the presence of nodal metastases
- Poorly differentiated tumors

For type of adjuvant chemotherapy see stage 3 section below.

Stage 3

Surgical resection cures approximately half of patients with stage 3 colon cancer. Patients with N1 disease can expect a cure rate with surgery alone of approximately 60–70%. Patients with N2 disease can expect a cure rate of 30% with surgery alone. Adjuvant chemotherapy is recommended for all patients with stage 3 colon cancer at improved overall survival.

Standard treatment can consist of 6 months of 5-fluorouracil (5FU) and leucovorin. Six months of capecitabine, an oral fluoropyrimidine, has equivalent efficacy to intravenous 5FU and leucovorin. Recently, the addition of oxaliplatin to intravenous 5FU and leucovorin has been associated with an improved disease-free survival compared with 5FU and leucovorin for patients with stage

Table 48-2

Major Phase 3 Studies in Stage 4 Colon Cancer

Common title	Regimen	No. of patients	Median survival (months)
Saltz study (8)	IFL	221	14.8
	5FU/LV	236	12.6
			$p = 0.04$
N9741 (9)	FOLFOX	264	19.5
	IFL	267	15.0
			$p = 0.0001$
Tournigand study (10)	FOLFOX	111	21.5
	FOLFIRI	109	20.4
			$p = 0.9$
Bevacizumab study (11)	IFL	411	20.3
	IFL/Bevacizumab	402	15.6
			$p = 0.00004$

IFL = irinotecan, 5FU, leucovorin.
FOLFOX = infusional + bolus 5FU, leucovorin, oxaliplatin.
FOLFIRI = infusional + bolus 5FU, leucovorin, irinotecan.

2 and 3 colon cancer. Subset analysis of patients with stage 2 disease did not reveal a statistically significant advantage in disease-free survival for patients receiving FOLFOX compared with 5FU and leucovorin.

Stage 4

All patients with isolated liver or lung metastases should be evaluated by a surgical specialist for consideration of resection of the metastases. Approximately 30% of patients undergoing complete resection of isolated liver or lung metastases will be cured (7).

For patients in whom a curative resection cannot be done, the median survival is approximately 6–8 months without chemotherapy and 2 years with chemotherapy. Approximately 10% of patients who undergo aggressive chemotherapy will live for 5 years.

Until 1997, 5FU was the only active chemotherapy. Studies demonstrated that the addition of folinic acid (leucovorin) to 5FU improved the response rates and time to tumor progression. Since 1997, irinotecan, oxaliplatin, bevacizumab, and cetuximab have been approved for use in patients with metastatic colon cancer. The major randomized studies are presented in Table 48-2.

First-line chemotherapy for patients with metastatic disease of consists of either FOLFOX (5FU, leucovorin, oxaliplatin) or FOLFIRI (5FU, leucovorin, irinotecan) with bevacizumab. Second-line chemotherapy typically consists of either an irinotecan-based regimen if FOLFOX was used as the first-line regimen, and an oxaliplatin-based regimen if FOLFIRI was used as the first-line regimen. Cetuximab is approved for use either alone or in combination with irinotecan for patients who had previously progressed on an irinotecan containing regimen. Capecitabine is often substituted for 5FU and leucovorin in the FOLFOX regimens. The median survival for patients with metastatic disease receiving all available therapy is approximately 2 years.

REFERENCES

1. Jemal A, Siegel R, Ward E, et al. Cancer statistics, 2006. CA Cancer J Clin. 2006; 56(2): 106–130.
2. Lynch HT, de la Chapelle A. Hereditary colorectal cancer. N Engl J Med. 2003; 348(10): 919–932.

3. Janne PA, Mayer RJ. Chemoprevention of colorectal cancer. N Engl J Med. 2000; 342(26): 1960–1968.

4. Winawer S, Fletcher R, Rex D, et al. Colorectal cancer screening and surveillance: clinical guidelines and rationale-update based on new evidence. Gastroenterology. 2003; 124(2): 544–560.

5. Imperiale TF, Wagner DR, Lin CY, Larkin GN, Rogge JD, Ransohoff DF. Risk of advanced proximal neoplasms in asymptomatic adults according to the distal colorectal findings. N Engl J Med. 2000; 343(3): 169–174.

6. Lieberman DA, Weiss DG, Bond JH, Ahnen DJ, Garewal H, Chejfec G. Use of colonoscopy to screen asymptomatic adults for colorectal cancer. Veterans Affairs Cooperative Study Group 380. N Engl J Med. 2000; 343(3): 162–168.

7. Fong Y, Fortner J, Sun RL, Brennan MF, Blumgart LH. Clinical score for predicting recurrence after hepatic resection for metastatic colorectal cancer: analysis of 1001 consecutive cases. Ann Surg. 1999; 230(3): 309–318; discussion 18–21.

8. Saltz LB, Cox JV, Blanke C, et al. Irinotecan plus fluorouracil and leucovorin for metastatic colorectal cancer. Irinotecan Study Group. N Engl J Med. 2000; 343(13): 905–914.

9. Goldberg RM, Sargent DJ, Morton RF, et al. A randomized controlled trial of fluorouracil plus leucovorin, irinotecan, and oxaliplatin combinations in patients with previously untreated metastatic colorectal cancer. J Clin Oncol. 2004; 22(1): 23–30.

10. Tournigand C, Andre T, Achille E, et al. FOLFIRI followed by FOLFOX6 or the reverse sequence in advanced colorectal cancer: a randomized GERCOR study. J Clin Oncol. 2004; 22(2): 229–237.

11. Hurwitz H, Fehrenbacher L, Novotny W, et al. Bevacizumab plus irinotecan, fluorouracil, and leucovorin for metastatic colorectal cancer. N Engl J Med. 2004; 350(23): 2335–2342.

RECTAL CANCER

EPIDEMIOLOGY

In 2005 there were approximately 145,000 Americans diagnosed with colon and rectal cancer. The American Cancer Society estimates that over 56,000 of these people will die of their disease. Approximately 2/3 will involve the colon and 1/3 the rectum. Epidemiological factors and pathogenesis are the same for rectal cancer as for colon cancer.

ANATOMY

The rectum is generally divided into three portions: lower rectum, mid-rectum, and upper rectum. The distances from the anal verge are approximations and may vary with flexible endoscopic techniques.

- Lower rectum: 4–8 cm from anal verge
- Mid-rectum: 8–12 cm from anal verge
- Upper-rectum: 12–16 cm from anal verge
- Anal canal: 4 cm in length

Important Landmarks

DENTATE LINE   The dentate line is the transition point between the squamous mucosa of the anus/perineum and the columnar mucosa of the rectum. Below the dentate line, the lymph drainage flows through the inguinal nodes and has implications for treatment.

RECTUM/SIGMOID BOUNDARY   In contrast to the sigmoid colon, peritoneum does not cover the circumference of the rectum. Rectal cancer has higher rates of local failure following surgery than colon cancer and requires aggressive local treatment.

Generally, rectal tumors should be no less than 6–7 cm from anal verge if a sphincter sparing operation is to be attempted in order to preserve muscle function while obtaining adequate margins.

DIAGNOSIS AND STAGING

Diagnosis

PRESENTING SYMPTOMS   The majority of patients diagnosed with rectal cancer present with symptoms, although many are nonspecific and this may lead to a delay in diagnosis. Common symptoms include bleeding (gross or occult), constitutional symptoms, abdominal pain, changes in stool caliber, and changes in bowel habits.

WORKUP   When cancer is in the differential diagnosis, the workup entails history and physical including digital rectal examination (DRE), complete blood count, liver and renal function tests, carcinoembryonic antigen (CEA), and endoscopy.

    DRE   DRE should be used to assess the location of the tumor in relation to the anal verge, the dentate line, and the anal sphincter. If possible, the tumor should be assessed with respect to anal sphincter involvement, circumferential extent, and possible fixation to normal structures. Baseline sphincter tone should be assessed.

Rigid proctosigmoidoscopy   This is used both to assess the location of the tumor (especially when nonpalpable), and to take biopsies for tissue diagnosis.

Staging

STAGING SYSTEM   Rectal cancer is staged using clinico-pathological parameters and classified using the AJCC TNM system (Table 49-1). Preoperative staging is used for prognostic purposes and to estimate the risk of recurrence after surgery to guide adjuvant therapy.

T AND N STAGE   Endorectal ultrasound and MRI are commonly used to assess the extent of the primary tumor. Nodal status can be determined using MRI, CT, and EUS, but may be difficult to assess radiographically.

ENDORECTAL ULTRASOUND (EUS)   EUS is able to distinguish the five layers of the rectal wall with good spatial resolution. The accuracy for T stage

Table 49-1

Colorectal Carcinoma Staging System of the American Joint Committee on Cancer, 6th Edition

Primary tumor (T)			
TX	Primary tumor cannot be assessed		
Tis	Carcinoma in situ		
T0	No evidence primary tumors		
T1	Tumor invades submucosa		
T2	Tumor invades muscularis propria		
T3	Tumor invades through the muscularis propria into the subserosa, or into nonperitonealized pericolic or perirectal tissues		
T4	Tumor directly invades other organs or structures, and/or perforates visceral peritoneum		
Lymph node (N)			
NX	Regional lymph nodes cannot be assessed		
N0	No regional lymph node metastases		
N1	Metastasis in 1 to 3 regional lymph nodes		
N2	Metastasis in 4 or more regional lymph nodes		
Distant metastasis (M)			
MX	Distant metastasis cannot be assessed		
M0	No distant metastasis		
M1	Distant metastasis		
Stage grouping			
Stage 0	Tis	N0	M0
Stage I	T1	N0	M0
	T2	N0	M0
Stage IIA	T3	N0	M0
Stage IIB	T4	N0	M0
Stage IIIA	T1-T2	N1	M0
Stage IIIB	T3-T4	N1	M0
Stage IIIC	Any T	N2	M0
Stage IV	Any T	Any N	M1

Used with the permission of the American Joint Committee on Cancer (AJCC), Chicago, IL. The original source for this material is the "AJCC Cancer Staging Manual," 6th edition, 2002, published by Springer-New York, www.springerlink.com.

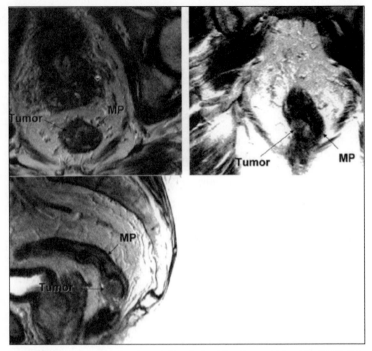

FIGURE 49-1 (Clockwise from lower left) sagittal, axial, and coronal T2 weighted MRI of the pelvis showing a rectal tumor invading through the muscularis propria (MP) making this a T3 lesion.

ranges from 67% to 97% with a propensity to overstage tumors as indicated by a reported specificity of 24% for peri-rectal penetration. EUS is operator dependent and associated with a fast learning curve (1, 2).

MAGNETIC RESONANCE IMAGING (FIGURE 49-1) When MRI is used for primary determination of T stage, a surface phased array coil is employed enabling differentiation of rectal wall layers. Accuracy is operator dependant with interrater accuracies in one study of 67% and 83%. MRI can also be used for preoperative assessment of the likely circumferential margin (CFM) following surgery. The accuracy of N stage evaluation is similar to that of CT in that both are based on size criteria (3).

ASSESSMENT OF METASTATIC DISEASE *Computed tomography (CT)* CT is used primarily for preoperative assessment of metastatic disease in the lungs, liver, or abdomen. It is less useful for the assessment of T stage with accuracy rates of only 33–77% resulting from the inability to distinguish layers of rectal wall. The sensitivity for detection of nodal disease ranges from 45 to 73% (1).

RESIDUAL OR RECURRENT DISEASE Positron emission tomography may be used for the assessment of residual or recurrent disease and may be helpful in areas of scarring or radiation changes (1).

TREATMENT

A general treatment algorithm is included in Figure 49-2.

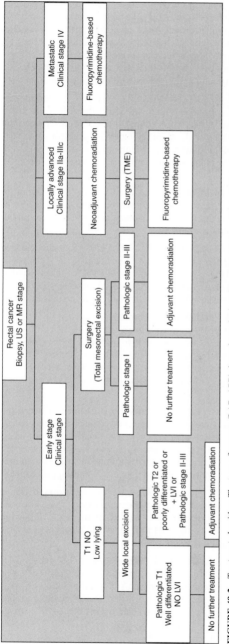

FIGURE 49-2 Treatment algorithm. The type of surgery (LAR, APR) depends on the location of the tumor and the ability to spare the anal sphincter while maintaining adequate surgical margins. Chemoradiation consists of 5FU given concurrently with radiation to a pelvic field.

Surgical Management

LOCAL EXCISION   A number of criteria must be met in order to proceed with local excision. These include T1 or T2 lesions without evidence of nodal disease, tumor within 8–10 cm of the anal verge, and involvement of less than 40% of circumference of bowel wall. Histopathological limitations include well to moderately differentiated histology and no evidence of lymphovascular invasion. Local excision techniques must be full-thickness excisions. These include transanal excision, posterior proctectomy, and transsphincteric excision.

ABDOMINAL PERINEAL RESECTION (APR)   An APR is a nonsphincter sparing operation requiring both an abdominal and perineal incision and a permanent colostomy. It is the standard procedure for tumor removal when the lower extent of the tumor does not allow for sphincter preservation with adequate tumor margins (traditional margin is 5 cm, although 2 cm margins have been used). The entire rectum along with the sphincter apparatus is removed through the perineum.

LOW ANTERIOR RESECTION (LAR)   LAR involves the mobilization of the entire rectum and complete resection of the involved segment of the rectum encompassing the tumor with a margin. The remaining ends are reanastomosed, so that no permanent colostomy is required.

TOTAL MESORECTAL EXCISION (TME)   Prior to TME, traditional surgical techniques invaded tissue planes during blunt dissection. The CFM status following surgery correlates with the risk of local recurrence. TME requires sharp dissection under direct visualization to remove the entire rectal mesentery along with the peri-rectal fat as one discrete unit. This procedure has improved outcomes (4).

COMBINED MODALITY THERAPY   Combined modality therapy is considered either when the risk of local recurrence is significant (stage II–III disease) or in an attempt to covert an APR to a sphincter sparing operation. When chemotherapy and radiation are used in addition to surgery for local disease control, fluoropyrimidine-based chemotherapy must be used for systemic therapy following surgery. Major adjuvant and neoadjuvant trials are listed in Table 49-2.

NEOADJUVANT THERAPY   Although survival was identical between the two arms, the Dutch Colorectal Cancer Group trial showed that in patients undergoing surgery with TME, preoperative radiation was associated with decreased rates of local recurrence (5). Trials with preoperative chemoradiation improved on the results of preoperative radiation. Chemoradiation has also been used preoperatively to convert tumors requiring APR into sphincter sparing procedures.

ADJUVANT THERAPY   In the mid-1980s, the Gastrointestinal Tumor Study Group (GITSG) showed that adjuvant chemoradiation was associated with a survival benefit when compared with no further treatment following surgery (6). This and other trials led the NIH to recommend adjuvant chemoradiotherapy for patients with stage II or III disease in 1990.

NEOADJUVANT VERSUS ADJUVANT THERAPY   The question of whether pre- or postoperative chemoradiation provided the most benefit was asked by the German Rectal Cancer Study Group. At 5 years of follow-up, preoperative chemoradiation was associated with a lower rate of local recurrence (6% versus 13%), a lower rate of grade 3 or 4 acute toxic effects (27% versus 40%), and lower rate of long-term toxic effects (14% versus 24%). There was no difference in overall survival. Preoperative chemoradiation also allowed for greater sphincter sparing (7). Standard preoperative chemoradiation includes 50.4 Gy in 1.8 Gy fractions given with continuous infusion 5FU (225 mg/m^2).

Table 49-2

Major Adjuvant and Neoadjuvant Trials

Study	Arms	Local control (%)	Overall survival (%)
		Pre-TME era	
GITSG (6, 8)	No adjuvant	55 (recurrence rate, med fu 80 mos)	27 (9 year)
	Adjuvant RT	48	
	Adjuvant chemo	46	
	Adjuvant chemo/RT	33	54 ($p = 0.01$)
Swedish Rectal Cancer Trial (9)	Surgery alone	73 (5 year)	48 (5 year)
	Neoadjuvant RT	89 ($p < 0.001$)	58 ($p = 0.004$)
		TME era	
Dutch Colorectal Cancer Study (3)	Surgery alone	91.8 (2 year)	82 (2 year)
	Neoadjuvant RT	97.6 ($p < 0.001$)	82 ($p = 0.84$)
German Rectal Cancer Study (7)	Neoadjuvant chemoradiation	94 (5 year)	76 (5 year)
	Adjuvant chemoradiation	87 ($p = 0.006$)	74 ($p = 0.8$)

UNRESECTABLE DISEASE   Neoadjuvant chemoradiation can be used to convert unresectable disease into resectable disease. If there is residual disease or if there is a strong possibility of positive margins, intraoperative radiation therapy (IORT) may be considered.

RECURRENT DISEASE   There are no clear data on the management of recurrent disease. If surgical resection is possible with negative margins, long-term survival is possible. Reirradiation can be associated with high rates of complications as a function of the radiation dose and time interval from prior treatment.

METASTATIC DISEASE   The foundation of the treatment of metastatic disease is fluoropyrimidine-based chemotherapy and is similar to the treatment of metastatic colon cancer (see chapter on colon cancer for details).

SURVEILLANCE AND FOLLOW-UP

2005 ASCO Guidelines

- *History and physical.* Every 3–6 months for the first 3 years, every 6 months for years 4 and 5, and at the discretion of the physician thereafter
- *Proctosigmoidoscopy.* Every 6 months for 5 years in patients not treated with radiation
- *CEA.* Every three months for 3 years; fluorouracil-based chemotherapy may cause false elevation
- *Pelvic CT* should be considered, especially in patients who have not received RT

REFERENCES

1.   Goh V, Halligan S, Bartram CI. Local radiological staging of rectal cancer. Clin Radiol. 2004; 59(3): 215–226.

2. Carmody BJ, Otchy DP. Learning curve of transrectal ultrasound. Dis Colon Rectum. 2000; 43(2): 193–197.

3. Beets-Tan RG, Beets GL, Vliegen RF, Kessels AG, Van Boven H, De Bruine A, von Meyenfeldt MF, Baeten CG, van Engelshoven JM. Accuracy of magnetic resonance imaging in prediction of tumour-free resection margin in rectal cancer surgery. Lancet. 2001; 357(9255): 497–504.

4. Bolognese A, Cardi M, Muttillo IA, Barbarosos A, Bocchetti T, Valabrega S. Total mesorectal excision for surgical treatment of rectal cancer. J Surg Oncol. 2000; 74(1): 21–23.

5. Kapiteijn E, Marijnen CA, Nagtegaal ID, Putter H, Steup WH, Wiggers T, Rutten HJ, Pahlman L, Glimelius B, van Krieken JH, Leer JW, van de Velde CJ. Preoperative radiotherapy combined with total mesorectal excision for resectable rectal cancer. N Engl J Med. 2001; 345(9): 638–646.

6. Thomas PR, Lindblad AS. Adjuvant postoperative radiotherapy and chemotherapy in rectal carcinoma: a review of the Gastrointestinal Tumor Study Group experience. Radiother Oncol. 1988; 13(4): 245–252.

7. Sauer R, Becker H, Hohenberger W, etal. Preoperative versus postoperative chemoradiotherapy for rectal cancer. N Engl J Med. 2004; 351(17): 1731–1740.

8. Gastrointestinal Tumor Study Group. Prolongation of the disease-free interval in surgically treated rectal carcinoma. N Engl J Med. 1985; 312(23): 1465–1472.

9. Swedish Rectal Cancer Trial. Improved survival with preoperative radiotherapy in resectable rectal cancer. N Engl J Med. 1997; 336(14): 980–987.

ANAL CANCER

Anal cancer is responsible for approximately 1.6% of digestive system malignancies with 3,990 new cases estimated in the United States in 2005 (1). Anal cancer was once believed to be caused by chronic inflammation of the anal canal and treated with abdominoperineal resection (APR). Research has now shown that the development of anal cancer is associated with human papillomavirus (HPV) infection and has a pathophysiology similar to that of cervical cancer. Concurrent chemotherapy and external beam radiation therapy (EBRT) regimens have essentially replaced APR as primary treatment and have allowed for a great majority of patients to be cured with preservation of the anal sphincter.

ANATOMY AND HISTOLOGY

The anal canal extends from the junction of the puborectalis portion of the levator ani muscle and the external anal sphincter to the anal verge. The length of the canal averages 4 cm. The anal canal is divided by the transitional zone, or dentate line, which represents the transition from squamous mucosa to glandular mucosa. There is no easily identifiable landmark between the rectum and anus, so clinicians should rely on the pathologic classification of tumors in this area rather than surgical or endoscopic classification. Anal cancers are primarily keratinizing or non-keratinizing squamous cell carcinomas. Adenocarcinomas of the anal canal comprise about 20% of anal tumors, and share the natural history of rectal adenocarcinomas and should be treated as such.

There are two sites of lymphatic drainage from the anal canal. Tumors above the dentate line drain to the perirectal and perivertebral nodes, while tumors below the denate line drain to the inguinal and femoral lymph nodes. For this reason, patients who present with anal masses should undergo examination of the inguinal lymph nodes, and patients who present with squamous cell cancers in the inguinal lymph nodes should be evaluated for primary anal tumors.

EPIDEMIOLOGY

The incidence of anal cancer has been rising in the United States. In a review of the SEER database from 1973 to 2000, the incidence of anal cancer in men and women has risen from 1.06 and 1.39 per 100,000 persons to 2.04 and 2.06 per 100,000 persons (2). Though the incidence of anal cancer has risen in both genders, the rate of rise for men is higher, particularly black men. This increase in incidence may be due to better screening techniques and an increased rate of risk factors for anal cancer within the US population that has occurred over time. Survival for patients with anal cancer is consistently worse for men compared to women and for black patients compared to white patients. Several risk factors have been associated with anal cancer:

- Human papillomavirus (HPV) infection
- History of genital warts
- Lifetime number of sexual partners
- Receptive anal intercourse
- History of cervical dysplasia or cancer
- History of previous sexually transmitted disease
- Human immunodeficiency virus (HIV) infection

- Cigarette smoking
- Chronic immunodeficiency

Anal cancer risk factors mirror risk factors of sexually transmitted diseases, and are due to the link between HPV and anal cancer. Similar to cervical dysplasia and cancer, HPV can cause premalignant anal squamous intraepithelial lesions (ASIL), which can be low grade (LSIL) or high grade (HSIL). Progression of ASIL to invasive anal cancer is influenced by HIV seropositivity, low CD4 count, infection with multiple HPV serotypes, serotype of HPV infection, and high levels of DNA of high-risk serotypes. As with cervical cancer, HPV type 16 is the most frequently isolated serotype in HSIL and invasive anal cancer, present in 30–75% of cases, and HPV types 6, 11, and 18 are present in 10% of cases.

Although not completely clear, there does seem to be a relationship between HIV infection and anal cancer. Multiple studies have suggested that anal cancer is increasingly prevalent in people with HIV infection (3). Studies have noted an increase in the incidence of HPV infection, ASIL, HSIL, and anal cancer in HIV positive patients compared to HIV negative patients. However, it is difficult to control for separate risk factors including receptive anal intercourse and prior HPV infection in these studies. Unlike traditional AIDS-related malignancies, risk of anal cancer in HIV positive patients does not seem to correlate with worsening immunosuppression. In addition, the incidence of anal cancer has continued to increase in the age of widespread use of highly active antiretroviral therapy (HAART) (3), while the incidence of AIDS-related malignancies such as Kaposi's sarcoma and non-Hodgkin's lymphoma has decreased. A possible explanation is that HAART allows for longer survival with HIV, but does not control HPV infection, allowing more time for HPV infection to create progressive dysplasia.

Individuals with non-HIV causes of chronic immunosuppression, such as renal transplant patients and patients on chronic glucocorticoid therapy, appear to be at an increased risk for ASIL and anal cancer, typically associated with persistent HPV infection. Several case-controlled studies have also noted an increased risk of anal cancer in smokers, particularly current smokers. Cigarette smoking is thought to act as a co-carcinogen.

SCREENING

Given the known high-risk groups for anal cancer, several studies have addresses screening in these populations. Similar to the cervical Papanicolaou smear, anal swabs for cytology are a possible screening method for ASIL and anal cancer. Sensitivity of anal cytology is in the range of 50–80%, with sensitivity being higher in the HIV positive population. Studies of the potential cost-effectiveness of screening have found that screening HIV positive and HIV negative homosexual and bisexual men every 2–3 years would be cost effective and have life expectancy benefits (4, 5). Other groups where possible benefit of screening has been suggested include all HIV positive individuals, women with a history of cervical dysplasia or cancer, and transplant recipients.

DIAGNOSIS

Diagnosis of anal cancer is based on clinical symptoms, physical exam, and biopsy. Patients can present with symptoms of pain, itching, bleeding, discharge, or anal irritation. Patients may also have tenesmus or, with larger tumors, obstructive-type symptoms. Physical exam should include rectal exam to fully assess the size and location of the tumor and inguinal lymph node exam. Biopsy confirmation to assess histology of the anal mass as well as fine needle aspiration of enlarged inguinal lymph nodes should also be performed. Transanal ultrasonography may be used to evaluate depth of tumor invasion.

CT scanning of the abdomen and pelvis can also be used to assess tumor size, invasion, lymph node involvement, and metastatic disease.

STAGING

The American Joint Committee on Cancer (AJCC) and the International Union Against Cancer have established a tumor-node-metastasis (TNM) staging system for anal cancer (Table 50-1). Since the primary treatment modality for anal cancer is non-surgical, staging is based on physical exam, fine needle aspiration of suspicious lymph nodes, and radiologic data. For this reason, the AJCC staging system is based on tumor size rather than depth of invasion. Patients with T1 or T2 lesions have an 80–90% 5-year survival rate, whereas patients with T4 lesions have less than a 50% 5-year survival rate. For patients with lymph node metastases,

Table 50-1

Anal Carcinoma Staging System of the American Joint Committee on Cancer, 2002

Primary tumor (T)

TX	Primary tumor cannot be assessed
Tis	No evidence primary tumors
T0	Carcinoma in situ
T1	Tumor 2 cm or less in greatest dimension
T2	Tumor more than 2 cm but not more than 5 cm in greatest dimension
T3	Tumor more than 5 cm in greatest dimension
T4	Tumor of any size invades adjacent organ(s), eg, vagina, urethra, bladder; Involvement of sphincter muscle(s) alone is not classified as T4

Lymph node (N)

NX	Regional lymph nodes cannot be assessed
N0	No regional lymph node metastases
N1	Metastasis in perirectal lymph node(s)
N2	Metastasis in unilateral internal iliac and/or ingional lymph node(s)
N3	Metastasis in perirectal and inguinal lymph nodes and/or bilateral internal iliac and/or inguinal lymph nodes

Distant metastasis (M)

MX	Presence of distant metastasis cannot be assessed
M0	No distant metastasis
M1	Distant metastasis

Stage grouping

Stage 0	Tis	N0	M0
Stage I	T1	N0	M0
Stage II	T2	N0	M0
	T3	N0	M0
Stage IIIA	T1	N1	M0
	T2	N1	M0
	T3	N1	M0
	T4	N0	M0
Stage IIIB	T4	N1	M0
	Any T	N2	M0
	Any T	N3	M0
Stage IV	Any T	Any N	M1

Source: Used with the permission of the American Joint Committee on Cancer (AJCC), Chicago, IL, USA. The original source for this material is the *AJCC Cancer Staging Manual*, Sixth Edition (2002) published by Springer, New York, http://www.springeronline.com.

the 5-year survival rate is significantly worse at 25–40%. At presentation, 50–60% of patients have a T1 or T2 lesion, and 12–20% are node-positive. The probability of nodal spread is directly related to tumor size and location.

TREATMENT

Before 1980, abdominoperineal resection (APR), a surgery removing the anorectum and creation of a permanent colostomy, was the treatment of choice for tumors of the anal canal. Surgical series prior to 1980 found the overall 5-year survival rate after an APR to range between 40% and 70%. Patients with large tumors and nodal metastases had poorer outcomes. In an attempt to improve surgical outcome, Nigro and colleagues at Wayne State evaluated pre-operative chemotherapy with 5-fluorouracil (5-FU) 1,000 mg/m^2 continuous infusion days 1–4 and 29–32 and mitomycin 10–15 mg/m^2 day 1 combined with EBRT to 30 Gy (6). Unexpectedly, the investigators found that the first three patients who received treatment achieved complete responses. Multiple confirmatory studies have found that combined chemoradiation therapy results in a 70–86% 5 year colostomy free survival rate and a 72–89% 5 year overall survival rate. (See Table 50-2 for suggested diagnosis and treatment options.)

Chemoradiation Versus Radiation Therapy Alone

Two phase III studies have evaluated the relative benefit of chemoradiation compared to radiation therapy alone.

- *UKCCCR*: The Anal Cancer Trial Working Party of the United Kingdom Coordination Committee on Cancer Research (UKCCCR) randomized 585 patients with anal cancer to external beam radiation therapy (45 Gy of EBRT with either a 15 Gy external beam boost or a 25 Gy brachytherapy boost) or the same radiation therapy in combination with concurrent 5-FU (1,000 mg/m^2 continuous infusion for 4 days or 750 mg/m^2 continuous infusion for 5 days during the first and last week of radiation therapy) and mitomycin (12 mg/m^2 day 1) (7). Chemoradiation improved local control (39% vs. 61%) and disease specific survival (28% vs. 39%), but 3 year overall survival was not statistically significantly different between the two arms (58% vs. 65%).
- *EORTC*: The European Organization for Research and Treatment of Cancer (EORTC) randomized 110 patients with anal cancer to radiation therapy (45 Gy of EBRT with either a 15 Gy or 30 Gy external beam boost) or the same radiation therapy in combination with concurrent 5-FU (750 mg/m^2 continuous infusion on days 1–5 and 29–33) and mitomycin (15 mg/m^2 day 1) (8). Similar to the UKCCCR study, the chemoradiation therapy improved local control (39% vs. 58%), with a 32% higher colostomy-free rate in the chemoradiation arm. However, 3 year overall survival was not statistically significantly different between the two groups (65% vs. 72%). In this study skin ulceration and nodal involvement were poor prognostic indicators, and women had better local control and survival than men.

These European trials showed that, compared to radiation therapy alone, chemoradiation offers patients a better chance of achieving local control, disease free survival, and colostomy free survival, but does not improve overall survival, possibly because of the impact of APR as salvage therapy. At present, combined modality therapy with chemoradiation is standard of care.

Role of Mitomycin

The Radiation Therapy Oncology Group (RTOG) and Eastern Cooperative Oncology Group (ECOG) have evaluated the role of mitomycin in the combined

Table 50-2

Suggested Diagnosis and Treatment Algorithm for Anal Cancer

Physical exam
> Assessment of primary tumor size
> Assessment of inguinal lymph nodes

Biopsy
> Anal tumor
> – If squamous cell cancer, proceed with algorithm
> – If adenocarcinoma, treat as rectal adenocarcinoma
> Inguinal lymph node(s)
> – If enlarged on physical exam or seen radiographically

Radiology
> Transanal ultrasound
> – Can evaluate tumor depth and local lymph nodes

> CT scan
> – Can evaluate tumor size, local and distant lymph nodes, metastases

Treatment
> Chemoradiation
> 5-FU 1,000 mg/m^2 continuous infusion days 1–4, 29–32
> Mitomycin 10 mg/m^2 days 1, 29
> EBRT 45–50 Gy total dose to primary tumor, with initial fields
> including the pelvis from S1 to S2 level, inguinal lymph nodes,
> and anus to 30–36 Gy

Post-treatment assessment
> Physical exam beginning 6–8 weeks after completion of
> chemoradiation
> Any remaining abnormalities 3 months after completion of treatment
> can be biopsied

Persistent/recurrent disease
> Salvage APR
> Salvage chemoradiation
> Salvage APR may be used for persistent/recurrent disease after
> salvage chemoradiation

Metastatic disease
> Systemic chemotherapy
> 5-FU/cisplatin
> Carboplatin
> Doxorubicin
> Possible utility of taxanes, gemcitabine, and irinotecan

modality regimen. Mitomycin is not a known radiation sensitizer, and its renal, pulmonary, and bone marrow toxicity have raised concerns about its safety. In this trial, 310 patients were randomized to EBRT (45–50.4 Gy) with either 5-FU (continuous infusion 1,000 mg/m^2 days 1–4 and 29–32) alone or the same 5-FU schedule with mitomycin 10 mg/m^2 for two doses (9). Patients who received mitomycin had significant improvements in colostomy free survival (59% vs. 71%) and disease free survival (51% vs. 73%), but not overall survival or disease specific survival. On subset analysis, the addition of mitomycin to patients with T3 or T4 tumors did not have a significant impact on outcome. Toxicity was higher in the mitomycin arm, with significantly increased Grade 4 and 5 toxicities (7% vs. 23%), with four patients in the mitomycin arm having fatal neutropenic sepsis versus 1 in the 5-FU only arm. From these results, the investigators concluded that despite the added toxicities, mitomycin plays a significant role in combined modality therapy for anal cancer. 5-FU, mitomycin, and EBRT remains the standard of care chemoradiation treatment for anal cancer.

Role of Cisplatin

Platinum compounds were not available when combination chemoradiation regimens were originally tested, but since have become an active component of chemotherapy regimens for squamous cell cancers. For this reason, they are being evaluated for treatment of anal cancers. Multiple preliminary studies have combined 5-FU, cisplatin, and EBRT in the treatment of anal cancers. Colostomy free survival rates range from 56 to 80%, disease free survival 67–94%, and overall survival 78–86%. Because of this impressive data, Intergroup trial RTOG 98-11 randomized 682 patients to either 5-FU 1,000 mg/m^2 days 1–4 and 29–32, mitomycin 10 mg/m^2 days 1 and 29, and EBRT or an induction course of chemotherapy with 5-FU 1,000 mg/m^2 on days 1–4 and 29–32 with cisplatin 75 mg/m^2 on days 1 and 29, with EBRT starting day 57 and 5-FU 1,000 mg/m^2 on days 57–60 and 85–88 and cisplatin 75 mg/m^2 on days 57 and 85 (10). For the 634 analyzable patients, the hazard ratio for disease free survival, which was the primary endpoint of the study, was 1.14 ($p = 0.34$), showing no difference between the two treatment arms. Overall survival was also no different between the two arms, but the colostomy rate was significantly higher for the cisplatin-treated patients than the mitomycin-treated patients (HR 1.63, $p = 0.04$). This study showed that despite encouraging data on the use of cisplatin in anal cancer patients, the combination of 5-FU, mitomycin, and radiation therapy remain standard of care.

Locally Advanced Tumors

Patients with larger tumors, T3/4 or with more extensive nodal metastases (N2/3) comprise a group of patients at higher risk for treatment failure. Only about 50% of these patients will be cured with standard therapy. The Cancer and Leukemia Group B (CALGB) evaluated the regimen of induction chemotherapy with 5-FU (1,000 mg/m^2 continuous infusion days 1–4 and 29–32) and cisplatin (75 mg/m^2 on days 1 and 29) followed by chemoradiation with 5-FU and mitomycin (DR52). An initial report of 45 patients treated with this regimen showed a 56% 21-month colostomy and disease free survival.

Treatment Complications

Complications of chemoradiation therapy for anal cancer include acute and chronic toxicities. Acute toxicities include diarrhea, desquamation and erythema, mucositis, pain, and myelosuppression. Late toxicities include anal ulcers, stricture/stenosis, fistulae, incontinence, and necrosis. Colostomy may be required for these late effects in 6–12% of patients. The risk of these complications increases with radiation dose.

Treatment of Patients with HIV

The combination of chemotherapy and radiation therapy is generally well tolerated and effective in HIV positive patients. However, treatment-related toxicity appears to be more common in these patients, particularly when radiation doses exceed 30 Gy. It is controversial whether CD4 counts correlate with increased toxicity. Occasionally, diverting colostomy or APR is used to manage local treatment toxicity in these patients. Blood counts should also be followed closely in these patients, with dose reductions or treatment breaks used as necessary.

Persistent or Recurrent Disease

Response to treatment is assessed approximately 6–8 weeks after completion of chemoradiation therapy. Whether the response to treatment should be assessed by physical exam alone or in combination with a biopsy is controversial. Squamous cell carcinomas tend to regress slowly over 3–12 weeks after the completion of therapy. In an Intergroup study evaluating the role of mitomycin in combination with 5-FU, patients had follow up biopsies 6 weeks after completion of therapy (9). Residual disease was found in % of patients. In this trial, patients with residual disease were treated with a salvage regimen of 5-FU plus cisplatin with 9 Gy of EBRT. Fifty-five percent of those patients achieved a complete response. It was unclear whether this high-salvage rate was due to the additional therapy or that the anal tumors in these patients were simply slower to regress after the completion of the original therapy. There is no consensus on the use and timing of biopsy in patients who have had a complete clinical response to therapy. It is, however, reasonable to biopsy persistent abnormalities at 3 months after the completion of chemoradiation at which point most tumors should be fully eradicated.

- *Persistent disease* – The treatment for persistent anal cancer is APR. In the UKCCCR trial, 29 patients who had achieved less than 50% response to primary therapy underwent salvage APR (7). Forty percent of the patients who underwent salvage APR eventually had local relapse.

  Salvage chemoradiation therapy has also been evaluated (9). Twenty-two patients on the Intergroup study evaluating the role of mitomycin C were labeled as having persistent disease. These patients received salvage 5-FU, cisplatin, and 9 Gy EBRT. Ten patients continued to have persistent disease and nine of the 10 underwent salvage APR. Six of the nine patients who underwent salvage APR eventually had disease recurrence. Of the 12 patients who were disease free after salvage chemoradiation, four required subsequent APR and remain disease free.

- *Recurrent disease* – The majority of patients who have recurrent disease recur locally. As with persistent disease, these patients are candidates for salvage APR or chemoradiation. Approximately 50% of patients with recurrent disease who undergo salvage APR will be rendered disease free. There have been no formal trials of salvage chemoradiation in the setting of recurrent disease, but the salvage chemoradiation regimen used to treat patients with persistent disease has been extrapolated to this setting by some practitioners.

Metastatic Disease

Distant recurrence occurs in 10–17% of patients who receive chemoradiation therapy. The most common site of distant metastasis is the liver. No known cure exists for metastatic anal cancer, and there is limited data on active regimens for these patients. Active regimens include: cisplatin plus 5-FU, carboplatin, doxorubicin, and semustine. There is little information about the response of metastatic anal cancer to more recent chemotherapy agents, such as taxanes, gemcitabine, or irinotecan.

CONCLUSIONS

Remarkable progress has been made in understanding the pathophysiology and treatment of anal cancer in the past 30 years. HPV has been clearly implicated in the development of the majority of anal cancers. Screening programs may allow for the diagnosis of anal dysplasia prior to progression to invasive cancer. The use of sphincter-sparing chemoradiation therapy has remarkably improved the quality of life and survival for patients with anal cancer. We await further data on the incorporation of cisplatin into the chemoradiation regimens.

REFERENCES

1. Jemal A, Murray T, Ward E, et al. Cancer statistics, 2005. CA Cancer J Clin. 2005; 55(1): 10–30.
2. Johnson LG, Medeleine MM, Newcomer LM, Schwartz SM, Daling JR. Anal cancer incidence and survival: the surveillance, epidemiology, and end results experience, 1973–2000. Cancer. 2004; 101(2): 281–288.
3. Chiao EY, Krown SE, Stier EA, Schrag D. A population-based analysis of temporal trends in the incidence of squamous anal canal cancer in relation to the HIV epidemic. J Acquir Immune Defic Syndr. 2005; 40(4): 451–455.
4. Goldie SJ, Kuntz KM, Weinstein MC, Freedberg KA, Welton ML, Palefsky JM. The clinical effectiveness and cost-effectiveness of screening for anal squamous intraepithelial lesions in homosexual and bisexual HIV-positive men. JAMA. 1999; 281(19): 1822–1829.
5. Goldie SJ, Kuntz KM, Weinstein MC, Freedberg KA, Palefsky JM. Cost-effectiveness of screening for anal squamous intraepithelial lesions and anal cancer in human immunodeficiency virus-negative homosexual and bisexual men. Am J Med. 2000; 108(8): 634–641.
6. Nigro ND, Vaitkevicius VK, Considine B, Jr. Combined therapy for cancer of the anal canal: a preliminary report. Dis Colon Rectum. 1974; 17(3): 354–356.
7. Epidermoid anal cancer: results from the UKCCCR randomised trial of radiotherapy alone versus radiotherapy, 5-fluorouracil, and mitomycin. UKCCCR Anal Cancer Trial Working Party. UK Co-ordinating Committee on Cancer Research. Lancet. 1996; 348(9034): 1049–1054.
8. Bartelink H, Roelofsen F, Eschwege F, et al. Concomitant radiotherapy and chemotherapy is superior to radiotherapy alone in the treatment of locally advanced anal cancer: results of a phase III randomized trial of the European Organization for Research and Treatment of Cancer Radiotherapy and Gastrointestinal Cooperative Groups. J Clin Oncol. 1997; 15(5): 2040–2049.
9. Flam M, John M, Pajak TF, et al. Role of mitomycin in combination with fluorouracil and radiotherapy, and of salvage chemoradiation in the definitive non-surgical treatment of epidermoid carcinoma of the anal canal: results of a phase III randomized intergroup study. J Clin Oncol. 1996; 14(9): 2527–2539.
10. Ajani JA, Winter KA, Gunderson LL, et al. Intergroup RTOG 98-11: A phase III randomized study of 5-fluorouracil (5-FU), mitomycin, and radiotherapy versus 5-fluorouracil, cisplatin, and radiotherapy in carcinoma of the anal canal. Proceedings of American Society for Clinical Oncology 318, 2006. Abstract 4009.

51	Pasi A. Jänne

MALIGNANT MESOTHELIOMA

BACKGROUND

Malignant mesothelioma is a rare malignancy arising from the mesothelial cells of the pleural or peritoneal surfaces. Mesothelioma can arise from the pleura (pleural mesothelioma), peritoneum (peritoneal mesothelioma), pericardium (pericardial mesothelioma) or *tunica vaginalis* (testicular mesothelioma). In the United States, there are approximately 3,000 new cases of mesothelioma reported annually. Approximately 80% of these occur as pleural mesothelioma. As this is the most common form of mesothelioma, this chapter will focus on malignant pleural mesothelioma.

The development of mesothelioma is most clearly associated with prior asbestos exposure (1). Asbestos was (and continues to be in some parts of the world) an important and affordable industrial resource due to its resistance to heat and combustion. Asbestos was used in shipbuilding, car brakes, in the production of cement, and as insulation. There are two main forms of asbestos known as amphiboles and chrysotile. Amphiboles are long thin asbestos fibers and are felt to be the most carcinogenic of the asbestos fibers. Chrysotile asbestos has also been associated with mesothelioma although the frequency may be less than with amphibole asbestos (1). The latency period between the time of asbestos exposure to development of mesothelioma can be 20–40 years. These unique features reflect the population of patients who develop mesothelioma including asbestos miners, plumbers, pipefitters or those who worked in shipbuilding industries. In the United States, mesothelioma is a disease of Caucasian men reflecting the population of asbestos workers in the 1960s and early 1970s. The median age of patients diagnosed with mesothelioma is in the mid 60s although in the surveillance epidemiology and end results (SEER) database from the United States the median age is over 70. Approximately 80% of patients who develop mesothelioma are men. Women who develop mesothelioma also may have worked in industries that used asbestos although there are reports of secondary exposure for example from clothing of spouses who worked directly with asbestos (2). The estimated incidence of mesothelioma worldwide also reflects the use of asbestos in different regions of the world. It is estimated that the cumulative worldwide the incidence of mesothelioma will not peak for another 10–20 years. However, in the United States some estimates suggest that this may have already occurred while in Europe, Australia, and Japan, where common asbestos use occurred until much later than in the United States, the incidence may not peak for another 15–20 years (3). In addition, asbestos is still extensively used in many developing countries suggesting that the worldwide incidence of mesothelioma will continue to rise.

A second, but very controversial factor thought to play a role in the development of mesothelioma is simian virus 40 (SV40). SV40 is an oncogenic polyoma virus in human cells and its infection leads to inactivation of tumor suppressor genes p53 and the retinoblastoma gene (Rb) (4). SV40 may have been transmitted to humans inadvertently as a contaminant in the polio vaccine 30–40 years ago. However, epidemiologic studies have not found a greater incidence of mesothelioma in those who received the polio vaccine during that time period (5). Although SV40 viral sequences have been detected in mesotheliomas (and not in normal adjacent lung tissues), this has not been a consistent finding and as suggested by some investigators may even be a false positive finding (6). Additional studies are underway to define the role of SV40 in the development of mesothelioma. Other etiologic factors leading to mesothelioma include prior ionizing radiation and rare familial forms reported to occur in Cappadocia, Turkey (7, 8).

CLINICAL PRESENTATION

The most common clinical presentation of malignant pleural mesothelioma includes dyspnea on exertion and shortness of breath. These clinical symptoms often lead physicians to obtain a chest X-ray where a unilateral pleural effusion is noted (Figure 51-1). Mesothelioma is rarely an incidental finding on a routine chest X-ray. Patients can also present with non-pleuritic chest pain. This symptom is important to elicit from patients as those who present with chest pains often have disease extending into the chest wall and thus they

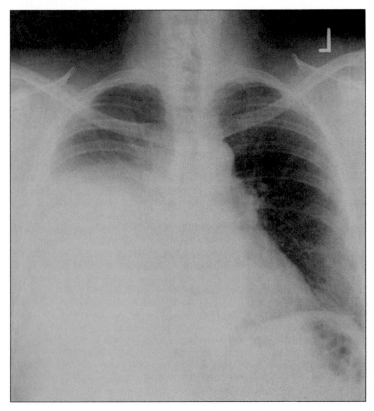

FIGURE 51-1 Anterior–Posterior chest radiograph of a patient with newly diagnosed malignant mesothelioma. A large right sided pleural effusion can be appreciated in this chest x-ray.

Table 51-1

Signs and Symptoms of Malignant Mesothelioma

Mesothelioma related	Constitutional
Dyspnea	Weight joss
Chest pain	Anorexia
Discordant chest wall expansion	Night sweats
Palpable chest wall mass	

The constitutional symptoms are often associated with mesothelioma, but are not specific to the disease.

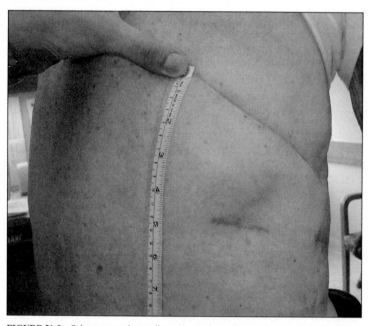

FIGURE 51-2 Subcutaneous chest wall mass in a patient with mesothelioma. This painful subcutaneous mass appeared a few months following surgical exploration.

are clearly not surgical candidates. Other presenting signs and symptoms include discordant chest wall expansion, weight loss, night sweats, and the presence of a palpable subcutaneous mass (Table 51-1 and Figure 51-2).

DIAGNOSTIC EVALUATION

The presentation of a patient with a new pleural effusion often leads to a thoracentesis to evaluate the nature of the effusion. The pleural effusions in mesothelioma are often cytologically negative and patients frequently undergo repeated thoracenteses in order to establish the diagnosis of mesothelioma. Due to frequent nature of cytologically negative effusions, cytology is not a reliable method to diagnose mesothelioma. In addition, cytologic specimens are often insufficient to determine the histologic subtype of mesothelioma which itself provides prognostic information.

The diagnostic procedure of choice for mesothelioma is a thoracoscopic biopsy. There are several advantages to this approach. First, it provides the surgeon the ability to assess the extent of tumor on the visceral and parietal pleura. Second, a biopsy of the involved area can be obtained under direct visualization. This is critical to able to make an accurate histologic diagnosis. Finally, thoracoscopy provides the ability to also perform a pleurodesis, which can help control recurrent pleural effusions. It is important to note that mesothelioma can grow along and through previous biopsy sites (for example see Figure 51-2). Thus if a patient is being considered for future a pneumonectomy it will be important to mark and excise en bloc the prior biopsy site.

The pathologic evaluation of malignant mesothelioma can be challenging and the disease can sometimes be confused pathologically with adenocarcinoma of the lung. However, several tumor markers can help distinguish adenocarcinoma from malignant mesothelioma (Table 51-2). Unlike adenocarcinomas, mesotheliomas do not express thyroid transcription factor 1 (TTF-1) or carcioembryonic antigen (CEA). In contrast, mesotheliomas do express the wilms tumor protein (WT-1) and calretinin which are not expressed by lung adenocarcinomas (9, 10). In addition to pathologic diagnosis of mesothelioma, it is important to distinguish the histologic subtype of mesothelioma. The most common histologic subtype is epithelial mesothelioma and accounts for approximately 60% of all mesotheliomas. Other subtypes of mesothelioma include sarcomatoid mesothelioma and mixed (containing components of both epithelial and sarcomatoid) type mesothelioma. The main reason to determine the histologic subtype of mesothelioma is that patients with sarcomatoid mesothelioma often have much worse prognosis than those with epithelial mesothelioma and may not be ideal candidates for aggressive surgical resection.

Two serum markers, osteopontin and soluble mesothelin-related (SMR) proteins, have also recently emerged as potential diagnostic markers in mesothelioma (11, 12). Osteopontin is protein that mediates cell–matrix interactions and cell signaling. It binds both integrin and CD44. In animal models of mesothelioma, osteopontin levels are upregulated in response to asbestos exposure. When osteopontin levels were examined in patients with and without documented asbestos exposure there were no differences in mean serum osteopontin levels (11). However, serum osteopontin levels were significantly higher in patients whose duration of asbestos exposure was >10 years compared to those with <10 years of asbestos exposure. In addition, serum osteopontin levels were significantly higher in patients with radiographic evidence of asbestos exposure (presence of pleural plaques and fibrosis) than in those with normal chest x-rays (11). Given that mesothelioma is often difficult to diagnose at an early stage, patients with elevated serum osteopontin levels and radiographic abnormalities may be appropriate

Table 51-2

Immunohistochemical Markers Used to Distinguish Malignant Mesothelioma from Lung Adenocarcinoma

	Mesothelioma	Adenocarcinoma
Cytokeratin	Positive	Positive
CEA	Negative	Positive
TTF-1	Negative	Positive
Calretinin	Positive	Negative
WT-1	Positive	Negative

CEA, carcinoembryonic antigen; TTF-1, thyroid transcription factor 1; WT-1, wilms tumor antigen.

candidates for additional radiographic and/or invasive studies to determine whether they in fact have mesothelioma. The second potential tumor marker is mesothelin. This is a cell surface protein present on mesothelial cells. It can remain membrane bound or be shed into the serum (soluble mesothelin-related proteins; SMR) and be detected using an ELISA assay (12). In a study using this assay, 37/44 (84%) of patients with mesothelioma had elevated levels or SMR compared to 3/160 (2%) of patients with other lung or pleural diseases. In addition, seven of 40 patients exposed to asbestos had elevated levels of SMR. Interestingly within 1–5 years, three of the seven patients developed mesothelioma suggesting that SMR may also serve as a screening test for asbestos exposed individuals. Additional clinical studies using both osteopontin and SMR are currently underway.

Three main imagine modalities, computed tomorgraphy (CT), positron emission tomography (PET), and magnetic resonance imagine (MRI), are used to evaluate patients with newly diagnosed mesothelioma. Contrast enhanced CT scanning often reveals a thickened lobulated circumferential pleural rind (Figure 51-3) with or without the presence of a concurrent pleural effusion. CT scanning can also help identify presence of pleural plaques, a sign of previous asbestos exposure, and whether the disease extends into the intralobular fissures. However, CT scanning is not very accurate in determining chest wall invasion or transdiaphragmatic extension of mesothelioma. These features are important to determine especially if the patient is being considered for surgery as treatment for mesothelioma. MRI is often used in this situation and can identify chest wall invasion (Figure 51-4) as well as transdiaphragmatic invasion of mesothelioma (13). FDG-PET scanning has also recently been evaluated for its clinical utility as most mesothelioma's are PET avid. Analogous to lung cancer, FDG-PET scanning can identify occult metastatic disease in patients that are otherwise potential surgical candidates (14). However, its utility in defining locoregional disease and the role of FDG-PET scanning in advanced mesothelioma remains to be determined.

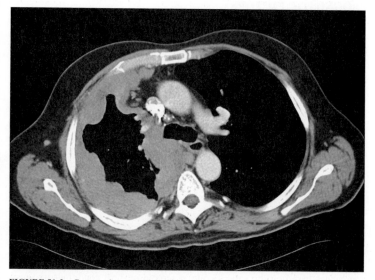

FIGURE 51-3 Computed tomography (CT) appearance of mesothelioma. A thickened circumferential pleural rind is seen on chest CT in this patient with epithelial mesothelioma.

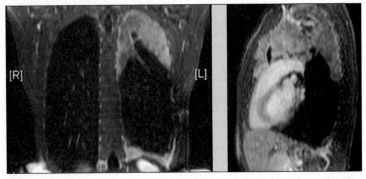

FIGURE 51-4   Coronal (*left*) and sagital (*right*) MRI images of the left hemithorax of a patient with newly diagnosed malignant mesothelioma. The MRI images help to define mesothelioma invading into the chest wall on the lateral side in the left hemithorax.

STAGING

There are multiple staging systems that have been described for pleural mesothelioma while there is no staging system for peritoneal mesothelioma. The goal of staging is to stratify prognosis and to identify patients that are potential candidates for surgery. The most commonly and widely accepted staging system is the International Mesothelioma Interest Group (IMIG) system which is modified tumor-node-metastases (TNM) staging system (15). Mesothelioma is a difficult disease to accurately stage based on radiographic imaging and often staging is only possible at the time of surgery. Some staging systems, such as the Brigham and Women's Hospital staging system, are based solely on findings at the time of surgery (16).

PROGNOSTIC FACTORS

There is no known curative treatment modality for mesothelioma. The median survival of newly diagnosed patients ranges from 6 to 18 months. The disease course (even untreated) can be highly variable and thus several prognostic systems have been developed in order to identify patients subsets with different prognoses. The two main prognostic systems are the Cancer and Leukemia Group B (CALGB) prognostic groups and the European Organization for Research and Treatment of Cancer (EORTC) prognostic factors and prognostic scores (17, 18). Patients with sarcomatoid mesothelioma, those with a poor performance status and those who present with chest pain (indicative of disease invasion into the chest wall) are ones with a poor prognosis. In addition, patients with evidence of a systemic inflammatory response to their mesothelioma manifested by either as an increased white blood cell (WBC) or platelet counts also tend to have a poorer prognosis.

TREATMENT

There is no standard therapeutic approach for malignant mesothelioma. One of the limitations in this disease is the lack of randomized clinical trials comparing different treatment modalities. Treatment approaches to mesothelioma vary significantly and range from palliative care to chemotherapy to aggressive surgical approaches based on the patient's age, comorbid medical conditions and performance status.

IMPACT OF TREATMENT

The true impact of any therapeutic modality in malignant mesothelioma is presently undefined. Some of the reasons behind this include the rarity of the disease, the paucity of randomized studies, the lack of uniform staging, heterogeneity within the pathologic subclasses of mesothelioma, imbalance of prognostic factors and difficulties in assessing response to therapy using computed tomography, and other radiographic imaging modalities. It is presently not clear whether any therapy prolongs survival in patients with mesothelioma compared to supportive care alone. There has never been a clinical trial comparing a treatment modality to best supportive care alone. The natural history of mesothelioma can be variable and thus benefits seen in clinical trials may be biased by patient selection. Many patients require control of their pleural effusion without the need of immediate systemic or local treatment. The impact of treatment compared to supportive care is presently being evaluated in a series of ongoing clinical trials described in the following sections.

SURGERY

Surgery is a therapeutic option for some patients with malignant mesothelioma. One of the rationales for performing surgery is that mesothelioma is a disease that tends to spread locally into adjacent structures such as the chest wall and the mediastinum before spreading to systemic sites. Thus local treatments such as surgery may offer therapeutic and palliative benefits to patients. Two main surgical approaches, an extrapleural pneumonectomy (EPP) and a pleurectomy/decortication (P/D), have been used to treat mesothelioma (19). An EPP is an en bloc resection of the parietal pleura, lung, pericardium, and diaphragm (20). The diaphragm and pericardium is then reconstructed with the use of a gortex patch. In contrast, a P/D is a resection of the parietal and mediastinal pleura and involved visceral and diaphragmatic pleura and pericardium. The lung however remains in place. It is unclear if either operation adheres to the principles of oncology surgery as no margin of uninvolved tissue is typically resected.

There are several controversies that exist regarding surgery for mesothelioma. The first is whether surgery improves survival or quality of life in patients with malignant mesothelioma. This very question is being tested in two ongoing clinical trials being conducted in the United Kingdom. The first is the mesothelioma and radical surgery (MARS) trial. In this trial patients with potentially respectable mesothelioma are offered chemotherapy followed by randomization to or not to receive and EPP. The primary endpoint of this trial is overall survival and will determine not only the impact on survival of doing an EPP, but also its effects on the quality of life of the patients undergoing this operation. The second trial called the MesoVATS trial will randomize patients with newly diagnosed mesothelioma with a pleural effusion to effusion control alone (with a talc pleurodesis) or to a video assisted thoracoscopic surgery (VATS) of their pleura (a pleurectomy). Endpoints of this trial include a comparison of survival at 1-year, control of effusion and of quality of life in the two different treatment arms. Both studies will help answering critical components of the contribution of surgery to the management of patients with malignant mesothelioma.

A second surgical dilemma is how to best identify patients benefiting from surgery and to choose the most appropriate operation for those patients (21). There have been no randomized studies comparing the two different surgical approaches. The patients most likely to benefit from an EPP are those with epithelial histology mesothelioma with negative resection margins in whom there is no N2 lymph node involvement (19). In general patients who are eligible for this operation are younger with appropriate cardiopulmonary reserve. Patients who undergo a P/D are often older with other co-morbid medical illnesses. In addition, patients with minimal pleural disease and those whose tumors do not extend into the interlobular pleural surfaces may be more appropriate candidates for a P/D operation.

Despite surgery mesothelioma recurs in most individuals. The pattern of recurrence depends to some degree on the type of operation. For patients who have undergone an EPP local recurrences (within the operated thoracic cavity) do occur although systemic recurrences begin to predominate. In contrast in patients who have undergone a P/D, local recurrences are the most common site of mesothelioma recurrence (22). Efforts to decrease both local and systemic recurrences have included the use of photodynamic therapy, intracavitary chemotherapy and neo-adjuvant, and adjuvant systemic chemotherapy.

CHEMOTHERAPY

Until recently mesothelioma was considered a disease refractory to systemic chemotherapy. In fact most if not all chemotherapy agents have been tested in clinical trials for patients with mesothelioma (23). The agents with the most consistent single agent anti-tumor activity include antifolates, platinum agents (cisplatin and carboplatin), vinorelbine, and gemcitabine. The largest (and only adequately powered) phase III clinical trial in mesothelioma compared the combination of cisplatin and pemetrexed to cisplatin alone as initial treatment for patients with malignant mesothelioma. This study demonstrated a response rate of 41% and a median survival of 12.1 months for the combination arm which were significantly better than in the cisplatin alone arm (16.7% and 9.3 months, respectively) (24). This trial was the basis for the FDA approval of cisplatin/pemetrexed in malignant mesothelioma and helped establish this combination as one standard treatment approach for mesothelioma patients. Alternative antifolates such as raltitrexed (cisplatin/raltitrexed), antimetabolites (gemcitabine; cisplatin/gemcitabine) and platinum agents (carboplatin; carboplatin/pemetrexed) have also been studied and are active combination treatment regimens for this disease (25–27). There is virtually no data on second line treatment of mesothelioma and this remains an active area of investigation.

In addition to chemotherapy many targeted agents have been investigated in mesothelioma. Both epidermal growth factor receptor (EGFR) inhibitors (gefitinib and erlotinib) and platelet derived growth factor receptor (PDGFR) inhibitors (imatinib) are inactive in this disease (28, 29). Mesotheliomas are very angiogenic tumors and angiogenesis inhibitors including SU5416, thalidomide and PTK787 have all demonstrated single agent activity in this disease (30). In addition, a large randomized phase II clinical trial evaluating bevacizumab (anti-VEGF antibody) has been performed but the outcome is presently not known.

RADIATION

Radiation has a limited therapeutic role for most patients with mesothelioma. Radiation is often used either in the palliative setting or to decrease the likelihood of tumor invasion into surgical or biopsy sites. In addition for patients who undergo an EPP radiation is used in the post-operative treatment of the hemithorax (31). Since the surgical margins following EPP are often involved with mesothelioma (or in very close proximity), radiation provides an opportunity to decrease local recurrence. Patients treated with early-stage mesothelioma and hemithorax radiation have a low chance of recurrence within the operated thoracic cavity, but a much greater chance of systemic recurrence. Many such patients are often treated with the combination of surgery, chemotherapy, and radiation.

REFERENCES

1. Hodgson JT, Darnton A. The quantitative risks of mesothelioma and lung cancer in relation to asbestos exposure. Ann Occup Hyg. 2000; 44: 565–601.

2. Miller A. Mesothelioma in household members of asbestos-exposed workers: 32 United States cases since 1990. Am J Ind Med. 2005; 47: 458–462.

3. Robinson BW, Lake RA. Advances in malignant mesothelioma. N Engl J Med. 2005; 353: 1591–1603.

4. De Luca A, Baldi A, Esposito V, et al. The retinoblastoma gene family pRb/p105, p107, pRb2/p130 and simian virus-40 large T-antigen in human mesotheliomas. Nat Med. 1997; 3: 913–916.

5. Strickler HD, Goedert JJ, Devesa SS, et al. Trends in U.S. pleural mesothelioma incidence rates following simian virus 40 contamination of early poliovirus vaccines. J Natl Cancer Inst. 2003; 95: 38–45.

6. Lopez-Rios F, Illei PB, Rusch V, Ladanyi M. Evidence against a role for SV40 infection in human mesotheliomas and high risk of false-positive PCR results owing to presence of SV40 sequences in common laboratory plasmids. Lancet. 2004; 364: 1157–1166.

7. Weissmann LB, Corson JM, Neugut AI, Antman KH. Malignant mesothelioma following treatment for Hodgkin's disease. J Clin Oncol. 1996; 14: 2098–2100.

8. Roushdy-Hammady I, Siegel J, Emri S, Testa JR, Carbone M. Genetic-susceptibility factor and malignant mesothelioma in the Cappadocian region of Turkey. Lancet. 2001; 357: 444–445.

9. Ordonez NG. Value of calretinin immunostaining in differentiating epithelial mesothelioma from lung adenocarcinoma. Mod Pathol. 1998; 11: 929–933.

10. Amin KM, Litzky LA, Smythe WR, et al. Wilms' tumor 1 susceptibility (WT1) gene products are selectively expressed in malignant mesothelioma. Am J Pathol. 1995; 146: 344–356.

11. Pass HI, Lott D, Lonardo F, et al. Asbestos exposure, pleural mesothelioma, and serum osteopontin levels. N Engl J Med. 2005; 353: 1564–1573.

12. Robinson BW, Creaney J, Lake R, et al. Mesothelin-family proteins and diagnosis of mesothelioma. Lancet. 2003; 362: 1612–1616.

13. Stewart D, Waller D, Edwards J, Jeyapalan K, Entwisle J. Is there a role for preoperative contrast-enhanced magnetic resonance imaging for radical surgery in malignant pleural mesothelioma? Eur J Cardiothorac Surg. 2003; 24: 1019–1024.

14. Flores RM, Akhurst T, Gonen M, Larson SM, Rusch VW. Positron emission tomography defines metastatic disease but not locoregional disease in patients with malignant pleural mesothelioma. J Thorac Cardiovasc Surg. 2003; 126: 11–16.

15. Rusch VW. A proposed new international TNM staging system for malignant pleural mesothelioma. From the International Mesothelioma Interest Group. Chest. 1995; 108: 1122–1128.

16. Sugarbaker DJ, Strauss GM, Lynch TJ, et al. Node status has prognostic significance in the multimodality therapy of diffuse, malignant mesothelioma. J Clin Oncol. 1993; 11: 1172–1178.

17. Herndon JE, Green MR, Chahinian AP, et al. Factors predictive of survival among 337 patients with mesothelioma treated between 1984 and 1994 by the Cancer and Leukemia Group B. Chest. 1998; 113: 723–731.

18. Curran D, Sahmoud T, Therasse P, et al. Prognostic factors in patients with pleural mesothelioma: the European Organization for Research and Treatment of Cancer experience. J Clin Oncol. 1998; 16: 145–152.

19. Sugarbaker DJ, Flores RM, Jaklitsch MT, et al. Resection margins, extrapleural nodal status, and cell type determine postoperative long-term survival in trimodality therapy of malignant pleural mesothelioma: results in 183 patients. J Thorac Cardiovasc Surg. 1999; 117: 54–63; discussion 63–55.

20. Sugarbaker DJ, Jaklitsch MT, Bueno R, et al. Prevention, early detection, and management of complications after 328 consecutive extrapleural pneumonectomies. J Thorac Cardiovasc Surg. 2004; 128: 138–146.

21. Maziak DE, Gagliardi A, Haynes AE, Mackay JA, Evans WK. Surgical management of malignant pleural mesothelioma: a systematic review and evidence summary. Lung Cancer. 2005; 48: 157–169.

22. Janne PA, Baldini EH. Patterns of failure following surgical resection for malignant pleural mesothelioma. Thorac Surg Clin. 2004; 14: 567–573.

23. Janne PA. Chemotherapy for malignant pleural mesothelioma. Clin Lung Cancer. 2003; 5: 98–106.

24. Vogelzang NJ, Rusthoven JJ, Symanowski J, et al. Phase III study of pemetrexed in combination with cisplatin versus cisplatin alone in patients with malignant pleural mesothelioma. J Clin Oncol. 2003; 21: 2636–2644.

25. van Meerbeeck JP, Gaafar R, Manegold C, et al. Randomized phase III study of cisplatin with or without raltitrexed in patients with malignant pleural mesothelioma: an intergroup study of the European Organisation for Research and Treatment of Cancer Lung Cancer Group and the National Cancer Institute of Canada. J Clin Oncol. 2005; 23: 6881–6889.

26. Ceresoli GL, Zucali PA, Favaretto AG, et al. Phase II study of pemetrexed plus carboplatin in malignant pleural mesothelioma. J Clin Oncol. 2006; 24: 1443–1448.

27. Nowak AK, Byrne MJ, Williamson R, et al. A multicentre phase II study of cisplatin and gemcitabine for malignant mesothelioma. Br J Cancer. 2002; 87: 491–496.

28. Govindan R, Kratzke RA, Herndon JE, II, et al. Gefitinib in patients with malignant mesothelioma: a phase II study by the Cancer and Leukemia Group B. Clin Cancer Res. 2005; 11: 2300–2304.

29. Mathy A, Baas P, Dalesio O, van Zandwijk N. Limited efficacy of imatinib mesylate in malignant mesothelioma: a phase II trial. Lung Cancer. 2005; 50: 83–86.

30. Dowell JE, Kindler HL. Antiangiogenic therapies for mesothelioma. Hematol Oncol Clin North Am. 2005; 19: 1137–1145, viii.

31. Yajnik S, Rosenzweig KE, Mychalczak B, et al. Hemithoracic radiation after extrapleural pneumonectomy for malignant pleural mesothelioma. Int J Radiat Oncol Biol Phys. 2003; 56: 1319–1326.

NON-SMALL CELL LUNG CANCER

INTRODUCTION

Epidemiology

Lung cancer is the most common cause of cancer mortality in the US for both men and women, with an estimated 166,000 deaths per year. The median age at diagnosis is 70 years and it affects men more often than women (ratio 1.6:1). Cigarette smoking is the strongest risk factor for developing lung cancer. Smoking and exposure to environmental tobacco smoke account for 90% of lung cancer cases and smokers have a 20-fold increased risk of death from lung cancer compared to non-smokers. Other risk factors include asbestos exposure, ionizing radiation, and exposure to carcinogenic chemicals and minerals. Research is ongoing regarding dietary and genetic risk factors.

Non-small cell lung cancer (NSCLC) is associated with a variety of molecular and genetic changes that affect cell cycle biology and apoptosis. These include mutations or overexpression of the oncogenes *ras, c-erbB-2, bcl-2,* and *myc* and loss of the tumor suppressor genes p53, RB, and p16. Acquisition of telomerase activity, expression of tyrosine kinase receptors such as EGFR, HER2/neu, and PDGFR, and pro-angiogenic factors such as vascular endothelial growth factor (VEGF) are important in the transformation and proliferation of NSCLC.

Over 80% of lung cancers are classified as NSCLC, a histopathologic designation that includes adenocarcinoma, squamous cell carcinoma (SqCC), and large cell carcinoma. SqCC was historically the most frequent type of NSCLC, but over the last 35 years adenocarcinoma has become twice as common as SqCC, likely due to changes in cigarette composition. Bronchioloalveolar cell carcinoma (BAC) is a well-differentiated form of adenocarcinoma associated with improved survival. The rising incidence of BAC and tumors with BAC features is thought to account for much of the increase in adenocarcinoma diagnoses.

Presentation

The majority of patients have symptoms at the time of presentation with NSCLC. Symptoms vary depending on the location and size of the tumor, and presence and location of metastases. The most common symptoms arising from the primary tumor are cough, dyspnea, blood-tinged sputum, and chest pain. Local extension of the tumor within the chest can cause pleural or pericardial effusions, hoarseness, brachial plexopathy, Horner's syndrome, and superior vena cava syndrome. Metastatic disease may present with weight loss, neurologic symptoms or bony pain. Paraneoplastic syndromes are more commonly associated with small cell lung cancer, but NSCLC may be associated with hypercalcemia of malignancy or hypertrophic pulmonary osteoarthropathy.

Staging and Prognosis

The primary determinant of prognosis in NSCLC is stage at diagnosis. All NSCLC patients should undergo a contrast-enhanced chest CT scan extending through the liver and adrenal glands, as well as a whole body PET scan to look for occult metastases. CT or MRI of the brain is also encouraged. If there is a suspected metastasis at presentation, biopsy of that site can yield both diagnosis and stage.

Stage is defined by the size of the primary tumor and involvement of regional lymph nodes and metastatic sites via the American Joint Committee on Cancer TNM system (Table 52-1). In the absence of metastatic disease, the N (nodal) status is the most important determinant of overall stage and therefore of prognosis. Thus, management decisions often depend on N staging. Nodal involvement may be assessed by clinical means such as CT and PET scan, or more accurately by pathologic evaluation via biopsy. The average 5-year overall survival (OS) for NSCLC decreases with increasing stage (Table 52-2). OS is better, stage for stage, when N status is determined pathologically because clinical staging can falsely imply that involved lymph nodes are negative. CT scan only has a sensitivity of 61% and a specificity of 79% for evaluation of mediastinal nodes in NSCLC, while PET scan is slightly better with a sensitivity of 85% and a specificity of 90% (1). Still, in the absence of obvious metastatic

Table 52-1

TNM Staging for NSCLC

Primary tumor (T)

TX	Primary tumor cannot be assessed, or tumor proven by the presence of malignant cells in sputum or bronchial washings but not visualized by imaging or bronchoscopy
T0	No evidence of primary tumor
Tis	Carcinoma in situ
T1	Tumor <3 cm in greatest dimension, surrounded by lung or visceral pleura, without bronchoscopic evidence of invasion more proximal than the lobar bronchus* (i.e., not in the main bronchus)
T2	Tumor with any of the following features of size or extent: .3 cm in greatest dimension
	Involves main bronchus <2 cm distal to the carina
	Invades the visceral pleura
	Associated with atelectasis or obstructive pneumonitis that extends to the hilar region, but does not involve the entire lung.
T3	Tumor of any size that directly invades any of the following: chest wall (including superior sulcus tumors), diaphragm, mediastinal pleura, parietal pericardium; or tumor in the main bronchus <2 cm distal to the carina, but without involvement of the carina; or associated atelectasis or obstructive pneumonitis of the entire lung
T4	Tumor of any size that invades any of the following: mediastinum, heart, great vessels, trachea, esophagus, vertebral body, carina; or tumor with a malignant pleural or pericardial effusion,† or with satellite tumor nodule(s) within the ipsilateral primary-tumor lobe of the lung

Regional lymph nodes (N)

NX	Regional lymph nodes cannot be assessed
N0	No regional lymph node metastasis
N1	Metastasis to ipsilateral peribronchial and/or ipsilateral hilar lymph nodes, and intrapulmonary nodes involved by direct extension of the primary tumor
N2	Metastasis to ipsilateral mediastinal and/or subcarinal lymph node(s)
N3	Metastasis to contralateral mediastinal, contralateral hilar, ipsilateral or contralateral scalene, or supraclavicular lymph node(s)

Distant metastasis (M)

MX	Presence of distant metastasis cannot be assessed
M0	No distant metastasis
M1	Distant metastasis present‡

Stage grouping

Stage	T	N	M
Occult carcinoma	Tx	N0	M0
0	Tis	N0	M0
IA	T1	N0	M0
IB	T2	N0	M0
IIA	T1	N1	M0
IIB	T2	N1	M0
	T3	N0	M0
IIIA	T3	N1	M0
	T1	N2	M0
	T2	N2	M0
	T3	N2	M0
IIIB	T4	N0	M0
	T4	N1	M0
	T4	N2	M0
	T1	N3	M0
	T2	N3	M0
	T3	N3	M0
	T4	N3	M0
IV	Any T	Any N	M1

*The uncommon superficial tumor of any size with its invasive component limited to the bronchial wall, which may extend proximal to the main bronchus, is also classified T1.

†Most pleural effusions associated with lung cancer are due to tumor. However, there are a few patients in whom multiple cytopathologic examinations of pleural fluid show no tumor. In these cases, the fluid is non-bloody and is not an exudate. When these elements and clinical judgment dictate that the effusion is not related to the tumor, the effusion should be excluded as a staging element and the patient's disease should be staged T1, T2, or T3. Pericardial effusion is classified according to the same rules.

‡Separate metastatic tumor nodule(s) in the ipsilateral nonprimary-tumor lobe(s) of the lung also are classified M1.

Used with the permission of the American Joint Committee on Cancer (AJCC), Chicago, Illinois. The original source for this material is the AJCC Cancer Staging Manual, Sixth Edition (2002) published by Springer-New York, http://www.springeronline.com.

Table 52-2

Five-Year Overall Survival by Clinical and Pathologic Stage

Stage	Clinical survival (%)	Pathologic survival (%)
IA	61	67
IB	38	57
IIA	34	55
IIB	24	39
IIIA	13	23
IIIB	5	6
IV	<1	<1

Data from Mountain, CF. Revisions in the International System for Staging Lung Cancer. Chest 1997 Jun; 111(6): 1710–1717. Retrieved from http://www.ncbi.nlm.nih.gov/entrez/query.fcgi? db=pubmed&cmd=Retrieve&dopt=AbstractPlus&list_uids=9187198&query_hl=9&itool=pubmed _docsum.

disease, mediastinoscopic biopsy is a vital component of NSCLC staging and remains the gold standard for determining N status.

In addition to stage, other major indicators of poor prognosis in NSCLC include poor performance status (PS), hypercalcemia, weight loss, symptomatic presentation, and anemia.

EARLY STAGE NSCLC

Surgery

Surgical resection of the tumor and draining lymph nodes is the cornerstone of therapy for stages I–IIIA NSCLC and provides the greatest likelihood of cure. The type of surgery performed depends on the tumor size, location, overall health of the patient, and local practice standards. Pulmonary resections are classified as anatomic if they encompass the draining lymphovascular structures, as in pneumonectomy, lobectomy and segmentectomy, or non-anatomic, as in wedge resection. Resections can be performed through a standard thoracotomy incision, or in some cases through a smaller incision with video thoracoscopic assistance. Complete resection with a clean margin is the strongest predictor of cure after NSCLC surgery; hence, the location and size of the tumor partially dictate the required operation.

An additional consideration is the amount of lung parenchyma to be resected and the resultant morbidity and mortality (Table 52-3). A randomized study of peripheral stage IA NSCLC tumors treated with lobectomy versus a limited surgery (segmentectomy or wedge) found that limited surgery was associated with an increased risk of local recurrence and a trend towards inferior survival, although the methodology of this study has been criticized (2). Hence, lobectomy is the preferred operation for NSCLC unless tumor characteristics or patient comorbidities dictate otherwise. Hospital surgical volume also correlates inversely with peri-operative mortality.

Table 52-3

Relative Advantages and Disadvantages of Various Operations for NSCLC

Resection	Advantages	Disadvantages
Pneumonectomy	Adequate margins for large and central tumors	Mortality[*] 6–26%[†]
	Anatomic resection	Substantial reduction in lung function
Lobectomy	Adequate margins for most tumors	Mortality 3–4%
	Anatomic resection	
Segmentectomy	Parenchymal sparing	Concern over adequate margins
	Anatomic resection	
	Mortality only 1.5%	
Wedge resection	Ultra parenchymal sparing	Mortality no better than segmentectomy
		Non-anatomic resection
		Concern over adequate margins

[*]All mortalities reported are deaths at 30 days post-operation.

[†]Upper range of pneumonectomy mortality reflects the combined mortality of surgery with chemotherapy and radiation, as is often required for larger tumors.

Medically Inoperable Patients

Patients with early stage NSCLC and excessive surgical risk due to medical comorbidities are deemed "medically inoperable." Characteristics such as current smoking, poor exercise capacity, weight loss, and severe COPD are associated with high-surgical risk. Patients with abnormal (<40–60% of predicted) FEV1 or DLCO on pulmonary function testing require an estimation of post-operative cardio-pulmonary reserve with a quantitative V/Q scan, exercise tolerance testing, or exercise physiology testing. Advanced age alone should not preclude an otherwise fit patient from surgery as retrospective analyses suggest survival among elderly patients is similar to younger patients after resection of early stage NSCLC. Because of the accompanying heart disease and other comorbidities in smokers, 10–20% of patients presenting with early stage NSCLC are medically inoperable.

Options for medically inoperable patients include radiation therapy (RT) with curative intent, radiofrequency ablation (RFA), and watchful waiting with a plan for palliative treatment if symptoms arise. Standard RT yields about one-third the cure rate achieved surgically, with a 5-year OS of 20–30% for stage I NSCLC. The cure rate may be even higher with modern RT techniques, though no large series to demonstrate this are mature. While the operative risks are avoided with RT, patients are still vulnerable to radiation pneumonitis and esophagitis, fatigue, and other side effects. However, RT is the recommended standard of care treatment for medically inoperable early stage NSCLC.

RFA is a minimally invasive technology that lacks long-term follow-up data, though early reports are promising. An RFA needle electrode is inserted directly into the tumor mass via percutaneous CT-guidance. Radiofrequency energy is then converted into heat energy to cause cell death and necrosis in a spherical shape about the electrode, with minimal damage to surrounding tissue. Tumors must be 5 cm or less in diameter and approachable by needle. Pneumothorax is the most common treatment complication.

Adjuvant Treatment

Despite surgery, 50–60% of patients with early stage NSCLC will relapse and die from their lung cancer. Post-operative, or adjuvant, chemotherapy and RT aim to decrease the risk of local and distant recurrence. Adjuvant RT can decrease local recurrence rates, but does not impact overall survival. A large meta-analysis even suggested adjuvant RT could increase the risk of death for stages I and II patients (3). In general, adjuvant RT is not standard of care treatment, but it may be considered for specific patients with positive or close surgical margins or with stage III disease.

In 2004, an international multicenter randomized trial with nearly 2,000 patients demonstrated a 4% absolute improvement in 5-year OS for stages I, II, and III NSCLC patients treated with cisplatin-based adjuvant chemotherapy (4). Since that time, several other randomized trials have confirmed a 3–15% improvement in survival with platinum-based adjuvant chemotherapy. This benefit is most evident in patients with stages IB, II, and IIIA disease treated with cisplatin-based regimens. Given the consistency of these results, adjuvant cisplatinum-based combination chemotherapy is now considered the standard of care treatment for resected stages IB, II, and IIIA NSCLC.

Stage III NSCLC

Stage III NSCLC, or locally advanced disease, encompasses a heterogeneous collection of TNM stages. Cure rates vary substantially within the stage III classification. Treatment of IIIB tumors will be discussed first, as it is more uniform. IIIB tumors are by definition unresectable, because involvement of vital structures, spread to the contralateral lymphatic system, or malignant pleural effusion (MPE) seeding the thoracic cavity. Patients with stage IIIB disease are treated "definitively," meaning with curative intent, using chemotherapy and RT, except in the case of a MPE, termed "wet IIIB." The biology of wet IIIB NSCLC is more similar to stage IV NSCLC and treatment is therefore palliative in nature, usually with chemotherapy only, see "Advanced NSCLC" section.

Cisplatin-based chemotherapy given concurrently with RT has been shown to improve survival for stage IIIB NSCLC compared to the two given sequentially and compared to RT alone (5, 6). Hence, for patients with a good PS, concurrent cisplatin-based chemoradiation is the recommended treatment for unresectable stage III NSCLC. The best survival with definitive treatment of stage IIIB patients was achieved in the SWOG 9504 trial, a phase II study of concurrent chemotherapy with RT, followed by consolidation chemotherapy (7). Median survival in this cohort was 27 months, an improvement compared to prior definitive treatment regimens yielding median survivals of 15–17 months. Phase III trials using this regimen are underway.

Optimal management of stage IIIA NSCLC is a controversial topic. Stage IIIA tumors are variable in their resectability, and surgical practice patterns are divergent by region and by hospital volume. The vast majority of IIIA cases are so designated because of N2 lymphadenopathy, meaning involvement of the ipsilateral mediastinal or subcarinal nodes. If the N2 status is clinically obvious by CT or PET scan (Figure 52-1), the surgical cure rate is only half that when N2 involvement is discovered incidentally at the time of biopsy or thoractomy (5-year OS 13% versus 23%, respectively). This discrepancy has generated two treatment strategies for clinically obvious N2 disease. The first is definitive chemoradiotherapy alone, as in treatment of unresectable IIIB NSCLC. The second strategy is pre-operative (neoadjuvant) chemoradiotherapy aimed at "sterilizing" the mediastinum, i.e., attempting to approximate the incidentally discovered N2 case before resection is performed.

The US Intergroup 0139 trial was designed to compare these strategies, and randomized 429 patients with N2 stage IIIA NSCLC to definitive cisplatin-based chemoradiotherapy or neoadjuvant chemoradiotherapy followed by surgery. At interim analysis, survival was not different between the arms, with median survival about 23 months (8). However, the definitive chemoradiotherapy arm had a higher rate of local recurrence while the surgical arm has more early deaths due to peri-operative complication, especially among patients requiring pneumonectomy. In fact, a subgroup analysis of the patients receiving lobectomy and matched non-surgical controls showed an increased median survival in the lobectomy group (34 months) compared to the definitive chemoradiotherapy group (22 months, $p = 0.002$). The interpretation of this data has been that tumors amenable to lobectomy likely benefit from neoadjuvant therapy, but tumors requiring pneumonectomy should be treated by definitive chemoradiotherapy without surgery. If there is progressive disease or clinical decline during the neoadjuvant treatment, the prognosis is poor and resection should no longer be considered.

Pancoast Tumors

Pancoast tumors, or NSCLC tumors located in the superior sulcus, make up only 5% of NSCLC cases, and are often considered as a single group although they encompass tumors of various stages, usually IIB (T3N0), IIIA (T3N1-2), and IIIB (T4anyN). They are frequently associated with arm pain, numbness, and weakness from involvement of the brachial plexus. Because the limited space in the superior sulcus makes surgical resection technically difficult, the historical treatment of Pancoast tumors was neoadjuvant RT followed by

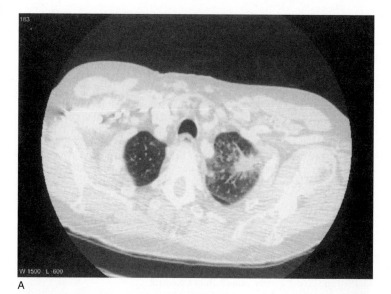

FIGURE 52-1   Clinically obvious stage IIIA NSCLC. Panel A shows a spiculated left upper lobe primary tumor. Panel B shows bulky ipsilateral mediastinal lymphadenopathy (*arrow*)

surgery, which yielded a 5-year OS of 30%. The success of neoadjuvant and definitive chemoradiotherapy in stage III NSCLC led to a phase II trial specific for Pancoast tumors with T2-4 and N0-1 status. A total of 110 patients received neoadjuvant chemoradiotherapy regimen, followed by surgery. Five-year OS was 41%, an improvement compared to historical findings with RT and surgery (9). Interestingly, the radiologic complete response rate to neoadjuvant therapy in this trial was 36%, yet at resection the pathologic complete and near-complete response rate was 65%, suggesting that there are often residual abnormalities on CT scan that do not contain viable tumor tissue.

ADVANCED NSCLC

Treatment Versus None

Forty-five percent of patients with NSCLC present with advanced NSCLC, meaning stage IV or wet IIIB. Advanced NSCLC is an incurable condition and the goals of treatment are palliative. The median survival is 6 months when treated with supportive measures only, and for many years it was thought that chemotherapy could not improve OS because few patients responded to treatment. Increased response to treatment was noted with the introduction of cisplatin in 1978 and taxanes in 1992. In 1995 a meta-analysis of 11 trials randomizing advanced NSCLC patients to cisplatin-based chemotherapy versus supportive care showed that treatment conferred an OS advantage [hazard ratio (HR) 0.73] (10). Several additional studies have now confirmed that chemotherapy improves median survival from 6 months to about 8 months and improves quality of life for patients with advanced NSCLC. An important caveat is that patients must have a good PS (0 or 1 on the ECOG scale) to receive chemotherapy, as patients with marginal or poor PS (≥ 2 on the ECOG scale) suffer increased toxicity and do not clearly benefit from treatment.

Local Therapies in Advanced NSCLC Patients

In certain cases of advanced NSCLC, it is appropriate to palliate a local complication prior to consideration of systemic chemotherapy. Patients with brain metastases are often treated with cranial RT prior to chemotherapy, even in the absence of neurologic symptoms, in an attempt to avoid a neurologic crisis from progressive disease, see Chapter 64. Patients with post-obstructive pneumonia have increased toxicity and death with chemotherapy; therefore, palliative RT to the obstructing tumor and antibiotics are often given before chemotherapy. Finally, for patients with uncontrollable painful bony metastases despite an attempt at medical analgesia or patients with unstable bony metastases in weight-bearing bones, palliative RT, or orthopedic surgical intervention should be attempted prior to systemic chemotherapy.

First-Line Chemotherapy for Advanced NSCLC

Many trials have been performed over the last decade in search of the optimal chemotherapy regimen for advanced NSCLC. Two-drug platinum-based combination regimens (doublets) are better than single agents, yet the addition of a third chemotherapeutic agent adds only toxicity without OS benefit. The doublets that are most efficacious with a reasonable toxicity profile in the treatment of advanced NSCLC are cisplatin/vinorelbine, cisplatin/paclitaxel, cisplatin/gemcitabine, cisplatin/docetaxel, carboplatin/paclitaxel, and carboplatin/gemcitabine. In general, there are no significant differences between these doublets with response rates of 20% and median survival approximately 8 months (11). Clinicians choose between regimens based on local practice patterns and patient preferences regarding side-effect profiles and schedules of administration.

In recent years as molecularly targeted agents have been developed for NSCLC, trials adding targeted agents to platinum-based doublets have been performed. At least 10 randomized trials of chemotherapy plus a promising targeted agent have failed to show a benefit over standard therapy (see Targeted Therapy for NSCLC, below). In 2005, the landmark ECOG 4599 trial was presented in abstract form, demonstrating an OS benefit with the addition of bevacizumab to carboplatin/ paclitaxel chemotherapy (12). Median survival was 10.2 months in the chemotherapy arm, somewhat higher than has been seen in other large randomized trials. Even so, the addition of bevacizumab, a monoclonal antibody against VEGF, improved median survival to 12.5 months. The population eligible for participation in ECOG 4599 was relatively selective, excluding patients with brain metastases, those with SqCC histology, and those with significant risks of bleeding or thrombosis. Nevertheless, ECOG 4599 represents a major advance in the primary treatment of NSCLC as it is the first randomized trial to show a median survival of greater than 1 year. The triplet regimen with bevacizumab is now considered standard of care treatment for patients that match the study eligibility criteria.

First-line chemotherapy should be discontinued at the time of disease progression. For patients that respond or have disease stabilization with chemotherapy, treatment beyond 4–6 cycles does not improve OS and only increases toxicity. Furthermore, while there seems to be a slight OS benefit to cisplatin-based regimens compared to carboplatin-based regimens in NSCLC, this difference is clinically significant only in the treatment of early stage disease, when cure is possible. In the United States, most clinicians prefer to use carboplatin-based regimens for advanced disease because of their more favorable side-effect profiles and to avoid the need for significant intravenous fluid administration with cisplatin.

Second- and Third-Line Treatment for NSCLC

All patients will eventually progress during or after first-line treatment for advanced NSCLC; however, if they have a reasonable PS second-line treatment can be considered. The expected response rate to second-line therapy is only 10%, approximately half that of first-line therapy. There are currently three single-agent treatments approved for second-line NSCLC therapy: docetaxel, pemetrexed, and erlotinib. Both docetaxel and erlotinib treatment confer an OS benefit compared to supportive care in this setting, and pemetrexed outcomes are equivalent to docetaxel with a better toxicity profile (13–15). A fourth agent, gefitinib, did not improve survival over supportive care in the second-line setting, although this study has not yet been published (Table 52-4). All published studies have found that patients that responded to first-line therapy are more likely to benefit from second-line therapy compared to primary refractory patients. The current practice after progression on first-line therapy is to

Table 52-4

Randomized Trials of Second-Line Single-Agent Treatments in Advanced NSCLC

Author	Treatment	MS (months)	p-value	ORR (%)
Shepherd	Docetaxel	7.0	0.047	6
	BSC	4.6		0
Shepherd	Erlotinib	6.7	<0.001	9
	BSC	4.7		0
Hanna	Pemetrexed	8.3	NS	9
	Docetaxel	7.9		9
Thatcher	Gefitinib	5.6	NS	–
	BSC	5.1		–

MS = median survival, ORR = objective response rate, BSC = Best supportive care, NS = Not significant, – = Not reported treat with sequential single agents if the patient is an appropriate candidate for active treatment. When available, patients should be considered for participation in clinical trials. When PS drops below three on the ECOG scale, patients should be treated with supportive care only.

Targeted Therapy for NSCLC

The most recent trend in clinical oncology is the development of therapeutic agents designed to affect molecular targets within the cancer cell. These targets are rationally chosen for their purported central role in maintaining cancer cell growth and immortality. In NSCLC, the two pathways that have been targeted with the most success thus far are those driven by epidermal growth factor receptor (EGFR), a transmembrane ErbB family protein that directs cell growth via intracellular signaling, and VEGF, a major regulator of angiogenesis. Several other molecular pathway targets are undergoing earlier stages of clinical and pre-clinical investigation.

Gefitinib and erlotinib are oral small molecule tyrosine kinase inhibitors (TKIs) that target EGFR. Both agents were active in the second- and third-line setting for advanced NSCLC in phase II trials, with response rates of 10–20% and median survival of 8–9 months. In 2003, gefitinib received accelerated FDA approval for third-line treatment of NSCLC based on these phase II data. When novel agents are promising in the salvage setting, they are often even more efficacious in primary therapy. However, four separate randomized trials comparing platinum-based doublet first-line chemotherapy to the same regimen combined with a TKI failed to show an OS benefit with the addition of the EGFR-targeted agent.

Nevertheless, it became clear as thousands of patients were treated with gefitinib and erlotinib that adenocarcinoma histology, non-smoking history, female gender and Asian race all predicted increased benefit from the EGFR TKIs. In 2004, somatic mutations in the *EGFR* gene were discovered that were associated with these clinical characteristics and with increased responsiveness to TKI therapy (16). Experimental models verified that *EGFR* mutations confer significantly increased sensitivity to TKIs in vitro. Retrospective analyses now suggest that response rates to TKI treatment in patients harboring *EGFR* mutations are as high as 60–80%.

Meanwhile, phase III studies to determine the effectiveness of TKIs as second-line therapy were ongoing. In 2004, the large randomized BR.21 trial examining second-line erlotinib versus supportive care showed an OS benefit with erlotinib and the drug subsequently gained FDA approval for this indication (15). Shortly thereafter the corresponding ISEL trial comparing second-line gefitinib to supportive care was negative, which led the FDA to restrict the use of gefitinib to clinical trials and to patients previously benefiting from therapy. It is likely that ISEL failed to show an OS benefit because a much lower biologically active dose of gefitinib was administered compared to the dose prescribed for erlotinib in BR.21. Clinical trials are now evaluating the appropriate use of *EGFR* mutation testing and other biomarkers in the selection of patients for TKI therapy. Novel agents that target EGFR, including monoclonal antibodies to the receptor, are also under investigation.

VEGF plays a central role in promoting aberrant angiogenesis in NSCLC tumors and contributes to the ability to grow and metastasize. Bevacizumab is a humanized monoclonal antibody that binds and neutralizes free VEGF. As discussed above, bevacizumab improves OS when added to first-line chemotherapy in a restricted patient population with advanced NSCLC (12). The safety of bevacizumab in the general population and the utility of other novel angiogenesis inhibitors are under active investigation.

SPECIAL CONSIDERATIONS IN NSCLC MANAGEMENT

Malignant Pleural Effusion

NSCLC is the most common cause of MPE and symptomatic effusions have a major impact on patient quality of life. MPE is associated with a poor prognosis and, even in the absence of metastatic disease, disqualifies patients from consideration of RT or surgery with curative intent. If the patient is asymptomatic, no specific management for MPE is indicated. Patients may present with dyspnea or chest pain, and initital management options include thoracentesis, chest tube drainage with talc slurry pleurodesis, or thoracoscopy with talc poudrage pleurodesis. Thoracentesis should be attempted first in all patients, and is appropriate definitive management for MPE in debilitated patients without a long-predicted survival as MPE invariably recurs within 1 month. In patients with a good PS that have relief of symptoms after thoracentesis, pleurodesis will provide more effective long-term palliation. Chest tube drainage requires a 3–6 day hospital stay and can be performed at the bedside. After the majority of the MPE is drained, talc slurry is inserted through the tube to promote pleurodesis. The success of this method depends on full lung re-expansion and the absence of a loculated effusion, but may be as high as 70% at 1 month. For patients with loculated MPE, intra-operative drainage and thoracoscopic poudrage (spraying talc over the surface of the pleura) may lead to slightly higher-success rates. Patients may have low-grade fever and chest pain for a few days after pleurodesis. Long-term indwelling catheters or pleuroperitoneal shunts can be considered for patients with persistent difficulties from MPE.

Oligometastatic Disease

One percent of NSCLC cases present with "oligometastatic NSCLC," meaning a primary lung tumor that meets criteria for resection in conjunction with a solitary and resectable metastatic site, most commonly in the brain or adrenal gland. Highly selected patients may achieve long-term disease control by an aggressive approach including surgical resection of both the primary and metastatic disease. Patients selected for such an approach should have a good PS and are often treated initially with chemotherapy to demonstrate disease response or stability before proceeding with surgery. Whole brain RT is usually indicated after resection of a solitary metastasis.

Elderly Patients

Those over the age of 70 make up half the NSCLC patient population. Lack of participation of older patients in clinical trials and biases in physician treatment patterns against aggressive treatment for the elderly have led to overall poorer outcomes for this population. Recently, an increased interest in studying elderly cancer patients has generated an extensive literature suggesting that "fit" elderly NSCLC patients derive equivalent benefit as younger patients from cancer treatment. The challenge is to determine which elderly patients are "fit." No standard measure of fitness exists, but a patient with a good PS, a limited number of comorbidities, who is living independently, and has the ability to perform the activities of daily living should generally be managed as per the standard of care for younger patients. Elder-specific clinical trials have also confirmed the benefit of single-agent chemotherapy in this population, with improvement in survival and quality of life compared to supportive care alone (17).

PS2 Patients

Patients who are confined to a bed or chair for at least 50% of their waking hours are given a PS score of 2 or worse. This is one of the strongest predictors

Table 52-5

Summary of Standard Treatment for NSCLC, by Stage

Stage	Treatment
IA	Surgery
IB, IIA, IIB	Surgery and adjuvant platinum-based chemotherapy
IIIA	If lobectomy possible, neoadjuvant chemoradiotherapy and surgery
	If lobectomy not possible, definitive chemoradiotherapy
IIIB	Definitive chemoradiotherapy
Wet IIIB, IV	Palliative systemic therapy of choice

of poor prognosis in NSCLC and also predicts for increased toxicity with chemotherapy treatment. The optimal therapy for such patients is unclear, as they have been excluded from participation in most clinical trials. For patients with advanced NSCLC, single-agent chemotherapy treatment or supportive care alone are reasonable options.

Women

Paralleling the change in smoking prevalence among women, the death rate from lung cancer in US women has risen by 600% since 1930. While the incidence of lung cancer in men is declining, it is projected to continue to increase in women. There is some evidence suggesting women are more predisposed to carcinogenic damage from cigarettes compared to men, and that women are more likely to get non-smoking related NSCLC than men, perhaps because of increased estrogen levels. Outcome with NSCLC also differs by gender. Women have improved survival compared to men after both surgery for early stage disease and chemotherapy for advanced disease. Women also have an increased response rate to EGFR TKI agents.

SUMMARY

NSCLC is a common and aggressive cancer. Treatment has advanced over the last decade and promising novel therapies are in development. A summary of standard treatment recommendations by stage can be found in Table 52-5.

REFERENCES

1. Gould MK, Kuschner WG, Rydzak CE, et al. Test performance of positron emission tomography and computed tomography for mediastinal staging in patients with non-small-cell lung cancer: a meta-analysis. Ann Intern Med. 2003; 139(11): 879–892.
2. Ginsberg RJ, Rubinstein LV. Randomized trial of lobectomy versus limited resection for T1 N0 non-small cell lung cancer. Lung Cancer Study Group. Ann Thorac Surg. 1995; 60(3): 615–622; discussion 622–613.
3. Postoperative radiotherapy in non-small-cell lung cancer: systematic review and meta-analysis of individual patient data from nine randomised controlled trials. PORT Meta-analysis Trialists Group. Lancet. 1998; 352(9124): 257–263.
4. Arriagada R, Bergman B, Dunant A, Le Chevalier T, Pignon JP, Vansteenkiste J. Cisplatin-based adjuvant chemotherapy in patients with completely resected non-small-cell lung cancer. N Engl J Med. 2004; 350(4): 351–360.
5. Dillman RO, Seagren SL, Propert KJ, et al. A randomized trial of induction chemotherapy plus high-dose radiation versus radiation alone in stage III non-small-cell lung cancer. N Engl J Med. 1990; 323(14): 940–945.

6. Furuse K, Fukuoka M, Kawahara M, et al. Phase III study of concurrent versus sequential thoracic radiotherapy in combination with mitomycin, vindesine, and cisplatin in unresectable stage III non-small-cell lung cancer. J Clin Oncol. 1999; 17(9): 2692–2699.

7. Gaspar L, Gandara D, Chansky K, et al. Consolidation docetaxel following concurrent chemoradiotherapy in pathologic stage IIIb non-small cell lung cancer (NSCLC) (SWOG 9504): patterns of failure and updated survival. Paper Presented at American Society of Clinical Oncology, San Francisco, CA, 2001.

8. Albain KS, Swann RS, Rusch V, et al. Phase III study of concurrent chemotherapy and radiotherapy (CT/RT) vs. CT/RT followed by surgical resection for stage IIIA(pN2) non-small cell lung cancer (NSCLC): outcomes update of North American Intergroup 0139 (RTOG 9309). Paper Presented at American Society of Clinical Oncology, Orlando, FL, 2005.

9. Rusch V, Giroux M, Kraut J, et al. Induction chemoradiotherapy and surgical resection for non-small cell lung carcinomas of the superior sulcus (pancoast tumors): mature results of Southwest Oncology Group trial 9416 (Intergroup trial 0160). Paper Presented at American Society of Clinical Oncology, Chicago, IL, 2003.

10. Chemotherapy in non-small cell lung cancer: a meta-analysis using updated data on individual patients from 52 randomised clinical trials. Non-small Cell Lung Cancer Collaborative Group. BMJ. 1995; 311(7010): 899–909.

11. Schiller JH, Harrington D, Belani CP, et al. Comparison of four chemotherapy regimens for advanced non-small-cell lung cancer. N Engl J Med. 2002; 346(2): 92–98.

12. Sandler A, Gray R, Brahmer J, et al. Randomized phase II/III trial of paclitaxel (P) plus carboplatin (C) with or without bevacizumab (NSC #704865) in patients with advanced non-squamous non-small cell lung cancer (NSCLC): an Eastern Cooperative Oncology Group (ECOG) Trial—E4599. Paper Presented at Amercian Society of Clinical Oncology, Orlando, FL, 2005.

13. Shepherd FA, Dancey J, Ramlau R, et al. Prospective randomized trial of docetaxel versus best supportive care in patients with non-small-cell lung cancer previously treated with platinum-based chemotherapy. J Clin Oncol. 2000; 18(10): 2095–2103.

14. Hanna N, Shepherd FA, Fossella FV, et al. Randomized phase III trial of pemetrexed versus docetaxel in patients with non-small-cell lung cancer previously treated with chemotherapy. J Clin Oncol. 2004; 22(9): 1589–1597.

15. Shepherd FA, Rodrigues Pereira J, Ciuleanu T, et al. Erlotinib in previously treated non-small-cell lung cancer. N Engl J Med. 2005; 353(2): 123–132.

16. Lynch TJ, Bell DW, Sordella R, et al. Activating mutations in the epidermal growth factor receptor underlying responsiveness of non-small-cell lung cancer to gefitinib. N Engl J Med. 2004; 350(21): 2129–2139.

17. Gridelli C. The ELVIS trial: a phase III study of single-agent vinorelbine as first-line treatment in elderly patients with advanced non-small cell lung cancer. Elderly Lung Cancer Vinorelbine Italian Study. Oncologist. 2001; 6(Suppl)1: 4–7.

REVIEW OF CLINICAL TRIALS IN THYMOMA

INTRODUCTION

Thymoma is a rare disease, with an incidence of only 0.15 per 100,000 person-years. However, it is the most common tumor of the anterior mediastinum, representing approximately 30% of anterior mediastinal lesions and 20% of all mediastinal tumors in adults. Based on Surveillance, Epidemiology, and End Results (SEER) data from 1973 to 1998, the incidence is higher in males than in females ($p = 0.007$). The median age at presentation is 52 years. Approximately one-third of patients are asymptomatic at presentation, one-third have symptoms from local extent of their tumor and one-third present with paraneoplastic syndromes, typically myasthenia gravis.

HISTOLOGIC CLASSIFICATION

Thymomas are tumors derived from the thymic epithelium. In 1989, Muller-Hermelink and Kirchner proposed a classification based on the similarity of the morphologic appearance of the tumor to normal thymic compartments. This classification subdivided tumors into medullary, mixed, predominantly cortical, cortical, and well-differentiated thymic carcinoma.

In an attempt to standardize the histologic diagnosis of thymoma, the World Health Organization (WHO) published its own classification in 1999, which subdivided tumors into six types: A, AB, B1, B2, B3, and C. Type A tumors have neoplastic cells with spindle or oval appearance, whereas type B tumors have cells with an epithelioid or dendritic appearance. Types B1, B2, and B3 correspond to the predominantly cortical, cortical, and well-differentiated thymic carcinoma. Tumors combining type A and type B1 or rarely B2 features are classified as type AB. Type C tumors correspond to the thymic carcinomas according to older classifications, which include tumors with histology foreign to thymic tissues (such as squamous cell carcinomas, mucoepidermoid, basaloid carcinoma, etc.). The 2004 WHO classification update encompassed neuroendocrine carcinomas within type C tumors.

Thymic carcinomas have distinct morphology and immunophenotype, they present at more advanced stages, and have a significantly inferior prognosis compared to other thymoma types. For that reason, some authors propose that well-differentiated thymic carcinomas should be designated as "atypical thymomas," not to be confused with type C tumors. Thymic carcinomas will not be considered in this review.

STAGING

The most widely used staging system was introduced by Masaoka in 1981, and was modified in 1994 allowing microscopic invasion into, but not through, the capsule to be classified as stage I (Table 53-1). Another staging system used by French groups, the GETT classification (Groupe d'Etudes des Tumeurs Thymiques) is based on extent of disease, but also on extent of surgical resection (complete, partial, or biopsy). Both staging systems have been shown to be prognostic of overall survival in multiple studies. In a study of 149 patients with non-metastatic thymomas staged both with the Masaoka and GETT systems, there was an 88% concordance between the two systems.

Table 53-1

Masaoka Clinical Staging of Thymoma

Stage	Description
I	Macroscopically and microscopically completely encapsulated (tumor invading into but not through the capsule is also included)
II	A. Microscopic transcapsular invasion B. Macroscopic invasion into surrounding fatty tissue or grossly adherent to but not through mediastinal pleura or pericardium
III	Macroscopic invasion into neighboring organs (i.e., pericardium, great vessels, or lung)
IV	A. Pleural or pericardial dissemination B. Lymphogenous or hematogenous metastasis

MYASTHENIA GRAVIS

Myasthenia gravis (MG) is the most common paraneoplastic disease associated with thymoma. Evoli reported on 207 patients with MG from Italy. Of the 188 patients with tumor that could be classified, 87% had type B thymomas (B1 in 22.3%, B2 in 55.3%, B3 in 3.1%, and combined B2/B3 in 6.3%), which is similar to findings from other authors showing that MG is primarily associated with thymoma of cortical histology. Interestingly, 13 patients developed MG 0.5–10 years following thymectomy. Out of 189 patients with adequate follow up only 17 patients had achieved drug free remission. As a result, some patients with thymoma succumb to complications of MG, rather than their malignant disease. In the study by Evoli et al. eight deaths were attributed to MG and seven deaths to progression of thymoma (1). Similarly, in a series from Mayo Clinic 13% of patients died of thymoma and 16% of myasthenia. Despite its contribution to the morbidity and mortality of thymoma patients, MG is not an independent predictor either of recurrence or survival.

OTHER PARANEOPLASTIC SYNDROMES

Up to 50% of patients with pure red cell aplasia (PRCA) have thymoma, whereas less than 10% of patients with thymoma have PRCA. In 17 cases reported by Masaoka et al., who were treated with resection of their tumor, six patients benefited from surgery. More recently, the combination of octreotide and prednisone has also been found to be effective in the treatment of PRCA. Hypogammaglobulinemia is an uncommon complication of thymoma, but up to 10% of patients with acquired hypogammaglobulinemia will have an associated thymoma (Good syndrome). Unfortunately, surgery does not reliably return immunoglobulin levels to normal levels.

TREATMENT

Resectable Disease

Surgery remains the only known curative therapy for thymoma. The definition of resectable thymomas includes not only early stage disease (stages I and II), but also more advanced cases where the bulk of the tumor can be removed. Obviously, criteria for unresectability vary among different centers, but extensive mediastinal infiltration or significant bilateral pleural based tumor would be considered inoperable by most surgeons.

Rates of complete resection based on Masaoka stage and WHO classification are shown in Tables 53-2 and 53-3. Long-term outcome for resected thymomas

Table 53-2

Rates of Complete Resection According to Masaoka Stage

Author	N	Stage I (%)	Stage II (%)	Stage III (%)	Stage IV (%)
Blumberg	118	100.0	73.0	56.0	78.0
Nakahara	141	100.0	100.0	73.0	0.0
Kondo	1049	100.0	100.0	84.6	41.6
Okumura	194	100.0	100.0	89.2	0.0

Table 53-3

Rates of Complete Resection According to WHO Classification Type

Author	N	WHO A (%)	WHO AB (%)	WHO B1 (%)	WHO B2 (%)	WHO B3 (%)
Kondo	100	100.0	100.0	100.0	100.0	92.0
Kim	108	100.0	88.0	100.0	90.6	55.0
Okumura	273	100.0	98.7	94.5	90.7	92.3
Park	150	100.0	92.3	100.0	90.0	65.2

is dependent both on Masaoka stage and WHO classification. Multivariate analyses in various studies have inconsistently shown that additional factors can have independent prognostic value, such as tumor size, incomplete resection, and invasion of great vessels for stage III patients.

In evaluating the effectiveness of therapy, long-term follow-up is paramount given the risk of late recurrences. Additionally, disease specific survival, rather than overall survival, should be the primary end-point, since death from thymoma can account for as low as 21% of all causes of death in large studies.

Stage I tumors have an exceptionally favorable outcome following surgery, with 5-, 10-, and 20-year survivals in the 90–100% range. Survival decreases for more advanced tumors, with the most significant difference usually manifested between stages II and III. Similarly, survival is excellent for WHO types A and AB, while survival rates drop significantly for types B2 and B3. WHO type B1 seems to have an intermediate prognosis (Tables 53-4 and 53-5).

Adjuvant Therapy

It is widely accepted that the cure rate of patients with encapsulated thymomas is excellent with surgery alone. However, in more advanced disease, the results reported in surgical series have included a variable percentage of patients undergoing adjuvant therapy, primarily radiation. Several institutions have consistently prescribed radiation therapy for all invasive tumors (stages II and above), while others have selected patients for additional therapy based on the judgment of the thoracic surgeon or the radiation oncologist. Retrospective comparisons of patients who did and did not receive adjuvant therapy are therefore subject to selection bias and cannot be considered conclusive.

Curran et al. showed that following complete resection, 6/18 patients with stage II and 2/3 patients with stage III thymomas recurred in the absence of radiation, whereas none of five patients with radiation experienced a recurrence. However, only one patient in the radiation group had stage II disease. In a review of the literature up to that date, the authors demonstrated a 28% recurrence in the absence of radiation and a 5% recurrence rate when radiation was administered (2). In another study of 241 patients with thymoma from the

Table 53-4

Ten-Year Survival of Patients with Thymoma According to Masaoka Stage

Author	N	I (%)	II (%)	III (%)	IV (%)
Kim	108	95.0	81.3	46.2	N/A
Park[*]	150	100.0	88.2	63.0	22.5
Rea	132	84.0	82.0	51.0	0.0
Kondo[*]	1320	100.0	98.4	88.7	70.6
Nagawaka	130	100.0	100.0	76.0	47.0
Okumura[†]	243	89.0	91.0	49.0	0.0
Blumberg[*]	118	95.0	70.0	50.0	100.0
Maggi	241	86.9	64.3	59.9	39.6
Nakahara	141	100.0	84.4	77.2	46.6
Rena	178	94.0	88.0	66.0	N/A

[*]Five-year survival data.

[†]20-year survival data.

N/A: not available.

Table 53-5

Ten-Year Survival of Patients with Thymoma According to WHO Classification

Author	N	A (%)	AB (%)	B1 (%)	B2 (%)	B3 (%)
Fang	204	68.5	68.5	68.5	36.7	36.7
Kondo	100	100.0	100.0	83.1	83.1	35.7
Park[*]	150	100.0	93.2	88.9	82.4	71.3
Rea	132	100.0	90.0	78.0	33.0	35.0
Nagawaka	130	100.0	100.0	86.0	85.0	38.0
Okumura[†]	243	100.0	87.0	91.0	59.0	36.0
Rena	178	95.0	90.0	85.0	71.0	40.0

[*]Five-year survival data.

[†]20-year survival data.

University of Torino, Italy, Maggi et al. reported that 11 of 55 patients with invasive thymoma and no adjuvant therapy recurred, compared to three of 21 with adjuvant therapy (mostly radiation therapy) (3).

However, subsequent studies have shown little benefit for postoperative radiation therapy.

In the largest retrospective study reported to date, 1,320 patients from 115 Japanese centers were reviewed. Complete resection was performed in 247 stage II and in 170 stage III patients, and adjuvant radiation therapy was given to 43.3% and 74.5% of stages II and III patients, respectively. Recurrence rates for patients with and without radiation therapy were 4.7% versus 4.1% in stage II and 23% versus 26% for stage III patients (4).

In a series of patients with stage III thymomas from Massachusetts General Hospital (MGH), 54% of recurrences occurred in the pleura (5). Similarly, in a study by Nakagawa et al. six out of 12 recurrences occurred in the pleura. Given the high propensity for such pleural dissemination, Haniuda et al. reviewed the efficacy of adjuvant radiation therapy in 70 patients undergoing complete resection of thymoma based on the degree of "pleural factor" defined as follows: p0, no adhesion to mediastinal pleura; p1, fibrous adhesion to the mediastinal pleura without tumor invasion; and p2, microscopic invasion of the mediastinal pleura. In p0 stage II patients no recurrence was observed regardless of radiation therapy. However, in p2 stage II tumors three out of four patients recurred, even in the presence of adjuvant radiation. Radiation appeared to be helpful in stage II p1 tumors, where none of six patients undergoing adjuvant therapy relapsed, compared to four out of 11 patients treated with surgery alone (6).

Ogawa et al. examined the results of 103 patients with completely resected thymoma treated with adjuvant radiation therapy. The pleura was the most common site of recurrence, which was seen in 12 of 17 patients with relapsed disease. While no pleural recurrences were seen among the 70 patients without pleural invasion in their surgical specimen, 12 out of 38 patients with pleural invasion experienced such a recurrence (7). Therefore, it appears that radiation therapy cannot adequately treat tumors at high risk for the most common site of recurrence.

Newer studies have also evaluated the role of WHO classification in determining risk of relapse following adjuvant therapy. Ströbel et al. reported on 228 thymoma patients treated with primary surgery with or without adjuvant therapy (8). The study also included a small proportion of type C tumors with squamous cell histology (4.8%). Postoperative therapy was quite uncommon in WHO type A thymomas (three out of 20), but was very frequent in type B3 (15 out of 22). The main finding of the study was that recurrences following complete resection were rare among tumors of type A, AB, or B1, even in stages II and III (two out of 33), while they were more frequent in stage III tumors of types B2 and B3 (five out of 18). These results are also supported by data from MGH, which showed no recurrences among 73 patients with types A and AB thymoma (9). How to approach early stage unfavorable histology thymomas is a more difficult issue. Chen identified WHO types B2, B3, and C as independent poor prognostic categories within stages I and II tumors. He observed four deaths among 24 patients, compared to only two deaths in 78 patients with types A, AB, and B1. However, it is known that type C tumors have distinct natural history and a worse prognosis compared to "pure" thymomas (10). Results in patients with B2 and B3 histology alone are more encouraging: there was only one recurrence out of 37 stage I/II patients in a recent study from Germany.

Exploring the role of adjuvant therapy in tumors of cortical histology (B2 and B3), Ströbel et al. showed that in stage II tumors there were no tumor relapses among those patients who received adjuvant radiation versus one relapse in 16 patients without further treatment. The relapse rate for stage III patients was 0% for the five patients who underwent adjuvant therapy, compared to 33% for the patients without adjuvant treatment (8).

Chen also reported that adjuvant therapy did not improve survival for types A, AB, and B1, whereas it had a statistically significant benefit for types B2, B3, and C (5-year survival 85.5% versus 48.3%).

Given the independent prognostic value of stage and WHO classification several authors have proposed treatment algorithms and risk stratification schemes following primary surgery, which take both parameters into consideration.

Unresectable Disease

When complete, or near complete, resection cannot be performed surgical procedures have ranged from biopsy alone to a variable degree of debulking approaches. Some studies have shown that debulking is superior to biopsy, but other studies have found no difference in survival. It is clear however, that patients can still experience long-term survival when treated with radiation therapy with or without the addition of chemotherapy.

Ninety patients from 10 French centers were treated with partial resection (31 patients), biopsy (55 patients), or complete resection (four patients with stage IVa disease and pleural implants). Radiation dose ranged from 30 to 70 Gy with a median dose of 50 Gy. Sequential platinum-based chemotherapy was added to 59 patients, while three patients received preoperative radiation and chemotherapy. The 5- and 10-year disease free survival was 60% and 36% for partial resection, compared to 38% and 31% for biopsy alone (11).

An American Intergroup study evaluated the combination of CAP (cyclophosphamide, doxorubicin, and cisplatin) followed by radiation therapy at a dose of 54 Gy in 23 patients with limited-stage unresectable thymoma, including two patients with thymic carcinoma. All, but one, of the patients had gross residual disease postoperatively. The overall response rate to induction chemotherapy was 69.6% (CR: five patients, PR: 11 patients) and the 5-year overall survival was 52.5% (12).

Based on the encouraging results of radiation and radio-chemotherapy, many centers have approached unresectable or borderline resectable thymic tumors with a multimodality treatment plan.

Kim et al. from the M.D. Anderson Cancer Center treated 22 patients deemed to be unresectable with neoadjuvant chemotherapy, followed by surgery, postoperative radiation, and consolidation chemotherapy. Eleven patients had stage III, 10 patients had stage IVa, and one patient had stage IVb thymoma. The induction program consisted of cyclophosphamide, doxorubicin via continuous infusion, cisplatin, and prednisone, and it resulted in an overall response rate of 77% (CR: three patients, PR: 14 patients). Radiation dose for 16 patients was 60 Gy, and for the remaining patients it was 50 Gy. Twenty-one patients underwent surgery and 16 (76%) had a complete resection. Six of these patients had a more than 80% necrosis in the surgical specimen. The progression-free survival at 7 years was 77%. Only one patient died of progressive thymoma with a median follow-up of 50.3 months (13).

Bretti et al. reported their results with neoadjuvant therapy in 33 patients who could not undergo upfront surgery for stage III–IV thymoma. Eight patients received radiation at a dose of 30 Gy in 15 fractions (24 Gy if more than 30% of the lung volume had to be included). The remaining patients received four cycles of chemotherapy, either ADOC (doxorubicin 40 mg/m^2, cisplatin 50 mg/m^2 on day 1, vincristine 0.6 mg/m^2 on day 2, and cyclophosphamide 700 mg/m^2 on day 4) or cisplatin and VP-16 (100 mg/m^2 on day 1 and 100 mg/m^2 on days 1–3, respectively). Surgery could be attempted on 17 patients and a total of 12 patients were able to have a complete resection following induction treatment (one patient post radiation, 11 patients post chemotherapy). These patients had shorter progression free survival (56.9 months versus not reached yet), but similar overall survival compared to a cohort of 20 patients with stage III–IV thymoma, which could be completely resected at the time of diagnosis. The patients who could not be resected were given 50–60 Gy postoperatively, but had a 5-year PFS of only about 10% (14).

Venuta et al. treated patients with stage III disease on a multimodality program: 30 patients with resectable disease underwent adjuvant chemotherapy and radiation (40 Gy for complete resection and 50–60 Gy for incomplete resection), while 15 patients judged to be unresectable were given neo-adjuvant cisplatin-based chemotherapy. Eleven patients out of the 45 had thymic carcinoma. Overall, ten patients had a response to the induction regimen (CR: two patients, PR: eight patients, overall RR 67%). Complete resection was possible in 87% of patients, however only one patient had a complete pathologic response (7%). Interestingly, the 10-year overall survival of patients receiving induction treatment was 90%, compared with 71% for patients considered initially resectable (15).

Table 53-6

Results for Patients Presenting with Unresectable Thymoma Treated Either with Definitive Radiation (or Chemo-Radiation) or with Induction Chemotherapy

Author	N	Compl res (%)	5-Year OS (%)	10-Year OS (%)	5-Year DFS (%)	10-Year DFS (%)
Definitive therapy						
Mornex	90	4.4	51	39	–	–
Ciernik	31	0.0	45	28	–	–
Loehrer	23	0.0	52.5	–	54.3	–
Urgesi	44	0.0	–	–	–	–
Krueger	12	8.3	57.0	–	–	–
Induction therapy						
Macchiarini	7	57	80 (2-year)	–	–	–
Bretti	33	36	–	–	–	–
Venuta	15	87	–	90 (9-year)	–	–
Rea	16	68.7	70 (3-year)	–	–	–
Kim	22	72.7	95	79 (7-year)	77	77 (7-year)

Compl res: complete resection; OS: overall survival; DFS: disease specific survival.

From the above studies it is reasonable to recommend an initial chemotherapy or chemo-radiation approach for patients who present with unresectable thymomas (Table 53-6).

Recurrent or Metastatic Disease

Recurrent disease amenable to re-operation should be approached surgically. Although there are no large comparative studies, there is evidence of long-term disease-free survival following aggressive therapy of recurrent tumors.

Systemic therapy is the only option for patients with extrathoracic disease, or with tumors that have progressed despite all available local measures (Table 53-7).

Multiple case reports and small series have demonstrated that thymoma is a responsive malignancy to single-agent chemotherapy.

Interestingly, significant responses have also been observed with the use of steroids, even in cases unresponsive to other modalities. Although it is widely accepted that steroids act mainly on the lymphoid population of the tumor, responses have been seen in primarily epithelial thymomas as well. Steroids may be even more efficacious in combination with octreotide. In a study by Palmieri et al., 16 patients with chemotherapy refractory thymoma were given prednisone (0.6 mg/kg/day for 3 months, 0.2 mg/kg/day during follow-up) and octreotide (1.5 mg/day or 30 mg every 14 days for the long-acting analog lanreotide). Six patients had thymic carcinoma, and half of them had progressive small cell neuroendocrine carcinoma. The response rate was 37%, including one patient with complete response. The median time to progression was 14 months, and the median survival time for the group was 15 months. The estimated 2-year survival is approximately 30% (16). Response to therapy did not appear to correlate with histology.

Table 53-7

Results of Chemotherapy in Patients with Advanced Thymoma

Author	Therapy	N	Carcinoma (%)	Chemo naïve (%)	RR (%)	MST (mos)	2-Year OS (%)	5-Year OS
Palmieri	Octreotide prednisone	16	37.5	0.0	37.0	15.0	~30	N/a
Loehrer	Octreotide prednisone	38	16.0	0.0	30.3	N/a	75.7	N/a
Fornasiero	ADOC	37	0.0	97.2	91.8	15.0	N/a	N/a
Loehrer	CAP	30	3.3	100.0	50.0	37.7	64.5	32.0%
Loehrer	VIP	28	29.0	100.0	32.0	31.6	70.0	N/a
Chahinian	Various	9	0.0	N/a	44.4	N/a	N/a	N/a
Göldel	Various	22	N/a	100.0	50.0	N/a	N/a	N/a
Giaccone	EP	16	0.0	100.0	56.0	51.6	N/a	50.0%
Kurup	Iressa	26	27.0	0.0	3.8	N/a	N/a	N/a

N/a: Not available; RR: Response rate; MST: Median survival time; OS: Overall survival; ADOC: Doxorubicin, cisplatin, vincristine, cyclophosphamide; CAP: cyclophosphamide, doxorubicin, cisplatin; VIP: etoposide, ifosfamide, cisplatin; EP: etoposide, cisplatin.

The Eastern Cooperative Oncology Group (ECOG) designed a study with the same combination therapy, but evaluated single agent octreotide initially (at a dose of 1.5 mg/kg daily) and only added prednisone (at a dose of 0.6 mg/kg daily) for patients with stable disease after 2 months of octreotide therapy. The study accrued 38 assessable patients with thymoma (32 patients), thymic carcinoma (5 patients), or thymic carcinoid (1 patient). At the end of the 2 months there were four partial responses, but the addition of prednisone resulted in six additional partial responses and two complete responses for an overall response rate of 30.3% for the combination. Only patients with typical histology responded to therapy. The 2-year overall survival was 75.7% (17). It appears therefore, that steroids add to the activity of octreotide. In an case report, a patient with type B3 thymoma progressive after 6 months of octreotide treatment was given prednisone 50 mg/day in addition to long-acting octreotide. After 7 months of combination therapy the patient achieved a complete remission.

EGFR immunoreactivity is observed in thymomas, and overexpression of EGFR is associated with more aggressive thymic tumos (B2 and B3). Based on this observation, 26 patients with previously treated thymoma or thymic carcinoma were treated with gefitinib at a dose of 250 mg daily. Only one response was seen, which lasted for 5 months. None of the five patients who underwent DNA sequencing, including the patient who responded, harbored an EGFR mutation (Kurup ProcASCO 2005).

Combination chemotherapy has been studied extensively in the treatment of advanced thymoma. More commonly, patients received cisplatin-based regimens, however responses have been reported with other regimens, such as cyclophosphamide, doxorubicin, vincristine (CAV), or CAV with the addition of prednisone ± bleomycin (CAVP ± Bleo). In a retrospective review of 123 patients treated on five ECOG trials, combination chemotherapy was associated with a higher response rate ($p < 0.0001$) and survival ($p = 0.035$) compared to single-agent cisplatin.

Fornasiero et al. reported on 37 patients treated with ADOC (cisplatin 50 mg/m^2 and doxorubicin 40 mg/m^2 on day 1, vincristine 0.6 mg/m^2 on day 3, and cyclophosphamide 700 mg/m^2 on day 4) over a period of 13 years. The overall response rate was impressive at 92%, with 43% complete remission rate. Seven patients were confirmed to have complete response pathologically following thoracotomy. The median duration of response was 12 months, and the median survival was 15 months (18). A similar regimen, CAP (cisplatin 50 mg/m^2, doxorubicin 50 mg/m^2, and cychophosphamide 500 mg/m^2), was given to 30 patients with advanced thymoma. Although the response rate was lower than ADOC at 50%, the median survival time was much more impressive (37.7 months), questioning the value of vincristine in this setting (19). Successful re-treatment with the same regimen in two patients relapsing 14 and 60 months after completion of initial therapy has been reported.

Based on the promising activity demonstrated by single-agent ifosfamide, 28 evaluable patients were treated with VIP (etoposide 75 mg/m^2, ifosfamide 1.2 g/m^2, and cisplatin 20 mg/m^2 days 1–4). Unfortunately, response rate and survival statistics did not appear superior to previous regimens (RR 32%, response duration 11.9 months, median survival time 31.6 months, and 2-year overall survival of 70%) (20).

The European Organization for the Research and Treatment of Cancer (EORTC) evaluated the combination of cisplatin (60 mg/m^2 day 1) and etoposide (120 mg/m^2 days 1–3) on 16 chemotherapy-naive patients. The observed response rate was 56%, the duration of response was 40 months, the median survival time was 51.6 months, and the 5-year overall survival was 50% (21).

CONCLUSIONS

Thymoma is a rare disease, but highly curable with surgery when complete resection can be achieved. Even for unresectable patients, long-term survival is feasible with the combination of chemotherapy and radiation. There is considerable excitement about the use of neo-adjuvant approaches in marginally resectable patients, but more studies are required in this group of patients. Metastatic disease should be treated with cisplatin-based regimens, but no "standard" therapy exists, and new agents need to be evaluated. The standardization of pathology has provided valuable prognostic information, but more refined prognostic and predictive markers, including molecular markers, are desperately needed.

REFERENCES

1. Evoli A, Minisci C, Di Schino C. Thymoma in patients with MG: characteristics and long-term outcome. Neurology. 2002; 59(12): 1844–1850.
2. Curran WJ, Jr, Kornstein MJ, Brooks JJ. Invasive thymoma: the role of mediastinal irradiation following complete or incomplete surgical resection. J Clin Oncol. 1988; 6(11): 1722–1727.
3. Maggi G, Casadio C, Cavallo A. Thymoma: results of 241 operated cases. Annl Thorac Surg. 1991; 51(1): 152–156.
4. Kondo K, Monden Y. Therapy for thymic epithelial tumors: a clinical study of 1,320 patients from Japan. Annl Thorac Surg. 2003; 76(3): 878–884; discussion 884–885.
5. Myojin M, Choi NC, Wright CD. Stage III thymoma: pattern of failure after surgery and postoperative radiotherapy and its implication for future study. Intl J Radiat Oncol Biol Phys. 2000; 46(4): 927–933.
6. Haniuda M, Morimoto M, Nishimura H. Adjuvant radiotherapy after complete resection of thymoma. Annl Thorac Surg. 1992; 54(2): 311–315.
7. Ogawa K, Uno T, Toita T. Postoperative radiotherapy for patients with completely resected thymoma: a multi-institutional, retrospective review of 103 patients. Cancer. 2002; 94(5): 1405–1413.
8. Strobel P, Bauer A, Puppe B. Tumor recurrence and survival in patients treated for thymomas and thymic squamous cell carcinomas: a retrospective analysis. J Clin Oncol. 2004; 22(8): 1501–1509.
9. Wright CD, Wain JC, Wong DR. Predictors of recurrence in thymic tumors: importance of invasion, World Health Organization histology, and size. J Thorac Cardiovasc Surg. 2005; 130(5): 1413–1421.
10. Chen G, Marx A, Wen-Hu C. New WHO histologic classification predicts prognosis of thymic epithelial tumors: a clinicopathologic study of 200 thymoma cases from China. Cancer. 2002; 95(2): 420–429.
11. Mornex F, Resbeut M, Richaud P. Radiotherapy and chemotherapy for invasive thymomas: a multicentric retrospective review of 90 cases. The FNCLCC trialists. Federation Nationale des Centres de Lutte Contre le Cancer [erratum appears in Int J Radiat Oncol Biol Phys 1995 33(2): 545]. Intl J Radiat Oncol Biol Phys. 1995; 32(3): 651–659.
12. Loehrer PJ, Sr, Chen M, Kim K. Cisplatin, doxorubicin, and cyclophosphamide plus thoracic radiation therapy for limited-stage unresectable thymoma: an intergroup trial. J Clin Oncol. 1997; 15(9): 3093–3099.
13. Kim ES, Putnam JB, Komaki R. Phase II study of a multidisciplinary approach with induction chemotherapy, followed by surgical resection, radiation therapy, and consolidation chemotherapy for unresectable malignant thymomas: final report. Lung Cancer. 2004; 44(3): 369–379.
14. Bretti S, Berruti A. Loddo C. Multimodal management of stages III–IVa malignant thymoma. Lung Cancer. 2004; 44(1): 69–77.
15. Venuta F, Rendina EA, Longo F. Long-term outcome after multimodality treatment for stage III thymic tumors. Annl Thorac Surg. 2003; 76(6): 1866–1872; discussion 1872.

16. Palmieri G, Montella L, Martignetti A. Somatostatin analogs and prednisone in advanced refractory thymic tumors. Cancer. 2002; 94(5): 1414–1420.
17. Loehrer PJ, Sr, Wang W, Johnson DH. Octreotide alone or with prednisone in patients with advanced thymoma and thymic carcinoma: an Eastern Cooperative Oncology Group Phase II Trial [erratum appears in J Clin Oncol. 2004; 22(11): 2261]. J Clin Oncol. 2004; 22(2): 293–299.
18. Fornasiero A, Daniele O, Ghiotto C. Chemotherapy for invasive thymoma. A 13-year experience. Cancer. 1991; 68(1): 30–33.
19. Loehrer PJ, Sr, Kim K, Aisner SC. Cisplatin plus doxorubicin plus cyclophosphamide in metastatic or recurrent thymoma: final results of an intergroup trial. The Eastern Cooperative Oncology Group, Southwest Oncology Group, and Southeastern Cancer Study Group. J Clin Oncol. 1994; 12(6): 1164–1168
20. Loehrer PJ, Sr, Jiroutek M, Aisner S. Combined etoposide, ifosfamide, and cisplatin in the treatment of patients with advanced thymoma and thymic carcinoma: an intergroup trial. Cancer. 2001; 91(11): 2010–2015.
21. Giaccone G, Ardizzoni A, Kirkpatrick A. Cisplatin and etoposide combination chemotherapy for locally advanced or metastatic thymoma. A phase II study of the European Organization for Research and Treatment of Cancer Lung Cancer Cooperative Group. J Clin Oncol. 1996; 14(3): 814–820.

SMALL CELL LUNG CANCER

EPIDEMIOLOGY

Lung cancer is the leading cause of cancer-related mortality in the United States with over 172,000 new cases and over 163,000 deaths in 2005. Approximately 15% of lung cancers diagnosed in 2005 were small cell lung cancer (SCLC), with the remainder being various subtypes of non-small cell lung cancer (NSCLC) such as adenocarcinoma, squamous cell, and large cell, among others. The proportion of new lung cancers diagnosed that are SCLC has been declining over the past few decades. The reasons for this are unclear but may relate at least in part to the changing composition of cigarettes and inhalation patterns.

SCLC is associated with cigarette smoking in the vast majority of cases. Both duration of smoking and number of cigarettes per day are directly correlated with lung cancer risk. Patients who quit smoking decrease their lung cancer risk, although not to never-smoking levels (1).

PATHOLOGY

SCLC is a type of high-grade neuroendocrine lung cancer. The neuroendocrine lung tumors encompass a diverse spectrum that ranges widely in prognosis, from low-grade typical carcinoids and intermediate-grade atypical carcinoids, to the higher-grade cancers including large cell neuroendocrine cancer and SCLC. SCLC and large cell neuroendocrine cancer behave similarly and have similar prognoses.

Pathologically, SCLC is defined as "a proliferation of small cells (<4 lymphocytes in diameter) with unique and strict morphologic features, scant cytoplasm, ill-defined borders, finely granular salt and pepper chromatin, absent or inconspicuous nucleoli, frequent nuclear molding, and a high mitotic count" (2). Immunohistochemical staining is generally positive for epithelial cell markers such as keratin and epithelial membrane antigen. In addition, neuroendocrine markers such as chromogranin A and synaptophysin are positive in the majority of SCLCs.

CLINICAL PRESENTATION

Most patients present with symptoms that are related to the intrathoracic bulk of disease or widespread dissemination. Cough, dyspnea, weight loss, and weakness are the most common presenting symptoms (3).

In addition, a variety of paraneoplastic syndromes are observed with SCLC. The ectopic production of hormones is a common culprit for the endocrine paraneoplastic disorders, which include hyponatremia (due to ectopic production of antidiuretic hormone), Cushing's syndrome (ectopic corticotropin production), and acromegaly (ectopic growth hormone releasing hormone). Neurologic paraneoplastic syndromes such as Lambert–Eaton myasthenic syndrome are caused by autoantibody-mediated damage to the nervous system. Treatment of the underlying tumor can help control these paraneoplastic syndromes; in addition, medical management of symptoms may be indicated (see Table 54-1).

Table 54-1

Clinical Presentation

Symptoms and signs	%
Local	
Cough	50
Dyspnea	40
Chest pain	35
Hemoptysis	20
Hoarseness	10
Distant	
Weight loss	50
Weakness	40
Anorexia	30
Paraneoplastic syndromes	15
Fever	10
Paraneoplastic syndromes	
Hyponatremia	15
Ectopic corticotropin	2–5
Acromegaly	<1
Lambert–Eaton	3
Encephalitis/subacute sensory neuropathy	<1
Cancer-associated retinopathy	<1

Adapted from (3).

DIAGNOSIS AND STAGING

Radiographically, SCLCs tend to present as central hilar masses with bulky mediastinal lymphadenopathy. Given the central location of most SCLCs, the diagnosis is usually made by pathologic analysis of a bronchoscopic biopsy sample. Alternatively, percutaneous CT-guided biopsies provide another means of obtaining tissue for diagnosis.

Once the diagnosis of SCLC is made, accurate staging is important for treatment planning. Unlike NSCLC, where the TNM staging system is used, SCLC is categorized into either limited stage or extensive stage disease, as described by the Veteran's Administration Lung Group. Limited stage is typically defined as disease that involves one hemithorax, or disease that is encompassable within one radiotherapy port. Extensive stage is any disease that extends beyond these parameters. The majority of patients present with extensive stage disease.

The staging work-up is designed to establish whether a patient has metastatic disease, since this will substantially alter both the prognosis and treatment plan. The work-up should include a CT of the chest with extension into the abdomen to evaluate the liver and adrenals, which are common sites of metastasis. Brain imaging should be performed since the CNS is a frequent site of spread. Both head CT and brain MRI are commonly used, but MRI is preferred for its greater sensitivity for detecting metastatic disease. Bone scan should be performed to assess for bony metastases. PET scans are increasingly being used for staging purposes but its exact role is not yet clearly defined.

TREATMENT FOR LIMITED STAGE SCLC

Limited stage SCLC is treated with a combination of chemotherapy and radiation, which typically yields a response rate of greater than 80% (complete response 40–60%) and median survival of 14–20 months. Surgery is not typically attempted due to the high early dissemination rate and poor overall survival at 5 years. Occasionally, patients present with a T1-2N0M0 cancer that is surgically resected on the presumption of NSCLC. These patients still need adjuvant chemotherapy after resection with appropriate SCLC regimens.

Combination chemotherapy and radiation remain the standard of care for limited stage SCLC. In terms of chemotherapy, cisplatin and etoposide is the standard regimen used. A randomized phase III trial demonstrated better survival among limited stage SCLC patients treated with cisplatin and etoposide in combination with radiation compared with the regimen of cyclophosphamide, epirubicin, and vincristine with radiation (4). As the cisplatin/etoposide regimen is easily combined with radiation, with little mucosal toxicity and less hematologic toxicity than other regimens, it remains the standard of care.

The addition of radiation to chemotherapy improves survival, and approximately 5% more patients are alive at 2 and 3 years when treated with combination chemoradiation versus chemotherapy alone (5). The early incorporation of radiation appears to yield better results than waiting until later in the treatment course. Several trials have addressed the timing of thoracic radiation. The National Cancer Institute of Canada randomized 308 patients receiving chemotherapy to (1) early thoracic radiation (starting with the second cycle of chemotherapy) versus (2) late thoracic radiation (starting with the sixth cycle). There was no difference in the total cumulative chemotherapy dose delivered between the two arms, but both progression-free survival and overall survival were improved in the early radiation arm (6). A meta-analysis of seven trials investigating early versus late radiation showed benefit with early RT (7).

Hyperfractionated radiation also appears to improve outcomes. Turrisi et al. randomized 417 patients with limited SCLC to cisplatin/etoposide given with either daily (qd) radiation (45 Gy total, 1.8 Gy fractions) or twice-daily (bid) radiation (45 Gy total, 1.5 Gy fractions). Patients on the bid dose schedule had better median survival (23 months for bid, versus 19 months for qd), and 5-year survival (26% versus 16%). Significantly worse toxicities were noted with the bid regimen, including Grade III esophagitis which occurred in 27% of this population versus 11% of the qd dosed population.

Not all centers have adopted the hyperfractionated dosing, however, the question of whether hyperfractionation or total dose of radiation is more important remains debated. Choi et al. tested escalating radiation doses in both the qd and bid schedules. The bid total dose was limited to 55 Gy while the qd dose went up to 70 Gy. In long-term follow up, both median survival (24 months versus 29.8 months) and 5-year survival (20% versus 36%) favored qd dosing (8).

Current NCCN guidelines recommend that radiation be delivered concurrently with chemotherapy in limited stage SCLC, starting within the first two cycles of chemotherapy. Either twice-daily dosing of radiation (to a total dose of 45 Gy in 1.5 Gy fractions) or once-daily dosing (to a total dose of at least 50 Gy in 1.8 Gy fractions) is acceptable (9).

PROPHYLACTIC CRANIAL IRRADIATION

Prophylactic cranial irradiation should be considered in both limited and extensive stage disease where there has been response.

PCI has been shown to improve overall survival at 3 years by approximately 5% (from 15.3% to 20.7%). In addition, PCI decreases the incidence of future brain metastases by approximately 25% (from 58.6% without PCI to 33.3% with PCI) (10) even in extensive stage disease, PCI appears to improve survival outcomes (11). Typical doses range from 25 Gy to 36 Gy.

Fractions greater than 3 Gy seem to be associated with late neurocognitive deficits and should be avoided.

TREATMENT FOR EXTENSIVE STAGE SCLC

Chemotherapy is the mainstay of treatment for extensive stage SCLC. As in limited stage SCLC, the combination of cisplatin and etoposide is one of the most widely used regimens in the United States. Response rates range from 60% to 70%, but the overall survival remains poor, with less than 5% of extensive SCLC patients alive at 2 years. Median survival is between 9 and 11 months.

A recent phase III trial in Japan raised a great deal of interest in a new combination of cisplatin and irinotecan for treatment of extensive SCLC, showing a significant improvement in median survival among patients treated with cisplatin/CPT11 versus cisplatin/etoposide (12.8 months versus 9.4 months) (12). However, a follow-up US study failed to show a significant difference in response or survival between the two regimens (13).

Numerous studies have attempted to alternate chemotherapy regimens or add a third agent, but none of these strategies have proven more effective than the doublet of cisplatin/etoposide. In addition, attempts to administer high-dose therapy with autologous bone-marrow transplantation have not shown a significant benefit in the phase III setting.

Therefore, cisplatin/etoposide remains the standard regimen in extensive SCLC. A total of four to six cycles are usually delivered, as prolonged maintenance chemotherapy has not shown any significant survival benefit and increases the toxicity risk. Since chemotherapy in the extensive stage setting is palliative in nature, carboplatin is often substituted for cisplatin to minimize toxicity. One small study compared EC versus EP and found similar response rates and survival times, with less toxicity in the EC regimen (14).

TREATMENT FOR REFRACTORY OR RELAPSED SCLC

Patients whose disease recurs within 3 months of completing initial chemotherapy or who have progressive disease during treatment are considered to have "refractory" disease. Patients whose disease recurs beyond 3 months of initial therapy are considered to have "relapsed" disease. Although refractory and relapsed patients are generally treated with similar second-line regimens, their prognoses are significantly different: patients with refractory disease have much poorer response to additional therapies.

Median survival after SCLC recurrence ranges from 2 to 6 months. Therefore the goals of salvage chemotherapy and a focus on palliation must be carefully discussed with patients and families.

For patients who have failed carboplatin/etoposide or cisplatin/etoposide, topotecan is commonly used as second-line therapy. In a phase II trial administering single agent topotecan to patients who progressed after first-line chemotherapy, overall response rate was 22%. Patients who had relapsed disease had higher complete and partial response rates (13% CR, 24% PR) compared with patients who had refractory disease (2% CR, 4% PR) (15). Other agents with activity include irinotecan, taxanes, and gemcitabine. Single agent therapy is generally preferred over combination therapies, as minimizing toxicities in this palliative setting is important. Enrollment on clinical trials is encouraged as none of the above regimens are extremely successful.

REFERENCES

1. Alberg AJ, Samet JM. Epidemiology of lung cancer. Chest. 2003; 123: 21S–49S.
2. Brambilla E, Travis WD, Colby TV, Corrin B, Shimosato Y. The new World Health Organization classification of lung tumours. Eur Respir J. 2001; 18: 1059–1068.
3. Jackman DM, Johnson BE. Small-cell lung cancer. Lancet. 2005; 366: 1385–1396.
4. Sundstrom S, Bremnes RM, Kaasa S, et al. Cisplatin and etoposide regimen is superior to cyclophosphamide, epirubicin, and vincristine regimen in small-cell lung cancer: results from a randomized phase III trial with 5 years' follow-up. JCO. 2002; 20: 4665–4672.
5. Pignon JP, Arriagada R, Ihde DC, et al. A meta-analysis of thoracic radiotherapy for small-cell lung cancer. NEJM. 1992; 327: 1618–1624.
6. Murray N, Coy P, Pater JL, et al. Importance of timing for thoracic irradiation in the combined modality treatment of limited stage small cell lung cancer. The National Cancer Institute of Canada Clinical Trials Group. JCO. 1993; 11: 336–344.
7. Fried DB, Morris DE, Poole C, et al. Systemic review evaluating the timing of thoracic radiation therapy in combined modality therapy for limited stage small cell lung cancer. JCO. 2004; 22: 4837–4845.
8. Choi NC, Herndon JE, Rosenman J, et al. Phase I study to determine the maximum-tolerated dose of radiation in standard daily and hyperfractionated-accelerated twice-daily radiation schedules with concurrent chemotherapy for limited-stage small-cell lung cancer. JCO. 1998; 16: 3528–3536.
9. National Comprehensive Cancer Network. Clinical Practice Guidelines in Oncology version 1. 2006.
10. Auperin A, Arriagada R, Pignon JP, et al. Prophylactic cranial irradiation for patients with small cell lung cancer in complete remission. NEJM. 1999; 341: 476–484.
11. Slotman B et al. A randomized trial of prophylactic cranial irradiation in small cell lung cancer after a response to chemotherapy. JCO Asco Ann Proceedings part 1. 2007; 25 (18S).
12. Noda K, Nishiwaki Y, Kawahara M, et al. Irinotecan plus cisplatin compared with etoposide plus cisplatin for extensive stage small cell lung cancer. NEJM. 2002; 346: 85–91.
13. Hanna NH, Einhorn L, Sandler A, et al. Randomized, phase III trial comparing irinotecan/cisplatin (IP) with etoposide/cisplatin (EP) in patients (pts) with previously untreated, extensive-stage (ES) small cell lung cancer (SCLC). Proc ASCO. 2005; Abstr 7004.
14. Skarlos DV, Samantas E, Kosmidis P, et al. Randomized comparison of etoposide-cisplatin vs. etoposide-carboplatin and irradiation in small-cell lung cancer: A Hellenic Co-operative Oncology Group study. Ann Oncol. 1994; 5: 601–607.
15. Ardizzoni A, Hansen H, Dombernowsky P, Gamucci T, et al. Topotecan, a new active drug in the second-line treatment of small cell lung cancer: a phase II study in patients with refractory and sensitive disease. JCO. 1997; 15: 2090–2096.

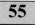

Richard T. Penson

OVARIAN CANCER

INTRODUCTION

Ovarian cancer remains the most lethal of gynecologic malignancies in developed countries. Growing awareness of this malignancy, and understanding of genetic predispositions has lead to successful prophylactic oophorectomy in high-risk populations and intraperitoneal chemotherapy in optimally surgically cytoreduced patients increases the cure rate from a quarter to one-third of patients. Adequate surgical staging and debulking should be attempted in all patients able to tolerate a laparotomy, followed by chemotherapy with paclitaxel and a platinum analog. Sequential palliative chemotherapy has enabled women to live with recurrent disease for years before suffering and dying with bowel obstruction. Despite advances, effective screening and cure remains elusive for most women.

INCIDENCE

Epithelial cancer of the ovary is the fifth most common solid tumor of women in the United States after cancer of the breast, colon, lung, and endometrium. It is the most lethal gynecologic malignancy, with approximately 24,000 cases and 16,000 deaths each year (1). One in 70 of American women will develop ovarian cancer sometime during their lifetime. In premenopausal women ovarian cancer is uncommon and found in less than 5% of adnexal masses, indeed, only 30% of adnexal masses are malignant in postmenopausal women.

EPIDEMIOLOGY OF EPITHELIAL OVARIAN CANCER

The majority of ovarian cancer presents in postmenopausal women with only 10–15% of cancers occurring in premenopausal patients. Median age at diagnosis is commonly reported between 60 and 65 years. Possible risk factors identified in case controlled studies, include white race, nulliparity, infertility, high-fat diet, lactose, paracetamol, and asbestos contaminated talc. Oral contraceptives, pregnancy, tubal ligation, and lactation reduce the risk. The association with early menarche, late menopause, and nulliparity suggests that uninterrupted "incessant" ovulation may predispose to malignancy. The oral contraceptive pill may offer some protective benefit in preventing ovarian cancer in high-risk populations. However, hormone replacement therapy appears to double the risk of death from ovarian cancer. Initial reports of very high risks from fertility drugs have not been confirmed.

FAMILIAL OVARIAN CANCER

The vast majority of ovarian cancer is sporadic in nature. However, a family history of ovarian cancer increases the risk of developing ovarian cancer two to threefold and it is estimated that 5% of all epithelial ovarian cancer cases result from hereditary predisposition. Approximately 75% of these families are linked to the breast ovarian cancer syndrome with loss of function of the tumor suppressor genes BRCA1 and BRCA2, involved in DNA repair, and inherited in an autosomally dominant fashion. Hereditary breast ovarian cancer syndrome (HBOC) accounts for 65–75% of all hereditary ovarian cancer cases, and is defined variably but typically with at least three cases of early onset (<60 years) breast or ovarian cancer. Mutations in BRCA1 (located on chromosome 17q) and BRCA2 (13q) are associated with a 16–44% and a 10% lifetime risk of ovarian cancer risk, respectively. The founder mutations 185delAG, and 5382insC in BRCA1, and 6174delT in BRCA2 are present in 2.5% of Ashkenazi women.

Hereditary non-polyposis colon cancer syndrome (HNPCC, Lynch syndrome (type II)) results from mismatch repair (MSH2, MLH1, and PMS2) genes defects, low penetrance allele and modifier gene defects. The American founder mutation is deletion of exons 1–6 of MSH2. HNPCC accounts for approximately 10–15% of all hereditary ovarian cancer cases. A diagnosis of HNPCC can be made using the Amsterdam Criteria (Colon cancer diagnosis in ≥3 relatives, one of whom is a first-degree relative of the other two, and one diagnosis before age 50). In a subsequent meeting the Bethesda Criteria were adopted to include the extracolonic tumors (e.g., endometrial) seen in HNPCC kindreds. The risk of developing ovarian cancer associated with HNPCC appears to be associated with an approximately 3.7-fold increase in lifetime risk of developing ovarian cancer. Hereditary site-specific ovarian cancer is defined as a family with three or more cases of invasive epithelial ovarian cancer at any age and no case of breast cancer diagnosed before age 50. The inherited predisposition syndromes are summarized in Table 55-1.

Women from high-risk families should have genetic counseling, and gene testing. At the present time a similar number of women elect biannual pelvic examinations, trans-vaginal ultrasound, and CA-125 with no proven effect on mortality, as we have a prophylactic risk reducing salpingoophorectomy (RRSO) which reduces the lifetime risk of ovarian cancer by 95% (2).

BIOLOGY

The common primary ovarian tumors are derived from the coelomic epithelium of the ovary. Though commonly termed "epithelial" the embryologic origin of ovarian cancer is mesodermal, from the peritoneal surface of the ovary. Increasing evidence points to subepithelial inclusion cysts that form after ovulation, as the initial focus of dyplastic change. Some series suggest that 5–10% of "ovarian" tumors may be primarily from the peritoneum (primary peritoneal cancer),

Table 55-1

Genetic Predisposition Syndromes

	Incidence	Lifetime risk and genes	
Sporadic	95% of ovarian cancer	1/70 lifetime	p53, K-ras, PTEN, myc, akt
HBOC	5% of ovarian cancer	BRCA1 16–44%	Chromosome 17q
		BRCA2 10%	Chromosome 13q
HNPCC	Rare	3.5 × increase	MSH2, MLH1, PMS2

HBOC: Hereditary Breast Ovarian Cancer syndrome, HNPCC: Hereditary non-polyposis colon cancer syndrome.

and fallopian tube carcinoma behaves in an identical fashion. The surface glycoprotein CA125 (Gene MUC-16) is found at elevated levels in the blood of >80% of patients with epithelial ovarian cancer (3). CA125 monitoring has not as yet been shown to be useful in screening for occult carcinoma, but blood concentrations typically correlate very well with disease bulk and response to treatment and it is an excellent tumor marker commonly used to assist physicians in treatment decisions. Array analysis has identified gene signatures predictive of survival and operability. These have confirmed some genes known to be important in ovarian tumor carcinogenesis (p53, PTEN, K-ras, myc, akt) and identified new candidates (CD9, MUC-1, epcam, HE4, SLP1, Mesothelin, CD24).

Tumor cells typically spread transcelomically to the pelvic structures, exfoliating and follow the circulation of the peritoneal fluid throughout the abdomen. Cells also metastasize by lymphatic and hematogenous routes. Extraperitoneal metastases are rare, but with increasing number of patients living for a protracted time, up to two-fifths of patients will develop metastases in the liver, lung, or the central nervous system during the later stages of their disease.

The majority of epithelial cancers are serous or papillary with a similar appearance to the lining of the fallopian tube (4). Endometrioid carcinoma is associated with synchronous endometrial carcinoma and endometriosis, and therefore more commonly present early, and have a better prognosis. Clear cell tumors have a particularly poor prognosis, are commonly associated with thromboses, and have distinct genetics that link the disease with other clear cell tumors. Mucinous tumors are more commonly bilateral and can be associated with pseudo-myxoma peritonei and mucocele of the appendix. The least common histological subtype, Brenner's tumor, has a histologic pattern similar to transitional cell carcinoma. Molecular evidence has confirmed that malignant mixed Müllerian tumors (carcinosarcomas) have a clonal proliferation of the epithelial element rather than being collision tumors and are treated as epithelial cancers. In women under the age of 40, but rarely in older patients, 60–70% of non-benign ovarian neoplasms are borderline tumors, a neoplasm that has distinctly malignant cytological features without invasion, which is treated surgically. Ovarian tumor pathology is summarized in Table 55-2.

NON-EPITHELIAL OVARIAN MALIGNANCIES

Non-epithelial ovarian cancer accounts for <10% of ovarian tumors. The commonest of these, germ cell tumors represent almost 70% of ovarian tumors in the first two decades of life, and one-third of these are malignant. These rare tumors disseminate early and the doubling time of the tumor can be very short. All patients should be treated in a specialist center because of continuing controversies in treatment. The tumor markers βHCG, αFP, and LDH are invaluable in the treatment and surveillance of germ cell tumors. Dysgerminoma, essentially the female equivalent of testicular seminoma, is exquisitely sensitive to platinum, and this is now favored over the tradition treatment of radiotherapy. Teratoma is probably most effectively treated with combination platinum-based chemotherapy such as BEP (bleomycin, etoposide, and cisplatin) and surgical removal of residual masses. Yolk sac, embryonal, and choriocarcinoma subtypes are rarer, curable, and require specialized care.

Sex-cord-stromal tumors account for even fewer ovarian malignancies. Granulosa cell tumors are typically relatively low grade, secrete estrogen and tumors in juveniles may be associated with sexual pseudo-precocity. The tumors secrete estradiol, Müllerian inhibiting substance, and dimeric inhibin, which serve as tumor markers. Sertoli–Leydig tumors are associated with the production of androgens. Thecomas and fibromas are also considered in this category.

Table 55-2

Ovarian Cancer Pathology

Histologic subgroup	Histologic subtype
Epithelial ovarian cancer	Serous papillary (70%)
	Endometrioid (20%)
	Clear cell (mesonephroid) (5%)
	Mucinous (2%)
	Brenner (transitional cell)
	Malignant mixed Müllerian tumor (MMMT carcinosarcoma)
Metastatic	Krukenberg (breast, colorectal, and gastric)
Sex-cord-stromal	Granulosa
	Sertoli–Leydig
	Thecoma-fibroma
Germ cell	Dysgerminoma (seminoma)
	Teratoma
	Yolk sac, embryonal, and choriocarcinoma
Benign	Epithelial or dermoid
Borderline	Tumor of low-malignant potential, micro-invasion

DIAGNOSIS

The presentation of ovarian cancer is typically subtle, "whispering," requiring a high index of suspicion, and delaying diagnosis. Although no symptoms are pathognomonic, persistent (>2 weeks) abdominal or pelvic pain, bloating, change in bowel habit, urinary, and constitutional symptoms are typical of peritoneal involvement by advanced disease and early stage, surgically curable, ovarian cancer is generally asymptomatic (Table 55-3). Unfortunately, most symptomatic women do not have a prompt diagnosis and indeed it is not uncommon for these women to be assigned erroneous diagnoses of irritable bowel syndrome, hiatal hernia, diverticulosis, or endometriosis. Pelvic examination remains an essential part of the examination of women complaining of abdominal symptoms.

The diagnosis and initial management of ovarian cancer is essentially surgical (Figure 55-1). Premenopausal women with a smooth, unilateral, mobile, cystic adnexal masses up to 8 cm in size can be managed conservatively with the use of oral contraceptives and serial ultrasound, typically performed at 6 weeks and at a different time of the menstrual cycle, as luteal cysts are common. In postmenopausal women cystic masses larger than 5 cm in diameter warrant an exploratory laparotomy. In postmenopausal women with a CA125 greater than 35 U/ml, adnexal masses are malignant in 80% of cases although this should not be confused with the finding of a raised CA125 in an asymptomatic postmenopausal woman, as perhaps only one in seven will have ovarian cancer. Occasionally there is uncertainty about the site of the primary and colonoscopy and mammography are appropriate. As early disease is typically asymptomatic, over 75% of tumors present as advanced stage disease (FIGO (International Federation of Gynecology and Obstetrics) stage III/IV) (Table 55-4).

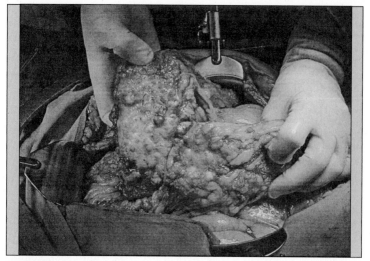

FIGURE 55-1   Advanced ovarian cancer (Courtesy of Dr. Arlan Fuller).

Table 55-3

Classical Presentations

Late
Adnexal mass (solid, complex, CA125>65)
Ascites
Pleural effusion, adnexal mass, and adenocarcinoma of unknown primary
Screening
Sister Mary Joseph's nodule (umbilical metastasis)
Paraneoplastic syndrome: Trousseau's syndrome (thrombosis), cerebellar
    degeneration, dermatomyositis, Leser-Trélat (seborrheic keratoses),
    palmer fasciitis Krukenberg's tumor (breast, gastric, or colorectal primary)

Table 55-4

Ovarian Cancer Staging (FIGO 1987)

Stage I: Limited to ovaries (10%)
IA.   One ovary, no ascites, intact capsule, no tumor on external surface.
IB.   Both ovaries, no ascites, intact capsule, no tumor on external surface.
IC.   One or both ovaries with capsular involvement, ruptured capsule, ascites,
        or positive peritoneal washings.

Stage II: Pelvic extension (5%)
IIA.   To uterus or Fallopian tubes.
IIB.   To other pelvic organs (e.g., bladder, rectum or vagina).
IIC.   Pelvic extension with factors as in IC.

Stage III: Upper abdominal involvement and/or positive lymph nodes (70%)
IIIA.   Microscopic seeding outside of pelvis with negative lymph nodes.
IIIB.   Gross deposits less than 2 cm with negative lymph nodes.
IIIC.   Gross deposits greater than 2 cm and/or positive lymph nodes.

Stage IV: Distant metastases (pleural effusion, liver parenchyma, etc.) (15%)

The differential diagnosis of adnexal masses includes simple of hemorrhagic physiologic cysts (follicular or corpus luteal), endometrioma, theca luteal cysts, benign, malignant or metastaic tumors, and extraovarian masses such as paraovarian or peritoneal cysts and pedunculated fibroids, extopic pregnancy, hydrosalpinx, tuboovarian, diverticular, or appendiceal abscesses.

SCREENING

Screening for ovarian cancer is an attractive proposition because of the significant morbidity and mortality associated with advanced disease, the availability of apparently sensitive and specific diagnostic tests (Ultrasound and CA125) and the better outcome for patients with early stage disease. However, there is continuing uncertainty about whether screening improves survival, and could be cost effective. The serum marker CA125 has been shown to be elevated in only 50% of patients with stage I disease, compared with 90% of stage II–IV ovarian cancers. CA125 has a sensitivity of 20–58% and a specificity of 97–99%. With a 1/70 lifetime risk, ovarian cancer is present in 1/2,000 postmenopausal women and therefore the false positive rate (1–3%) for CA125 may be unacceptably high, given the morbidity of laparotomy. In the largest study reported to date in 21,935 UK postmenopausal healthy women, the death rate was apparently halved by screening (18 of 10,977 vs. 9 of 10,958). However, this was not statistically significant ($p = 0.083$) (5).

The massive US study, PLCO (Prostate, Lung, Colorectal, and Ovary Cancer Screening Trial) will enroll 150,000 subjects and there continues to be speculation about whether the sensitivity of screening can be improved by the use of a panel of markers, ROCA (Rise of CA125 Algorithm), or proteinomics. At the present time, screening is only recommended in high-risk populations (+ve family history).

MANAGEMENT OF EARLY OVARIAN CANCER

Approximately 2,000 to 3,000 patients a year in the United States will have disease confined to pelvis. While this group accounts for only 15% of ovarian cancer cases, approximately one-third to one-half of all cured patients come from this group. Although different features confer significantly different prognoses within stage I, it is likely that grade is more significant than the extent of disease, very dense local adhesions should probably be considered stage II. Adequate staging requires that a surgeon with subspecialty expertise perform an exploratory laparotomy, total abdominal hysterectomy and bilateral salpingo-oophorectomy, omentectomy, careful examination of the peritoneal surfaces of the liver, diaphragm, pericolic gutters, and pelvic sidewalls with multiple biopsies and sampling of ascitic fluid and peritoneal washings with para-aortic and pelvic lymph node sampling. Patients diagnosed with apparently early stage ovarian cancer without adequate staging should undergo re-exploration for definitive staging.

The overall 5-year survival of patients with apparent stage I epithelial cancer was about 60% in earlier reports. With accurate staging, and migration of patients with clinically occult nodal or omental metastases to stage III, survival of stage I patients is now commonly reported as ≥90%. In a series of 656 accurately staged patients no patient with stage I grade I cancer died of their disease. Approximately 30–46% of cancers that appear to be confined to the pelvis (stage I and II) have occult metastatic disease in the upper abdomen or lymph nodes (stage III). In patients with stage IA and IB disease of low grade no adjuvant treatment is warranted. For all other patients and those with high-risk histology, adjuvant treatment is recommended with platinum-based chemotherapy based on ICON I (International Collaboration in Ovarian Neoplasia) and the EORTC's (European Organization for the Research and Treatment of Cancer) ACTION study (6).

GOG 157 (Gynecologic Oncology Group—US NCI funded cooperative research group) compared #3 with #6 cycles of carboplatin and paclitaxel in early stage disease. While more cycles were associated with more toxicity, based on a non-statistically significant superior outcome in this population with few events (recurrences or deaths) most patients receive six cycles of chemotherapy if tolerated.

MANAGEMENT OF ADVANCED OVARIAN CANCER

The principle of therapy for patients with advanced ovarian cancer is to cytoreduce with surgery and chemotherapy to a state of minimal residual disease. For some patients this will translate into cure, but for the majority of patients it delays symptomatic relapse. Current standard of care has been defined as cytoreductive surgery and six cycles of a taxane with either cisplatin or carboplatin chemotherapy. Five-year survival rates for patients treated with platinum-based regimens are approximately 20–40%. Even after a CR (complete response) to first-line therapy with no clinical or aradiologic evidence of disease and a normal CA125, only approximately 50% of patients with negative second look operations are cured. Figure 55-2 illustrates a treatment algorithm for advanced ovarian cancer.

Cytoreductive Surgery

Griffith is credited with the concept that successful surgical debulking to a residual tumor size of ≤1.5 cm maximum diameter results in superior survival.

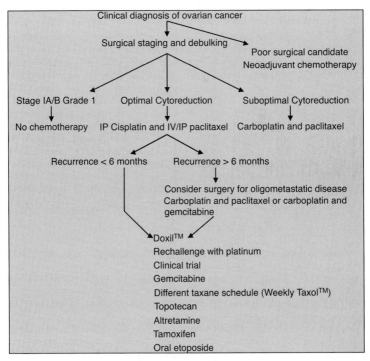

FIGURE 55-2 Treatment algorithms for ovarian cancer.

More contemporary studies now strive for even smaller tumor volumes (<1 cm). Surgical cytoreduction (debulking) has two main advantages. First, it improves physiology with the immediate correction of the functional disorders and pain associated with bowel and ureteral obstruction, as well as improving the profound protein loss associated with exudative ascites. Second, optimal debulking can remove 90% to many logs of tumor cells thereby reducing the volume of residual disease to be treated by systemic or intraperitoneal chemotherapy. In theory cytoreduction may remove de novo chemotherapy-resistant clones and facilitate drug delivery having removed tumor with a compromised blood supply. Several studies have demonstrated that patients with tumors that can be cytoreduced to minimal residual disease survive longer. However, this may simply reflect the biology of the tumor.

Van der Burg reported a 33% reduction in the risk of death ($p = 0.008$) in a phase III study of interval cytoreduction (after #3 cycles of chemotherapy) in patients with initially suboptimally cytoreduced disease (>1 cm). However, this advantage cannot be replicated if the initial attempt at debulking was performed by a gynecologic oncologist who has already made a maximal attempt at cytoreduction (7). The role of debulking for stage IV disease remains controversial, and the once common practice of second look laparotomy, which gives important prognostic information, only has a role in a research setting as it has no therapeutic benefit, and at the present time no consolidation strategy, that it might indicate, is associated with an overall survival advantage.

Follow up for patients should include a pelvic examination and CA125, initially every 3 months.

Platinum-Based First-Line Chemotherapy

Chemotherapy plays an essential role in advanced stage ovarian cancer. Over the last 30 years, tumor response rates (shrinkage of the tumor by more than 50%) have increased from the 20% range with single agent melphalan used in the 1970s to 75% in recent studies using platinum with a taxane. Although overall survival has improved very little, median survival time has significantly increased over the last few decades, and the overall median survival of patients with suboptimally debulked advanced stage disease has nearly tripled over the past quarter century coincident with an almost fourfold improvement in combined response rates. While some of this benefit is certainly due to improvements in supportive care and improved surgical staging, the primary reason for this improvement is modern chemotherapy which is both less toxic and more effective. Following the model of Hodgkin's disease, combination therapy logically followed single agent therapy with cyclophosphamide-based combinations, which produced response rates of approximately 35%. In the 1980s, cisplatin and subsequently carboplatin, non-classical alkylators were demonstrated to have very significant activity in ovarian carcinoma with response rates of approximately 60%, thus redefining the combinations of chemotherapy used for advanced disease, with a significant survival advantage proven in 1986. Meta-analysis of randomized trials prior to 1991 concluded that cisplatin regimes were superior to non-cisplatin regimes, cisplatin combinations were superior to cisplatin alone, and that cisplatin and carboplatin were equally effective.

Paclitaxel (Taxol™), initially derived from the Western Pacific yew tree (*Taxus brevofolia*), inhibits microtubule depolymerization and demonstrated significant activity in patients with ovarian cancer refractory to platinum chemotherapy. Following the introduction of pre-medication that prevented a hypersensitivity reaction, McGuire reported a response rate of 24% using paclitaxel in heavily pretreated patients whose tumors were resistant to platinum. McGuire reported a substantial survival advantage replacing cyclophosphamide with paclitaxel, in 410 randomly assigned women with suboptimally debulked advanced ovarian cancer (GOG 111). Cisplatin 75 mg/m^2 and paclitaxel 135 mg/m^2 over 24 h was associated with more alopecia, neutropenia, fever, and allergic reactions, but improved median overall survival from 24 to 38 months ($p < 0.001$) (8). This result was confirmed by OV10, which also demonstrated that combining a 3-h infusion of 175 mg/m^2 paclitaxel with cisplatin produced unacceptable neurotoxicity. Two subsequent studies GOG 132 and ICON II suggested that platinum alone of sequential platinum and paclitaxel may be equally effective. The present standard of care was defined in GOG 158, which compared cisplatin and paclitaxel with carboplatin and paclitaxel. Six cycles of carboplatin AUC 7.5 and paclitaxel 175 mg/m^2 over 3 h was a convenient out patient regimen which produced less gastrointestinal, renal, and metabolic toxicity, and leukopenia, and a similar degree of peripheral neuropathy with a median overall survival of 57 months. As this regimen is associated with greater thrombocytopenia the AUC (area under the concentration time curve) dosing, based on renal function is now typically targeted at 5 or 6, and based on the Calvert formula (Total dose (mg) = target AUC(mg/ml/min) $\times$ (CrCl + 25) (ml/min)). The moderate increases in platinum dose that can be achieved by 'high dose' chemotherapy, or more cycles of chemotherapy (# 10 vs. 5, or #12 vs. 6) do not improve outcomes.

The integration of gemcitabine, liposomally encapsulated doxorubicin hydrochloride (Doxil™), and topotecan with carboplatin and paclitaxel as first-line therapy is being widely investigated. However, we appear to be a symptotically the ceiling of benefit for combination platinum based therapy. The SCOTROC study demonstrated that Docetaxel (Taxotere™) was significantly less neurotoxic than paclitaxel and equally effective in combination with carboplatin, and is a valid, but less used alternate to paclitaxel.

In patients with suboptimally debulked disease, who are destined to have relapse, maintenance therapy is a rational strategy. GOG 178 compared 1 year with 3 months of monthly single agent paclitaxel, and appeared to delay the time to recurrence by 7 months for 9 months more toxicity, and is not a standard of care but provoked GOG 212, which investigates a potentially less neurotoxic agent, polyglutamated paclitaxel (Xyotax™) (9). Consolidation with other agents such as topotecan have been shown not to improve survival.

GOG 218 investigates the integration of bevacizumab (Avastin™) in to the upfront treatment of advanced ovarian cancer administered with carboplatin and paclitaxel and as consolidation. Bevacizumab is a particularly promising agent as the response rate is highest in ovarian cancer compared with any other solid tumor. Toxicities in patients with recurrent disease have included hypertension, proteinuria, arterial thromboses, and one study was halted with five of 44 patients developing bowel perforations.

Intraperitoneal Chemotherapy

The debate about whether total dose or dose intensity of chemotherapy is most important in the treatment of ovarian cancer continues to be explored. One way to achieve high concentrations of cytotoxics is regional administration. Intraperitoneal (IP) infusion lends itself to this approach with a very high ratio of IP drug concentration that bathes the tumor in comparison to systemic concentrations (Platinum 10$\times$, paclitaxel 1000$\times$).

Alberts initially reported a randomized trial of cyclophosphamide intravenously with either intraperitoneal or intravenous cisplatin (GOG 104), with an 8-month median survival advantage. Markman reported a second phase III study (GOG 114), which included intravenous paclitaxel with intraperitoneal cisplatin, but also included two initial cycles of moderate dose carboplatin as "medical" cytoreduction, and had more toxicity, but an 11-month survival advantage. The third study (GOG 172) has led to an NCI alert about the potential advantage of intraperitoneal therapy in patients with optimally debulked ovarian cancer because of an unprecedented 16-month survival advantage (10). Armstrong's regimen of paclitaxel 135 mg/m^2 over a 24-h period (to reduce neurotoxicity) followed by intraperitoneal cisplatin 100 mg/m^2 on day 2 with intraperitoneal paclitaxel 60 mg/m^2 on day 8 given every 3 weeks for six cycles was associated with more fatigue, hematologic, gastrointestinal, metabolic, and neurologic toxicity, with significantly worse quality of life, but an improvement in median duration of overall survival from 50 to 66 months ($p = 0.03$).

Ongoing studies are examining consolidation intraperitoneal cisplatin and intraperitoneal carboplatin. Some concerns remain given that intraperitoneal chemotherapy may not reach subperitoneal disease, lymphnodes, or areas walled off by adhesions. The biggest concerns remain catheter complications (infection, pain, and blockage), which are serious in a quarter of patients and prevented 58% of patients completing intraperitoneal-therapy in GOG 172, and these challenges remain a barrier to its use in some settings.

RECURRENT DISEASE

The majority of patients who achieve a complete remission with first-line platinum-based chemotherapy will ultimately develop recurrent disease. More than 40% of women with ovarian cancer survive longer than 5 years. Recurrent ovarian cancer is often considered a chronic disease, since active chemotherapy agents allow patients to live for years with their disease, and quality of life is one of the most important considerations. There are now standardized scales and approximately 10% of all randomized cancer trials include health related QOL as one of the main end points.

The definition of relapse is important as a rising CA 125 typically has a lead-time of 2–4 months before symptoms develop. Patients with an asymptomatic rising marker can be managed expectantly, as palliative chemotherapy has toxicities. However, patients and clinicians often treat patients before they have bulk disease (>5 cm), which is associated with a poorer response to chemotherapy. The most important factor associated with poor prognosis at time of relapse is a short disease- and treatment-free interval. Disease relapsing more than 2 years after last being treated with a platinum is two to three times as likely to respond to rechallenge with platinum compared with disease that relapses within a year. Potentially platinum resistant disease is arbitrarily defined as disease that relapses within 6 months of platinum, and platinum sensitive disease after more than 6 months. Rechallenge with a platinum and taxane combination is appropriate with a platinum-free interval of at least 6 months or a year, with ICON 4 demonstrating an absolute improvement in the 1-year progression-free survival of 10% and 18% reduction in risk of death ($p = 0.02$) (11). An AGO study demonstrating a PFS advantage for carboplatin and gemcitabine over carboplatin alone, and this combination is also an option for platinum sensitive disease.

Continual sequential single agent palliative chemotherapy is the mainstay of treatment for recurrent disease. CA125 may better predict response to treatment and outcome than CT scans of measurable disease. Outside of the setting of a clinical trial there are a number of active single agents to use including Doxil, rechallenge with platinum, gemcitabine, different taxane schedule (weekly taxol), topotecan, altretamine, tamoxifen and oral etoposide. Hormonal therapy, often tamoxifen, can be effective in ER +ve tumors. The role of surgery is controversial. Many patients are appropriate for clinical trials, and an exciting number of agents are being investigated.

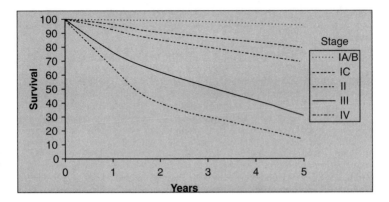

FIGURE 55-3 Overall survival for patients with ovarian cancer.

Obstructive symptoms typically herald the last chapter of patients' lives. The constellation of difficult to treat symptoms requires multi-professional care. Surgery should be limited to patients with chemotherapy responsive disease, and for others a G-tube (Gastric venting tube) alleviates vomiting. Total parenteral nutrition does not substantially alter the clinical course. Steroids and Otreotide™ may provide symptom relief, and attending to end of life issues is a vital part of holistic care.

PROGNOSIS

With modern surgical cytoreduction followed by as little as 18 weeks of chemotherapy, overall survival rates at 5 years exceed 40%. Stage, grade, histologic subtype, age, and whether the patient can be optimally surgically cytoreduced predict prognosis. Although the ultimate long-term prognosis of patients with advanced disease remains poor, current therapy often provides excellent palliation for these women for many years. Figure 55-3 illustrates the overall survival of patients with ovarian cancer. Table 55-5 lists some

Table 55-5

Novel Therapies in Randomized Clinical Trials for Epithelial Ovarian Cancer

Class	Targets	Agents
Antiangiogenic	VEGF	Bevacizumab (Avastin™)
	Multiple	Thalidomide (GOG 198)
	VEGFR-2/RAF kinase	Sorafenib (Nexavar ™)
Cytotoxic	Glutathione-*S*-transferase	Telcyta™ (TLK-286)
Sensitizer	Antiapoptotic protein XIAP	Phenoxodiol
Growth factor inhibitors	EGFR	Erlotinib (Tarceva™)
Minor groove binder	DNA	Yondelis™ (ET-743)
Monoclonal antibodies	CA125	Orgovomab (OvaRex™)
	EGFR/HER-2/neu	Pertuzumab (Omnitarg™)
Cytokine	Immune system	IFNγ (GRACES)
CAM		Acupuncture, Essiac

Table 55-6

Key Points

1. The presentation of ovarian cancer is often subtle and a low index of suspicion is necessary.
2. A strong family history should prompt consideration of gene testing and risk reducing salpingoophorectomy.
3. Surgical staging and cytoreduction is essential in the successful management of ovarian cancer and should be undertaken by a trained gynecologic oncologist.
4. Combination taxane and platinum chemotherapy is standard and should be delivered intraperitoneally in patients with optimally cytoreduced disease.
5. Chemotherapy provides effective palliation with an increasing number of therapeutic options.

exciting new agents in late stages of development, with the hope that the impact of novel biologics will more than match the improvement in outcomes with radical surgery and the introduction of platinum and Table 55-6 provides chapter key points.

REFERENCES

1. Cannistra SA. Cancer of the ovary. N Engl J Med. 2004; 351: 2519–2529.
2. Kauff ND, Satagopan JM, Robson ME, et al. Risk-reducing salpingo-oophorectomy in women with a BRCA1 or BRCA2 mutation. N Engl J Med. 2002; 346: 1609–1615.
3. Bast RC Jr, Klug TL, St John E, et al. A radioimmunoassay using a monoclonal antibody to monitor the course of epithelial ovarian cancer. N Engl J Med. 1983; 309: 883–887.
4. Young RH, Scully RE. Differential diagnosis of ovarian tumors based primarily on their patterns and cell types. Semin Diagn Pathol. 2001; 18: 161–235.
5. Jacobs IJ, Skates SJ, MacDonald N, et al. Screening for ovarian cancer: a pilot randomised controlled trial. Lancet. 1999; 353: 1207–1210.
6. Colombo N, Guthrie D, Chiari S, et al. International Collaborative Ovarian Neoplasm trial 1: a randomized trial of adjuvant chemotherapy in women with early-stage ovarian cancer. J Natl Cancer Inst. 2003; 95: 125–132.
7. Rose PG, Nerenstone S, Brady MF, et al. Secondary surgical cytoreduction for advanced ovarian carcinoma. N Engl J Med. 2004; 351: 2489–2497.
8. McGuire WP, Hoskins WJ, Brady MF, et al. Cyclophosphamide and cisplatin compared with paclitaxel and cisplatin in patients with stage III and stage IV ovarian cancer. N Engl J Med. 1996; 334: 1–6.
9. du Bois A, Quinn M, Thigpen T, et al. 2004 consensus statements on the management of ovarian cancer: final document of the 3rd International Gynecologic Cancer Intergroup Ovarian Cancer Consensus Conference (GCIG OCCC 2004). Ann Oncol. 2005; 16(Suppl 8): viii7–viii12.
10. Armstrong DK, Bundy B, Wenzel L, et al. Intraperitoneal cisplatin and paclitaxel in ovarian cancer. N Engl J Med. 2006; 354: 34–43.
11. Parmar MK, Ledermann JA, Colombo N, et al. Paclitaxel plus platinum-based chemotherapy versus conventional platinum-based chemotherapy in women with relapsed ovarian cancer: the ICON4/AGO-OVAR-2.2 trial. Lancet. 2003; 361: 2099–2106.

PRIMARY SQUAMOUS CARCINOMA OF THE UTERINE CERVIX: DIAGNOSIS AND MANAGEMENT

INTRODUCTION

Squamous cell carcinoma of the uterine cervix comprises and estimated 80% of all cervical cancers. The other histologies include adenocarcinoma (15%), and adenosquamous carcinomas (3–5%), with only a small fraction of all cervical cancers having neuroendocrine or small cell histology. This chapter will focus on the diagnosis and management of primary squamous cell carcinoma of the uterine cervix. Cervical carcinoma of the uterine cervix is the second most common cause of cancer-related death among women worldwide, with over 500,000 new cases diagnosed annually and a 50% mortality rate (1). In the United States, approximately 10,370 new cases of invasive cervical cancer are diagnosed annually, with and estimated 3,710 deaths from the disease, making it the sixth most common cause diagnosed malignancy among American women (1). An estimated 79% of these cases occur in developing countries (1). The worldwide discrepancy in both the incidence and mortality from cervical cancer can be explained as the result of the widespread implementation of cervical cancer prevention programs in developed countries. In these countries, there has been a 75% decrease in the incidence and mortality of cervical cancer over the past 50 years. In contrast, approximately 60% of women diagnosed with cervical cancer in the developing countries have either never been screened or have not been screened in the 5 years antecedent their diagnosis (2). This worldwide discrepancy in cervical cancer incidence and mortality is also notable among different racial groups in the United States. Lastly, although cervical cytology is an excellent screening instrument for pre-invasive disease, the false negative rate for detecting invasive carcinoma is relatively high, reportedly 50%.

Incidence

The incidence of invasive cervical cancer is related to age, with a mean age at the time of diagnosis of 47 years in the United States (3). From 1995 to 1999, the incidence of cervical cancer in the United States in girls under 20 years of age was 0/100,000/year (3). In women ages 20–24, this incidence is reported to be 1.7/100,000/year, peaking in women ages 45–49 at 16.5/100,000/year, with only 10% of cases seen in women age 75 or older (3).

Epidemiology

Patients with squamous cell carcinoma of the cervix share the same risk factors as patients with cervical intraepithelial neoplasia or dysplasia (4). These factors include:

- Early onset of sexual activity
- Multiple sexual partners
- High-risk sexual partners
- History of sexually transmitted diseases
- Tobacco use
- Multiparity
- Low socio-economic status
- Immunosuppression
- Previous history of vulvar or vaginal dysplasia

Perhaps the most significant risk factor for developing squamous cell cervical cancer is lack of cervical cytological screening. It is critical to underscore that infection with certain subtypes of the human papillomavirus (HPV) has been identified as the central causative factor in the development of cervical neoplasia (4). High-risk oncogenic types can be detected in almost all cervical cancers (4). Although most HPV infections are transient, chronic persistent HPV infection with the oncogenic subtypes is the central causative factor in the development of cervical neoplasia. The virus alone, however, is not sufficient to cause cervical neoplasia or cancer (4).

CLINICAL MANIFESTATIONS

Symptoms

Because early cervical cancer is usually asymptomatic, screening is critical. Common symptoms, when they occur, include abnormal vaginal bleeding, bleeding after intercourse, and a vaginal discharge (watery, mucoid, malodorous, or even purulent). In the setting of advanced disease, patients may complain of back pain radiating to the lower extremities or pelvic pain. Other symptoms seen in the setting of advanced disease include bowel and urinary symptoms, such as hematuria, hemotochezia, or stool/urine passage *per* vagina.

Physical Examination

Findings at the time of physical examination may range from a normal appearing cervix to a grossly abnormal cervix with an exophytic, plaque-like, indurated, ulcerated, or endophytic lesion. Findings encountered in patients with regionally advanced stage disease include parametrial, paracervical, or vaginal involvement, lower extremity edema, and inguinal adenopathy. Distant disease may be manifest in ascites, pleural effusions, and supraclavicular adenopathy.

PATTERNS OF SPREAD

Squamous cell carcinoma of the cervix may spread via direct extension, lymphatic and hematogenous dissemination. It can spread directly to the parametria, the uterine corpus, the vagina, bladder, rectum, and peritoneal cavity. Although prior dictum described a predictable pattern of lymphatic spread, sentinel node mapping has demonstrated that the first site of metastasis may involve any one of the pelvic lymph node chains.

DIAGNOSIS

Squamous cell carcinoma of the uterine cervix is staged clinically based on the criteria delineated by the International Federation of Gynecology and Obstetrics (FIGO) (Table 56-1).

Clinical Staging Procedures

After histological confirmation of an invasive cancer, a thorough physical examination is mandated. This survey should include careful inspection of the cervix, assessment of its size, and careful examination of the entire vagina. Cervical tumor size and parametrial involvement are best evaluated through a rectovaginal examination. The inguinal and supracervical regions should be inspected for the presence of adenopathy. It is reasonable to arrange for an examination under anesthesia in order to better appreciate the

Table 56-1

Staging of Cervical Cancer Based on Criteria from the International Federation of Gynecology and Obstetrics (FIGO)

Stage	Definition
Stage IA_1	Microscopic tumor $\leq$3 mm in depth and $\leq$7 mm horizontal spread
Stage IA_2	Microscopic tumor 3.1–5.0 mm in depth and $\leq$7 mm horizontal spread
Stage IB_1	Clinical tumor $\leq$4.0 cm in diameter
Stage IB_2	Clinical tumor >4.0 cm in diameter
Stage IIA	Extension to the proximal 2/3 of the vagina
Stage IIB	Parametrial extension
Stage IIIA	Extension to the distal 1/3 of the vagina
Stage IIIB	Sidewall extension, hydronephrosis, or non-functioning kidney
Stage IVA	Extension to bladder/rectal mucosa*
Stage IVB	Distant metastasis

*Bullous edema alone is not sufficient.

extent of local disease and to facilitate patient comfort. The following studies and procedures are allowed by FIGO as part of the staging of cervical cancer:

- Chest x-ray
- Intravenous pyelogram
- Barium enema
- Skeletal x-rays
- Colposcopy/biopsies
- Cervical conization
- Cystoscopy
- Proctoscopy

Other optional studies and procedures that can be obtained, but which cannot alter FIGO staging, include the following:

- Computed tomography
- Magnetic resonance imaging
- Ultrasonography
- Radionucleotide scanning
- Laparoscopy
- Laparotomy

PROGNOSIS

Prognosis for squamous cell carcinoma of the uterine cervix is influenced by numerous tumor-related factors, including stage, tumor volume, depth of invasion, lymph node involvement, lymph-vascular space involvement, histologic subtype, and tumor grade. FIGO tumor stage correlates with 5-year survival (Table 56-2) (5). Lymph nodal status is also an important prognostic factor. Five-year survival in the presence of pelvic lymph node involvement is 45–60% (6). Five-year survival in the setting of para-aortic lymph node involvement is estimated to be 15–30% (7). The number of involved lymph nodes also plays a critical role. In the presence of one involved pelvic lymph node, the recurrence risk in 35% (7). When two or three pelvic lymph nodes are involved, the risk of recurrence is 59–69%, respectively (7).

Table 56-2

Five-Year Survival for Squamous Cell Carcinoma of the Uterine Cervix Based on FIGO Staging

FIGO stage	Five-year survival (%)
IA	98
IB$_1$	90
IB$_2$	80
IIA	73
IIB	67
IIIA	45
IIIB	36
IVA	4

Adapted from information contained in (5).

TREATMENT

Treatment options for squamous cell carcinoma of the uterine cervix include surgery and radiation therapy. Both surgical intervention and definitive radiation therapy with concomitant chemotherapy are appropriate alternatives for the treatment of early stage cervical cancer, including FIGO stage IIA (8).

Surgery

For women with stage IA$_1$ lesions, surgical treatment may be in the form of a loop electrosurgical excision procedure (LEEP) or cervical conization (if they desire to preserve fertility) or an extra-fascial hysterectomy (8). For certain selected patients who want to preserve fertility and with Stage IA$_2$/IB$_1$ lesions, a radical trachelectomy with lymphadenectomy may be an alternative to a radical hysterectomy. A radical trachelectomy involves removal of the entire cervix and the parametria, with placement of a cerclage in order to allow preservation of the uterine corpus with a competent vaginal-uterine junction (8). The radical trachelectomy can be performed abdominally or vaginally, and combined with a laparoscopic or open therapeutic lymphadenectomy. The radical trachelectomy appears to be a reasonable alternative for women with Stage IA$_2$/IB$_1$ lesions desiring fertility preservation with tumors less than 2 cm in size, absence of lymph vascular space involvement and absence of lymph nodal disease. The experience with this procedure indicates that it results in a similar oncologic outcome as a radical hysterectomy, allowing for the possibility of future pregnancies.

For patients with Stage IA$_2$ lesions, surgical treatment may be in the form of a Type II or modified hysterectomy (8). During this type of hysterectomy, the uterine artery is ligated where it crosses over the ureter, the uterosacral and the cardinal ligaments are divided midway towards their attachment to the sacrum and the pelvic sidewall, respectively, and the upper one-third of the vagina is resected. For Stage IB$_1$, IB$_2$, and IIA lesions, the recommended surgical treatment is a Type III or radical hysterectomy. During this procedure, the uterine artery is ligated at its origin from the internal iliac artery. The uterosacral and the cardinal ligaments are divided at their insertion into the sacrum and the pelvic sidewall, respectively, and the upper one-half of the vagina is divided.

In pre-menopausal women, the surgery, as compared to radiation therapy as the alternative treatment modality, offers the advantage of ovarian preservation and may avoid vaginal stenosis. It also allows for "debulking" of enlarged lymph nodes and may allow for the individualization and tailoring of the radiation treatment fields.

Part of the surgical treatment of cervical cancer for Stage IA_2–IIA includes a lymphadenectomy. For women with Stage IA_2 and small IB_1 tumors, a pelvic lymphadenectomy should be performed at the time of hysterectomy (8). For those with enlarged lymph nodes, macroscopic Stages IB_1, IB_2, or IIA tumors, or those with histologic confirmation of metastatic nodal disease at the time of frozen section, the surgical intervention should include both a pelvic and para-aortic lymphadenectomy.

Primary Radiation Therapy

Since the oncologic results are similar, radical surgery, and definitive radiation therapy are acceptable treatment modalities for stage IA, IB, and non-bulky IIA lesions (8). For women undergoing definitive treatment with radiation therapy, the use of concomitant cisplatin-based chemotherapy is also recommended. The progression-free survival and overall survival advantage of concomitant chemoradiotherapy ovary radiation alone in patients with early and locally advanced cervical cancer has been demonstrated in at least five randomized, controlled clinical trials and a meta-analysis.

Radiation therapy can be delivered in the form of external beam radiation or brachytherapy. Brachytherapy allows for treatment of centrally located disease, primarily the cervix, the vagina, and the parametria. It can be delivered via an intracavitary or interstitial needle system. The intracavitary systems include uterine tandems, vaginal colpostats, and vaginal cylinders. External beam radiation therapy involves radiation of the entire pelvis, with doses ranging from 4,500 to 5,000 cGy, given in daily fractions over several weeks (usually 180 cGy/fraction). As noted earlier, radiation therapy is administered with concomitant chemotherapy using cisplatin (40 mg/m^2/week) (8).

Adjuvant Chemoradiotherapy

Patients with localized cervical cancer treated primarily with surgery and who have tumors with either intermediate or high-risk factors for disease recurrence should receive adjuvant chemoradiotherapy (9). High-risk factors include positive or close resection margins, positive lymph nodes, and microscopic parametrial involvement (9). Intermediate risk factors for disease recurrence include tumor size, deep stromal invasion, or the presence of lymph vascular space involvement (9). The recommended regimen includes radiation therapy with the use of concomitant cisplatin (40 mg/m^2/week) (8, 9).

POST-TREATMENT SURVEILLANCE

After completion of their treatment plan, patients should be evaluated every 3 months for the first 2 years, every 6 months for the subsequent 3 years, and annually thereafter. Evaluation should include a thorough review of systems and physical examination and a Pap smear at the time of each surveillance visit. Most vaginal recurrences are asymptomatic and may be only recognized through a Pap smear. For women with Stage IIB or greater, an annual chest x-ray is recommended. Any palpable mass needs to be biopsied to rule out the presence of recurrent disease.

CONCLUSIONS

Squamous cell cancer of the cervix is staged clinically and can be treated through primary surgical therapy or radiation therapy with concomitant chemotherapy. The choice of treatment modality depends on numerous factors including the patient's general condition, stage of disease, and desire for fertility preservation. Stage IA_1 tumors may be treated with a cervical conization or

LEEP or with an extrafascial hysterectomy. Stage IA_2 lesions may be treated with a modified radical hysterectomy and pelvic lymphadenectomy. The surgical treatment of choice for Stages IB_1, IB_2, and small IIA lesions is a radical hysterectomy with a pelvic lymphadenectomy. Chemoradiation therapy may be offered to these patients instead of primary surgical therapy. Patients with Stages IIB–IV disease should be treated with chemoradiation therapy. It is estimated that approximately 50% of recurrences from squamous cell carcinoma of the cervix occur within a year of completing treatment. Treatment options for recurrent disease depend on the modality of therapy utilized in the primary setting. Women treated surgically may be candidates for radiation therapy or systemic chemotherapy. Women treated initially with chemoradiation may be candidates for surgical resection or systemic chemotherapy at the time of disease recurrence. The choice of surgical treatment in the recurrent setting is generally limited to those women who are candidates for exenterative surgery. These patients are limited to those who have a central recurrence following primary treatment, in the absence of distant metastasis.

REFERENCES

1. Jemal A, Murray T, Ward E, et al. Cancer statistics. CA Cancer J Clin. 2005; 55: 10–30.
2. Parkin DM, Bray F, Ferlay J, et al. Global cancer statistics, 2002. CA Cancer J Clin. 2005; 55: 74–108.
3. Franco EL, Schlecht NF, Saslow D. The epidemiology of cervical cancer. Cancer J. 2003; 9: 349–359.
4. Castle PE, Wacholder S, Lorincz AT, et al. A prospective study of high-grade cervical neoplasia risk among human papillomavirus-infected women. J Natl Cancer Inst. 2002; 94: 1406–1414.
5. Benedet JL, Odicino F, Maisonneuve P, et al. Carcinoma of the cervix uteri. J Epidemiol Biostat. 2001; 6: 7–43.
6. Averette HE, Nguyen HN, Donato DM, et al. Radical hysterectomy for invasive cervical cancer: a 25-year prospective experience with the Miami technique. Cancer 1993; 71: 1422–1437.
7. Tanaka Y, Sawada S, Muratta T. Relationship between lymph node matastases and prognosis in patients irradiated postoperatively for carcinoma of the uterine cervix. Acta Radiol Oncol. 1984; 23: 455–459.
8. Committee on Practice Bulletins-Gynecology. Diagnosis and treatment of cervical carcinomas, number 35, May 2002. Obstet Gynecol. 2002; 99: 855–867.
9. Peters WA III, Liu PY, Barrett RJ II, et al.. Concurrent chemotherapy and pelvic radiation therapy compared with pelvic radiation therapy alone as adjuvant therapy after radical surgery in high-risk early-stage cancer of the cervix. J Clin Oncol. 2000; 18: 1606–1613.

UTERINE CANCER

INCIDENCE AND EPIDEMIOLOGY

Uterine corpus malignancies represent the fourth most common malignancy and eighth most common cause of cancer death in US women in 2005, with 40,880 new cases and 7,210 deaths (1). Uterine cancer can be broadly divided into two basic types: endometrial adenocarcinoma, which arises from the endometrium (lining of the uterus) and uterine sarcoma, in which the cells of origin are from the myometrium (uterine muscle wall) or other non-epithelial structures, such as stromal cells. Endometrial cancer is the most common of the gynecologic malignancies, comprising 6% of all female cancers. It most often presents early, in stages I and II, when it is confined to the corpus and is usually curable with either surgery alone or surgery plus radiotherapy. By contrast, uterine sarcomas are extremely rare, representing only about 4% of uterine cancers, and often present in advanced stages. The rarity of these tumors has hampered our understanding of their biology and optimal treatment.

EPIDEMIOLOGY OF ENDOMETRIAL CANCER

Epidemiology and presentation divide endometrial cancer into two types: those that arise related to estrogen stimulation and those that develop unrelated to estrogen.

- Type I endometrial cancer, which comprises 80% of cases, is estrogen-related. This is typically a cancer of the post-menopause and tends to be associated with atypical endometrial hyperplasia (a precursor condition). It most often presents as a low-grade, early stage, endometrioid tumor. The risk factors for this type of endometrial cancer include obesity, nulliparity, estrogen excess (endogenous or exogenous), hypertension and diabetes mellitus.
- Type II endometrial cancer is unrelated to estrogen or endometrial hyperplasia, and accounts for 20% of endometrial cancer. These patients typically present with more advanced disease, higher-grade tumors and/or poor prognostic histologic subtypes, such as clear cell or papillary serous tumors.

Risk Factors

There is an increased risk in women with familial predispositions, including the Lynch II syndrome, or HNPCC (Hereditary non-polyposis colorectal cancer) which is associated with extracolonic cancers including endometrial cancer, and cancers of the stomach, hepatobiliary tract, upper renal tract and ovary. The development of endometrial cancers may precede colon cancer. While it is not clear if individuals with BRCA 1 and 2 mutations have increased risk, there does seem to be higher risk for patients with breast cancer, perhaps because of shared risk factors. Other than these genetic conditions, the known risk factors only identify women at risk for type I disease. The cause of this type of cancer is excess estrogen, either endogenous or exogenous.

ENDOGENOUS ESTROGEN   Excess estrogen may be produced from functional ovarian tumors, i.e., granulosa cell tumors. Endogenous conversion of adrenal precursors into estrogen by adipose tissue. This accounts for the higher incidence of endometrial cancer in obese women, who have higher levels of estrogen due to the conversion of androstenedione to estrone and the aromatization of androgens to estradiol, a process which occurs in peripheral adipose tissue. Diabetes and hypertension are both linked to obesity, but may also be independent risk factors. Increased age is associated with increasing incidence of endometrial cancer. Chronic anovulation is also associated with excess endogenous estrogen, for instance, as in polycystic ovary syndrome (PCOS).

Exogenous Estrogen

TREATMENT OF POST-MENOPAUSAL WOMEN WITH ESTROGEN-ONLY THERAPY   Endometrial hyperplasia arises in 20–50% of women receiving unopposed estrogen within 1 year, and both case control and prospective studies demonstrate an increased risk of endometrial cancer, with the relative risk ranging from 3.1 to 15. Both the dose and duration of therapy are correlated with risk (2). This risk is substantially lowered by combining the estrogens with progestins.

Tamoxifen, used as adjuvant therapy in breast cancer, as treatment for metastatic disease and as a breast cancer protectant in high-risk individuals, also contributes to excess exogenous estrogens. It is a competitive inhibitor of estrogen, but it also has partial agonist activity at certain binding sites, including the endometrium.

Pathogenesis of Endometrial Cancer

There is no single molecular event that gives rise to endometrial cancer. Endometrioid hyperplasia and carcinoma are associated with multiple genetic abnormalities, including K ras and PTEN mutations, microsatellite instability and defects in mismatch repair genes. P53 mutations typically occur late in type I lesions and earlier in type II lesion. Type II cancers are often found to be HER-2/neu overexpressors and nondiploid.

HISTOPATHOLOGY OF ENDOMETRIAL CANCER

Endometrial cancers are graded by the World Health Organization scheme. Endometrial cancers are graded 1–3, but all serous and clear cell cancers are considered to be high grade. Most of these histologies are treated identically, with the possible exceptions of serous and clear cell cancers. By contrast, uterine sarcomas have quite different natural histories and treatment paradigms.

Endometrioid is the most common type of endometrial cancer, comprising 75–80%. The majority are well-differentiated; these tumors demonstrate back-to-back glands, with little intervening stroma; worsening differentiation is evidenced by increasing solid components as well as increasing nuclear atypia.

Papillary serous, which accounts for 5–10% of endometrial cancer and clear cell cancer, 1–5% of endometrial cancers, are more aggressive subtypes, which often present at later stages and are always considered to be high grade.

Squamous cancer, and mucinous cancer are both quite rare, each accounting for only 2% endometrial cancers.

CLINICAL PRESENTATION

The typical presenting sign of endometrial cancer is abnormal uterine bleeding. Any woman with post-menopausal bleeding requires evaluation for endometrial cancer. Pre-menopausal women with menometrorrhagia also need evaluation.

Diagnosis

The initial diagnostic test for the evaluation of endometrial cancer is office endometrial biopsy using a Pipelle (a thin, flexible curette), reserving with dilatation and curettage (D&C) for those who are unable to tolerate Pipelle sampling, or for non-diagnostic specimens. Limitations of this procedure are that only a small fraction of the endometrium is sampled, and thus up to 70% of the samples are non-diagnostic, thus dictating additional assessment. It may be combined with hysteroscopy and directed biopsy. Transvaginal ultrasound is used to measure the thickness of the endometrium, with the incidence of endometrial cancer increasing as the thickness reaches 20 mm.

Preoperative evaluation should include a complete blood count, and chemistry tests, including a CA125, which is often useful as a marker of extra-uterine disease. Chest x-ray is routine. CT is unnecessary unless extra-uterine disease is strongly suspected, as it rarely alters treatment and is not useful in assessing myometrial depth of invasion, nodal status, or cervical involvement.

STAGING OF ENDOMETRIAL CANCER

Endometrial cancer is staged surgically according to the joint International Federation of Gynecology and Obstetrics (FIGO)/American Joint Committee on Cancer (AJCC) classification system (see Table 57-1). This operation represents the primary therapy for patients with operable disease. These patients are usually operated on by a Gynecologic Oncologist, who is trained in the specialized surgery needed. Complete surgical staging includes:

1. Upon entering the abdomen peritoneal cytology should be collected (peritoneal washings). These are most commonly positive with extra-uterine disease.
2. Abdominal exploration with biopsy of any suspicious areas.
3. Total abdominal hysterectomy and bilateral salpingo-oophorectomy (TAH-BSO). The removal of the ovaries is necessary to remove micrometastases, synchronous endometrial and ovarian cancers that occur between 5% and 10% of the time, as well as removing a source of estrogen in pre-menopausal women.

The uterine specimen is bivalved in the operating room to assess extent of myometrial invasion, and guide the surgeon in extent of surgical staging necessary. If any features indicate high risk for nodal disease, including clear cell or serous histology, high-grade tumor, greater than 50% myometrial invasion, cervical or lower uterine segment involvement, tumor >2 cm, adnexal or pelvic disease or clinically enlarged or suspicious nodes, full lymph node resection including pelvic and paraortic lymph nodes should be performed. Lymph nodes need to be investigated visually and by palpation, with any suspicious nodes

Table 57-1

Surgical/Pathologic Staging

- IA—limited to endometrium
- IB—<1/2 of myometrium
- IC—1/2 or more of myometrium
- II—invades cervix
  IIA—glandular epithelium of endocervix
  IIB—stroma of cervix
- IIIA—involves serosa and/or adnexa (direct extension or mets) and/or ascites or positive peritoneal washings
- IIIB—vaginal involvement (direct extension or mets)
- IIIC—LN+
- IVA—bladder or bowel
- IVB—distant mets

removed. Some surgeons believe that all endometrial cancers necessitate lymph node sampling, if not complete lymphadenectomy.

Prognostic Factors

The primary prognostic factors are:

- disease stage (see Table 57-2)
- histologic subtype
- grade

Together these features are used to divide women with early stage disease into low-, intermediate- and high-risk groups and determine post-operative therapy. Molecular markers, including PTEN status, p53 and p16 overexpression, as well as hormonal status, may soon provide further information regarding prognosis and may help direct post-operative treatment.

POST-OPERATIVE TREATMENT FOR EARLY-STAGE DISEASE

The recommendations for post-operative treatment, based on the prognostic factors above, are predicated on the risk of recurrent disease, and divide women into three categories of risk.

- *Low risk*: There patients have grade 1 or 2 histology, without myometrial invasion (stage IA) or invasion into less than one-half of the myometrium (stage IB), or grade 3 histology without myometrial invasion. Their tumor must not show lymphovascular space invasion and have no lymph node involvement. These low-risk patients are adequately treated with surgery alone. Brachytherapy is administered to the vaginal vault in the case of grade 3 histology.
- *Intermediate risk*: These patients have a grade 1 or 2 tumor involving greater than one-half of the myometium (stage IC) or involving the cervix (stage II). There should be no lymphovascular space involvement and no evidence of nodal or distant disease. These patients are usually treated with brachytherapy and in some instances pelvic external beam radiation therapy (EBRT). This is a complicated issue and the reader is referred to three seminal studies for details of this decision-making process. These include GOG 99, the PORTEC study and results from the Norwegian Radium Hospital (4–6). The studies differ as to the patients included and the completeness of operative staging, but they clearly show that adjuvant RT reduces pelvic recurrences. It is not clear if RT improves survival, nor do these trials help us decide

Table 57-2

Uterine Cancer by FIGO Stage 1996–1998

Stage	n	Overall survival (%)		
		1 Year	2 Years	5 Years
IA	1063	98.5	96.8	91.1
IB	2735	98.2	96.1	89.7
IC	1219	97.6	92.3	81.3
IIA	364	95.8	90.3	78.7
IIB	426	97.4	87.5	71.4
IIIA	484	89.9	77.3	60.4
IIIB	73	70.6	51.7	30.2
IIIC	293	85.7	70.7	52.1
IVA	47	65.6	39.4	14.6
IVB	160	51.1	38.6	17.0

Adapted from (3).

which patients need brachytherapy alone, and which patients need EBRT to the pelvis. More recent retrospective studies suggest that completely staged patients may not need pelvic RT. The efficacy of chemotherapy to replace RT in this group is under debate, though a recent study comparing the two showed no difference in PFS or OS (7). Current guidelines from the NCCN recommend that women with stages I and II endometrial cancer receive RT.

- *High Risk*: This group of patients includes all grade 3 histology, grade 2 histology with myometrial involvement extending into the outer half (stage IB) and cervical or vaginal involvement, lymphovascular space involvement or adnexal or pelvic metastases. They may be further divided into those with *organ-confined disease* and those with *extra-uterine disease*. The latter will be discussed separately below. In general patients with high-risk organ-confined disease should receive adjuvant therapy, though the optimal regimen is not clear, as in the intermediate risk group.

POST-OPERATIVE TREATMENT FOR ADVANCED STAGE DISEASE (EXTRA-UTERINE DISEASE)

Stage III patients as well as stage IV patients were recently randomized on the GOG 122 study which compared whole abdominal irradiation (WAI) to chemotherapy with doxorubicin and cisplatin (AP) in patients in 422 patients. Chemotherapy was found to significantly improve progression-free survival and overall survival in comparison to WAI at 5 years with greater acute toxicity seen in the AP arm (8). Based on this publication, most women with stage III disease receive chemotherapy, though trials with combined chemoradiotherapy indicate that this may be feasible. The precise regimen of chemotherapy administered is in flux, as discussed in the section on chemotherapy below.

Systemic Therapy

Systemic therapy is the treatment of choice for patients with patients with advanced extra-uterine disease and metastatic disease, as well as many cases of recurrent disease.

Hormonal Therapy

As the majority of women with endometrial cancer have type I cancers triggered by overexposure to estrogens, most of these tumors express estrogen and progesterone receptors and are sensitive to hormonal manipulation. Hormonal agents are appealing options for the treatment of endometrial cancer because of their attractive side-effect profiles.

Progestins.   Endometrial cancer, particularly tumors which are ER and/or PgR positive, of low grade histology, and having a long treatment free interval may respond to progestin therapy. Many different progestins have been used. Megace (megestrol acetate) at 160 mg per day is generally well-tolerated.

Other Hormonal Agents.   Tamoxifen, a selective estrogen modulator (SERM), has activity in advanced endometrial cancer, with response rates ranging between 10% and 22%. Aromatase inhibitors, including Arimidex, and GnRH agonists also have some activity.

CHEMOTHERAPY

High-risk extra-uterine disease including peritoneal, extensive nodal or distant metastases, either primarily or after a trial of hormonal therapy, may be treated with systemic chemotherapy. Many oncologists have already adopted the taxol and carboplatin regimen as their standard, though it is currently being compared to cisplatin, doxorubicin, and taxol. A prior GOG study 184 showed superiority of the cisplatin, doxorubicin, and paclitaxel combination over cisplatin and doxorubicin alone (9). Single agents with activity in this disease include cis-platin and carboplatin, cyclophosphamide, doxorubicin, topotecan, with responses between 20% and 28%. Paclitaxel is probably the single most active agent in this disease.

TREATMENT OF PAPILLARY SEROUS AND CLEAR CELL CANCERS

Even well-staged stage I disease of aggressive histology has a 20–30% relapse rate (10). Because of this, these patients are typically treated with adjuvant chemotherapy, though there are little data to show an improved outcome with this approach. Most commonly they are treated like advanced ovarian cancer, with platinum and taxane combinations. Papillary serous tumors often overexpress HER-2/neu, and traztuzumab (Herceptin) may prove to be a useful therapy for some of these patients.

TREATMENT OF METASTATIC DISEASE AND RECURRENT ENDOMETRIAL CANCER

Treatment of recurrent disease depends on multiple factors including:

- initial treatment
- hormonal status
- site and extent of recurrence.

The majority of recurrences occur in the vaginal vault and these may be salvaged with radiation. There are rare, isolated central pelvic recurrences, and some of these patients may be salvaged with pelvic exenteration. Localized recurrences, such as confined lymph node sites are occasionally treated with radiotherapy or surgery followed by extended radiation. More distant disease, such as pulmonary, or widespread peritoneal disease, or disease in previously irradiated areas, are typically treated with systemic chemotherapy or hormonal therapy.

UTERINE SARCOMA

Epidemiology of Uterine Sarcoma

Uterine sarcoma is a disease of middle age, most often affecting women ages 40–60 years. In the United States, some histologies including leiomyosarcoma and carcinosarcomas, are more common among African-Americans as compared to Caucasians. Long-term use of tamoxifen is associated with a higher incidence of sarcomas, particularly carcinosarcomas, though the absolute risk is still small (11). Pelvic irradiation is a predisposing factor in 5–10% of patients.

HISTOPATHOLOGY OF UTERINE SARCOMA

The GOG classifies these tumors into five categories:

1. Mixed homologous mullerian sarcomas.
2. Mixed heterologous mullerian sarcomas— Mixed malignant mullerian tumors (MMMTs) or carcinosarcomas are the most common type of uterine sarcoma, and as the name suggests, contain both epithelial (carcinoma) and mesenchymal (sarcoma) elements. They are believed to represent dedifferentiation of a carcinoma.
3. Leimyosarcoma— Leiomyosarcoma arise from the myometrium, and account for about one-third of uterine sarcomas.
4. Endometrial stromal sarcoma— Endometrial stromal sarcomas, the third most common type of uterine sarcoma, arise from stromal cells within the endometrium.
5. Other, including liposarcoma, chondrosarcoma, rhabdomyosarcoma.

PRESENTATION, DIAGNOSTIC EVALUATION, AND STAGING

Presentation

The most common presenting symptom is vaginal bleeding, sometimes accompanied by malodorous discharge, pelvic pain, and enlarged uterus.

Diagnostic Evaluation

Radiography is useful in demonstrating an abnormality, but cannot distinguish between benign leimyomata (fibroids), sarcoma and other types of uterine pathology. These patients eventually come to surgical exploration.

Staging

There is no separate staging system for uterine sarcomas and the FIGO staging classification for endometrial cancer is used. Surgical procedure usually involves TAH BSO, biopsy of any suspicious areas and removal of suspicious lymph nodes. Full lymph node dissection is usually not important. Surgical debulking is appropriate if the tumor can be completely removed without undue morbidity.

TREATMENT OF UTERINE SARCOMA

These tumors tend to be aggressive and primary treatment is surgical. For early stage disease this may be the only treatment necessary. Adjuvant pelvic irradiation has been shown to improve local control but has no effect on overall survival. There is no role for adjuvant chemotherapy. Metastatic or recurrent disease treatments are not standardized. Carcinosarcomas act and are often treated like endometrial cancer or ovarian cancer, with nodal and or peritoneal dissemination most commonly. Leiomyosarcomas tend to early hematogenous dissemination, often spreading to the lungs. Endometrial stromal sarcomas tend to be the least aggressive of the group, with local recurrence more common than distant disease. These recurrences may be treated with repeat surgical excisions if feasible. This tumor also tends to be hormonally responsive. Given the poor response of these tumors to standard therapies, treatment on clinical trials is appropriate.

REFERENCES

1. Jemal A, Murray T, Ward E, et al. Cancer Statistics, 2005. CA Cancer J Clin. 2005; 55: 10–30.
2. Persson I, Adami HO, Bergkvist L, et al. Risk of endometrial cancer after treatment with oestrogens alone or in conjunction with progestins: results of a prospective study. BMJ. 1989; 298(6667): 147–151.
3. Creasman WT, Odicino F, Maisonneuve P, et al. Carcinoma of the corpus uteri: FIGO annual report. Int J Gynaecol Obstet. 2003; 83: 79–118.
4. Keys HM, Roberts JA, Brunetto VL, et al. A phase III trial of surgery with or without adjunctive external pelvic radiation therapy in intermediate risk endometrial adenocarcinoma: a Gynecologic Oncology Group study. Gynecol Oncol. 2004; 92(3): 744–751.
5. Creutzberg CL, van Putten WL, Koper PL, et al. Surgery and postoperative radiotherapy versus surgery alone for patients with stage-1 endometrial carcinoma: multicentre randomised trial. PORTEC Study Group. Post Operative Radiation Therapy in Endometrial Carcinoma. Lancet. 2000; 355(9213): 1404–1411.
6. Aalders J, Abeler V, Kostad P, Onsrud M. Postoperative external irradiation and prognostic parameters in stage I endometrial carcinoma: clinical and histopathologic study of 540 patients. Obstet Gynecol. 1980; 56(4): 419–427.

7. Sagae S, Udagawa Y, Susumu N, et al. Randomized phase III trial of whole pelvic radiotherapy vs cisplatin-based chemotherapy in patients with intermediate risk endometrial carcinoma. J Clin Oncol. 2005; 23: 455 (suppl; abstr 5002).

8. Randall ME, Filiaci VL, Muss H, et al. Randomized phase III trial of whole-abdominal irradiation versus doxorubicin and cisplatin chemotherapy in advanced endometrial carcinoma: a Gynecologic Oncology Group Study. J Clin Oncol. 2006; 24: 36–44.

9. Fleming, G, Brunetto,V, Cella D, et al. Phase III trial of doxorubicin plus cisplatin with or without paclitaxel plus filgrastim in advanced endometrial carcinoma: a gynecologic oncology group study. J Clin Oncol. 2004; 22: 2159–2166.

10. Creasman WT, Kohler MF, Odincion F, et al. Prognosis of papillary serous, clear cell, and grade 3 stage I carcinoma of the endometrium. Gynecol Oncol. 2004; 95: 593.

11. Wickerham, DL, Fisher, B, Wolmark, N, et al. Association of tamoxifen and uterine sarcoma. J Clin Oncol. 2002; 20: 2758–2760.

58	Tessa Cigler, Paula D. Ryan

BREAST ONCOLOGY: CLINICAL
PRESENTATION AND GENETICS

EPIDEMIOLOGY

Breast cancer is the most commonly diagnosed cancer among women and second only to lung cancer as the leading cause of cancer-related deaths in women (1). It is estimated that 212,920 women in the United States were diagnosed with breast cancer in 2006, and that 14,970 women died of the disease (1). Breast cancer occurs approximately 150 times more frequently in women than in men, with 1,720 cases of male breast cancer diagnosed in 2006 (1). Approximately 13.22% of women born in the United States will be diagnosed with breast cancer during their lifetime, translating into a lifetime probability of one in eight (2). Since 1990 mortality from breast cancer appears to be decreasing, thought to be due to both increased usage of screening mammograms, which allow for detection of cancers at earlier stages, as well as advances in adjuvant therapy.

RISK FACTORS

It is estimated that 50% of women diagnosed with breast cancer have identifiable risk factors besides age and gender. Certain hormonal and reproductive factors as well as certain lifestyle, diet, and environmental factors are associated with increased breast cancer risk. In addition to a personal or family history of breast cancer, a history of benign breast disease is another predisposing risk factor.

Endogenous Estrogen Exposure/ Reproductive Factors

Breast cancer is believed to be hormone dependent, with increasing levels and duration of estrogen exposure associated with increasing risk. In post-menopausal women, for example, higher serum levels of estrogen correlate with increased breast cancer risk. Certain hormonal and reproductive factors are known to confer increased risk. These include early menarche, late menopause, and nulliparity or greater than 30 years of age at birth of first child (3). Higher bone mineral density and increased mammographic breast density, perhaps surrogates for increased long-term exposure to endogenous estrogen, have also been associated with increased breast cancer risk. Breastfeeding is believed to confer a protective effect on breast cancer risk.

Exogenous Estrogen Exposure

The role of exogenous estrogen on breast cancer risk is complicated and has been extensively studied. It is generally accepted that past oral contraceptive (OC) use does not result in any significant increase in breast cancer risk in women over 40 years of age. There is a suggestion however, that current OC use confers a slightly increased risk of breast cancer. Since current OC users tend to be young, the rise in absolute risk is very small.

Studies of estrogen replacement therapy (ERT) in postmenopausal women support a modestly increased associated risk of breast cancer. Risk appears to rise with increasing duration of use. Short-term use of ERT (less than 4–5 years), however, has not been definitively associated with increased breast cancer risk. In addition, women who have stopped ERT for more than 5 years appear not to be at increased risk compared with never users. The risk of breast cancer seems to be higher with combination estrogen and progestin therapy compared with estrogen alone.

Lifestyle

Obesity has been demonstrated to affect breast cancer risk differentially in pre- and postmenopausal women. In premenopausal women, obesity is associated with longer menstrual cycles and increased anovulatory cycles, resulting in less total estrogen exposure and a lower risk of breast cancer. In postmenopausal women, in whom the primary source of estrogen is metabolism in peripheral tissues, obesity is associated with higher serum concentrations of bioavailable estrogen, and an increased risk of breast cancer. The relationship between exercise and breast cancer risk remains unsettled. Some data suggest that increased activity levels among postmenopausal women confer a reduced risk of breast cancer. This may be due to the reduction in BMI or the reduced serum estrogen levels associated with exercise.

Diet

Alcohol is perhaps the best-established dietary risk factor for breast cancer. Moderate alcohol intake, which increases endogenous estrogen levels, is associated with increased breast cancer risk. Studies examining fat consumption and breast cancer risk have yielded mixed results, with several case control and cohort studies suggesting a modest increase in risk with increased dietary fat consumption.

Environmental

The strongest known environmental risk factor for breast cancer is ionizing radiation. Moderate to high doses of ionizing radiation to the chest at a young age such as that given for treatment of Hodgkins disease is a significant risk factor for the development of breast cancer later in life. The highest risk of breast cancer appears to be in individuals exposed during pre-pubertal and pubertal years.

Benign Breast Disease

Benign breast diseases are classified as proliferative or non-proliferative lesions. Non-proliferative lesions are not associated with increased breast cancer risk. Proliferative lesions without atypia such as hyperplasia, sclerosing adenosis, diffuse papillomatosis, radial scar, and complex fibroadenomas are believed to result in a small increase in relative risk estimated between 1.5 and 2.0. Proliferative lesions with atypia, either ductal or lobular, confer an increased risk of invasive breast cancer of approximately four-fold.

RISK ASSESSMENT

Two useful models to assess breast cancer risk in women not suspected of having a hereditary predisposition to breast cancer (see Breast Cancer Genetics), include the Gail model and the Claus model (4). The Gail model derives age-specific breast cancer risk estimates for women based on their age at menarche, age at first live birth, number of previous breast biopsies, presence of atypical hyperplasia in prior breast biopsy, and number of first-degree relatives with breast cancer. By including only first-degree relatives, the Gail model tends to underestimate risk in women with strong family histories of breast cancer. A breast cancer risk assessment tool based on the Gail model can be accessed at http://www.cancer.gov/bcrisktool. The Claus model derives age-specific breast cancer risk estimates for women with at least one relative with breast cancer.

BREAST CANCER GENETICS

While 20–30% of women with breast cancer have at least one relative with a history of breast cancer, only 5–10% of women with breast cancer have an identifiable hereditary predisposition. Most of the known hereditary breast cancers are due to mutations in the BRCA 1 or BRCA 2 genes, which also predispose to ovarian cancer. Rare mutations in other genes including PTEN, p53, MLH1, MLH2, and STK 11 are also associated with increased breast cancer risk (Table 58-1).

BRCA 1 and BRCA 2

BRCA 1 and 2 genes were cloned in 1994 and 1995, respectively. BRCA 1 and 2 are autosomal dominant genes that are believed to act as tumor suppressor genes. They play a role in cellular response to DNA damage and are involved with double-stranded DNA repair (5). BRCA 1 maps to chromosome 17q21 whereas BRCA 2 maps to chromosome 11. The prevalence of mutations in either BRCA 1 or BRCA 2 varies among ethnic groups. A noticeably higher frequency of about one in 50 has been observed among individuals of Ashkenazi Jewish ancestry. Increased frequency of mutations has also been observed in individuals from Iceland, Poland Sweden, and the Netherlands.

Inherited mutations in either BRCA 1 or BRCA 2 predispose male carriers to breast cancer and female carriers to breast and ovarian cancer. Pancreatic cancer, prostate cancer, and melanoma can also be seen in BRCA 1 or BRCA 2 mutation carriers. In general, it is estimated that the lifetime risks of developing breast cancer varies between 50% and 80% for a woman carrying either a BRCA 1 or BRCA 2 mutation and between 5% and 10% for a male mutation carrier. The lifetime risk of ovarian cancer among female BRCA 1 carriers is

Table 58-1

Breast Cancer Susceptibility Genes

Gene	Syndrome	Associated malignancies
BRCA1	Hereditary breast and ovarian cancer	Breast and ovarian cancer
BRCA2	Hereditary breast and ovarian cancer	Breast and ovarian cancer
TP53	Li–Fraumeni syndrome	Soft tissue and osteosarcomas, breast cancer, brain tumors, adrenal cortical carcinoma, leukemia
PTEN	Cowden's	Hamartomas, benign and malignant tumors of the thyroid, breast, and endometrium
STK11	Peutz–Jeghers	Breast, gastrointestinal, ovarian, testicular, uterine, endometrial cancers
MLH1/MSH2	Muir–Torre	Skin tumors, benign and malignant tumors of the gastrointestinal and genitourinary tracts, breast cancer
CHEK2	–	Breast cancer

estimated to be between 30% and 45%, while that of female BRCA 2 carriers ranges from 10 to 20%. BRCA1 associated breast cancers are usually high grade, stain negative for estrogen receptor and progesterone receptor proteins and do not overexpress HER2/neu. BRCA 2-associated breast cancers appear similar to that of sporadic breast cancers.

GENETIC TESTING FOR BRCA 1 AND BRCA 2 MUTATIONS

Whether to undergo testing for BRCA 1 or 2 mutations is a complex decision that has implications for both the individual as well as his or her family members. Individuals are usually offered testing if their risk of carrying a deleterious mutation is reasonable which has generally been considered to be at least 10%. BRCAPRO is a predictive algorithm frequently used in high-risk clinics. It can be downloaded from http://www3.utsouthwestern.edu/cancergene.

While there are no standardized criteria, family histories suggestive of the presence of BRCA 1 or 2 mutations include two or more relatives affected with breast cancer, usually with a predominance of early onset cases (less than 50 years of age), ovarian cancer, male breast cancer, and evidence of transmission in two or more generations or through male relatives. A personal history of breast cancer diagnosed at age less than 40, invasive ovarian cancer, bilateral breast cancer, or both breast and ovarian cancer are also characteristic of BRCA 1 or 2 mutations carriers. In addition, individuals of Ashkenazi Jewish ancestry with breast cancer and relatives of known mutation carriers are at increased risk of carrying a BRCA 1 or 2 mutation and should be considered for testing (6).

The United States Preventive Services Task Force recommends that individuals without a diagnosis of breast or ovarian cancer, who are not of Ashkenazi Jewish descent, be offered testing if their family history includes two first-degree relatives with breast cancer, one of whom received the diagnosis at age 50 years or younger; a combination of three or more first or second-degree relatives with breast cancer regardless of age at diagnosis; a combination of both breast and ovarian cancer among first and second-degree relatives; a first-degree relative with bilateral breast cancer; a combination of two or more first or second-degree relatives with ovarian cancer regardless of age at diagnosis; a first or second-degree relative with both breast and ovarian cancer at any age; or a history of breast cancer in a male relative. For unaffected individuals of Ashkenazi Jewish heritage, any first-degree relative or two second-degree relatives on the same side of the family should prompt consideration of BRCA mutation testing (7).

Before undergoing genetic testing, individuals must receive careful counseling regarding the potential clinical, psychological, and legal ramifications associated with testing. The implications of both a positive and negative test result should be reviewed carefully. At risk family members based on family pedigree should be identified and, individuals with a positive test result should be encouraged to share this information with their relatives.

MANAGEMENT OF BRCA MUTATION CARRIERS

Several strategies exist for risk reduction among BRCA mutation carriers. Bilateral prophylactic mastectomy, the most effective method to reduce breast cancer risk among carriers, should be offered to all women with BRCA 1 or 2 mutations. Residual breast cancer risk following surgery is <10%. Prophylactic bilateral salpingoooophorectomy (BSO) should also be offered to women with BRCA 1 or 2 mutations. In addition to reducing risk of ovarian cancer by 90%, BSO has been shown to reduce the risk of breast cancer by approximately 50% in premenopausal mutation carriers who have not undergone prophylactic surgery.

Women who elect not to undergo prophylactic mastectomies need to be closely screened for breast cancer. In general, guidelines for mutation carriers suggest annual screening mammograms beginning at 25–30 years of age, clinical breast exams twice a year, and monthly self-breast examinations. Breast MRI has recently been demonstrated to be more sensitive than mammograms in detecting breast cancers in high-risk women at the cost of a higher false positive rate (8). The American Cancer Society guidelines for breast screening recommend annual MRI screening as an adjunct to mamography in BRCA mutation carriers (9).

For those women who elect not to undergo prophylactic BSO, ovarian cancer screening with twice yearly transvaginal ultrasounds and measurements of CA-125 tumor marker is recommended. It is cautioned, however, that these measures are of unproved efficacy.

BREAST CANCER SCREENING IN GENERAL POPULATION

Most North American expert groups recommend breast cancer screening with mammography with or without clinical breast examination every year for women over age 50 and every 1–2 years for women aged 40–49. Although clinical breast examination (CBE) is generally recommended, its independent role is difficult to determine as most studies included both mammography and CBE. There are few randomized trials to date to guide recommendations regarding breast self-examination (BSE). Limited data suggest that BSE may aid in the diagnosis of cancers at early stages when tumors are more amenable to conservative local therapy. Correct technique of BSE appears to be an important factor. While there is some belief that women with first-degree relatives with histories of breast cancer, particularly premenopausal breast cancer, should undergo screening at an earlier age, mortality data to support this recommendation does not yet exist. BRCA 1 and 2 carriers are advised to undergo more intensive screening as detailed above.

DIAGNOSIS

Breast cancer is most often diagnosed by biopsy of a palpable breast mass or biopsy of a mammographic abnormality. Definitive diagnostic workups should be promptly initiated for any breast abnormality and pursued until resolution. It is important to remember that unilateral lesions in men should be evaluated similarly to those in women and that dominant masses in a pregnant or lactating woman should not be automatically attributed to hormonal changes and should undergo prompt diagnostic evaluation. In the presence of a persistent breast nodule, physical examination alone or a normal mammogram cannot exclude malignancy. It is generally recommended that mammography be included as part of the evaluation of a palpable breast mass in any woman of age 30 or older in order to evaluate the mass in question as well as to evaluate for other clinically occult lesions in either breast.

Palpable Breast Mass

In women 30 years or older, most experts agree that any dominant mass should be evaluated by physical exam, mammography, and ultrasound. Imaging guided core needle biopsy can be performed if the lesion is suspicious and visible on an imaging study. If it is not easily targeted, then it should be referred to a surgeon for definitive diagnosis. Surgical evaluation usually entails FNA, core needle biopsy, or excisional biopsy of the suspicious lesion. It is important to note that negative mammogram does not exclude breast cancer.

For women younger than 30 years, initial evaluation is typically by physical exam and ultrasound followed by ultrasound guided biopsy or surgical referral for definitive diagnosis. Although some believe that benign solid masses can be distinguished from malignant solid masses using ultrasound, many feel that these should be evaluated with needle or excisional biopsy. Palpable lesions can be aspirated under clinical guidance and if fluid is drained and the mass resolves this is good evidence of a simple cyst. If ultrasound demonstrates a simple cyst no further intervention is needed. Symptomatic cysts can be aspirated to provide symptomatic relief although they often recur. Non-simple cysts (complex) that appear to contain both fluid and solid tissue should undergo excisional biopsy following needle localization in order to evaluate the entire cyst. Alternatively, consideration can be given to ultrasound guided biopsy, but if this is performed a clip should be placed so that if additional evaluation is needed there is a marker to guide further intervention since the biopsy may render it difficult to visualize the lesion. In cases where physical exam and breast imaging are consistent with fibrocystic breast tissue, an FNA may be considered. Whether or not FNA is performed, all such patients should be seen in follow-up at 2 months to ensure stability.

Abnormal Mammogram

Women who present with an abnormal screening mammogram in the absence of a palpable breast mass also require prompt evaluation. The work up usually depends on the recommendation of the radiologist interpreting the mammogram. The degree of abnormality is categorized using the Breast Imaging and Reporting Data System (BI-RADS).

STAGING SYSTEM

Breast cancer is most commonly staged according to the TMN staging system. The staging system, published by the American Joint Committee on Cancer (AJCC), was modified in 2002 (Table 58-2) (10). Five-year survival rates are highly correlated with tumor stage, ranging from 99% for women with Stage 0 disease to 14% for women with Stage IV disease.

STAGING EVALUATION

Initial evaluation of any woman with newly diagnosed breast cancer should include a thorough physical exam with meticulous palpation of each breast, skin, lymph nodes and abdomen, bilateral mammograms, and routine blood tests including a complete blood count and liver function tests. Abnormal lab values or signs or symptoms of metastatic disease should prompt further evaluation with chest x-ray, CT scan of the chest, abdomen, and pelvis, and bone scan.

For asymptomatic women with early stage breast cancer (stages I and II), radiographic studies such as chest x-ray, CT scan of the chest, abdomen and pelvis, and bone scan have been shown to have a low-diagnostic yield and are not generally recommended. In contrast, all women with stage III disease should undergo evaluation with chest x-ray, CT scan of the chest, abdomen and pelvis, and bone scan. While PET scans can identify sites of metastatic breast cancer, their role in the diagnostic work up of breast cancer has not yet been clearly established.

Table 58-2

TMN Staging System for Breast Cancer

Primary tumor (T)

TX—Primary tumor cannot be assessed
T0—No evidence of primary tumor
Tis—Carcinoma in situ
  Tis (DCIS)—Intraductal carcinoma in situ
  Tis (LCIS)—Lobular carcinoma in situ
  Tis (Paget's)—Paget's disease of the nipple with no tumor; tumor-
    associated Paget's disease is classified according to the size of the
    rimary tumor
T1—Tumor 2 cm or less in greatest dimension
  T1mic—Microinvasion 0.1 cm or less in greatest dimension
  T1a—Tumor more than 0.1 but not more than 0.5 cm in greatest dimension
  T1b—Tumor more than 0.5 cm but not more than 1 cm in greatest
    dimension
  T1c—Tumor more than 1 cm but not more than 2 cm in greatest
    dimension
T2—Tumor more than 2 cm but not more than 5 cm in greatest dimension
T3—Tumor more than 5 cm in greatest dimension
T4—Tumor of any size with direct extension to (a) chest wall or (b) skin, only
  as described below:
  T4a—Extension to chest wall
  T4b—Edema (including peau d'orange) or ulceration of the breast skin,
    or satellite skin nodules confined to the same breast
  T4c—Both (T4a and T4b)
  T4d—Inflammatory carcinoma

Regional lymph nodes: clinical classification (N)

NX—Regional lymph nodes cannot be assessed (e.g., previously removed)
N0—No regional lymph node metastases
N1—Metastasis to movable ipsilateral axillary lymph nodes(s)
N2—Metastasis to ipsilateral axillary lymph node(s) fixed or matted, or in
  clinically apparent ipsilateral internal mammary nodes in the absence of
  evident axillary node metastases
  N2a—Metastasis to ipsilateral axillary lymph node(s) fixed to one
    another (matted) or to other structures
  N2b—Metastasis only in clinically apparent ipsilateral internal mammary
    nodes in the absence of evident axillary node metastases
N3—Metastasis to ipsilateral infraclavicular lymph node(s) with or without
  clinically evident axillary lymph nodes, or in clinically apparent ipsilateral
  internal mammary lymph node(s) and in the presence of cliniucally evident
  axillary lymph node metastases, or metastasis in ipsilateral supraclavicular
  lymph nodes with or without axillary or internal mammary nodal involvement
  N3a—Metastasis to ipsilateral infraclavicular lymph node(s)
  N3b—Metastasis to ipsilateral internal mammary lymph node(s) and
    clinically apparent axillary lymph nodes
  N3c—Metastasis in ipsilateral supraclavicular lymph nodes with or
    without axillary or internal mammary nodal involvement

Regional lymph nodes: pathologic classification (pN)

*Classification is based on axillary lymph node dissection (ALND) with or
without sentinel lymph node dissection (SLND). Classification based solely on
SLND without ALND should be designated (sn) [e.g., pN0 (i +) (sn)].*

                                                            (continued)

Table 58-2 (*Continued*)

TMN Staging System for Breast Cancer

pNX—Regional lymph nodes cannot be assessed (e.g., previously removed, or not removed for pathologic study)

pN0—No regional lymph node metastasis; no additional examination for isolated tumor cells (ITCs, defined as single tumor cells or small lusters not greater than 0.2 mm, usually detected only by immunohisto-chemical or molecular methods but which may be verified on hematoxylin and eosin (H&E) stains. ITCs do not usually show evidence of malignant activity [e.g., proliferation or stromal reaction])

> pN0 (i-)—No histologic nodal metastases, and negative by immunohis-tochemistry (IHC)
>
> pN0 (i+)—No histologic nodal metastases but positive by IHC, with no cluster greater than 0.2 mm in diameter
>
> pN0 (mol-)—No histologic nodal metastases and negative molecular findings (by reverse transcriptase polymerase chain reaction, RT-PCR)
>
> pN0 (mol+)—No histologic nodal metastases, but positive molecular findings (by RT-PCR)

pN1—Metastasis in 1–3 ipsilateral axillary lymph node(s) and/or in internal mammary nodes with microscopic disease detected by SLND but not clinically apparent

> pN1mi—Micrometastasis (greater than 0.2 mm, none greater than 2.0 mm)
>
> pN1a—Metastasis in 1–3 axillary lymph nodes
>
> pN1b—Metastasis to internal mammary lymph nodes with microscopic disease detected by SLND but not clinically apparent
>
> pN1c—Metastasis in 1–3 ipsilateral axillary lymph node(s) and in internal mammary nodes with microscopic disease detected by SLND but not clinically apparent. If associated with more than three positive axillary nodes, the internal mammary nodes are classified as N3b to reflect increased tumor burden.

pN2—Metastasis in 4–9 axillary lymph nodes or in clinically apparent internal mammary lymph nodes in the absence of axillary lymph nodes

> pN2a—Metastases in 4–9 axillary lymph nodes (at least one tumor deposit >2 mm) pN2b—Metastasis in clinically apparent internal mammary lymph nodes in the absence of axillary lymph nodes

pN3—Metastasis in 10 or more axillary lymph nodes, or in infraclavicular lymph nodes, or in clinically apparent ipsilateral internal mammary lymph nodes in the presence of one or more positive axillary nodes; or in more than three axillary lymph nodes with clinically negative microscopic metastasis in internal mammary nodes; or in ipsilateral supraclavicular lymph node(s)

> pN3a—Metastasis in 10 or more axillary lymph nodes (at least one tumor deposit greater than 2.0 mm), or metastasis to the infraclavicular lymph nodes
>
> pN3b—Metastasis in clinically apparent ipsilateral internal mammary lymph nodes in the presence of one or more positive axillary nodes; or in more than three axillary lymph nodes with microscopic metastasis in internal mammary lymph nodes detected by SLND but not clinically apparent
>
> pN3c—Metastasis in ipsilateral supraclavicular lymph node(s)

Distant metastasis (M)

MX—Distant metastasis cannot be assessed

M0—No distant metastasis

M1—Distant metastasis

TMN stage groupings for breast cancer

Stage 0—Tis N0 M0
Stage I—T1 N0 M0 (including T1mic)
Stage IIA—T0 N1 M0; T1 N1 M0 (including T1mic); T2 N0 M0
Stage IIB—T2 N1 M0; T3 N0 M0
Stage IIIA—T0 N2 M0; T1 N2 M0 (including T1mic); T2 N2 M0; T3 N1 M0;
   T3 N2 M0
Stage IIIB—T4 Any N M0
Stage IIIC—Any T N3 M0
Stage IV—Any T Any N M1

Used with the permission of the American Joint Committee on Cancer (AJCC), Chicago, Illinois. The original source for this material is the AJCC Cancer Staging Manual, Sixth Edition (2002) published by Springer-Verlag, New York, www.springeronline.com.

REFERENCES

1. Jemal A, Siegel R, Ward E, et al. Cancer statistics, 2006. CA Cancer J Clin. 2006; 56: 106–130.
2. Ries LAG, Melbert D, Krapcho M, et al. SEER cancer statistics Review, 1975–2004. National Cancer Institute, Bethesda, MD, http:seer.cancer.gov/csr/1975–2004/, based on November 2006 SEER datasubmission, posted to the SEER website, 2007.
3. Clemons M, Goss P. Estrogen and the risk of breast cancer. N Engl J Med. 2001; 344(4): 276–285.
4. Armstrong K, Eisen A, Weber B. Assessing the risk of breast cancer. N Engl J Med. 2000; 342(8): 564–571.
5. Narod SA, Foulkes WD. BRCA1 and BRCA2: 1994 and beyond. Nat Rev Cancer. 2004; 4(9): 665–676.
6. Narod SA, Offit K. Prevention and management of hereditary breast cancer. J Clin Oncol. 2005; 23(8): 1656–1663.
7. Genetic risk assessment and BRCA mutation testing for breast and ovarian cancer susceptibility: recommendation statement. U.S. preventive services Task force. Ann Intern Med. 2005; 143: 355–361.
8. Liberman L. Breast cancer screening with MRI—what are the data for patients at high risk? N Engl J Med. 2004; 351(5): 497–500.
9. Saslow D, Boetes C, Burke W, et al. for American Cancer Society Breast Cancer advisory group. CA Cancer J Clin 2007; 57: 75–89.
10. AJCC (American Joint Committee on Cancer) Cancer Staging Manual. In FL Greene, DL Page, ID Fleming, et al. (eds.), Springer-Verlag, New York, 2002, pp. 223–240.

LOCALIZED BREAST CANCER

Breast cancer is usually considered "localized" if it is technically possible to surgically remove all cancerous tissue, if the tumor does not involve the skin or structures deep to the breast, and if the tumor has not metastasized beyond the axillary or internal mammary lymph nodes.

A variety of prognostic and predictive factors influence the treatment of localized breast cancer because they have a bearing on both prognosis and selection of adjuvant treatment. The most important factors are the presence or absence of cancer in the axillary lymph nodes, tumor size, hormone receptor status, HER2/neu status, and a woman's age or menopausal status.

PROGNOSTIC AND PREDICTIVE FACTORS

Lymph Node Involvement

Fluid from the breast tissue normally drains into lymph nodes located in the axilla, and cancerous involvement of these nodes is an indication of the likelihood that breast cancer has spread and could grow in other organs. Women with node-positive breast cancer are generally offered chemotherapy, hormone therapy, or both after local treatment, even if the tumor was completely removed. The type of systemic treatment that is recommended depends upon whether the breast cancer expresses hormone receptors and/or the protein HER2/neu.

Size and Extent of the Tumor

In addition to lymph node status, the prognosis of a breast cancer depends upon its size, since larger tumors recur more often. In some cases, chemotherapy may be given before surgery to shrink a large tumor or one that has grown into the chest wall.

Histology

There are several histologic types of breast cancer. However, from the standpoint of treatment, the most important distinction is between invasive and noninvasive (in situ) breast cancer. The surgical treatment of in situ cancers is similar to that of invasive cancers, but axillary nodal dissection is generally not recommended.

Hormone Receptor Status

Estrogen receptor (ER) and progesterone receptor (PR) assays are routinely performed by pathologists on tumor material. Women with hormone receptor-positive tumors benefit from postoperative endocrine treatments such as tamoxifen, or in postmenopausal women, the aromatase inhibitors (anastrozole, letrozole, or exemestane). For premenopausal women, ovarian ablation or suppression can be considered but is controversial. Hormone therapy is not beneficial for women with hormone receptor-negative tumors.

HER2/Neu Status

Assays for HER2/neu status are routinely performed on the tumor material. Recent studies have shown that women with invasive tumors that overexpress

HER2/neu benefit from postoperative trastuzumab, a monoclonal antibody directed at HER2/neu.

Age and/or Menopausal Status

Women who are under the age of 50 or premenopausal at the time of breast cancer diagnosis derive more benefit from adjuvant systemic chemotherapy than postmenopausal women. Postmenopausal women have a lesser absolute benefit in reduction of recurrence risk than premenopausal women but still can have some benefit from adjuvant chemotherapy.

SURGERY FOR LOCALIZED BREAST CANCER

Generally, surgical options for women with localized breast cancer include breast conserving therapy (BCT) and mastectomy.

BCT

BCT offers women the option of preserving the breast without compromising survival. The tumor is surgically removed without removing excess amounts of normal breast tissue. BCT is followed by radiation therapy (RT), either to the entire breast or just to the original tumor site (partial breast irradiation) to eradicate residual disease. BCT plus radiation provides a surgery equivalent to mastectomy but allows women to preserve the breast. An overview of completed trials shows equivalent survival with BCT as compared to mastectomy (1).

Absolute contraindications to BCT:

- Persistently positive resection margins after re-excision attempts.
- Multicentric disease with two or more primary tumors in separate breast quadrants.
- Diffuse malignant-appearing microcalcifications on mammography confirmed by biopsy.
- History of prior RT to the breast or chest wall that precludes further RT.
- Inflammatory breast cancer.

Relative contraindications to BCT:

- History of connective tissue disease (particularly scleroderma) because RT is generally tolerated poorly.
- Large tumor +/− small breast that would lead to a significantly poor cosmetic outcome.

Mastectomy

Mastectomy refers to the surgical removal of the breast. There are several different types of mastectomy.

RADICAL MASTECTOMY   Radical mastectomy is the most extensive surgical procedure and is no longer routinely performed nor is it indicated. The breast is removed along with the pectoralis major and minor muscles and some overlying skin (at least 4 cm on each side of the tumor biopsy site), and there is an en bloc resection of all axillary contents, including lymph nodes beyond the subclavian vein.

MODIFIED RADICAL MASTECTOMY   Modified radical mastectomy removes the entire breast and includes an axillary dissection, in which the level I and II axillary lymph nodes are also removed. Most women who have mastectomies today for invasive breast cancer have modified radical mastectomies.

SIMPLE OR TOTAL MASTECTOMY   Simple or total mastectomy removes the entire breast and a small amount of skin but does not remove the axillary lymph nodes. A total mastectomy is appropriate for women with ductal carcinoma in situ (DCIS), and for women seeking prophylactic mastectomies, that is, breast removal in order to prevent any possibility of breast cancer occurring.

MANAGEMENT OF THE REGIONAL LYMPH NODES

Axillary Lymph Node Dissection (ALND)

ALND has traditionally been used to manage localized breast cancer both to prevent an axillary recurrence and to provide prognostic information. Axillary metastases are an important indicator of the need for adjuvant systemic therapy and postmastectomy RT. ALND is the standard of care for patients with palpable axillary lymphadenopathy. Complications of ALND include:

- Injury or thrombosis of the axillary vein
- Injury to the motor nerves
- Severe lymphedema
- Seroma formation
- Shoulder dysfunction
- Loss of sensation
- Mild edema of the arm and breast.

Sentinel Node Biopsy (SLNB)

SLNB is routinely used for women with breast cancer without palpable axillary lymphadenopathy. SLNB is possible because breast tumor cells migrating from a primary tumor drain to one or a few axillary lymph nodes before involving other axillary nodes. Injection of a vital blue dye and/or radioactive colloid in the breast area permit intraoperative identification of the sentinel lymph node(s). The status of the SLN accurately predicts the status of the remaining regional nodes (2).

RADIATION THERAPY (RT) FOR LOCALIZED BREAST CANCER

RT is delivered after BCT and may also be indicated after mastectomy. The intent of RT is to eradicate subclinical residual disease and to minimize local recurrence rates. RT is indicated in virtually all subgroups of women with breast cancer. Even in the lowest risk disease with the most favorable prognostic features (e.g., low grade tumor, ER+, small size), whole breast RT demonstrates a significant reduction (about 75%) in the rate of local recurrence regardless of the use of adjuvant therapy (3). Common side effects of RT include fatigue and skin toxicity. Rare side effects include pulmonary toxicity, cardiac toxicity, increased risk of coronary artery disease, and increased risk of developing a secondary malignancy, such as radiation-induced sarcoma. RT after BCT may possibly avoided in two circumstances:

- Elderly women taking hormonal therapy for ER+ breast cancer—In women over age 70 with ER+ tumors no larger than 2 cm, RT decreased the rate of in-breast recurrence by 75% but the overall rate of local recurrence in these women taking tamoxifen is so low that very few actually benefit from RT (4).
- Well-differentiated DCIS—If the resection margins are adequate, it is possible that RT can be avoided but this is very controversial.

Postmastectomy RT in women with larger (≥5 cm) tumors or axillary lymph node-positive disease reduces the risk of locoregional recurrence, increases disease-free survival, and reduces a woman's risk of dying from breast cancer. Women with ≥5 cm tumors or ≥4 positive axillary lymph nodes are routinely offered postmastectomy RT. The benefit of RT for women with 1–3 positive lymph nodes is uncertain. The treatment field usually includes the chest wall and supraclavicular and infraclavicular regions.

ADJUVANT SYSTEMIC THERAPY

Adjuvant systemic therapy is the administration of hormonal therapy, chemotherapy, and/or trastuzumab (a humanized monoclonal antibody directed against HER2/neu) after definitive local therapy for breast cancer. Adjuvant therapy significantly reduces the risk of both recurrence and death from breast cancer.

HORMONAL THERAPY

Hormonal therapy is directed toward preventing estrogen from stimulating the growth of cancer cells that require estrogen to proliferate. Hormone receptor (ER and/or PR)-positive breast cancer requires estrogen to grow while hormone receptor-negative breast cancers are not dependent on estrogen for growth. Therefore, hormonal therapy is only effective in hormone receptor-positive breast cancers.

Hormonal therapies include:

- *Tamoxifen*—an oral selective estrogen receptor modulator.
- *Aromatase inhibitors*—only for postmenopausal women. In premenopausal women, inhibition of aromatase results in reduced feedback of estrogen to the hypothalamus and pituitary, leading to increased gonadotropin secretion, which stimulates the ovary.
- *Fulvestrant* an intramuscularly injectable pure anti-estrogen.
- *Ovarian function suppression or ablation*—via surgical removal of the ovaries, irradiation of the ovaries, or use of luteinizing hormone releasing hormone analogs (e.g., goserelin or leuprolide).

Benefits of Hormonal Therapy

Data from the Early Breast Cancer Trialists' Collaborative Group (EBCTCG) showed that 5 years of tamoxifen reduces the annual risk of breast cancer recurrence by about 40% and decreases the annual risk of death by about 35% (5). Adjuvant tamoxifen for 5 years is one of the standard options for *postmenopausal* women with ER-positive localized breast cancer and is the *only* standard option for *premenopausal* women ER-positive localized breast cancer.

Aromatase Inhibitors for Postmenopausal Women

Several randomized clinical trials of postmenopausal women with localized hormone receptor-positive breast cancer have shown that adjuvant use of aromatase inhibitors, either used upfront or sequenced after tamoxifen, is superior to tamoxifen alone or placebo in terms of disease-free survival and rates of contralateral breast cancer (6–8). An aromatase inhibitor should be considered either upfront or sequenced after tamoxifen in all postmenopausal women with hormone receptor-positive breast cancer (9).

Side effects of hormonal therapy generally include vasomotor complaints and vaginal discharge and/or atrophy. Although rare, tamoxifen is also associated with an increased risk of uterine cancer, thromboembolic events, and cerebral vascular accidents. Aromatase inhibitors are also associated with loss of bone density, increased risk of bone fractures, musculoskeletal aches, and modestly increased cholesterol.

Chemotherapy

Adjuvant chemotherapy benefits both premenopausal and postmenopausal women, although the absolute magnitude of benefit is greater in younger as compared to older women. The EBCTCG 2000 overview (5) concluded that adjuvant administration of two or more chemotherapy agents:

- For women under age 50, chemotherapy reduces the risk of relapse by 37% and death by 30%. This results into a 10% absolute improvement in 15-year survival.
- For women ages 50–69, chemotherapy reduces the risk of relapse by 19% and death by 12%. This results in a 3% absolute improvement in 15-year survival.
- For women over age 70, the benefits of chemotherapy are uncertain because few studies include women in this age group.

In the United States and other parts of the world, adjuvant chemotherapy is generally recommended for women with hormone receptor-negative breast cancer, particularly if they have positive lymph nodes, larger tumors, or other adverse features. Adjuvant chemotherapy is also generally recommended for women with node-positive breast cancer, regardless of hormone receptor-status. The benefit of adding chemotherapy to hormonal therapy for women with hormone receptor-positive, node-negative breast cancer is unclear.

There are many choices of adjuvant chemotherapy regimens. There is a modest but significant benefit for anthracycline-containing regimens compared to nonanthracycline-containing regimens (such as cyclophosphamide, methotrexate, plus fluorouracil, or CMF). A taxane-containing chemotherapy regimen is often considered for premenopausal and postmenopausal women with node-positive breast cancer. Chemotherapy regimens commonly used as adjuvant therapy for breast cancer are listed in Table 59-1.

SIDE EFFECTS OF CHEMOTHERAPY   Acute side effects include temporary hair loss, nausea, vomiting, fatigue, mucositis, and diarrhea. Cardiomyopathy caused by anthracyclines is rare and increases in frequency at higher cumulative doses of the drug. All chemotherapy agents are also potential carcinogens and can rarely cause secondary leukemias.

Trastuzumab

Approximately 20% of breast cancers overexpress the HER2/neu protein. Trastuzumab is a humanized anti-HER2/neu monoclonal antibody and improves response rate and survival in women with HER2/neu overexpressed metastatic breast cancer. The addition of trastuzumab to adjuvant chemotherapy has also been shown to significantly improve disease-free survival and overall survival in women with localized HER2/neu overexpressed breast cancer (10). However, combined trastuzumab and chemotherapy treatment regimens are associated with a small but significant increase in cardiotoxicity. Trastuzumab is generally recommended in addition to an anthracycline and taxane-based regimen for women with node-positive breast cancer. The benefit of trastuzumab in women with high-risk, node-negative breast cancer is more controversial but is also generally recommended. Trastuzumab should be not be given concurrently with an anthracycline outside of a clinical trial due to excessive cardiotoxicity risks.

Table 59-1

Common Adjuvant Chemotherapy Regimens for Early Stage Breast

Regimen	Cycle number and duration (days)	Cytoxan (mg/m²)	Methotrexate (mg/m²)	5-FU (mg/m²)	Doxorubicin/epirubicin (mg/m²)	Paclitaxel/docetaxel (mg/m²)
Oral CMF	6 × 28	100, PO days 1–14	40, IV days 1, 8	600, IV days 1, 8	—	—
IV FAC	6 × 28	400, IV day 1	—	400, IV days 1, 8	40, IV day 1	
CAF	6 × 21	500, IV day 1	—	500, IV day 1	50, IV day 1	
AC	4 × 21	600, IV day 1	—	—	60, IV day 1	
AC-T	4(AC), 4(T) × 21	600, IV day 1	—	—	60, IV day 1	P: 175, IV day 1
Dose dense AC-T	4(AC), 4(T) × 14	600, IV day 1	—	—	60, IV day 1	P: 175, IV day 1
TAC	6 × 21	500, IV day 1	—	—	50, IV day 1	D: 75, IV day 1
Oral CEF	6 × 28	75, PO days 1–14	—	500, IV days 1, 8	Epirubicin 60, IV days 1, 8	—
IV FEC	6 × 21	500, IV day 1	—	—	Epirubicin 100, IV day 1	—

REFERENCES

1. Fisher B. Twenty-year follow-up of a randomized trial comparing total mastectomy, lumpectomy, and lumpectomy plus irradiation for the treatment of invasive breast cancer. N Engl J Med. 2002; 347: 1233.

2. Lyman GH. American Society of Clinical Oncology guideline recommendations for sentinel lymph node biopsy in early-stage breast cancer. J Clin Oncol. 2005; 23: 7703.

3. Early Breast Cancer Trialists' Collaborative Group. Effects of radiotherapy and surgery in early breast cancer. An overview of the randomized trials. N Engl J Med. 1995; 333: 1444.

4. Hughes KS. Lumpectomy plus tamoxifen with or without irradiation in women 70 years of age or older with early stage breast cancer. N Engl J Med. 2004; 351: 971.

5. Early Breast Cancer Trialists' Collaborative Group. Effects of chemotherapy and hormonal therapy for early breast cancer on recurrence and 15-year survival: an overview of the randomized trials. Lancet. 2005; 365: 1687.

6. Howell A. Results of the ATAC (Arimidex, Tamoxifen, Alone or in Combination) trial after completion of 5 years' adjuvant treatment for breast cancer. Lancet. 2005; 365: 60.

7. Goss PE. A randomized trial of letrozole in postmenopausal women after five years of tamoxifen therapy for early-stage breast cancer. N Engl J Med. 2003; 349: 1793.

8. Coombes RC. A randomized trial of exemestane after two to three years of tamoxifen therapy in postmenopausal women with primary breast cancer. N Engl J Med. 2004; 350: 1081.

9. Winer EP. American Society of Clinical Oncology technology assessment on the use of aromatase inhibitors as adjuvant therapy for postmenopausal women with hormone receptor-positive breast cancer: status report 2004. J Clin Oncol. 2005; 23: 619.

10. Romond E. Doxorubicin and cyclophosphamide followed by paclitaxel with or without trastuzumab as adjuvant therapy for patients with HER-2 positive operable breast cancer. American Society of Clinical Oncology, Orlando, FL, May 16, 2005.

METASTATIC BREAST CANCER

INTRODUCTION

Since 1990, the annual rate of breast cancer death has been decreasing by approximately 2.1% per year (1). Historically, median survival of patients with metastatic breast cancer (MBC) was estimated to be 18–30 months. Many experts agree that median survival has improved in recent years beyond 30 months, though definitive data are lacking. Newer active agents include taxanes, third generation aromatase inhibitors, and biologic agents such as trastuzumab and bevacizumab. Despite these advances, breast cancer remains the second leading cause of cancer death in women in the United States, with 40, 910 women estimated to die of breast cancer in 2007 (1).

Prognosis

Several factors contribute to predicting an individual patient's course of disease:

- Prolonged relapse-free survival of more than 5 years is more favorable.
- Isolated chest wall or ipsilateral nodal recurrence predicts better outcome than visceral disease.
- Bone and soft-tissue recurrence is more favorable than visceral or central nervous system disease.
- The prognostic value of HER2, status on MBC, especially with the advent of trastuzumab and lapatinib is not established.
- A prognostic index predicts median overall survival of 50, 23, and 11 months for low-, intermediate-, and high-risk groups, respectively (Figure 60-1) (2).
- Up to 2–3% of patients with favorable characteristics may be long-term survivors with over 20-year survival. Such patients tend to be young, have limited disease, and have a complete response to initial therapy.

Goals of Treatment

Metastatic breast cancer is not considered curable. Therefore, the goals of treatment must carefully balance the risks of treatment-induced toxicity with the expected clinical benefit. Accepted clinical endpoints in the treatment of MBC include prolonged overall survival, improved quality of life (QOL), progression-free survival, and cancer-related symptom control.

DIAGNOSTIC EVALUATION

Most patients with MBC present with a recurrence following treatment for early stage breast cancer. Less than 10% of patients present with MBC at the time of initial diagnosis. The most common sites of metastatic recurrence are bone, lungs, liver, and the central nervous system. Up to 50–75% of patients with MBC will have single organ involvement. Local recurrence after mastectomy usually involves the chest wall or overlying skin. In such cases, distant metastatic disease is present in 25–30% of cases.

Evaluation of patients presenting with recurrent or MBC includes (3):

- History and Physical exam
- Complete blood count
- Liver function tests

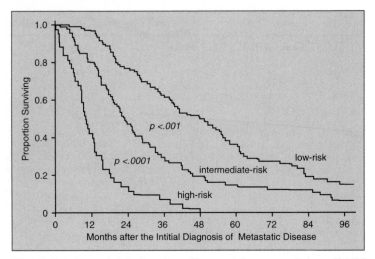

FIGURE 60-1 Prognostic index for patients with metastatic breast cancer. Patients with MBC were stratified into risk groups based on the total sum of individual prognostic factors as follows: (1) adjuvant chemotherapy—add 1 point if received; (2) distant lymph node metastates—add 1 point if present; (3) liver metastases—add 1 if present; (4) lactate dehydrogenase—add 1 point if >1× normal; (5) Disease free interval—add two points if <24 months. Low-risk group ≤1 point, intermediate group = 2–3 points, high risk ≥4 points. Source: adapted from (2) with permission.

- Chest radiograph and/or CT
- CT (or MRI) evaluation of abdomen and pelvis
- Positron emission tomography (PET) scan (optional)
- Bone scan, with subsequent radiographs of areas of concern for fracture
- Biopsy to confirm first metastatic recurrence, with determination of hormone receptor and HER2 status if not done previously

Biopsy proven confirmation of the first metastatic recurrence is preferred. The presence of estrogen receptor (ER), progesterone receptor (PgR), and HER2/Neu overexpression in tumors will influence the selection of therapy. Therefore, biopsy of initial metastatic recurrence is increasingly clinically indicated to confirm ER, PgR, and HER2 status. In addition, patient with a history of breast cancer are at increased risk for secondary non-breast cancers which may affect treatment selection.

TREATMENT

Overview

A treatment algorithm for MBC is shown in Figure 60-2. Selection of initial and subsequent treatment requires consideration of multiple factors:

- Patient goals
- Social support
- ER, PgR, and HER2 status
- Sites of disease
- Comorbid conditions
- Performance status (ECOG or Karnofsky)
- Toxicities of treatments
- Pace of disease progression
- Previous treatment and responses

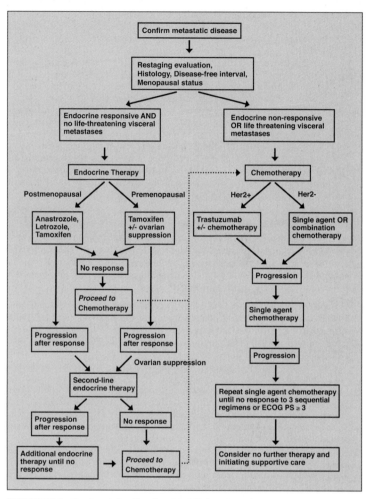

FIGURE 60-2 Treatment algorithm for metastatic breast cancer.

- Need for concurrent localized therapy (e.g., radiotherapy or surgery for bone or CNS disease)
- Likelihood of response to treatment

Monitoring Treatment

Treatment may be followed by periodic evaluation of the following:

- History and physical exam—Monthly evaluation for patients with MBC is reasonable to assess for progression and toxicities of treatment.
- Serum tumor markers: CA15-3, CA27.29, and CEA—The serum markers CA15-3 and CA 27.29 correlate with the course of disease in 60–70% of patients, and carcinoembryonic antigen (CEA) levels correlate in 40%. Elevated serum markers prior to treatment initiation allow periodic monitoring of marker levels during the course of treatment. A "flare" reaction often

occurs causing a rise in serum markers in the first month of treatment. The only recommended use of serum tumor markers is to monitor patients with MBC, according to an expert panel convened by the American Society of Clinical Oncology (4).

- Radiographic studies: CT, MRI, PET, bone scans, plain films—Standardized guidelines for radiographic monitoring of patients with MBC are not established and monitoring must be individualized for each patient. Periodic scans in the absence of rising tumor markers or changing symptoms is unlikely to affect survival. Radiographic evaluation is appropriate if symptoms change or tumor markers rise. CT scans are useful to establish a new baseline after maximum response to a given therapy is achieved. PET scans are currently approved for MBC for staging and monitoring response to therapy. However, its value in clinical decision making is not established. Routine use of MRI or CT scans to monitor the central nervous system is not recommended unless a patient has known CNS disease or presents with symptoms suggestive of CNS involvement.

Endocrine Therapy

Endocrine therapy is preferred for most patients with hormone receptor positive MBC. Hormonal agents used in MBC are listed in Table 60-1. The mechanism of action and toxicities are described in more detail in Chapter 12 "Hormonal Agents: Anti-Estrogens." The following general guidelines apply to selection of hormonal therapy for MBC (Figure 60-2):

- Endocrine therapy should be initial treatment for patients with hormone receptor positive tumors without symptomatic visceral metastases or rapidly progressive disease.
- The response rates to hormonal therapy for ER+/PgR+, ER+/PgR-, ER-/PgR- are 70%, 40%, and 10%, respectively.
- Patients with primary endocrine resistance generally should proceed directly to chemotherapy.
- Patients who respond to initial endocrine therapy may proceed to additional lines of endocrine therapy until no further response is attained or visceral metastases develop requiring rapid and more effective response. The response rate to second line endocrine therapy is up to 33% in patients who initially responded to tamoxifen and 15% in patients who had no initial response.
- Tamoxifen is commonly used as first-line hormonal therapy in both pre- and postmenopausal women with MBC. Response rates are as high as 50–60% and may last on average over 12 months. A "tamoxifen flare" can result in bone pain and increased metastatic skin lesions in up to 13% of patients. Withdrawal of tamoxifen can induce a secondary withdrawal response.
- Anastrozole and letrozole are third-generation aromatase inhibitors (AIs) approved for first-line use in postmenopausal women with MBC and as second-line use after tamoxifen failure. Letrozole is more potent than anastrozole but results in no difference in overall survival.
- Direct comparison of tamoxifen to AIs as first-line therapy in three large randomized studies showed no statistically significant difference in median overall survival (5, 6). However, letrozole produced a longer time to progression (TTP) and a higher overall response rate (6). As a result, AIs are often preferred over tamoxifen as first-line therapy in postmenopausal women with MBC.
- Exemestane is approved for second-line therapy in postmenopausal women with MBC. Exemestane may induce responses in patients with primary resistance to tamoxifen. Preliminary data suggest exemestane results in prolonged progression free survival (PFS) compared to tamoxifen for first-line therapy. Although not approved in the United States for first-line therapy in MBC, it is a reasonable choice.

Table 60-1

Hormonal Agents Used in MBC

Agent	Regimen
• *Partial antiestrogens*	
– Tamoxifen	20 mg PO daily
– Toremifine	60 mg PO daily
• *Non-steroidal Aromatase Inhibitors**	
– Anastrozole	1 mg PO daily
– Letrozole	2.5 mg PO daily
• *Steroidal aromatase inhibitors**	
– Exemestane	25 mg PO daily
• *Pure antiestrogens**	
– Fulvestrant	250 mg IM monthly
• *LHRH-agonists†*	
– Goserelin	3.6 mg SC every 28 days
– Leuprolide	7.5 mg IM every 28 days
– Triptorelin	3.75 mg IM every 28 days
• *Progestin*	
– Megestrol acetate	40 mg PO four times daily
• *Androgens*	
– Fluoxymestrone	10–40 mg PO daily, in divided doses
• *High-dose estrogen*	
– Ethinyl estradiol	1 mg PO three times daily

*Therapy is appropriate for postmenopausal women only or premenopausal women receiving concurrent ovarian suppression.

†Therapy is appropriate for premenopausal only.

- Fulvestrant is approved for postmenopausal MBC and results in similar median survival and TTP as tamoxifen (7, 8). Fulvestrant is similar in efficacy and safety to exemestane following progression on a non-steroidal aromatase inhibitor.
- Ovarian suppression (OvS) with the leutinizing hormone-releasing hormone (LHRH) agonists (goserelin, triptorelin, and leuprolide) has equal efficacy to surgical OvS for premenopausal women with MBC. LHRH agonists may cause a flare reaction similar to tamoxifen. Combined tamoxifen and OvS results in higher response rates than OvS alone (39% vs. 30%), without clear survival benefit over sequential therapy.
- Megestrol acetate may have a role in patients who progress on previous therapies but has largely been replaced by the anti-estrogens and AIs.

Chemotherapy

A treatment algorithm is shown in Figure 60-2 and representative common chemotherapy regimens for MBC are shown in Tables 60-2–60-4 (3, 9–14). The mechanism of action and toxicities of specific chemotherapies are described in more detail Section 2 "Classes of Drugs." The following are guidelines for chemotherapy treatment in MBC:

- Patients with visceral metastases, rapidly progressive disease, or hormone-refractory disease may be treated with chemotherapy.
- First-line chemotherapy results in response rates of 30–60% and improved QOL.
- Combination chemotherapy has higher response rates but more toxicity and no survival benefit over sequential single agents. Second-line chemotherapy should use single agents except in selected patients.

Table 60-2

Single Agent Chemotherapy Regimens for Metastatic Breast Cancer

Regimen	Agent	Cycle length
Doxorubicin	60 mg/m^2 IV day 1	21 days
Doxorubicin—weekly	20 mg/m^2 IV	7 days
Pegylated liposomal doxorubicin	50 mg/m^2 IV day 1	28 days
Paclitaxel	175 mg/m^2 IV	21 days
Paclitaxel—weekly	80 mg/m^2 IV	7 days
Nanoparticle albumin-bound paclitaxel	260 mg/m^2 IV day 1	21 days
Docetaxel	100 mg/m^2 IV	21 days
Docetaxel-weekly	40 mg/m^2 IV day 1, 8, 15, 22, 29, 36	48 days
Vinorelbine	30 mg/m^2 IV	7 days
Capecitabine	1,250 mg/m^2 PO twice daily days 1–14	21 days
Gemcitabine	1,200 mg/m^2 IV days 1,8,15	28 days

Table 60-3

Combination Chemotherapy Regimens for Metastatic Breast Cancer

Regimen	Agent	Cycle length
CAF	Cyclophosphamide 100 mg/m^2 PO days 1–14 Doxorubicin 30 mg/m^2 IV days 1, 8 5-Fluorouracil 500 mg/m^2 IV days 1, 8	28 days
FAC	5-Fluorouracil 500 mg/m^2 IV days 1, 8 Doxorubicin 50 mg/m^2 IV day 1 Cyclophosphamide 500 mg/m^2 IV day 1	21 days
AC	Doxorubicin 60 mg/m^2 IV day 1 Cyclophosphamide 600 mg/m^2 IV day 1	21 days
CMF	Cyclophosphamide 100 mg/m^2 PO days 1–14 Methotrexate 40 mg/m^2 IV days 1, 8 5-Fluorouracil 600 mg/m^2 IV days 1, 8	28 days
Docetaxel/ Capecitabine	Docetaxel 75 mg/m^2 IV day 1 Capecitabine 950 mg/m^2 PO twice daily days 1–14	21 days
Docetaxel/ Carboplatin	Docetaxel 75 mg/m^2 IV day 1 Carboplatin AUC 6 IV day 1	21 days
GT	Paclitaxel 175 mg/m^2 IV day 1 Gemcitabine 1250 mg/m^2 IV day 1, 8	21 days
FEC	5-Fluorouracil 500 mg/m^2 IV days 1, 8 Epirubicin 50 mg/m^2 IV day 1, 8 Cyclophosphamide 400 mg/m^2 IV days 1, 8	28 days
Paclitaxel/ Bevacizumab	Paclitaxel 90 mg/m^2 days 1, 8, 15 Bevacizumab 10 mg/kg IV days 1, 15	28 days

- Factors predicting resistance to chemotherapy include relapse within 12 months of adjuvant chemotherapy, progression on a prior chemotherapy regimen, poor performance status, and multiple sites of visceral disease.

Table 60-4

HER2-Directed Chemotherapy Regimens

Agent	Regimen	
Single agents		
Paclitaxel*	175 mg/m^2 IV days 1,8,15, every 21 days or 80 mg/m^2 IV weekly	
Docetaxel*	80 mg/,2 IV day 1, every 21 days or 35 mg/m^2 IV weekly	
Vinorelbine*	25 mg/m^2 IV weekly	
Trastuzumab	4 mg/kg IV day 1, followed by 2 mg/kg IV weekly or 8 mg/kg IV day 1, followed by 6 mg/kg IV every 3 weeks	
Capecitabine/ Lapatinib	Capecitabine 2000 mg/m^2 PO days 1–14 21 days Lapatinib 1250 mg PO daily	

Regimen	Agent	Cycle length
Combination regimens		
PCH*	Carboplatin AUC of 6 IV day 1 Paclitaxel 175 mg/m^2 IV day 1	21 days
TCH*	Paclitaxel 80 mg/m^2 IV day 1, 8, 15 Carboplatin AUC of 2 IV days 1, 8, 15	28 days

*Each chemotherapy regimen listed may be used with either weekly or every three week dosing schedule of trastuzumab as shown for trastuzumab monotherapy.

- Concurrent chemotherapy and hormonal therapy for MBC is generally avoided.
- Anthracyclines, taxanes, and capecitabine are all reasonable first-line agents.
- Liposomal doxorubicin has equal efficacy to standard doxorubicin (10) but allows for increased cumulative dosing.
- Paclitaxel and docetaxel may be given on weekly or every three-week schedules. Response rates may be higher with weekly dosing, but overall survival is similar and neurotoxicity is significantly worse. Patients who progress on paclitaxel may respond to docetaxel. Docetaxel is also active as first-line therapy.
- Nanoparticle albumin-bound (nab)-paclitaxel is approved for treatment of MBC. Benefits include treatment without steroid premedication, shorter infusion times, higher effective administered paclitaxel dose, and lower hematologic toxicity. Direct comparison of standard versus nab-paclitaxel showed a higher response rate (33% vs. 19%), longer TTP (23 vs. 17 weeks), and less grade 4 neutropenia for nab-paclitaxel (14).
- Bevacizumab is a monoclonal antibody against vascular endothelial growth factor (VEGF). First-line therapy using paclitaxel plus bevacizumab compared to paclitaxel monotherapy showed a significant improvement in PFS (11.4 vs. 6.1 months) (11). No difference in overall survival has yet been observed. The role of bevacizumab in MBC is not yet clear, but its use with paclitaxel as first-line chemotherapy is reasonable.
- Capecitabine, an oral 5-FU derivative, has response rates up to 28% as monotherapy. The combination of capecitabine and docetaxel showed improved survival (14.5 vs. 11.5 months) compared to single agent docetaxel in patients who progress after anthracycline therapy (12). 5-Fluorouracil is used in many of the common combination regimens for MBC but rarely as a single agent.
- Single agent vinorelbine has response rates up to 25–50% and is particularly well tolerated in elderly patients.

- Single agent gemcitabine is well tolerated and has response rates up to 40% in chemotherapy naïve patients. Combination with cisplatin, vinorelbine, or paclitaxel results in higher response rates. Single agent or combination therapy may have a role in third-line therapy and beyond.
- Supportive measures should be considered in patients with an ECOG performance status ≥ 3 or after lack of response to three successive single agent chemotherapy regimens.

HER2-Directed Therapy

First-line treatment of HER2+ disease should include trastuzumab-based therapy as shown in Table 60-4.

Trastuzumab monotherapy has a response rate of at least 35% and 18% as first- and second-line treatment, respectively, in HER2+ patients with 3+ overexpression by immunohistochemistry. Trastuzumab combination therapy with a taxane, platinum, or vinorelbine has higher response rates than monotherapy. Paclitaxel and trastuzumab had higher response rates (41% vs. 17%), TTP (6.9 vs. 3.0 months) and a trend toward overall survival (22.1 vs. 18.4 months) compared to paclitaxel alone (9). Doectaxel combined with trastuzumab has also been shown to be superior to docetaxel alone in HER2+ patients.

Single agent trastuzumab has not been directly compared to combinations with taxanes leaving combination regimens as the preferred choice. Impressive activity with response rates over 50–60% has also been shown in combinations of trastuzumab with vinorelbine or with paclitaxel and carboplatin, and these are reasonable choices for first-line therapy. Continued use of trastuzumab following disease progression is safe and may provide some benefit.

Patients treated with trastuzumab may have a higher incidence of brain metastases due to the lack of CNS penetration of the drug despite effective systemic disease control elsewhere.

Concurrent administration of trastuzumab and anthracyclines is contraindicated due to cardiotoxicity (9). Trastuzumab following anthracycline treatment also increases the risk of cardiotoxicity that is often reversible and can be managed medically.

The novel oral agent lapatinib is a HER2 and TTP receptor dual kinase inhibitor that was shown in a phase III study to improve TTP in combination with capecitabine compared to capecitabine alone from 4.4 to 8.4 months in women who progressed after anthracycline, taxane, and trastuzumab therapy (15).

TREATMENT OF THE ELDERLY

The treatment of women over 65 with MBC is similar to younger women with some exceptions. The elderly are at increased risk for reduced social support structures, reduced tolerance to chemotherapy, and cognitive impairment. Elderly women without visceral disease or rapid progression may warrant a trial of hormonal therapy, regardless of hormone receptor status, as response rates up to 20% have been reported in elderly patients with hormone receptor negative tumors. AIs may have higher response rates in the elderly. Cardiac toxicity from doxorubicin is increased in women over 70, but is uncommon with liposomal doxorubicin. Methotrexate and capecitabine should be dose-adjusted because of declining renal function. Sequential chemotherapy is preferable because of lower toxicity than combination regimens. Agents that are particularly well tolerated in the elderly include capecitabine, vinorelbine, trastuzumab, and the taxanes.

LOCAL THERAPY IN MBC

In selected patients, specific organ-directed therapy may improve QOL or survival.

Surgery has a limited role in MBC. Patients with a solitary metastasis or oligometastatic disease may be candidates for metastatectomy. Observational studies suggest surgery may improve survival in selected cases.

Up to 10–24% of patients with MBC will develop disease limited to the lung. Surgical resection may improve survival in such patients. More than 50% of solitary pulmonary nodules in MBC represent a primary lung cancer.

Malignant pleural effusions commonly develop in patients with MBC. Talc pleuradesis may help provide temporary symptomatic relief for patients with recurrent effusions. Therapeutic paracentesis may provide symptomatic relief for patients with malignant ascites. Radiofrequency ablation or surgery is an option in selected patients with limited liver disease.

Up to one-third of the patients who develop brain metastases will have brain-only disease. Resection of solitary brain lesions may improve survival and QOL. The management of epidural spinal cord compression and central nervous system metastases is discussed in Chapter 64 "Metastatic Brain Tumors."

Bone is the most common site of metastatic disease in breast cancer. Patients with identified bone metastases should receive bisphosphonate therapy (zoledronic acid given as a 4 mg IV dose monthly) to reduce the risk of bone events. Radiotherapy is an effective approach to alleviate specific sites of painful bone metastasis. The management of bone metastases is discussed in detail in Chapter 17 "Bisphosphonates."

REFERENCES

1. Jemal A, Siegel R, Ward E, et al. Cancer statistics, 2007. CA Cancer J Clin. 2007; 57(1): 43–66.
2. Yamamoto N, Watanabe T, Katsumata N, et al. Construction and validation of a practical prognostic index for patients with metastatic breast cancer. J Clin Oncol. 1998; 16(7): 2401–2408.
3. Carlson RW, McCormick B. Update: NCCN breast cancer clinical practice guidelines. J Natl Compr Canc Netw. 2005; 3(suppl 1): S7–S11.
4. Bast RC Jr., Ravdin P, Hayes DF, et al. 2000 update of recommendations for the use of tumor markers in breast and colorectal cancer: clinical practice guidelines of the American Society of Clinical Oncolog. J Clin Oncol. 2001; 19(6): 1865–1878.
5. Bonneterre J, Buzdar A, Nabholtz JM, et al. Anastrozole is superior to tamoxifen as first-line therapy in hormone receptor positive advanced breast carcinoma. Cancer 2001; 92(9): 2247–2258.
6. Mouridsen H, Gershanovich M, Sun Y, et al. Phase III study of letrozole versus tamoxifen as first-line therapy of advanced breast cancer in postmenopausal women: analysis of survival and update of efficacy from the International Letrozole Breast Cancer Group. J Clin Oncol. 2003; 21(11): 2101–2109.
7. Howell A, Pippen J, Elledge RM, et al. Fulvestrant versus anastrozole for the treatment of advanced breast carcinoma: a prospectively planned combined survival analysis of two multicenter trials. Cancer. 2005; 104(2): 236–239.
8. Howell A, Robertson JF, Abram P, et al. Comparison of fulvestrant versus tamoxifen for the treatment of advanced breast cancer in postmenopausal women previously untreated with endocrine therapy: a multinational, double-blind, randomized trial. J Clin Oncol. 2004; 22(9): 1605–1613.
9. Slamon DJ, Leyland-Jones B, Shak S, et al. Use of chemotherapy plus a monoclonal antibody against HER2 for metastatic breast cancer that overexpresses HER2. N Engl J Med. 2001; 344(11): 783–792.

10. O'Brien ME, Wigler N, Inbar M, et al. Reduced cardiotoxicity and comparable efficacy in a phase III trial of pegylated liposomal doxorubicin HCl (CAE-LYX/Doxil) versus conventional doxorubicin for first-line treatment of metastatic breast cancer. Ann Oncol. 2004; 15(3): 440–449.

11. Miller KD, Wang M, Gralow J, et al. A randomized phase III trial of paclitaxel versus paclitaxel plus bevacizumab as first-line therapy for locally recurrent or metastatic breast cancer: a trial coordinated by the Eastern Cooperative Oncology Group (E2100). "San Antonio Breast Cancer Symposium," San Antonio, TX, 2005.

12. Miles D, Vukelja S, Moiseyenko V, et al. Survival benefit with capecitabine/docetaxel versus docetaxel alone: analysis of therapy in a randomized phase III trial. Clin Breast Cancer. 2004; 5(4): 273–278.

13. Hamilton A, Hortobagyi G. Chemotherapy: what progress in the last 5 years? J Clin Oncol. 2005; 23(8): 1760–1775.

14. Gradishar WJ, Tjulandin S, Davidson N, et al. Phase III trial of nanoparticle albumin-bound paclitaxel compared with polyethylated castor oil-based paclitaxel in women with breast cancer. J Clin Oncol. 2005; 23(31): 7794–7803.

15. Geyer CE, Forster J, Lindquist D, et al. Lapatinib plus capecitabine for HER2-positive advanced breast cancer. N Engl J Med. 2006; 355(26): 2733–2743.

61	Donald P. Lawrence, Krista M. Rubin MS, RN, FNP-c

MELANOMA

EPIDEMIOLOGY, RISK FACTORS, SCREENING, AND PREVENTION

Epidemiology

An estimated 62,190 new cases of cutaneous melanoma were diagnosed in the United States in 2006 and an estimated 7,910 deaths from melanoma occurred (1). The incidence has increased fivefold since 1950 and continues to rise more rapidly than that of any other cancer. Melanoma is currently the second leading cancer diagnosis among US women under 40 years of age, and the third leading cancer diagnosis among men in this age group. Five-year survival has increased from 80% in the period from 1975 to 1976 to 92% between 1995 and 2001 (2).

On a global basis, the incidence of melanoma varies widely, with the annual age-adjusted incidence rates of <1 per 100,000 persons in Japan and India, to 37.8 and 29.4 per 100,000 among Australian males and females, respectively. African Americans have a low risk of melanoma (1.3 and 0.8 per 100,000 for men and women, respectively, compared to 24 and 15.9 per 100,000 in US Caucasians) (3).

Risk Factors

Risk factors for melanoma include light complexion, poorly tanning skin, and blonde or red hair, which confer a relative risk of 1.3–4.1. Intense, intermittent sun exposure and a history of blistering sunburn appear to confer a greater risk than lower-level, continuous sunlight exposure. Both Ultraviolet A (UVA) and Ultraviolet B (UVB) radiation have been implicated in the pathogenesis of melanoma. Exposure to UV radiation via tanning booths, and, with psoralen, as a treatment for psoriasis, is associated with an increase in the risk of melanoma (4, 5).

Numerous common nevi are a marker of increased risk, as are atypical nevi. Large congenital nevi have a high risk of malignant transformation (lifetime risk 4–10%). Following the diagnosis of melanoma, the probability of developing a second primary melanoma has been estimated to be 5.34% over an interval of 20 years (6).

Melanoma in a first-degree relative confers an increased risk, and about 10% of individuals diagnosed with melanoma have an affected family member. However, the magnitude of the risk associated with family history is quite variable. Most families with multiple affected members have no identifiable genetic abnormality. Genes in which germline mutations or polymorphisms have been associated with an increased risk of melanoma include CDKN2A (7) and CDK4 (8), which encode cell cycle regulatory proteins, the melanocortin 1 receptor gene (9), and the breast cancer susceptibility gene, BRCA2 (relative risk for melanoma, 2.58) (10).

The dysplastic nevus syndrome is characterized by numerous atypical nevi, and the development of melanoma at an early age. The lifetime risk of melanoma approaches 100% in this syndrome. Its genetic basis remains unknown.

Screening

The majority of melanomas display at least one of the following features:

A: Asymmetry
B: Irregularity of borders
C: Color variegation
D: Diameter >6 mm
E: Enlargement or evolution

Melanoma is highly curable by surgical excision when detected at an early stage (i.e., less than 1 mm in thickness), whereas the risk of mortality rises sharply with thicker lesions. The American Academy of Dermatology has sponsored a screening program for over one million individuals. In a subgroup for which pathologic data were available, a presumptive diagnosis of melanoma was made in 0.8% and confirmed in 0.15%. The highest yield was among white males over the age of 50, a population that also has the highest risk for mortality from melanoma (11). While no survival data are available from this program, it lends support to the feasibility, and possibly the efficacy, of large-scale screening, as do similar programs in other countries. The overall benefit and cost-effectiveness of screening remains to be determined.

Prevention

The efficacy of topical sunscreens in the primary prevention of melanoma has not been rigorously demonstrated (12). This may be due to the fact that some commercially available sunscreens reduce exposure to UVB radiation but not to UVA, that they are inadequately applied, or that they provide a false sense of security leading to more prolonged sun exposure. Effective melanoma prevention strategies will probably involve a combination of education and behavior modification beginning at an early age. Such programs are underway in the United States, Australia, and other endemic areas, but their impact is difficult to gauge at this point.

PATHOLOGIC FEATURES OF MELANOMA

The likelihood of recurrence and death from melanoma is directly correlated with tumor thickness. Ulceration (the absence of an intact epidermal layer overlying the melanoma) is a powerful adverse prognostic feature. A high mitotic rate, vascular and neural invasion are also associated with a poor prognosis.

Melanoma may arise de novo, from a pre-existing nevus, or from melanoma in situ, in which the melanocytic proliferation is limited to the epidermis. Radial growth phase melanoma is confined in large part to the epidermis and has a low likelihood of dissemination. The vertical growth phase is characterized by prominent dermal invasion, and signals the acquisition of metastatic potential.

Several distinct growth patterns of melanoma are recognized. Superficial spreading melanoma is defined by the presence of both a radial and vertical growth phase, and accounts for up to 75% of melanomas. Nodular melanomas (15–25%) are vertical growth phase lesions, located exclusively or predominantly in the dermis. Lentigo maligna melanoma typically arises from a noninvasive precursor lesion (lentigo maligna, or lentigo maligna melanoma in situ) and occurs most frequently on the face, scalp, or neck in older individuals. Acral lentiginous melanoma accounts for only 5% of melanomas, but is the most common form in non-Caucasians. The most common sites are the palmar and plantar surfaces. It is characterized by the presence of nests of atypical melanocytes at the dermal–epidermal junction, with infiltration of single cells or nests into the dermis.

A minority of melanomas are amelanotic, lacking obvious pigmentation. Amelanotic melanoma may mimic a variety of benign entities, often leading to a delay in diagnosis. In other respects their behavior is similar to pigmented melanomas.

The detection of melanocyte-associated antigens by immunohistochemistry may suggest or support the diagnosis of melanoma in difficult cases, such as metastatic cancer of uncertain histogenesis. Immunohistochemistry may also detect small deposits of metastatic melanoma within lymph nodes that are not evident on routine microscopic examination. S-100 is expressed by cells of melanocytic lineage, but also by histiocytes and certain neural tumors. Melan-A is also somewhat non-specific. Antigens with a higher degree of specificity for melanocytes include tyrosinase, the microphthalmia transcription factor, and a protein in the premelanosome complex targeted by the monoclonal antibody HMB45. None of these antigens, however, can be used to distinguish melanoma from benign melanocytic proliferative processes.

STAGING AND PROGNOSTIC FACTORS

The American Joint Committee on Cancer staging system for cutaneous melanoma is based on an analysis of prognostic factors in 17,600 cases (13, 14). Melanomas without regional lymphatic spread are designated as stage I or II. The staging of node-negative melanomas is based on the thickness of the primary lesion, ulceration, and, for thin melanomas (≤ 1 mm), the anatomic depth of invasion (Table 61-1). While the majority of stage I and II melanomas are cured by surgery alone, even melanomas 1 mm or less in thickness, without ulceration or nodal involvement (T1aN0M0) may have metastatic potential, and are associated with a 10-year survival of under 90%. The 10-year survival in patients with thick melanomas (stages IIB and IIC) is 32.3–53.9%. Ulceration is associated with a relative risk of death of 1.9 in node-negative melanomas.

Table 61-1

Primary Tumor Stage, Cutaneous Melanoma

TX	Primary tumor cannot be assessed
T0	No evidence of primary tumor
Tis	Melanoma in situ
T1	≤ 1 mm in thickness*
T2	1.01–2 mm in thickness[†]
T3	2.01–4 mm in thickness[†]
T4	>4 mm in thickness[†]

[*]a: Non-ulcerated, invasion to anatomic level<IV; b: Ulcerated, or invasion to anatomic level IV or V.

[†]a: Non-ulcerated; b: Ulcerated.

Source: Adapted from (14).

Stage III is defined by the presence of satellite and/or in-transit metastases, and/or involvement of regional lymph nodes (Table 61-2). Lymphatic metastases within 2 cm of the primary lesion are designated satellite metastases; those located more than 2 cm from the primary melanoma, but before the first echelon of draining lymph nodes, are designated in-transit metastases. The burden of tumor in the lymph nodes is predictive of outcome, and is represented by the number of nodes involved, and whether the involvement is microscopic (clinically inapparent prior to surgery), or macroscopic (clinically apparent).

Table 61-2

Regional Nodal/Lymphatic Staging of Melanoma

NX	Regional lymph nodes cannot be assessed
N0	No regional lymph node/lymphatic metastases
N1a	Metastasis in one regional lymph node, clinically occult
N1a	Metastasis in one regional lymph node, clinically apparent
N2a	Metastases in 2–3 regional lymph nodes, clinically occult
N2b	Metastases in 2–3 regional lymph nodes, clinically apparent
N2c	In-transit/satellite metastases without nodal involvement
N3	Metastases in >4 regional lymph nodes, matted lymph nodes, or in-transit/satellite metastases with nodal involvement

Source: Adapted from (14).

Stage III melanomas are heterogeneous. Those with microscopic nodal involvement, and without ulceration of the primary tumor have a 10-year survival rate of 56.9–63.0%. For patients with clinically detectable lymphadenopathy, or with ulceration of the primary melanoma and any degree of nodal involvement, the 10-year survival ranges from 15% to 47.7%.

Stage IV melanoma represents distant metastatic spread, and is stratified according to sites of involvement and lactate dehydrogenase level (Table 61-3). Based on these T, N, and M criteria, patients can be grouped according to prognosis (Table 61-4).

Table 61-3

Staging of Melanoma, Distant Metastases

MX	Distant metastases cannot be assessed
M0	No distant metastases
M1a	Metastases to skin, subcutaneous sites, and/or distant lymph nodes
M1b	Metastases to lung only
M1c	Metastases to all other sites, or to any site with elevated serum lactate dehydrogenase (LDH)

Adapted from (14).

Table 61-4

Pathologic Stage Grouping and Prognosis in Melanoma

Stage	TNM	10-year survival (%)
Node/lymphatic negative		
IA	T1aN0M0	87.9 ± 1.0
IB	T1bN0M0	83.1 ± 1.5
	T2aN0M0	79.2 ± 1.1
IIA	T2bN0M0	64.4 ± 2.2
	T3aN0M0	63.8 ± 1.7
		(Continued)

Table 61-4 (*Continued*)

Stage	TNM	10-year Survival (%)
IIB	T3bN0M0	50.8 ± 1.7
	T4aN0M0	53.9 ± 3.3
IIC	T4bN0M0	32.3 ± 2.1
Node/lymphatic positive		
IIIA	T1-4aN1aM0	63.0 ± 4.4
	T1-4aN2aM0	56.9 ± 6.8
IIIB	T1-4bN1aM0	37.8 ± 4.8
	T1-4bN2aM0	35.9 ± 7.2
	T1-4aN1bM0	47.7 ± 5.8
	T1-4aN2bM0	39.2 ± 5.8
	T1-4(a or b)N2cM0	
IIIC	T1-4bN1bM0	24.4 ± 5.3
	T1-4bN2bM0	15.0 ± 3.9
	T(any)N3M0	18.4 ± 2.5
Metastatic		
IV	T(any)N(any)M1a	15.7 ± 2.9
	T(any)N(any)M1b	2.5 ± 1.5
	T(any)N(any)M1c	6.0 ± 0.9

Adapted from (13) & (14).

Stage-for-stage, advanced age and male sex are associated with a worse prognosis in melanoma. Melanomas of the extremities have a more favorable prognosis than those of the trunk. Head and neck melanomas, particularly those of the scalp and ears, have a worse prognosis than other sites.

SURGICAL MANAGEMENT

When melanoma is under consideration, biopsy techniques should be employed that preserve the pathologist's ability to assess the thickness and depth of invasion of the lesion, i.e., conservative excisional biopsy, or punch biopsy. Ablative procedures such as cryotherapy should be avoided.

Once the diagnosis of melanoma is established, wide local excision is the treatment of choice. Five randomized trials have assessed the effect of margins of resection on local recurrence (15–19). For melanomas ≤1 mm in depth, local recurrence was not significantly different with 1 or 3 cm margins; therefore, 1-cm margins are acceptable for thin melanomas. For melanomas greater than 1 mm, the data generally support margins of 2 cm.

Randomized studies have failed to demonstrate a survival benefit for elective lymph node dissection in patients without clinically apparent nodal involvement, and this approach has largely been abandoned. The procedure of sentinel lymph node mapping and selective lymphadenectomy is highly sensitive for the detection of microscopic nodal metastases, and has a high negative predictive value. Thus, patients without clinical evidence of nodal involvement (the majority) can be accurately staged without the morbidity of a complete nodal dissection, and patients harboring occult nodal disease can be identified. For patients with a positive sentinel node, a complete dissection of the involved lymph node basin(s) is usually recommended, although the benefit of this procedure has not been formally demonstrated. The detection of occult nodal metastases also identifies patients who may be candidates for adjuvant systemic therapy with interferon-alfa (INTRON A), or participation in clinical trials.

In the Multicenter Selective Lymphadenectomy Trial, 1,327 patients with melanomas 1.2–3.5 mm were randomized to wide excision with sentinel node mapping and biopsy, or wide excision followed by observation (20). Patients found to have positive sentinel nodes underwent completion node dissections. At a median follow-up of 59.8 months, the melanoma specific survival in the two groups was not significantly different (death from melanoma occurred in 13.8% of the observation group and 12.5% of the biopsy group). However, patients assigned to biopsy had statistically superior disease-free survival compared with those who were observed (78.3% vs. 73.1%), and patients with positive sentinel nodes who underwent completion node dissection had markedly superior survival when compared with patients on the observation arm who subsequently developed clinically apparent nodal metastases and had therapeutic nodal dissections (5-year survival 72.3% vs. 52.4%, hazard ratio for death 0.51, confidence interval 0.32–0.81). Although based on a subgroup analysis, this finding suggests that sentinel node biopsy may identify patients who derive a survival benefit from early lymphadenectomy.

ADJUVANT THERAPY FOR HIGH-RISK MELANOMA

The staging criteria described above identify patients at high risk for recurrence and death. Most studies of adjuvant therapies have focused on patients with thick primary melanomas (>4 mm), and/or those with nodal involvement (stages IIB, IIC, and III), a group with an expected survival rate of less than 50%. Attempts to identify effective adjuvant therapy have been hampered by the absence of systemic therapies that produce meaningful response rates in advanced melanoma.

High-dose Interferon alfa-2b (HDI) has been the subject of three phase III trials in high-risk, resected melanoma (21–23), yet controversy persists about its efficacy. A pooled, updated analysis of two of these trials showed a relapse-free survival advantage for HDI versus observation (HR = 1.30, $p < 0.006$) at a median follow-up of 7.2 years, but no benefit for HDI in terms of overall survival (24). In a third trial, 880 patients with stage IIB–III melanoma were randomized to HDI or to vaccination with GM2, an immunogenic ganglioside expressed by melanoma cells. At a median follow-up of 2.4 years, there was a statistically significant advantage for HDI in terms of relapse-free and overall survival (24).

The impact of HDI on the risk of relapse seems confined to 20–30% of patients, and its adverse effects are considerable. Recent investigations suggest a correlation between autoimmunity and a benefit from interferon. In a cohort of 200 patients receiving HDI, those who developed autoimmune manifestations (vitiligo, thyroid dysfunction, or autoantibodies) had dramatically better outcomes: 7/52 (13.5%) relapsed, and 2/52 (4%) died, as compared with 108/148 (73%) relapses and 80/148 (54%) deaths in patients without autoimmunity ($p < 0.001$) (25). Identifying genetic factors that predispose to autoimmunity may allow selection of patients more likely to benefit from interferon.

Lower dose interferon regimens have not demonstrated consistent benefits in relapse-free or overall survival. Various vaccination strategies have been studied in the adjuvant setting, including whole-cell lysates, cellular fractions, and defined melanoma antigens. As yet, no phase III data supports the use of these agents.

METASTATIC MELANOMA

The prognosis for patients with metastatic melanoma is poor, with 1-year survival rates of 59% in patients with involvement only of skin, subcutaneous sites and lymph nodes (M1a), 57% with lung involvement (M1b), and 41% in patients with metastases to other visceral sites, or with an elevated lactate dehydrogenase level (M1c). Melanoma disseminates widely, and frequently involves sites that are unusual in other cancers, such as the GI tract and the skin. Brain metastases are very common, and are associated with a median survival of less than 4 months. Central nervous system involvement contributes to the death of approximately 50% of patients with metastatic melanoma.

No treatment has been demonstrated to improve median survival in metastatic melanoma, and response rates to systemic therapies are low. Despite these grim statistics, there are occasional spontaneous regressions, and some long-term survivors, including up to 15% of patients with M1a metastases (13, 14).

Surgery and Limb Perfusion

A small and highly selected group of patients with advanced melanoma may achieve prolonged freedom from relapse after surgical resection of metastases. The patients that appear most likely to benefit are those with a solitary metastasis involving skin, lungs, distant lymph nodes, or the gastrointestinal tract, those with a long disease-free interval, and those in whom the metastatic focus can be completely resected. In these patients, 5-year survival rates of 4–35% have been reported (26–30).

Isolated limb perfusion with melphalan and moderate hyperthermia is an effective treatment for recurrent or unresectable in-transit metastases of an extremity. High concentrations of chemotherapy to the limb can be achieved without excessive systemic exposure by isolation of the circulation, leading to complete responses in greater than 50% of patients (31).

Chemotherapy and Immunotherapy

Melanoma is refractory to most standard cytotoxic agents. Objective response rates to single-agent chemotherapy are in the range of 10–23%, and are typically of brief duration. Response rates to combination chemotherapy are somewhat higher, but toxicity is increased with the use of multiple agents, and no survival advantage has been demonstrated. Dacarbazine (DTIC) has been considered a "standard" treatment, and temozolomide (Temodar), an oral methylating agent, is commonly used. In a randomized trial comparing these agents, response rates were similar (13.5% with temozolomide and 12.1% with DTIC). Progression-free survival was slightly longer in the temozolomide arm (1.9 months vs. 1.5 months), but there was no statistical difference in overall survival (7.7 and 6.4 months) (32).

Several lines of evidence suggest that melanoma is immunogenic. Lymphocytic infiltration and regression of primary cutaneous melanoma is common. Melanoma antigens with the capacity to induce host T-cell responses have been identified and cloned.

Interleukin-2 (IL-2) is a central regulator of the cellular immune response, inducing activation and proliferation of T-cells and NK-cells. In vitro, it stimulates the development of lymphokine-activated killer (LAK) cells, which can lyse autologous tumor cells. IL-2 (Proleukin) treatment has been evaluated extensively in patients with metastatic melanoma. The objective response rate to high-dose IL-2 was 16% and the complete response rate was 6% in an analysis of 270 patients. Twelve of the responding patients remained progression free, including 10 patients in continuous complete remission. Five other responding patients remained disease free after surgery or radiation for limited sites of progressive disease (33). Patients with metastases limited to skin and subcutaneous sites appear most likely to benefit (response rate 53.6%) (34). IL-2 treatment is associated with substantial toxicity, including a capillary leak syndrome, hemodynamic instability, and a high risk of infection.

IL-2 has been evaluated in various contexts: with adoptive cellular immunotherapy using autologous LAK cells or tumor-infiltrating lymphocytes, with other cytokines, and with chemotherapy agents and vaccines. To date, none of these approaches has demonstrated clear superiority compared to IL-2 as a single agent.

Other cytokines have been the subject of clinical trials in metastatic melanoma, as have vaccines of tumor cells engineered to secrete cytokines, dendritic cell vaccines, and vaccines consisting of defined tumor antigens. Despite the demonstration that these approaches can induce in vivo antitumor immune responses, objective tumor regression has been sporadic at best (35).

Recent investigations in immunotherapy have focused on overcoming barriers to generating a sustained and effective antitumor immune response. Cytotoxic T-lymphocyte-associated antigen-4 (CTLA-4) is expressed on activated T-cells. When CTLA-4 is engaged by its ligands on antigen presenting cells, the T-cell response is inhibited and anergy may result. Monoclonal antibodies that block the interaction of CTLA-4 with its ligands enhance antitumor immune responses. Complete responses and sustained partial responses have been reported in up to 13% of patients with metastatic melanoma treated with anti-CTLA-4 antibodies, but serious autoimmune toxicity, including enterocolitis and hyphophysitis, has also been observed (36, 37). There appears to be a positive correlation between autoimmune phenomena and response.

A second putative mechanism of resistance to immunotherapy is the activity of regulatory T-cells (Tregs), a relatively minor population of CD4+CD25+ lymphocytes that are essential for immune homeostasis and prevention of autoimmunity. Tregs inhibit antitumor immune responses in murine models (38). Strategies to circumvent the effects of Tregs are under investigation. Lymphodepleting chemotherapy is one approach that has shown promise. Lymphodepletion with cyclophosphamide and fludarabine, followed by adoptive transfer of tumor-infiltrating lymphocytes with interleukin-2, was associated with a 51% response rate in 35 patients who had progressed after treatment with IL-2 alone (39).

Targeted Therapy for Melanoma

Recent research has begun to elucidate the genetic abnormalities underlying dysregulated growth, resistance to apoptosis, invasion, and metastasis in melanoma. Substantial molecular heterogeneity has been discovered among melanomas, but a number of mutations occur with high frequency and appear to be critical for survival and growth. Activating mutations in mitogen-activated protein kinase (MAP kinase) signal transduction pathway are found in the large majority of melanomas, most frequently in the serine-threonine kinase BRAF, where a single amino acid substitution (V600E) is present in 26–70%. Activating mutations are found in N-RAS in 15–30% of cases (40). These mutations are mutually exclusive in the large majority of melanomas. Melanomas lacking mutations in N-RAS or BRAF have been found to harbor abnormalities in cell cycle regulatory genes that may obviate the requirement for an activated MAP kinase pathway, e.g., amplification of CCND1 or CDK4, or loss of the tumor suppressor gene CDKN2A (p16) (41).

The majority of acral lentiginous and mucosal melanomas express wild-type BRAF and N-RAS, but have more diffuse chromosomal gains and losses than other types of melanoma (41). Approximately one-third have mutations or amplification of the gene encoding the receptor tyrosine kinase c-kit. Small-molecule signal transduction inhibitors that target the MAP kinase pathway are being evaluated in clinical trials in advanced melanoma.

Other genes and signaling pathways that contribute to the pathogenesis of melanoma include vascular endothelial growth factor and its receptors, the PI-3-kinase/Akt signaling pathway, regulators of NF-kB, and the microphthalmia-associated transcription factor (MITF).

OCULAR AND MUCOSAL MELANOMA

Ocular Melanoma

The incidence of intraocular melanoma is <1% that of cutaneous melanoma. UV light exposure, fair skin and light eye color have been implicated as risk factors (42). The large majority of uveal melanomas arise in the choroid. Uveal melanomas are often diagnosed on routine funduscopic exam, or present with visual symptoms. Small uveal melanomas can be difficult to distinguish from benign nevi, and can be followed closely, since some will not progress. Enucleation is reserved for advanced lesions. The majority of uveal melanomas can be treated either by brachytherapy with implantation of radioactive plaques, or by charged particle (proton or helium ion) radiotherapy. Local recurrence rates with these modalities are low, and survival rates are similar to those obtained with enucleation (43).

Risk factors for metastatic spread of uveal melanoma include tumor diameter, ciliary body involvement, and scleral or extraocular extension. Uveal melanoma is an aggressive disease, with metastases developing in 34% of patients within 10 years (44). Dissemination tends to be hematogenous, and up to 90% of patients who develop metastases have liver involvement. The mortality rate for metastatic uveal melanoma is 80% 1 year after diagnosis and 95% within 2 years (44).

Mucosal Melanoma

Mucosal melanomas are uncommon and aggressive tumors. They typically present at an advanced stage, and are associated with a poor prognosis. The most common sites are the female genitalia, the head and neck (oral and nasal cavities and paranasal sinuses), and the anorectal region. In each of these sites, surgical resection is the mainstay of therapy, but the high risk of distant relapse must be weighed when considering radical surgery.

For anorectal melanomas, sphincter-sparing surgery followed by radiotherapy is a reasonable alternative to abdominoperineal resection. Vulvar melanomas tend to occur in older, Caucasian women. Prognostic factors are similar to those for cutaneous sites, and wide local excision, when feasible, appears to be associated with outcomes similar to radical vulvectomy. Reported 5-year survival rates range from 22% to 54% (45–47) . Melanomas of the vaginal mucosa have an extremely poor prognosis, with a reported 5-year survival rate of 14% (48).

For mucosal melanomas of the head and neck, the possibility of cure rests on adequate surgical control of the primary tumor. Even with radical surgery, however, most patients will subsequently relapse and die from their disease. Five-year survival rates of 20–50% have been reported. Postoperative radiotherapy may decrease the likelihood of local relapse but is unlikely to affect survival given the high incidence of distant metastases (49).

REFERENCES

1. Jemal A, Siegel R, Ward E, et al. Cancer statistics, 2006. CA Cancer J Clin. 2006; 56(2): 106–130.
2. Ries L, Eisner MP Kosary CL, et al. (eds.). "SEER Cancer Statistics Review, 1975–2002," National Cancer Institute, Bethesda, MD, 2005.

3. GLOBOCAN. International Agency for Research on Cancer, 2002.

4. Stern RS. The risk of melanoma in association with long-term exposure to PUVA. J Am Acad Dermatol. 2001; 44(5): 755–761.

5. Gallagher RP, Spinelli JJ, Lee TK. Tanning beds, sunlamps, and risk of cutaneous malignant melanoma. Cancer Epidemiol Biomarkers Prev. 2005; 14(3): 562–566.

6. Goggins WB, Tsao H. A population-based analysis of risk factors for a second primary cutaneous melanoma among melanoma survivors. Cancer. 2003; 97(3): 639–643.

7. Bishop DT, Demenais F, Goldstein AM, et al. Geographical variation in the penetrance of CDKN2A mutations for melanoma. J Natl Cancer Inst. 2002; 94(12): 894–903.

8. FitzGerald MG, Harkin DP, Silva-Arrieta S, et al. Prevalence of germ-line mutations in p16, p19ARF, and CDK4 in familial melanoma: analysis of a clinic-based population. Proc Natl Acad Sci USA. 1996; 93(16): 8541–8545.

9. Kanetsky PA, Rebbeck TR, Hummer AJ, et al. Population-based study of natural variation in the melanocortin-1 receptor gene and melanoma. Cancer Res. 2006; 66(18): 9330–9337.

10. The Breast Cancer Linkage Consortium. Cancer risks in BRCA2 mutation carriers. J Natl Cancer Inst. 1999; 91(15): 1310–1316.

11. Geller AC, Zhang Z, Sober AJ, et al. The first 15 years of the American Academy of Dermatology skin cancer screening programs: 1985–1999. J Am Acad Dermatol. 2003; 48(1): 34–41.

12. Dennis LK, Beane Freeman LE, VanBeek MJ. Sunscreen use and the risk for melanoma: a quantitative review. Ann Intern Med. 2003; 139(12): 966–978.

13. Balch CM, Soong SJ, Gershenwald JE, et al. Prognostic factors analysis of 17,600 melanoma patients: validation of the American Joint Committee on Cancer melanoma staging system. J Clin Oncol. 2001; 19(16): 3622–3634.

14. Balch CM, Buzaid AC, Soong SJ, et al. Final version of the American Joint Committee on Cancer staging system for cutaneous melanoma. J Clin Oncol. 2001; 19(16): 3635–3648.

15. Veronesi U, Cascinelli N, Adamus J, et al. Thin stage I primary cutaneous malignant melanoma. Comparison of excision with margins of 1 or 3 cm. N Engl J Med. 1988; 318(18): 1159–1162.

16. Khayat D, Rixe O, Martin G, et al. Surgical margins in cutaneous melanoma (2 cm versus 5 cm for lesions measuring less than 2.1-mm thick). Cancer. 2003; 97(8): 1941–1946.

17. Cohn-Cedermark G, Rutqvist LE, Andersson R, et al. Long term results of a randomized study by the Swedish Melanoma Study Group on 2-cm versus 5-cm resection margins for patients with cutaneous melanoma with a tumor thickness of 0.8–2.0 mm. Cancer. 2000; 89(7): 1495–1501.

18. Balch CM, Soong SJ, Smith T, et al. Long-term results of a prospective surgical trial comparing 2 cm vs. 4 cm excision margins for 740 patients with 1–4 mm melanomas. Ann Surg Oncol. 2001; 8(2): 101–108.

19. Thomas JM, Newton-Bishop J, A'Hern R, et al. Excision margins in high-risk malignant melanoma. N Engl J Med. 2004; 350(8): 757–766.

20. Morton DL, Thompson JF, Cochran AJ, et al. Sentinel-node biopsy or nodal observation in melanoma. N Engl J Med. 2006; 355(13): 1307–1317.

21. Kirkwood JM, Strawderman MH, Ernstoff MS, Smith TJ, Borden EC, Blum RH. Interferon alfa-2b adjuvant therapy of high-risk resected cutaneous melanoma: the Eastern Cooperative Oncology Group Trial EST 1684. J Clin Oncol. 1996; 14(1): 7–17.

22. Kirkwood JM, Ibrahim JG, Sondak VK, et al. High- and low-dose interferon alfa-2b in high-risk melanoma: first analysis of intergroup trial E1690/S9111/C9190. J Clin Oncol. 2000; 18(12): 2444–2458.

23. Kirkwood JM, Ibrahim JG, Sosman JA, et al. High-dose interferon alfa-2b significantly prolongs relapse-free and overall survival compared with the GM2-KLH/QS-21 vaccine in patients with resected stage IIB-III melanoma:

results of intergroup trial E1694/S9512/C509801. J Clin Oncol. 2001; 19(9): 2370–2380.

24. Kirkwood JM, Manola J, Ibrahim J, Sondak V, Ernstoff MS, Rao U. A pooled analysis of eastern cooperative oncology group and intergroup trials of adjuvant high-dose interferon for melanoma. Clin Cancer Res. 2004; 10(5): 1670–1677.

25. Gogas H, Ioannovich J, Dafni U, et al. Prognostic significance of autoimmunity during treatment of melanoma with interferon. N Engl J Med. 2006; 354(7): 709–718.

26. Wong JH, Skinner KA, Kim KA, Foshag LJ, Morton DL. The role of surgery in the treatment of nonregionally recurrent melanoma. Surgery. 1993; 113(4): 389–394.

27. Fletcher WS, Pommier RF, Lum S, Wilmarth TJ. Surgical treatment of metastatic melanoma. Am J Surg. 1998; 175(5): 413–417.

28. Karakousis CP, Velez A, Driscoll DL, Takita H. Metastasectomy in malignant melanoma. Surgery. 1994; 115(3): 295–302.

29. Leo F, Cagini L, Rocmans P, et al. Lung metastases from melanoma: when is surgical treatment warranted? Br J Cancer. 2000; 83(5): 569–572.

30. Agrawal S, Yao TJ, Coit DG. Surgery for melanoma metastatic to the gastrointestinal tract. Ann Surg Oncol. 1999; 6(4): 336–344.

31. Grunhagen DJ, de Wilt JH, van Geel AN, Eggermont AM. Isolated limb perfusion for melanoma patients—a review of its indications and the role of tumour necrosis factor-alpha. Eur J Surg Oncol. 2006; 32(4): 371–380.

32. Middleton MR, Grob JJ, Aaronson N, et al. Randomized phase III study of temozolomide versus dacarbazine in the treatment of patients with advanced metastatic malignant melanoma. J Clin Oncol. 2000; 18(1): 158–166.

33. Atkins MB, Lotze MT, Dutcher JP, et al. High-dose recombinant interleukin 2 therapy for patients with metastatic melanoma: analysis of 270 patients treated between 1985 and 1993. J Clin Oncol. 1999; 17(7): 2105–2116.

34. Phan GQ, Attia P, Steinberg SM, White DE, Rosenberg SA. Factors associated with response to high-dose interleukin-2 in patients with metastatic melanoma. J Clin Oncol. 2001; 19(15): 3477–3482.

35. Restifo NP, Rosenberg SA. Use of standard criteria for assessment of cancer vaccines. Lancet Oncol. 2005; 6(1): 3–4.

36. Attia P, Phan GQ, Maker AV, et al. Autoimmunity correlates with tumor regression in patients with metastatic melanoma treated with anti-cytotoxic T-lymphocyte antigen-4. J Clin Oncol. 2005; 23(25): 6043–6053.

37. Ribas A, Camacho LH, Lopez-Berestein G, et al. Antitumor activity in melanoma and anti-self responses in a phase I trial with the anti-cytotoxic T lymphocyte-associated antigen 4 monoclonal antibody CP-675,206. J Clin Oncol. 2005; 23(35): 8968–8977.

38. Shimizu J, Yamazaki S, Sakaguchi S. Induction of tumor immunity by removing CD25+CD4+ T cells: a common basis between tumor immunity and autoimmunity. J Immunol. 1999; 163(10): 5211–5218.

39. Dudley ME, Wunderlich JR, Yang JC, et al. Adoptive cell transfer therapy following non-myeloablative but lymphodepleting chemotherapy for the treatment of patients with refractory metastatic melanoma. J Clin Oncol. 2005; 23(10): 2346–2357.

40. Davies H, Bignell GR, Cox C, et al. Mutations of the BRAF gene in human cancer. Nature. 2002; 417(6892): 949–954.

41. Curtin JA, Fridlyand J, Kageshita T, et al. Distinct sets of genetic alterations in melanoma. N Engl J Med. 2005; 353(20): 2135–2147.

42. Tucker MA, Shields JA, Hartge P, Augsburger J, Hoover RN, Fraumeni JF, Jr. Sunlight exposure as risk factor for intraocular malignant melanoma. N Engl J Med. 1985; 313(13): 789–792.

43. Grin JM, Grant-Kels JM, Grin CM, Berke A, Kels BD. Ocular melanomas and melanocytic lesions of the eye. J Am Acad Dermatol. 1998; 38(5 Pt 1): 716–730.

44. Diener-West M, Reynolds SM, Agugliaro DJ, et al. Development of metastatic disease after enrollment in the COMS trials for treatment of choroidal melanoma: Collaborative Ocular Melanoma Study Group Report No. 26. Arch Ophthalmol. 2005; 123(12): 1639–1643.

45. Trimble EL, Lewis JL Jr, Williams LL, et al. Management of vulvar melanoma. Gynecol Oncol. 1992; 45(3): 254–258.

46. Davidson T, Kissin M, Westbury G. Vulvo-vaginal melanoma—should radical surgery be abandoned? Br J Obstet Gynaecol. 1987; 94(5): 473–476.

47. DeMatos P, Tyler D, Seigler HF. Mucosal melanoma of the female genitalia: a clinicopathologic study of forty-three cases at Duke University Medical Center. Surgery. 1998; 124(1): 38–48.

48. Creasman WT, Phillips JL, Menck HR. The National Cancer Data Base report on cancer of the vagina. Cancer. 1998;83(5):1033–1040.

49. Mendenhall WM, Amdur RJ, Hinerman RW, Werning JW, Villaret DB, Mendenhall NP. Head and neck mucosal melanoma. Am J Clin Oncol. 2005; 28(6): 626–630.

62

Sam S. Yoon, Francis J. Hornicek,
David C. Harmon, Thomas F. DeLaney

SOFT TISSUE AND BONE SARCOMAS

SOFT TISSUE SARCOMAS

Soft tissue sarcomas (STS) are uncommon malignancies with an estimated 9,530 newly diagnosed patients and 3,500 deaths in the United States in 2006. Although malignant tumors of soft tissue are scarce, benign tumors including lipomas are 100 times more common. STS occur at any age with a median age of around 50 years old, and are equally common in men and women.

STS constitute a highly heterogeneous group of tumors with respect to anatomical distribution, histologic subtype, and clinical behavior (1). STS occur throughout the body, but nearly one-half occur in the extremities, with about one-third occurring in the lower extremity and 15% occurring in the upper extremity. Another one-third of STS occur in the abdomen, and these are equally divided among intra-abdominal visceral sarcomas (primarily gastrointestinal stromal tumors and leiomyosarcomas) and retroperitoneal sarcomas. Other anatomic sites include the head/neck, trunk, and other miscellaneous sites (e.g., heart).

STS are comprised of all of the malignant tumors which arise from the mesodermal tissues (e.g., fat, muscle, connective tissue, and vessels) excluding bone and cartilage. In addition, malignant tumors of peripheral nerve sheaths are usually included despite being ectodermal in origin. There are over 50 different histologic subtypes of STS: most common are liposarcoma, malignant fibrous histiocytoma, and leiomyosarcoma. All suspected STS cases should be reviewed by a pathologist experienced in sarcomas given that about 10% of cases originally designated as STS are in fact not STS and about 20% are initially assigned the incorrect histologic subtype. While each histologic subtype may have certain specific clinical behaviors, all STS can generally be categorized into low, intermediate, and high-grade tumors. Low-grade tumors grow more slowly, can locally recur after resection, but have a low risk of distant metastases (about 5%). High-grade tumors tend to grow more rapidly, can recur locally, and have the added risk of distant metastasis that can approach 50% for large tumors.

The treatment of STS has advanced significantly over the past few decades. In particular, evidence has accumulated that in addition to surgery, there are important roles for radiation therapy and chemotherapy in the management of some STS patients. Optimal results from more conservative local treatment strategies require a multidisciplinary approach to the overall management of these patients. The team should include not only an experienced and specialized surgeon, but also a radiation oncologist, medical oncologist, pathologist, and diagnostic radiologist expert in the disease.

Etiology

The vast majority of STS occur as sporadic tumors in patients with no identified genetic or environmental risk factors. However, certain genetic syndromes are

Table 62-1

Soft Tissue Sarcoma Chromosomal Translocations and Genes Involved

Histologic subtype	Translocation	Genes involved
Alveolar rhabdomyosarcoma	t(2;13) (q35,q14)	PAX3, FKHR
	t(1;13) (p36;q14)	PAX7, FKHR
Alveolar soft part sarcoma	t(X;17) (p11;q25)	TFE2, ASPL
Clear cell sarcoma	t(12;22) (q13;q12)	ATF1; EWF
Dermatofibrosarcoma protuberans	t(17;22) (q22;q13)	COL1A1, PDGFB1
Desmoplastic small round cell tumor	t(11;22) (p13;q12)	WT1, EWS
Ewing's sarcoma/primitive neuroectodermal tumor	t(11;22) (q24;q12)	FLI1, EWS
	t(21;22) (q22;q12)	ERG ,EWS
	t(7;22) (p22;q12)	ETV1, EWS
	t(2;22) (q33;q12)	FEV, EWS
	t(17;22) (q12;q12)	E1AF, EWS
Extraskeletal myxoid chondrosarcoma	t(9;22) (q21–31;q12.2)	CHN, EWS
	t(9;17) (q22;q11)	CHN, RBP56
Myxoid/round cell liposarcoma	t(12;16) (q13;p11)	CHOP, TLS
	t(12;22) (q13;q11–q12)	CHOP, EWS
Synovial sarcoma	t(X;18) (p11.2;q11.2)	SSX1 or SSX2, SYT

Adapted from (2).

associated with an increased risk of developing sarcomas including neurofibromatosis 1 (NF1, von Recklinghausen's disease), hereditary retinoblastoma and Li-Fraumeni syndrome. Specific genetic abnormalities, evidenced by nonrandom chromosomal aberrations, are well established in certain STS histologic subtypes, and are often utilized in the definitive diagnosis (Table 62-1).

Radiation is recognized as capable of inducing sarcomas of bone and soft tissue. The frequency increases with radiation dose and with the post-radiation observation period. Chemotherapeutic agents are likewise associated with risks of sarcoma induction. Exposure to a few selected industrial chemicals may be followed by the appearance of sarcomas. STS (primarily lymphangiosarcomas) may be observed following massive and quite protracted edema after axillary lymphadenectomy (Stewart-Treves syndrome). Chronic irritation secondary to foreign bodies may be a factor in the induction of sarcomas. Trauma is rarely a factor in the development of these tumors with the exception of desmoid tumors.

Staging

The Task Force on STS of the American Joint Committee on Cancer (AJCC) Staging and End Result Reporting has established a staging system for STS which is an extension of the TNM system to include G for histological grade (Table 62-2). Grade, size, depth, and presence of nodal or distant metastases are the determinants of stage. Some institutions will assign grades 1–3, where grade 1 lesions are considered low grade with minimal metastatic potential and the intermediate grade 2 and high grade 3 lesions are considered high grade and capable of metastatic disease. Other institutions use a 2- or 4-tiered system.

Table 62-2

AJCC Staging System for Soft Tissue Sarcomas

Histological grade of malignancy
GX   Grade cannot be assessed
G1   Well differentiated
G2   Moderately differentiated
G3   Poorly differentiated
G4   Undifferentiated

T Primary tumor
TX   Primary tumor cannot be assessed
T0   No evidence of primary tumor
T1   Tumor 5 cm or less in greatest dimension
T1a   Superficial tumor
T1b   Deep tumor
T2   Tumor greater than 5 cm in greatest dimension
T2a   Superficial tumor
T2b   Deep tumor

N Regional lymph nodes
NX   Regional lymph nodes cannot be assessed
N0   No histologically verified metastases to regional lymph nodes
N1   Histologically verified regional lymph node metastasis

M Distant metastasis
MX   Distant metastasis cannot be assessed
M0   No distant metastasis
M1   Distant metastasis

Stage I	A	Low grade, small, superficial and deep	G1-2	T1a-1b	N0	M0
	B	Low grade, large, superficial	G1-2	T2a	N0	M0
Stage II	A	Low grade, large, deep	G1-2	T2b	N0	M0
	B	High grade, small, superficial and deep	G3-4	T1a-1b	N0	M0
	C	High grade, large, superficial	G3-4	T2a	N0	M0
Stage III		High grade, large, deep	G3-4	T2b	N0	M0
Stage IV		Any metastasis	any G	any T	N1	M0
			any G	any T	N0	M1

Used with the permission of the American Joint Committee on Cancer (AJCC), Chicago, Illinois. The original source for this material is the AJCC Cancer Staging Manual, Sixth Edition (2002) published by Springer-New York, www.springerlink.com.

EXTREMITY STS

Clinical Evaluation   The most frequent initial complaint is that of a painless mass for a few weeks to several months. Occasionally, pain or tenderness precedes the detection of a mass. With progressive growth of the tumor, symptoms appear which are usually secondary to infiltration of or pressure on adjacent structures. One should obtain a complete history and physical examination, with particular attention paid to the region of the primary lesion: definition of size, site of origin (superficial or deep, attached to or fixed to deep structures), involvement or discoloration of overlying skin, functional status of vessels and nerves, mass effect on adjacent organs and joints, and presence of distal edema. Laboratory studies need not go beyond a complete blood count and chemistry panel. There are no tumors markers for STS.

For the primary site, the radiographic evaluation should include a CT scan or MRI. The most useful radiologic study to evaluate an extremity or trunk primary site is the MRI, but CT scans can provide supplemental information. A chest CT should be obtained for high-grade tumors to evaluate for lung metastases. A chest X-ray is adequate for low-grade tumors. The role of PET scans has yet to be defined, but many primary and metastatic tumors do show increased FDG uptake.

An adequate biopsy is required to determine a histologic diagnosis as to tumor type and grade and to determine an optimal treatment strategy. In the majority of cases, the diagnosis can be established by core needle biopsy. Superficial lesions which are readily palpable can be directly biopsied without imaging, but for tumors which are located at depth, a CT-directed approach is advocated. Open biopsies should be reserved for the uncommon cases where core biopsy is not adequate. The incision for open biopsies should be oriented longitudinally such that it can be easily incorporated in the definitive resection. For tumors <3–5 cm in size, an excisional biopsy can be performed, and incisional biopsies can be performed for larger lesions. Care should be taken to minimize bleeding and contamination of surrounding tissues. Fine needle biopsy can be employed to confirm metastatic or recurrent tumor when the primary diagnosis is already established.

Surgery and Radiation Therapy   Several surgical principles should be followed when resecting STS. First, the pre-operative imaging studies should be carefully examined to identify the full extent of tumor penetration as well as the relationship of the tumor to adjacent structures. Second, tumors should be resected with about a 2 cm margin of normal tissue if this can be performed without severe morbidity. Third, some normal tissues such as fascia provide a better quality margin than other tissues such as fat and muscle. One can often accept a few millimeters of fascia margin but should be more concerned about a close margin of fat or muscle. Fourth, STS usually do not invade the peri-adventitial tissue of arteries or the periosteum of bone and can often be dissected along these planes. Surgeons must use considerable judgment in resecting STS. Positive microscopic margins are very strongly associated with an increased risk of local recurrence, and one should strive for negative microscopic margins in all cases unless this would create major or unacceptable morbidity. In such cases one may rely on adjuvant radiation therapy in order to reduce major surgical morbidity, given radiation can usually be delivered in doses to the extremity that can eradicate microscopic residual disease.

If STS are "shelled out" as is performed for benign tumors such as lipomas, the local recurrence will be up to 90% after surgery alone. Radical resection of tumors with a margin of normal tissue can decrease the local recurrence rate to 10–30%. However, many extremity STS grow adjacent to major blood vessels and bones, and the standard operation for many STS up until the early 1980s was amputation. Rosenberg SA et al. at the National Cancer Institute (NCI) published a randomized trial of amputation versus limb-sparing surgery and radiation (both groups received chemotherapy) in 1982 and demonstrated equivalent overall survival with a local recurrence rate of 0% versus 15% (3) Currently limb-sparing surgery can be performed in over 90% of patients with extremity STS, and overall local recurrence rates are often less than 10%.

Several studies have defined the essential role of radiation therapy in the local control of STS. Another NCI randomized trial published in 1998 comparing limb-spring surgery alone to surgery and external beam radiation (patients with high-grade tumors all received chemotherapy) demonstrated that radiation reduced local recurrence from 20–33% to 0–4% (4). The rate of distant recurrence was the same in both groups. Brachytherapy has also been used to deliver radiation. In a randomized trial of surgery alone versus surgery and brachytherapy, local recurrence for high-grade tumors was reduced from 30% to 5% with brachytherapy. At our institution, brachytherapy is usually reserved for patients who have a local recurrence after prior surgery and radiation, and this allows the delivery of additional radiation while minimizing morbidity. Brachytherapy or intra-operative radiation therapy can also be used to deliver a focal boost to areas of close or positive surgical margins.

The sequencing of radiation therapy in relation to surgery is a subject of debate between major sarcoma centers. One randomized trial by the Canadian NCI examined pre-operative and post-operative radiation therapy and found no difference in local control (5). Wound complications were twice as high in the pre-operative therapy group (35% vs. 17%), but tissue fibrosis and other late complications were more frequent in the post-operative radiation group.

There are certain situations such as difficult anatomical location (e.g., spine or base of skull) or major medical comorbidities in which a conservative surgical procedure cannot be performed and radiation alone is delivered. In one study from Memorial Sloan-Kettering, 25 patients were treated by radiotherapy alone, and local control was achieved in 14 of the 25 patients. To achieve a high probability of local control, high doses of 70–75 Gy are essential. Among patients receiving ≥ 63 Gy, Kepka et al. reported local control in 72% of patients with tumors ≥ 5 cm in size, 42% for lesions >5 cm but ≤ 10 cm , and only 25% for lesions >10 cm (6). Because high doses are required for control of these unresected lesions, special treatment techniques such as proton beam radiation may be required to deliver dose and stay within the constraints of normal tissue tolerance.

Patients with large (>8–10 cm), deep, high-grade sarcomas present more difficult problems in terms of local control and are at significant risk of distant metastasis. Some groups have combined chemotherapy with surgery and radiation therapy strategies. Eilber and Morton have been proponents of a program, which has consisted of intra-arterial doxorubicin followed by rapid fraction radiation therapy (3.5 Gy/fraction, 28 Gy total) and subsequent local excision. Their data have shown local recurrence rates of <10% with survival rates of 74% in Stage III tumors. Among these patients, there was a 5% amputation rate. They have since shown that it is not necessary to provide the doxorubicin by an intra-arterial route. Our institution has employed a regimen of pre-operative mesna, Adriamycin, ifosfamide, and dacarbazine (MAID) chemotherapy interdigitated with radiation therapy (44 Gy) followed by post-operative MAID chemotherapy for patients with >8 cm, high-grade STS (7). Five-year local control was 92% and 5-year overall survival was 87%. In experimental protocols, hyperthermic isolated limb perfusion (HILP) with chemotherapeutic agents (e.g., tumor necrosis factor alpha, melphalan, and interferon gamma) have been used to control large tumors that would otherwise require amputation because of proximity to nerve or blood vessels.

Adjuvant Chemotherapy   Although surgery and radiotherapy achieve control of the primary tumor in the majority of patients, many patients (especially those with large, high-grade tumors) develop and die of metastatic disease not evident at diagnosis. Doxorubicin and ifosfamide are the most active chemotherapy agents in metastatic STS. For doxorubicin, objective response rates between 20% and 40% have been reported. Several prospective studies using single agent doxorubicin failed to show an improvement in disease-free or overall survival in patients receiving post-operative chemotherapy compared with surgery alone. The large EORTC study of adjuvant chemotherapy employed CyVADic consisting of cyclophosphamide, vincristine, Adriamycin and DTIC found improved 7-year recurrence-free survival (56% vs. 43%) but no significant difference in overall survival (63% vs. 56%) (8). A meta-analysis of

14 randomized trials of doxorubicin-based adjuvant chemotherapy versus no chemotherapy in STS was performed in 1997 (9). The adjuvant chemotherapy group had a statistically significant higher rate of local recurrence-free survival (81% vs. 75%, $p = 0.016$), distant recurrence-free survival (70% vs. 60%, $p = 5$ 0.003), and overall-recurrence-free survival (55% vs. 45%, $p = 5$ 0.001). However, overall survival differed only by 4% (54% vs. 50%) and this difference did not attain statistical significance. The trend toward benefit in the few, under-powered studies done to date may favor the use of adjuvant chemotherapy for the highest risk patients. However, the toxicities associated with these chemotherapeutic agents dictate caution in generalizing adjuvant chemotherapy to all patients and favor continuing enrollment of patients in clinical trials.

Retroperitoneal STS   Approximately 10–15% of STS arise in the retroperitoneum. These tumors are usually asymptomatic until reaching large sizes and often identified on imaging studies for unrelated complaints. Patients may also present with a palpable abdominal mass or with symptoms such as abdominal pain or lower extremity neurologic symptoms. Since the retroperitoneum can often accommodate large tumors without symptoms, the average size of tumors in large series is often greater than 10 cm. Upon histologic examination, about two-thirds of tumors are either liposarcomas or leiomyosarcomas, with the remaining tumors distributed among a large variety of other histologic subtypes. Retroperitoneal liposarcomas are further classified into well-differentiated, de-differentiated, myxoid-round cell, and pleomorphic subtypes.

Most unifocal tumors in the retroperitoneum that do not arise from adjacent organs will be either benign soft tissue tumors (e.g., Schwannomas) or sarcomas. Other malignancies in the differential diagnosis include primary germ cell tumor, metastatic testicular cancer, and lymphoma. Following a careful history and physical examination, radiologic assessment of these tumors is usually performed with an abdominal and pelvic CT scan. Liposarcomas often have a characteristic appearance with large areas of abnormal appearing fat (well-differentiated liposarcoma) sometimes containing higher density nodules (de-differentiated liposarcoma). Patients with high-grade tumors should have a chest CT to evaluate for lung metastases. A chest x-ray is adequate for low-grade tumors.

The primary treatment for the local control of these tumors is surgical resection (10). The optimal goal of surgical resection, complete gross resection with microscopically negative margins, can be difficult to accomplish, and complete gross resection rates in large series are reported to be around 60%. In about three-quarters of cases, complete gross resection requires removal of adjacent viscera. The goal of obtaining negative microscopic margins for large retroperitoneal tumors is frequently not achieved. These tumors are surrounded by a pseudocapsule that often contains microscopic disease, and dissection with a normal tissue margin away from the pseudocapsule is difficult, especially along the posterior aspect of the tumor where it abuts the retroperitoneal fat and musculature. Controversy exists as to the optimal role of radiation therapy for local control of retroperitoneal sarcomas. Those who advocate radiation therapy usually prefer that radiation be delivered preoperatively. With the tumor still in place, normal organs are pushed away from the radiation field, the margin around the tumor at risk of local recurrence is more clearly defined, and the effective radiation dose required to control microscopic disease is likely lower.

In the extremity, the local control of sarcomas treated with total gross resection with positive microscopic margin and adjuvant radiation therapy is about 75%. Typically, positive microscopic margins are treated with a boost of post-operative radiation to a total dose of about 60–70 Gy. It is reasonable to assume that total gross resection of retroperitoneal tumors along with adequate doses of radiation could achieve local control rates similar to that seen for extremity tumors resected with positive microscopic margins. However, unlike the extremity, it is difficult to deliver high doses of radiation to the abdomen. The availability of intensity modulated radiation therapy, proton beam radiation, and intra-operative radiation therapy may facilitate the efficacy and minimize morbidity of adjuvant radiation therapy for these tumors. In a report from our institution, 29 patients were treated with pre-operative radiation to a median dose of 45 Gy and then underwent complete gross resection (11). Intra-operative radiation therapy (IORT) (10–20 Gy) was delivered to 16 of the 29 patients. Local control at 5 years was 83% for patients who received both pre-operative and intra-operative radiation therapy and 61% for those who received only pre-operative radiation. More recently, we have incorporated the use of pre-operative proton beam radiation therapy along with resection and intra-operative radiation therapy for retroperitoneal tumors to further minimize morbidity on adjacent structures.

Follow-up   The intensity of follow-up visits and imaging studies varies between institutions, and can also be varied according to tumor grade. At our institution, for low-grade and high-grade lesions, patients are evaluated by history and physical examination every 3 months for the first two years, every 6 months from years 2–5, and then yearly. Imaging of the primary tumor site depends on the location. For superficial tumors, physical examination is often sufficient. For deeper extremity tumors, CT scan or MRI may be performed with every other visit. For intra-abdominal or retroperitoneal tumors, CT scan are performed with every other visit for 5 years, and then yearly with each visit. For low-grade lesions, chest x-rays are obtained every other visit over the first 5 years and then yearly. For high-grade lesions, chest CT scans are obtained with every other visit over the first 5 years, and then a chest x-ray can be obtained yearly.

METASTATIC DISEASE

While local control of STS can be attained in >90% of patients, up to 50% of patients present with or develop metastatic disease. Median survival after the development of metastatic disease is 8–12 months. The most common site of metastatic disease for extremity and trunk STS is the lung. Intra-abdominal and retroperitoneal sarcomas metastasize with about equal frequency to the lung and liver. STS uncommonly metastasize to regional lymph nodes (about 5%) except for certain histologic subtypes including epithelioid sarcoma, rhabdomyosarcoma, hemangiosarcoma, and synovial sarcoma.

As noted above, doxorubicin and ifosfamide have been demonstrated to be the most active chemotherapy agents in widely disseminated soft tissue sarcoma (12). Response rates range from about 20–30%, and there is some evidence that higher doses can result in increased response rates. These two agents carry significant risks of toxicity: doxorubicin dosage is limited by cardiotoxicity and ifosfamide causes hemorrhagic cystitis and nephrotoxicity. Ifosfamide-induced hemorrhagic cystitis can be avoided by adding the protective agent mesna. Another agent with some activity against STS is dacarbazine (DTIC), with reported response rates around 20%. However for metastatic disease, complete responses are uncommon (<15% even with combination therapy), duration of response averages 8 months, and as yet the higher response rates seen with intense combination therapy have not been proven to provide a survival advantage over that conferred by sequential single agent treatment.

A variety of combination chemotherapy regimens for metastatic disease have been studied in randomized clinical trials. Most of these studies were small

Table 62-3

Selected Randomized Chemotherapy Trials for Metastatic Soft Tissue Sarcomas

Investigator/group (year)	Regimen	Patients (n)	Response rate (%)	Median survival (m)
Schoenfeld et al. ECOG (1983)	A	54	27	8.5
	CyAV	56	19	7.7
	CyActV	58	11	9.4
Borden et al. ECOG (1987)	A q 3 wks	94	18	8.0
	A q wk	89	16	8.4
	ADtic	92	30	8.0
Borden et al. ECOG (1990)	A	148	17	9.4
	AVd	143	18	9.9
Edmonson et al. ECOG (1993)	A	90	20	<9
	AI	88	34	11
	MAP	84	32	9
Santoro et al. EORTC (1995)	A	263	23	12.0
	AI	258	28	12.7
	CyVADtic	142	28	11.8
Antman et al. CALBG/ SWOG (1993)	AD	170	17	12
	AID	170	32	13
Nielsen et al. EORTC (1998)	A	112	14	10.4
	Epi	111	15	10.8
	Epi	111	14	10.4
EORTC meta-analysis (1999)	Any anthracycline-based regimen	2185	26	11.8

A, doxorubicin (adriamycin); Act, actinomycin; CALGB, Cancer and Leukemia and Group B; Cy, cyclophosphamid; Dtic, dacarbazine; Epi, epirubicin; I, ifosfamide; M, mitomycin C; P, Cisplatin; SWOG, Southwest Oncology Group; V, vincristine; Vd, vindesine.

Adapted from Brennan et al. (12).

and included mixed histologies (see Table 62-3). Most of these trials include doxorubicin (or epirubicin) and an alkylating agent. Overall survival for any combination chemotherapy regimen has not been clearly demonstrated to be superior to doxorubicin alone, but trials have been underpowered due to the rarity of this disease type. The most commonly used combination chemotherapy regimen is MAID (Mesna, Adriamycin, ifosfamide, and dacarbazine). In a large Phase II trial, this regimen achieved an overall response rate of 47%. When MAID was compared to the combination of Adriamycin and Dacarbazine in a randomized trial, the response rate was higher for MAID (32% vs. 17%). However, there were more toxic deaths in the MAID group and there was no survival advantage to MAID. Higher doses of chemotherapy can be given with better control of toxicity if GCSF is used.

There are ongoing trials evaluating the use of other chemotherapy agents such as taxotere, gemcitabine, vinorelbine, and topotecan. Some histologies may be particularly sensitive to specific agents, such as scalp angiosarcoma to Taxol. Another agent that has shown some promise in recent trials against STS is ET-743, which is also known as Yondelis or Trabectidin. This drug seems to have particular activity against myxoid liposarcomas but is not yet approved for marketing. Patients with metastatic disease should be strongly considered for enrollment in investigational trials.

Surgical resection has been performed for isolated STS metastases to the lung or liver. For select patients with STS metastases isolated to the lung, surgical resection (a.k.a. metastasectomy) can be performed, and 5-year survival can approach 20–30%. Intra-abdominal and retroperitoneal STS metastasize commonly to the liver as well as the lung. Isolated, resectable liver metastases from STS are less common than isolated, resectable lung metastases, but several small series have examined hepatectomy for these patients and 5-year survival can reach 30%.

GASTROINTESTINAL STROMAL TUMORS

Gastrointestinal stromal tumors (GIST) are the most common mesenchymal tumor of the gastrointestinal tract and are thought to originate from the interstitial cells of Cajal (13). Interstitial cells of Cajal and the vast majority of GIST express c-KIT, which is a 145 kD transmembrane glycoprotein that acts as the receptor for stem cell factor (SCF). Prior to the identification and availability of immunohistochemistry for c-KIT, the majority of GIST were thought to be of smooth muscle origin and termed leiomyomas, leiomyosarcomas, and leiomyoblastomas. It is now known that the majority of stromal tumors of the gastrointestinal tract are GIST. Ninety-five percent of GIST stain positive on immunohistochemistry for c-KIT, and the majority of GIST have a mutation in the c-KIT gene. Unlike most other cancers, GIST seem highly dependent on this single pathway for neoplastic growth.

GIST can occur at nearly all ages, with the median age being around 60. The incidence is roughly equal in men and women. There are roughly 5,000 cases per year in the United States. GIST are located most commonly in the stomach (60%) followed by the small intestine (30%), colon/rectum (5%), and esophagus (5%). These tumors can be found on upper endoscopy, where they appear as submucosal lesions. However, even large GIST of the stomach may not be seen on endoscopy if they are pedunculated or exophytic. Endoscopic biopsy can establish the diagnosis, especially following staining for c-KIT expression. For small bowel tumors, CT-guided biopsy poses the risk of inadequate tissue and spillage of tumor cells and is likely not necessary given most isolated small bowel tumors require resection. Staging workup should include an abdomen and pelvis CT scan to rule out intra-abdominal or liver metastases.

GIST can range from small, pedunculated lesions to large lesions with adherence or invasion of surrounding tissues and organs. Thus the surgical approach can be quite varied but certain principles should be followed. Upon surgical exploration, the liver and peritoneal cavity should be examined for possible metastatic disease. GIST uncommonly metastasize to lymph nodes so a regional lymphadenectomy is not required. Thus for a pedunculated gastric tumor, wedge resection of the gastric wall along with resection of the tumor is adequate. Some gastric tumors encompass a large portion of the stomach and a formal distal, subtotal, or even total gastrectomy may be required. For small bowel and colon tumors, segmental bowel resection can be performed. Small rectal GIST can be removed through transanal procedures while larger tumor may require low anterior resection or even abdominal-perineal resection. Some large GIST with significant necrosis are susceptible to tumor rupture and spillage, which can lead to intra-peritoneal spread of disease, and so these tumors should be manipulated carefully. For large GIST that invade adjacent organs, an en bloc resection of should be performed.

Risk of recurrence is most closely related to size and mitotic count. A surgical series from Memorial Sloan-Kettering found in 80 patients with resected GIST that size was the most important predictor of overall survival, with 5 year overall survival being 60% for tumors <5 cm, 45% for tumors 5–10 cm, and 20% for tumors >10 cm. The most common sites of metastasis are the liver and

Table 62-4

Imatinib Trials for Metastatic GIST

Trial	Phase	Patients	Dose	Follow-up	CR	PR	SD	PD
		(*n*)	(mg/day)	(months)	%	%	%	%
Demetri et al.	II	73	400	10	0	36	23	12
US and Finland		74	600		0	43	18	8
(2002)								
Verweij et al.	III	470	400	25	5	45	32	13
EORTC		472	800		6	48	32	9
(2004)								
Benjamin et al.	III	361	400	14	NR	43	32	NR
US Intergroup		360	800		NR	41	32	NR
(2003)								

Adapted from van der Zwan SM et al. (13).

CR, complete response; PR, partial response; SD, stable disease; PD, progressive disease; PFS, progression-free survival.

peritoneal cavity, and less common sites include the lung and bone. Prior to the introduction of imatinib (a.k.a. Gleevac), GIST were found to be highly resistant to chemotherapeutic agents. Imatinib inhibits both the c-KIT receptor and platelet-derived growth factor receptor (PDGFR) tyrosine kinases. Several large studies have shown imatinib to be highly effective against metastatic GIST, with a partial response rate of about 40% and stable disease rate of about 30% (see Table 62-4). The median time to progression is 19–24 months. Even tumors that are sensitive to imatinib may take months to show a decrease in tumor size on CT scans, and so PET scans have been employed to assess response. GIST are usually positive on PET scans, and response to imatinib as demonstrated by decrease in PET activity can frequently be seen after just 1–2 weeks and sometimes within a day. The role of imatinib in the adjuvant setting is currently being studied in large, multicenter trials in the United States and Europe.

The role of surgery for metastatic GIST has yet to be defined. Some investigators surgically resect or debulk imatinib-responsive disease to decrease tumor burden and hypothetically delay the development of imatinib resistance. When resistance to imatinib ultimately develops, the dose can be escalated or other newly targeted biologic agents, which have shown promise for imatinib-resistant GIST, may be considered. The most studied agent is SU11248, which targets not only c-KIT and PDGFR but also the VEGF receptors, fms-related tyrosine kinase (Flt3), and the Ret oncogene. In one study of 48 patients with imatinib-refractory GIST, SU11248 achieved stable disease or partial response in 42% and 13% of patients, respectively.

DESMOID TUMOR (AGGRESSIVE FIBROMATOSIS)

Desmoid tumors are benign, slowly growing neoplasms arising from fibroblastic stromal elements. Although neoplastic and locally aggressive, desmoids do not have the capacity to establish metastatic lesions. Desmoid tumors are uncommon (possibly about 1,000 per year in the United States), slightly more common in females than males, and occur predominantly in individuals of 15–60 years of age. There is no significant racial or ethnic distribution. The etiology of desmoid tumors is not known, but these tumors occur commonly in patients with Gardner's syndrome and occur more frequently at sites of trauma or surgery.

Desmoid tumors usually present as a painless or minimally painful mass with a history of slow growth, but can cause symptoms if they impinge on adjacent structures. Desmoid tumors occur at virtually all body sites; most commonly in the torso (shoulder girdle and hip-buttock region) and the extremities. The location is usually deep in the muscles or along fascial planes. Multiple lesions at distant sites are infrequent; however, additional lesions are not rare on the same extremity following the initial treatment.

The natural history of desmoids can be quite variable. They commonly grow relatively slowly, with periods of comparative stability or even temporary regression. Desmoid tumors can be locally progressive with infiltration of adjacent normal tissues and structures. They may become locally malignant and highly destructive of normal tissue leading to the death of the patient. Spontaneous regressions have been observed and re-growth is not observed in all patients following grossly incomplete surgical resection.

Desmoid tumors are usually treated by surgical resection with a wide margin when medically and technically feasible. Since these tumors are benign, treatments with potentially serious late sequelae should be avoided if at all possible. Radiation therapy is an effective option for patients who are not good surgical candidates or decline surgery and, as an adjunctive therapy, for patients with grossly or microscopically positive margins. While some advocate adjuvant radiation for primary disease, our institution generally reserves radiation for recurrent tumors given that this is a benign disease. Results from a number of centers demonstrate that radiation alone (50–60 Gy) or radiation combined with surgery in patients with positive margins achieves permanent control of desmoid tumors in approximately 70–80% of patients (14).

There is increasing evidence for a role for systemic therapy in patients whose desmoid tumors that cannot be controlled without morbid surgery and/or radiation (15). Increasing experience is accumulating with systemic agents in patients with advanced or recurrent disease, especially at intra-abdominal and abdominal wall sites. There are, for example, a number of anecdotal reports of excellent response to tamoxifen, the antiestrogen toremifine, and progestational agents. There are also documented responses to nonsteroidal anti-inflammatory drugs (NSAIDs, most often sulindac) alone or in combination with tamoxifen. Regression is usually partial and may take many months after an initial period of tumor enlargement. Low-dose chemotherapy based upon methotrexate and vinblastine has obtained worthwhile response rates in patients with desmoid tumors, particularly in children. The combination of methotrexate and vinorelbine may produce a similar response to methotrexate and vinblastine with less neurotoxicity. In addition, there are anecdotal reports of doxorubicin-based drug protocols with good responses. For patients with Gardner's syndrome and intra-abdominal desmoid tumor, one should often avoid aggressive surgery given the relatively poor results of surgery and the higher rate of recurrence. Such patients can be treated with tamoxifen, NSAIDs, or low-dose chemotherapy. Surgery is the second option if there is no response.

BONE SARCOMAS

Malignant tumors of the skeletal system are rare. There were an estimated 2,760 new bone sarcomas cases in the United States in 2006, with 1,260 deaths. The most common primary bone sarcoma is osteosarcoma, followed by chondrosarcoma and Ewing's sarcoma. Osteosarcoma and Ewing's sarcoma occur primarily in childhood and adolescence. Other primary bone sarcomas, including chondrosarcomas, fibrosarcoma, and MFH, occur primarily in adults. Malignant tumors of bone must be differentiated from benign bone and cartilage tumors such as osteochondroma, enchondroma, osteoid osteoma, osteoblastoma, and desmoplastic fibroma, and giant cell tumor of bone.

OSTEOSARCOMA

Osteosarcoma is the most common malignant bone tumor (16). Tumors are usually located in the metaphysis of long bone, especially the distal femur, proximal tibia, and proximal humerus. The most common presentation of patients with bone sarcomas is pain or swelling in a bone or near a joint. At the time of presentation, 10–20% of patients have macroscopic metastatic disease and over 80% of patients likely harbor micrometastatic disease. Osteosarcomas metastasize primarily to the lung (90%) and less commonly to other bone sites (10%). On pathologic analysis, the characteristic feature of osteosarcoma is the presence of tumor cell produced osteoid. Several histologic subtypes of osteosarcomas exist: conventional (including osteoblastic, chondroblastic, and fibroblastic), telangiectatic, parosteal (arising from bone cortex), and periosteal (arising just below periosteum).

Diagnosis and Staging

The radiologic appearance of osteosarcomas and other malignant bone tumors are usually quite different from that of benign tumors. Benign tumors usually have well-circumscribed borders with no cortical destruction or periosteal reaction. Malignant tumors often have irregular borders, bone destruction, periosteal reaction, and soft tissue extension. Patients should be fully evaluated by history and physical examination, plain radiographs, MRI and CT scan of the primary tumor site, chest CT, and bone scan. The diagnosis can usually be established by CT guided core biopsy. Often there exists an associated soft tissue component that can be biopsied. For uncommon cases in which this modality is nondiagnostic, an open biopsy can be performed. The most commonly used staging system was developed by Enneking et al. and is outlined in Table 62-5 (17).

Surgery and Radiation

About 90% of osteosarcomas can be removed using limb-sparing surgery, although amputation is sometimes necessary to achieve a negative surgical margin. Limb-sparing surgery is divided into three components:

1. Resection of tumor—tumors are ideally removed with a rim of normal tissues to obtain a negative gross and microscopic margin.
2. Skeletal reconstruction—the skeletal defect created by the resection can be reconstructed using a variety of techniques including autologous bone graft, allograft, endoprosthesis, and rotationplasty.
3. Muscle and soft tissue coverage—local muscle, fat, and skin can be mobilized to cover the tumor resection bed and skeletal reconstruction. For larger defects, rotational or free flaps may be required.

Osteosarcomas are relatively resistant to radiation. Radiation therapy is generally not used in the primary treatment of most patients osteosarcomas, but is reserved for patients who refuse definitive surgery, have no good surgical option (i.e., base of skull), have grossly or microscopically positive resection margins, have less than wide resection margins and poor histologic response, have primary lesions in sites with high rates of relapse after surgery including head and neck, spine, or pelvis, present with a pathologic fracture and might be at higher risk of local recurrence, or require palliation. Retrospective reports suggest potential benefit for the addition of radiation therapy in these settings (18). For osteosarcomas in patients with extremity lesions who refused amputation, a

Table 62-5

Musculoskeletal Tumor Society Staging System for Bone Sarcomas

Histological Grade(G)	G1	Low grade
	G2	High grade
Site (T)	T1	Intracompartmental*
	T2	Extracompartmental*
Metastases	M0	No lymphatic or distant metastases
	M1	Lymphatic or distant metastases
Stage I A (G1, T1, M0)		Low-grade tumor, intracompartmental lesion without metastases
Stage IB (G1, T2, M0)		Low-grade tumor, extracompartmental lesion without metastases
Stage IIA (G2, T1, MO)		High grade, intracompartmental lesion without metastases
Stage IIB (G2, T2, M0)		High-grade tumor, extracompartmental lesion without metastases
Stage IIIA (G1/G2, T1, M0)		Any grade tumor, intracompartmental lesion with metastases
Stage IIIB (G1/G2, T2, M0)		Any grade tumor, extracompartmental lesion with metastases

Adapted from (17).

*Compartment is defined as an anatomic structure or space bounded by natural barriers for tumor extension.

A compartment can includes any individual bone, intra-articular spaces, and any clearly identified facially enclosed space.

combination of chemotherapy and primary radiation therapy (median dose 60 Gy) has been reported to obtain a 5-year local control of 56% in 31 patients; local control was 11/11 in selected patients who had a good response based on imaging and normalization of alkaline phosphatase. However, at our institution, surgical resections of osteosarcomas even in difficult locations requiring internal hemipelvectomy have been performed with acceptable morbidity, and local recurrence risk is substantially decreased.

Chemotherapy

In the 1970s prior to the use of adjuvant chemotherapy, <20% of osteosarcoma patients treated with surgery alone lived over 5 years. With the introduction of adjuvant chemotherapy (high-dose methotrexate), five-year survival rates rose to 40–60%. Prospective randomized trials performed in the 1980s confirmed the utility of adjuvant chemotherapy. Effective agents include high-dose methotrexate, doxorubicin, bleomycin, cyclophosphamide, dactinomycin, vincristine, cisplatin, ifosfamine, and etoposide (Pediatric Oncology Group, POG 8651). Neoadjuvant chemotherapy was originally introduced at Memorial Sloan-Kettering in concert with increased utilization of limb-sparing surgery. Chemotherapy was delivered to patients prior to surgery while awaiting creation of custom prosthetics, and retrospective analysis suggested these patients fared better than those that received post-operative chemotherapy alone. A randomized trial of comparing alternating course of high dose methotrexate with leucovorin rescue, cisplatin and doxorubicin, and bleomycin, cyclophosphamide, and dactomycin given before or after surgical resection showed equivalent 5 year relapse free survival (61% vs. 65%) and limb salvage rates (50% vs. 55%).

Currently about 65% of osteosarcoma patients treated with adjuvant chemotherapy attain long-term survival. Most centers deliver chemotherapy in the neoadjuvant setting, and this has several theoretical advantages: (1) early delivery of treatment for micrometastases, (2) increase in limb-salvage rates, and (3) assessment of tumor response. Tumor response to neoadjuvant chemotherapy (>90% tumor necrosis) is the most important prognostic factor for survival, and poor responders can be switched to alternative post-operative chemotherapy regimens. There exists some controversy as to the benefits of switching to alternative chemotherapy regimens in patients with <90% tumor necrosis.

The optimal chemotherapy regimen is still controversial. Many centers offer children, adolescents and younger adults treatment similar to the POG regimen described above in the neoadjuvant setting. Ifosfamide and etoposide are used in some regimens. Older adults may not tolerate doxorubicin and cisplatin for more than six cycles. However, high-dose methotrexate and ifosfamide can also be used for most adults.

Recurrent and Metastatic Disease

Patients with metastatic osteosarcoma have long-term survival ranging from 10 to 40% with chemotherapy and surgery and in some cases radiation therapy. Patients with isolated lung metastases have a more favorable prognosis than those with bone metastases. The most active single agents are high-dose methotrexate, doxorubicin, cisplatin, and ifosfamide, with response rates ranging between 20% and 40%, and a variety of combination regimens have been used. Patients who recur following initial treatment with adjuvant chemotherapy and surgery tend to have chemotherapy-resistant disease. For isolated lung metastases that are few in number and do not invade the pleura, complete resection of all lesions can result in 5-year survival up to 35%. Unresectable metastatic disease can be treated with alternative chemotherapy regimens. Most patients who have already received doxorubicin and cisplatin (with or without high-dose methotrexate) can receive etoposide and ifosfamide with or without carboplatin, and such patients should be considered for enrollment in clinical trials.

EWING'S SARCOMA FAMILY OF TUMORS

Ewing's sarcoma was initially described by James Ewing as a tumor that was responsive to radiation treatment, and are rare tumors that arise in bone and less commonly in soft tissue. There is currently a spectrum of neoplastic diseases known as the Ewing's sarcoma family of tumors, which includes Ewing's sarcoma, primitive neuroectodermal tumors (PNET), adult neuroblastoma, malignant small cell tumor of the thoracopulmonary region (Askin's tumor), paravertebral small cell tumor, and atypical Ewing's sarcoma. These tumors are thought to be derived from a common cell of origin, share pathologic characteristics, and often have common chromosomal translocations (Table 62-1). As with osteosarcomas, these tumors primarily occur in adolescents and young adults and present with pain or swelling in a bone or joint. They usually involve flat bones or the diaphysis of tubular bones. While less than 25% of patients present with overt metastases, the majority of patients likely harbor micrometastatic disease, and the common sites of metastasis are the lung, bone, and bone marrow. Workup and diagnosis are performed in a way similar to that for patients with osteosarcoma, except that bone marrow biopsy may be useful.

The surgical principles used for these tumors are similar to those for osteosarcoma.

Ewing's sarcoma/PNET are relatively sensitive to radiation which is often applied to patients with positive surgical margins. Primary radiation therapy may be used in cases where surgery would be highly morbid. Selection factors make it difficult to determine whether primary radiotherapy results in as good local control as surgery alone or as surgery combined with radiation therapy. The major concern with the use of radiation therapy is the potential for late radiation induced malignancies.

For Ewing's sarcoma/PNET, standard chemotherapy includes vincristine, doxorubicin, and cyclophosphamide with or without actinomycin D (VDCA or VDC) alternating with ifosfamide and etoposide (IE). Usually at least a few of the cycles are given pre-operatively. With modern multimodality treatment, long-term survival can be achieved in 70–80% of patients with nonmetastatic disease.

For patients with metastatic disease, high-dose chemotherapy with or without whole body radiation and autologous hematopoietic stem cell support has been used. Patients with metastatic disease have a better prognosis when the lung is involved compared to bone and bone marrow. With chemotherapy, 5-year survival can be 20–40%. Low dose bilateral lung radiation can also be used, and isolated lesions in other locations can be controlled with radiation.

CHONDROSARCOMAS

Chondrosarcomas are the second most common malignant bone tumor and occur in patients usually in their third to fifth decade of life (19). The most common anatomic locations are the pelvis (31%), femur (21%), and shoulder girdle (13%). They occur in five primary types: 75% are "conventional" chondrosarcomas of either central (arising within a bone) or peripheral (arising from a bone surface) types and 25% are chondrosarcoma variants (mesenchymal, differentiated, and clear cell). The central and peripheral types of chondrosarcoma can be primary tumors or arise secondary to an underlying neoplasm such as benign cartilage tumors. Most chondrosarcomas are grade I or II and uncommonly metastasize, but grade III lesions have the same metastatic potential as osteosarcomas. In a large single institution series of 344 chondrosarcomas, overall 5-year survival was 77% (20). Local recurrence developed in 20% and distant metastases in 14%. Local recurrence was higher for shoulder and pelvis tumors, high-grade tumors, and tumors with intralesional or marginal resections. High-grade was also an important prognostic factor distant recurrence. These results are similar to those reported by our institution (21).

The primary treatment of chondrosarcomas is surgical resection. These tumors are highly resistant to chemotherapeutic agents, possibly due to their extracellular matrix. Intralesional excision of grade I tumors has been advocated due to their benign behavior, although tumors located in the spine and pelvis can have a more aggressive biology. Grades II and III tumors should be resected similarly to osteosarcomas. Although it has been stated repeatedly that chondrosarcoma is a radioresistant tumor, several recent reports have demonstrated the effectiveness of conventional radiation therapy for this histology. High rates of local control of these lesions in the base of skull/cervical spine and lower spine and sacrum with proton radiation therapy have been reported. The indications for radiation therapy for chondrosarcomas include unresectable or subtotally tumors, those resected with positive margins, and recurrent tumors. Because of the need for high radiation doses for control of these tumors and the proximity of radiosensitive critical structures in the skull base, spine, and pelvis, proton beam radiation, which has no exit dose beyond the target, is advantageous for treatment of tumors in these sites.

There is no standard chemotherapy for chondrosarcoma, but patients with metastatic disease should be considered for enrollment in clinical trials.

CHORDOMAS

Chordomas are rare tumors that arise from the notochordal remnant in the midline of the neural axis (19). They occur most commonly in the sacrococcygeal region and base of skull, but can occur in the thoracic and lumbar spine regions. Sacrococcygeal lesions usually present with local pain. Patient can also have constipation or urinary symptoms. Base of skull lesions usually present with headache, visual changes, or cranial nerve dysfunction. CT scans and MRI are used for radiologic evaluation. CT imaging of the liver and lung should be performed to rule out metastases, and CT guided biopsy usually establishes the diagnosis.

While these tumors uncommonly metastasize, the tumors are lethal due to their location adjacent to vital structures, locally aggressive behavior, and high rate of recurrence. Local control is difficult and local recurrence and complications often lead to death. The best chance at local control for these tumors is with the initial treatment, and such treatment should include aggressive surgical resection if feasible and radiation therapy when extraosseous extension is present. Even in small lesions after radical resection, recurrence rates are as high as 50–100% with local control and survival curves following a continuous downward slope. Salvage treatment after local failure rarely is curative. A possible dose–response relationship for conventional radiation treatment has been reported. One of the best results of conventional, postoperative radiation treatment was published by Keisch et al. The rate of actuarial disease-free survival at 5 years was significantly better for patients undergoing surgery and radiotherapy (60%) compared to that of patients undergoing surgery only (25%), although patients continued to recur beyond 5 years. Investigators at the Lawrence Berkeley Laboratory (LBL) and our institution have demonstrated promising results for chordomas at the base of skull and cervical spine using charged particle irradiation, although local control is less favorable than with chondrosarcomas. Munzenrider and Liebsch reported that the ten-year local control for skull base tumors was highest for chondrosarcomas, intermediate for chordomas in males, and lowest for chordomas in females (94%, 65%, and 42%, respectively). For cervical spine tumors, 10-year local control rates were not significantly different for chordomas and chondrosarcomas (54% and 48%, respectively), nor was there any significant difference in local control between males and females. Hug et al. reported five-year rates of local control and survival for lower spine and sacral chordomas of 53% and 50%, respectively, with a mean dose of 74.6 CGE (cobalt gray equivalent). A trend for improved local control was noted for primary lesions compared to recurrent tumors, with radiation doses of at least 77 CGE and less residual tumor burden.

There is no standard chemotherapy for chordomas, but for metastatic disease there is some evidence for the use of imatinib, and patients should be considered for enrollment in clinical trials.

REFERENCES

1. Brennan MF, Lewis JL. "Diagnosis and Management of Soft Tissue Sarcoma." Martin Dunitz, London, 2002.
2. Clark MA, Fisher C, Judson I, Thomas JM. Soft-tissue sarcomas in adults. N Engl J Med 2005; 353(7): 701–711.
3. Rosenberg SA, Tepper J, Glatstein E, Costa J, Baker A, Brennan M, et al. The treatment of soft-tissue sarcomas of the extremities: prospective randomized

evaluations of (1) limb-sparing surgery plus radiation therapy compared with amputation and (2) the role of adjuvant chemotherapy. Ann Surg. 1982; 196(3): 305–315.

4. Yang JC, Chang AE, Baker AR, Sindelar WF, Danforth DN, Topalian SL, et al. Randomized prospective study of the benefit of adjuvant radiation therapy in the treatment of soft tissue sarcomas of the extremity. J Clin Oncol. 1998; 16(1): 197–203.

5. O'Sullivan B, Davis AM, Turcotte R, Bell R, Catton C, Chabot P, et al. Preoperative versus postoperative radiotherapy in soft-tissue sarcoma of the limbs: a randomised trial. Lancet. 2002; 359(9325): 2235–2241.

6. Kepka L, DeLaney TF, Suit HD, Goldberg SI. Results of radiation therapy for unresected soft-tissue sarcomas. Int J Radiat Oncol Biol Phys. 2005; 63(3): 852–859.

7. DeLaney TF, Spiro IJ, Suit HD, Gebhardt MC, Hornicek FJ, Mankin HJ, et al. Neoadjuvant chemotherapy and radiotherapy for large extremity soft-tissue sarcomas. Int J Radiat Oncol Biol Phys. 2003; 56(4): 1117–1127.

8. Bramwell V, Rouesse J, Steward W, Santoro A, Schraffordt-Koops H, Buesa J, et al. Adjuvant CYVADIC chemotherapy for adult soft tissue sarcoma-reduced local recurrence but no improvement in survival: a study of the European Organization for Research and Treatment of Cancer Soft Tissue and Bone Sarcoma Group. J Clin Oncol. 1994; 12(6): 1137–1149.

9. Adjuvant chemotherapy for localised resectable soft-tissue sarcoma of adults: meta-analysis of individual data. Sarcoma Meta-analysis Collaboration. Lancet. 1997; 350(9092): 1647–1654.

10. Lewis JJ, Leung D, Woodruff JM, Brennan MF. Retroperitoneal soft-tissue sarcoma: analysis of 500 patients treated and followed at a single institution. Ann Surg. 1998; 228(3): 355–365.

11. Gieschen HL, Spiro IJ, Suit HD, Ott MJ, Rattner DW, Ancukiewicz M, et al. Long-term results of intraoperative electron beam radiotherapy for primary and recurrent retroperitoneal soft tissue sarcoma. Int J Radiat Oncol Biol Phys. 2001; 50(1): 127–131.

12. Brennan MF, Alektiar KM, Maki RG. Soft tissue sarcoma. In: DeVita VT, Hellman S, Rosenberg SA (eds.), "Cancer: Principles & Practice of Oncology," Philadelphia: Lippincott Williams & Wilkins, 2001, pp. 1841–1980.

13. van der Zwan SM, DeMatteo RP. Gastrointestinal stromal tumor: 5 years later. Cancer. 2005; 104(9): 1781–1788.

14. Nuyttens JJ, Rust PF, Thomas CR Jr., Turrisi AT, III. Surgery versus radiation therapy for patients with aggressive fibromatosis or desmoid tumors: a comparative review of 22 articles. Cancer. 2000; 88(7): 1517–1523.

15. Schlemmer M. Desmoid tumors and deep fibromatoses. Hematol Oncol Clin North Am. 2005; 19(3): 565–571.

16. Gebhardt MC, Hornicek FJ. Osteosarcoma and variants. In Bell MJ, Buckwalter J, Bulstrode C, Butcher I, Carr A, Fairbank J et al. (eds.), "Orthopaedics and Trauma," Oxford University Press, Oxford, 2002, pp. 224–238.

17. Enneking WF, Spanier SS, Goodman MA. A system for the surgical staging of musculoskeletal sarcoma. Clin Orthop Relat Res. 1980; 153: 106–120.

18. DeLaney TF, Park L, Goldberg SI, Hug EB, Liebsch NJ, Munzenrider JE, et al. Radiotherapy for local control of osteosarcoma. Int J Radiat Oncol Biol Phys. 2005; 61(2): 492–498.

19. Harsh GR, Janecka IP, Mankin HJ, Ojemann RG, Suit H. "Chordomas and Chondrosarcomas of the Skull Base and Spine,." Thieme Medical Publishers, New York, 2003.

20. Bjornsson J, McLeod RA, Unni KK, Ilstrup DM, Pritchard DJ. Primary chondrosarcoma of long bones and limb girdles. Cancer 1998; 83(10): 2105–2119.

21. Lee FY, Mankin HJ, Fondren G, Gebhardt MC, Springfield DS, Rosenberg AE, et al. Chondrosarcoma of bone: an assessment of outcome. J Bone Joint Surg Am. 1999; 81(3): 326–338.

| 63 | Andrew S. Chi, Tracy T. Batchelor |

PRIMARY BRAIN TUMORS

INTRODUCTION

There are over 100 different types of primary brain tumors, with heterogeneous biologies and divergent clinical outcomes (1). The incidence rate of all primary central nervous system (CNS) tumors in the United States is 14.8 cases per 100,000 person-years. The worldwide incidence rate of malignant primary CNS tumors is approximately 3 per 100,000 person-years. An estimated 43,800 primary CNS tumors were diagnosed in the United States in 2005. Approximately 18,500 of these tumors were malignant and this subgroup represented 1.35% of all malignant cancers diagnosed in the United States (2).

Although relatively uncommon, primary brain tumors cause a disproportionate morbidity and mortality. An estimated 12,760 deaths were attributed to malignant primary CNS tumors in the United States in 2005. The 5-year survival rate following diagnosis of a malignant primary CNS tumor is approximately 30%. In adults, malignant gliomas are the most common type of primary CNS tumor. Despite advances in research and treatment, malignant gliomas continue to carry a poor prognosis. In this chapter we review the clinical evaluation, biology, and management of various primary brain tumors.

DIAGNOSIS

Clinical Features

Patients with primary brain tumors can present suddenly with seizures or subacutely with progressive focal or non-focal neurological symptoms. Progressive focal neurological deficits may be referable to the growth of a tumor in a specific brain location. Non-focal symptoms include headache, vomiting, fatigue, mental status changes, mood disturbances, imbalance, and gait disorder, and may reflect elevated intracranial pressure (ICP). Less often, patients may present with an acute stroke-like neurological deficit caused by hemorrhage into a previously subclinical tumor. Headaches result from local irritation of pain-sensitive structures or from increased ICP. Headaches from increased ICP due to tumors are usually holocephalic, progressive, worse with recumbency, and may awaken a patient from sleep. They may be precipitated by Valsalva maneuvers or coughing. Systemic symptoms such as malaise, anorexia, weight loss, and fever are usually absent, and their presence suggests a metastatic rather than primary brain tumor.

Laboratory Evaluation

Primary brain tumors are not associated with serologic abnormalities, and no widely accepted primary brain tumor-specific systemic marker exists. Lumbar puncture (LP) for cerebrospinal fluid (CSF) analysis may be helpful for evaluating for metastatic disease from systemic cancers and for assessing

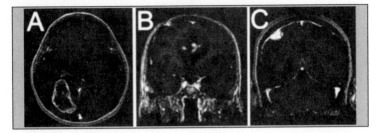

FIGURE 63.1   Magnetic resonance images of primary brain tumors. (a) Axial T1 contrast-enhanced sequence of a glioblastoma. A heterogeneous, peripherally enhancing, centrally necrotic lesion is centered in the right temporal-occipital region. There is mass effect on adjacent structures with midline shift of the midbrain. (b) Typical appearance of a primary CNS lymphoma. A T1 hypointense mass located in the left cingulate gyrus and subcortical area extends across the corpus callosum and contains several discrete areas of contrast enhancement. (c) Right parietal meningioma. Coronal T1 contrast-enhanced sequence shows a dural-based, extra-axial mass with intense contrast enhancement and adjacent T1 hypointensity in the brain parenchyma representing vasogenic edema.

leptomeningeal spread of certain primary brain tumors such as primary CNS lymphoma, primitive neuroectodermal tumors, and rarely astrocytomas. The CSF may demonstrate an elevated protein level and a mild lymphocytic pleocytosis. An LP may precipitate brain herniation if there is increased ICP, and should be performed only after reviewing cranial imaging and obtaining neurological consultation.

Neuroimaging

The diagnosis of a primary brain tumor is suggested by contrast-enhanced cranial imaging with either computerized tomography (CT) or magnetic resonance imaging (MRI). With the exception of skull bone evaluation, MRI is almost always superior to CT and is the imaging modality of choice. Abnormal enhancement after the administration of intravenous contrast material on either CT or MRI correlates with areas of blood-brain barrier disruption. On CT, tumors and associated vasogenic edema usually appear as regions of low attenuation. Areas of increased attenuation may indicate hemorrhage or calcification. On MRI, tumors often have low signal intensity on T1-weighted sequences and high signal intensity on T2-weighted and FLAIR sequences, although signal characteristics vary with specific tumor types (Figure 63-1). In general, contrast-enhancement is characteristic of higher grade tumors. Other technologies such as magnetic resonance spectroscopy and positron emission tomography are useful in specific situations such as surgical guidance and distinguishing between recurrent tumor and radiation necrosis. The gold standard for diagnosis, however, remains biopsy and histological analysis.

GLIOMAS

Classification

Gliomas are tumors with cells that display glial differentiation. They consist of a spectrum of cancers of varying grades of malignancy. Glial cells include astrocytes, oligodendrocytes, and ependymal cells, and gliomas comprise a group of tumor types that includes astrocytomas, oligodendrogliomas, mixed gliomas (oligoastrocytomas), ependymomas, choroid plexus tumors, and less common variants. Astrocytomas are the most common type of glioma and account for 75% of the total. Gliomas are most often supratentorial, although they may be located throughout the neuraxis.

The World Health Organization (WHO) classification, the most commonly accepted grading system, categorizes gliomas into four grades based upon their histology (1). Tumors are assessed for key histologic features, including cellularity, atypical cells, mitoses, microvascular proliferation, and necrosis. Grade I is reserved for specific histological variants such as juvenile pilocytic astrocytoma, pleomorphic xanthoastrocytoma, and dysembryoplastic neuroepithelial tumor, all of which are relatively benign, slow-growing tumors with an excellent prognosis after surgical resection. Gliomas that possess only one abnormal histological feature, usually atypical cells, are grade II. Low-grade glioma (LGG) refers to either grade I or grade II tumors. Tumors with two or more features are considered malignant or high-grade gliomas and are classified as grade III or grade IV tumors.

Low-Grade Gliomas

Most adult LGGs (grade II) can be categorized into three groups: astrocytoma, oligodendroglioma, and oligoastrocytoma. LGGs are relatively uncommon tumors that typically present between the second and fourth decades of life. They are highly infiltrative tumors that invade and expand contiguous brain tissue. Although initially slow growing, LGGs nearly always progress to higher-grade tumors which are invariably fatal. Outcome is variable with a median survival between 5 and 10 years (Table 63-1). Histological subtype is a critical determinant of outcome. Oligodendrogliomas have a more indolent course and better responsiveness to therapy than astrocytomas. Patients with oligoastrocytomas have an intermediate outcome. Genetic markers are helpful in predicting prognosis and response to treatment. Approximately 50–70% of low-grade oligodendrogliomas have combined loss of heterozygosity on chromosomes 1p and 19q, and loss of both markers correlates with chemosensitivity and longer survival. Proliferation indices such as the Ki-67 antigen or the MIB-1 antibody may be helpful, but there are conflicting opinions regarding the prognostic relevance of these mitotic markers.

Because patients at diagnosis are typically younger and have little or no neurological deficit, the management of LGG is controversial. Treatment options at diagnosis include observation, resection, radiation therapy (RT), or chemotherapy (3). Although no randomized data exist regarding the benefit of extensive resection of LGGs, a number of retrospective analyses suggest cytoreductive surgery improves outcome. The objective is to perform a gross total resection, however the invasiveness of LGGs and their frequent location near eloquent brain regions often precludes complete excision. The risk of creating neurological dysfunction from the surgery itself must be carefully weighed against the potential benefits

Table 63-1

Survival Rates for Selected Primary Brain Tumors (2)

Histology	10-year survival (%)
Astrocytic tumors	
Pilocytic astrocytoma (WHO grade I)	90
Diffuse astrocytoma (WHO grade II)	40
Anaplastic astrocytoma (WHO grade III)	20
Glioblastoma (WHO grade IV)	2
Oligodendroglial tumors	
Oligodendroglioma (WHO grade II)	50
Anaplastic oligodendroglioma (WHO grade II)	30
Primary CNS lymphoma	10

of resection. Surgery also has an important role in obtaining tissue for histological diagnosis and in providing relief from symptoms of increased ICP.

Radiation is a standard component of treatment for LGGs, but its timing remains controversial. Prospective, randomized data suggest that RT provided at the time of initial diagnosis delays time to tumor progression but does not prolong overall survival compared to deferral of RT until the time of tumor progression. Because patients with LGGs usually live for many years, the risk of developing radiation-related adverse effects including cognitive impairment (neurotoxicity) and endocrinopathy (pituitary dysfunction), must be carefully considered. Technical advances in imaging, computer optimization, and radiation delivery allow more accurate planning of target volumes and conformation of radiation beams, and may increase the effectiveness and minimize the long-term side effects of RT. However, future prospective studies of cognitive function are necessary to assess the risk of neurotoxicity with modern radiation techniques.

There is limited but emerging evidence that chemotherapy may be effective in treating LGGs, particularly oligodendrogliomas. Procarbazine, lomustine, and vincristine (PCV) combination therapy and temozolomide have activity in both newly diagnosed and progressive LGGs, although further investigation is required.

Because of these uncertainties, current management strategies vary. Typically, tumors that are completely resected and have a low mitotic

Table 63-2

Clinical Prognostic Factors for Survival in Selected Primary Brain Tumors

Prognostic factor	Favorable	Unfavorable
Low-grade glioma		
Age (years)	<40	>40
Largest diameter of the tumor	<6 cm	≥6 cm
Tumor crossing midline	No	Yes
Histology	Oligodendroglioma/ mixed glioma	Astrocytoma
Neurologic deficit	Absent	Present
High-grade glioma		
Age (years)	<45	>45
Histology	Oligodendroglioma/ mixed glioma	Astrocytoma
Functional status (KPS*)	>70	<70
Genetic markers (Oligodendrogliomas, oligoastrocytomas)	1p and 19q co-deletion	1p and 19q retention
Primary CNS Lymphoma (4)		
Age (years)	<60	>60
Functional status (KPS*)	>70	<70
Lactate Dehydrogenase (LDH)	Normal	Elevated
CSF protein concentration	Normal	Elevated
Area of brain involved	Superficial	Deep[†]

*Karnofsky Performance Status Scale.

[†]Periventricular, basal ganglia, brainstem, cerebellum.

labeling index are monitored closely with serial contrast-enhanced cranial MRI scans. Adjuvant radiation is often provided in the setting of incomplete resection and a high mitotic index. Therapeutic decisions are individualized and are based on a number of clinical prognostic factors, including histology, age, the size of the tumor, and presence of neurological deficits (Table 63-2).

Malignant Gliomas

Malignant gliomas (MG) include grade III tumors such as anaplastic astrocytoma (AA), anaplastic oligodendroglioma (AO), and anaplastic oligoastrocytoma (AOA), as well as grade IV gliomas (glioblastoma or GBM). Glioblastoma, the most common and the most malignant primary brain tumor, accounts for 60% of malignant gliomas. The average age at diagnosis of GBM is 64 years, although the range of ages at presentation is broad. Most GBMs arise as a result of genetic alterations involving tumor suppressor genes and proto-oncogenes within a progenitor cell. A rare subgroup of gliomas are associated with certain hereditary syndromes (Table 63-3).

At least two distinct clinical and genetic forms of GBM have been described (5). Primary GBMs, which account for the vast majority of cases, arise de novo typically in older patients. These tumors are associated with increased activity of the epidermal growth factor receptor (EGFR), inactivation of the phosphatase and tensin homolog deleted on chromosome 10 *(PTEN)* gene, and non-mutated *p53*. Secondary GBMs arise from prior low-grade astrocytomas which have undergone malignant transformation, and typically occur in younger patients. The genetic pathway to secondary GBM involves mutations of *p53* and overexpression of platelet-derived growth factor (PDGF) and its receptor (PDGFR) in low-grade astrocytomas. Progression to AA is associated with inactivation of the retinoblastoma gene *(RB1)* and increased activity of human double minute 2 *(HDM2)*, and subsequent progression to GBM involves loss of chromosome 10 among other changes. An increasing number of such molecular alterations associated with phenotypic features of malignancy are being characterized. These alterations primarily deregulate two cellular systems, the growth factor mediated signaling pathways and the cell cycle, and contribute to increased cell proliferation, inhibition of apoptosis, invasion, and angiogenesis (6). Increased knowledge of these underlying molecular pathways in MGs has presented an opportunity to exploit some as therapeutic targets.

Table 63-3

Hereditary Risk Factors for Gliomas

Hereditary syndromes	Gene
Neurofibromatosis type 1 (NF1)	*NF1*
Neurofibromatosis type 2 (NF2)	*NF2*
Tuberous sclerosis complex (TSC)	*TSC1; TSC2*
Nevoid basal cell carcinoma syndrome (NBCCS), Gorlin-Goltz syndrome	*PTC* *CH*
Li-Fraumeni syndrome	*TP53*
Brain tumor-polyposis syndrome (BTPS), hereditary non-polyposis colorectal cancer (HNPCC), Turcot syndrome	DNA mismatch repair *(MLH1, MSH2, MSH6, PMS1, and PMS2)*
Multiple endocrine neoplasia type 1 (MEN1), Wermer syndrome	*MEN1*

The prognosis of patients with malignant gliomas is poor: the median survival of patients with AA is 2–3 years, while the survival is 10–15 months for those with GBM. Only a small minority achieve long-term survival (Table 63-1). Improved outcomes are seen in patients with grade III tumors, oligodendrogliomas, younger age, and better performance status (Table 63-2). Patients with anaplastic oligodendrogliomas, particularly the 50–70% of patients whose tumors have 1p and 19q co-deletion, are more responsive to treatment and have a better prognosis than those with astrocytomas. In two randomized phase III trials of newly diagnosed anaplastic oligodendrogliomas, chemotherapy increased progression-free survival and combined 1p and 19q loss independently correlated with improved overall survival (7). Despite aggressive therapy nearly all MGs recur, and available salvage therapies are ineffective. Novel strategies targeting molecular alterations commonly observed in gliomas and tumor-induced angiogenesis promise to offer more effective therapeutics for patients with these deadly tumors (8).

TREATMENT OF NEWLY DIAGNOSED GBM Treatment of MGs requires supportive care and multimodality antitumor therapy (9). Supportive care requirements are considerable, and include management of cerebral edema, seizures, venous thromboembolism, infections, and cognitive dysfunction. Definitive antitumor therapy usually begins with maximal safe resection. Retrospective data suggest a survival benefit in patients undergoing maximal surgical resection. The decision between biopsy and resection depends on the proximity of the tumor to critical brain regions, the patient's age and functional status, and the degree of mass effect. Resection may also be indicated to relieve symptoms such as local compression or elevated ICP. Modern intraoperative imaging and physiological monitoring techniques may allow for more extensive resection of tumors located in or near eloquent brain regions. RT has long been the standard adjuvant therapy for newly diagnosed GBM. Focal conformal radiation, known as involved-field radiation therapy (IFRT), is directed at the tumor and a small surrounding margin. The radiation field is limited to prevent recurrent tumors that usually arise within 2 cm of the prior resection margin while minimizing the risk of neurotoxicity.

Currently, the standard-of-care in the adjuvant setting consists of IFRT with concurrent temozolomide (Temodar®; Schering-Plough, NJ, USA), a well-tolerated oral DNA methylating agent, followed by 6–12 months of post-radiation temozolomide. This standard was established by a European Organization for Research and Treatment of Cancer/National Cancer Institute of Canada randomized trial which demonstrated an increase in median survival by 2.5 months and an increase in 2-year survival rate from 10% to 26.5% in patients treated with concurrent radiation and temozolomide followed by six cycles of monthly temozolomide compared to patients treated with radiation alone (10).

Intratumoral or intracavitary administration of chemotherapy may increase the exposure of drug to the tumor with reduced systemic toxicity. Implantation of BCNU-impregnated wafers (Gliadel®; MGI Pharma, MN, USA) at the time of surgical resection is sometimes utilized in patients with newly diagnosed MG (11). This therapy has only modest activity, however, with a median survival of 13.9 months for patients treated with BCNU wafers versus 11.6 months for placebo-treated patients.

SALVAGE THERAPY Because of the limited efficacy of current salvage options, treatment decisions for patients with recurrent MG must be individualized (12). Tumor location, size, histology, prior therapy, and the general health of the patient must be considered. If surgically accessible, debulking may improve symptoms and allow time for additional therapy. Some evidence suggests that stereotactic radiosurgery (SRS), which delivers a high single dose of radiation to a small (<4 cm) treatment volume may be beneficial in recurrent MGs. A number of conventional chemotherapeutic agents, including BCNU, carboplatin, etoposide, irinotecan, and PCV combination therapy, are used as salvage agents although none significantly improves survival. In general, patients with recurrent disease should be considered for clinical trials.

EXPERIMENTAL THERAPY There has been a significant expansion in the number of clinical trials of experimental therapeutics against MGs. Several novel treatment strategies are being developed, including locoregional therapies, radiosensitizers, biological agents, and immunological therapy. A major focus of clinical development is on molecularly targeted inhibitors of components of aberrant signaling pathways (7). EGFR, PDGFR, vascular endothelial growth factor (VEGF), the RAS/MAP kinase signaling pathway, the PI3K/AKT signaling pathway, and tumor-associated angiogenesis are targeted due to the frequency of abnormalities observed in these systems. A number of small molecule tyrosine kinase inhibitors are in preclinical and clinical development for MGs.

Initial clinical trials with targeted agents in MGs were disappointing, with low response rates and no significant increases in survival (13). Many factors may have contributed to the limited activity observed, including inadequate intratumoral concentrations and increased metabolism of drugs due to concurrently administered cytochrome P450 3A4/5 inducing antiepileptics, although the most important may have been the genetic heterogeneity of MGs. The molecular diversity of MGs, even within a single tumor, suggests that any single drug will not be effective in most tumors. Nonetheless, subsets of responders were identified in some trials, suggesting increased efficacy with targeted agents may be derived with improved patient selection (14, 15, 16). Current clinical efforts are focused on improving molecular profiling of tumors, combination regimens of targeted agents, and combinations of molecularly targeted agents with cytotoxic therapies such as radiation or chemotherapy.

PRIMARY CENTRAL NERVOUS SYSTEM LYMPHOMA

Primary central nervous system lymphoma (PCNSL) is a rare form of non-Hodgkin lymphoma that presents within the CNS without evidence of systemic lymphoma. Most cases are high-grade B-cell lymphoma. PCNSL may affect the brain, spinal cord, leptomeninges, and eyes. They occur commonly in immunocompromised patients, including those with AIDS, autoimmune diseases, and iatrogenic immunosuppression for organ transplants. Tumor cells in immunocompromised patients are invariably associated with Epstein-Barr virus (EBV) infection. Immunocompetent patients with PCNSL usually present after the age of 60. Lesions are most often supratentorial and periventricular, and discrete masses characteristically span the corpus callosum. Immunocompetent patients most often have solitary lesions, whereas AIDS-associated PCNSL is often multicentric. Up to 40% of patients have leptomeningeal involvement, and 20% may have ocular disease. On MRI, lesions are typically hyperintense on T2-weighted or FLAIR images, exhibit diffusion-restriction, and markedly enhance after contrast administration (17).

Diagnostic evaluation includes physical examination, slit-lamp examination, serum lactate dehydrogenase levels, human immunodeficiency virus testing, CT scans of the chest/abdomen/pelvis, bone marrow biopsy, contrast-enhanced brain MRI, and LP (Table 63-2). Testicular ultrasonography and contrast-enhanced MRI of the entire spine should be considered if clinically indicated. Diagnosis is established by pathological analysis of CSF, vitreous fluid, or a brain biopsy specimen. CSF studies should include chemistry (glucose and protein), cell counts, cytology, flow cytometry, and PCR for clonal immunoglobulin gene rearrangements or EBV DNA. Brain biopsy remains the gold standard for diagnosis of mass lesions in the parenchyma.

Treatment consists of chemotherapy alone or in combination with whole-brain radiation therapy (WBRT) (18). High-dose methotrexate, with or without other agents, is the mainstay of chemotherapy and is the most effective drug against PCNSL. Although most patients eventually recur, salvage chemotherapy may be effective. Systemic chemotherapy has increased the overall survival from 18 months to up to 55 months (Table 63-1).

Due to the wide variety of reported regimens and the lack of randomized trials, the optimal treatment regimen and timing of WBRT remains controversial. WBRT is often deferred for patients over age 60 because of the risk of neurotoxicity. In younger patients, chemotherapy-only regimens are commonly used although these approaches may be associated with earlier relapse. High-dose chemotherapy followed by autologous stem cell rescue has been the subject of small, non-randomized trials. The initial results in both the newly diagnosed and relapsed setting have been encouraging.

MENINGIOMAS

Meningiomas arise from the meninges, originating from arachnoidal cap cells of the arachnoidal granulations. These tumors are typically located along the dura of the superior sagittal sinus. Other common locations include the cerebral convexities, base of the brain, sphenoidal ridges, and parasellar areas. Meningiomas are the most common intracranial non-glial tumor, and constitute up to 26% of all intracranial tumors. An estimated 2–3% of the population has an incidental asymptomatic meningioma. They occur mostly in middle-aged or elderly patients, with a female preponderance of 2:1 which recedes with age. Approximately one-third of meningiomas are asymptomatic, diagnosed incidentally or at autopsy. Patients usually present with slowly progressive symptoms due to compression of neighboring brain structures and less commonly with seizures or progressive hydrocephalus (19).

On contrast-enhanced cranial MRI meningiomas are characteristically extra-axial, dural-based masses with intense, uniform contrast enhancement. Meningiomas are usually low-grade (WHO grade I) tumors associated with long progression-free survival after gross total resection. Rarely, they have aggressive histopathological features and are classified as atypical (WHO grade II) or anaplastic (WHO grade III) meningiomas. These tumors have much higher rates of recurrence and may invade the brain or metastasize outside the CNS.

There are several options for management of a newly discovered presumed meningioma on MRI. Small, asymptomatic meningiomas may be observed with serial cranial imaging to monitor for tumor growth. Treatment, usually resection, is recommended if meningiomas are symptomatic and associated with worsening neurological function. Fractionated, three-dimensional conformal RT or SRS is used for subtotally resected tumors, atypical or malignant meningioma resection cavities, or tumors in close proximity to critical brain regions such as the optic apparatus or brainstem.

REFERENCES

1. Kleihues P, Cavenee WK (eds.): World Health Organization Classification of Tumours. Pathology and Genetics: Tumours of the Nervous System, Lyon, IARC Press, 2000.
2. CBTRUS. Statistical Report. Primary Brain Tumors in the United States, 2006, 1998–2002.

3. Lang FF, Gilbert MR. Diffusely infiltrative low-grade gliomas in adults. J Clin Oncol. 2006; 24: 1236–1245.

4. Ferreri AJ, Blay JY, Reni M, et al. Prognostic scoring system for primary CNS lymphomas: the International Extranodal Lymphoma Study Group experience. J Clin Oncol. 2003; 21: 266–272.

5. Kleihues P, Ohgaki H. Primary and secondary glioblastomas: from concept to clinical diagnosis. Neuro-oncology. 1999; 1: 44–51.

6. Maher EA, Furnari FB, Bachoo RM, et al. Malignant glioma: genetics and biology of a grave matter. Genes Dev. 2001; 15: 1311–1333.

7. Jaeckle KA, Ballman KV, Rao RD, et al. Current strategies in treatment of oligo-dendroglioma: evolution of molecular signatures of response. J Clin Oncol. 2006; 24: 1246–1252.

8. Sathornsumetee S, Rich JN. New treatment strategies for malignant gliomas. Expert Rev Anticancer Ther. 2006; 6: 1087–1104.

9. Stupp R, Hegi ME, van den Bent MJ, et al. Changing paradigms—an update on the multidisciplinary management of malignant glioma. Oncologist. 2006; 11: 165–180.

10. Stupp R, Mason WP, van den Bent MJ, et al. Radiotherapy plus concomitant and adjuvant temozolomide for glioblastoma. N Engl J Med. 2005; 352: 987–996.

11. Westphal M, Hilt DC, Bortey E, et al. A phase 3 trial of local chemotherapy with biodegradable carmustine (BCNU) wafers (Gliadel wafers) in patients with primary malignant glioma. Neuro-oncology. 2003; 5: 79–88.

12. Butowski NA, Sneed PK, Chang SM. Diagnosis and treatment of recurrent high-grade astrocytoma. J Clin Oncol. 2006; 24: 1273–1280.

13. Wen PY, Kesari S, Drappatz J. Malignant gliomas: strategies to increase the effectiveness of targeted molecular treatment. Expert Rev Anticancer Ther. 2006; 6: 733–754.

14. Mellinghoff IK, Wang MY, Vivanco I, et al. Molecular determinants of the response of glioblastomas to EGFR kinase inhibitors. N Engl J Med. 2005; 353: 2012–2024.

15. Haas-Kogan DA, Prados MD, Lamborn KR, et al. Biomarkers to predict response to epidermal growth factor receptor inhibitors. Cell Cycle. 2005; 4: 1369–1372.

16. Batchelor TT, Sorensen AG, di Tomaso E, et al. AZD2171, a pan-VEGF receptor tyrosine kinase inhibitor, normalizes tumor vasculature and allevi-ates edema in glioblastoma patients. Cancer Cell. 2007; 11(1): 83–95.

17. Eichler AF, Batchelor TT. Primary central nervous system lymphoma: presen-tation, diagnosis and staging. Neurosurg Focus. 2006; 21: E15.

18. Omuro AM, Abrey LE. Chemotherapy for primary central nervous system lymphoma. Neurosurg Focus. 2006; 21: E12.

19. Whittle IR, Smith C, Navoo P, et al. Meningiomas. Lancet. 2004; 363: 1535–1543.

METASTATIC BRAIN TUMORS

INTRODUCTION

Brain metastasis is a common complication of cancer. Recent population-based data suggest that up to 20% of adults with cancer will develop symptomatic brain metastases during life (1). Autopsy studies indicate that another 25–30% of patients with disseminated cancer have asymptomatic brain metastases at the time of death. The incidence of brain metastasis varies by primary cancer type, being highest for lung (20%) followed by melanoma (7%), renal (6.5%), breast (5%), and colorectal (1.8%). Prostate, gynecologic, head and neck, and non-melanomatous skin cancers involve the brain parenchyma infrequently. The prevalence of brain metastases has increased in the past three decades. Contributing factors may include more sensitive imaging techniques (gadolinium-enhanced MRI), lengthened survival due to more effective systemic therapies, and poor central nervous system (CNS) penetration of many chemotherapeutic agents.

CLINICAL MANIFESTATIONS

Common signs and symptoms of metastatic brain tumors can be classified as either focal or generalized (Table 64-1) (2). Focal symptoms, such as hemiparesis, aphasia, and visual field defects, vary according to location of the tumor. Generalized symptoms, such as headache, confusion, lethargy, nausea, and vomiting, result from increased intracranial pressure (ICP) or hydrocephalus. Metastatic deposits near the ventricular system can cause obstructive hydrocephalus by interruption of normal cerebrospinal fluid outflow pathways through the third and fourth ventricles. Obstructive hydrocephalus is of particular concern with posterior fossa tumors. Headaches caused by increased ICP and/or hydrocephalus may have the following characteristics:

- Worse in the morning and with recumbancy;
- Associated with nausea and vomiting;

Table 64–1

Symptoms and Signs of Brain Metastasis

Symptoms	%	Signs	%
Headache	49	Mental status change	58
Focal weakness	30	Hemiparesis	59
Mental disturbance	32	Sensory loss	21
Gait ataxia	21	Papilledema	20
Speech difficulty	12	Gait ataxia	19
Visual disturbance	6	Aphasia	18
Sensory disturbance	6	Visual field cut	7
Limb ataxia	6	Limb ataxia	6
		Depressed consciousness	4

Data from Cairncross JG, Kim J-H, Posner JB. Radiation therapy for brain metastases. Ann Neurol 7: 529–541, 1980 and Young DF, Posner JB, Chu F, et al: Rapid-course radiation therapy of cerebral metastases: Results and complications. Cancer 4: 1069–1076, 1974.

- Exacerbated by coughing or straining;
- Accompanied by confusion or lethargy.

The presence of papilledema is very suggestive of increased ICP, although its absence does not exclude it.

EVALUATION

Contrast-enhanced MRI has replaced CT as the study of choice for patients with suspected brain metastasis (Figure 64-1). MRI is more sensitive than CT for small lesions, particularly in the brain stem and posterior fossa (Figure 64-2). In addition, MRI is better able to distinguish metastatic lesions from alternative diagnoses such as abscess or stroke. All cancer patients with new neurological symptoms should be screened for brain metastases. In patients who cannot undergo MRI because of implanted hardware, morbid obesity, or extreme claustrophobia, a contrast-enhanced CT should be obtained instead. If leptomeningeal enhancement is present, lumbar puncture should be strongly considered to rule out leptomeningeal metastases. Lumbar puncture should not be performed in patients with increased intracranial pressure, from obstructive hydrocephalus, lateral shift of midline structures, or any evidence of mass effect in the posterior fossa.

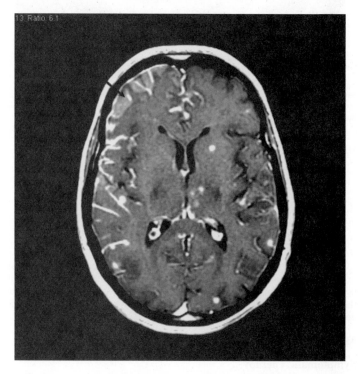

FIGURE 64-1   Gadolinium-enhanced T1-weighted MRI showing multiple small parenchymal metastases (*arrowheads*) and leptomeningeal enhancement (*arrow*) in a patient with non-small cell lung cancer. Spinal fluid was positive for malignant cells.

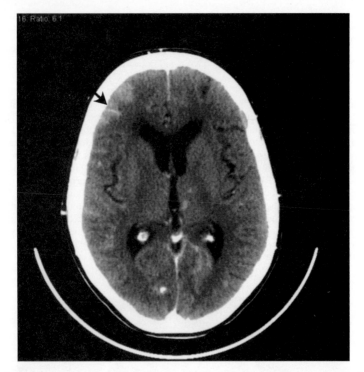

FIGURE 64-2   Contrast-enhanced CT in the same patient showing only two parenchymal lesions is (*arrowheads*) and faint leptomeningeal enhancement (*arrow*). This image demonstrates the lesser sensitivity of CT compared with MRI for detecting small metastases.

DIFFERENTIAL DIAGNOSIS

The differential diagnosis of a mass lesion in a patient with cancer is broad and includes:

- Primary brain tumor;
- Abscess (bacterial, mycobacterial, fungal, parasitic);
- Acute demyelinating plaque;
- Subacute cerebral infarction;
- Primary intracranial hemorrhage.

In a study of 54 patients with cancer who underwent biopsy of a single mass lesion, a diagnosis other than metastatic cancer was obtained in 11% (equally divided between primary brain tumor and infection) (3). This study highlights the importance of obtaining pathologic confirmation before proceeding with definitive therapy if the diagnosis is at all uncertain.

MANAGEMENT

Symptomatic Therapy

CORTICOSTEROIDS   Corticosteroids should be administered to patients with focal deficits, headache, or other symptoms resulting from peritumoral edema or increased ICP. Corticosteroids act to restore the integrity of the blood–brain barrier and thereby reduce cerebral edema. Dexamethasone is the most widely used corticosteroid for this purpose because of its long half-life and minimal mineralocorticoid effects. It is typically given as an intravenous 10 mg loading dose followed by 16 mg/day divided in two to four doses (either intravenous or oral). Symptoms should improve within 2–3 days, and higher doses may be required in some patients. Adverse effects of corticosteroids are dose-dependent, and therefore the dose should always be tapered to the lowest possible dose required to ameliorate symptoms. Patients taking daily steroids for longer than 2–4 weeks should receive prophylaxis for pneumocystis carinii, typically with trimethoprim/sulfamethoxazole.

ANTICONVULSANTS   Twenty to 40% of all brain tumor patients experience a seizure by the time their tumor is diagnosed. In these patients, the need for anticonvulsant therapy is clear. An additional 20–40% of patients will develop seizures as a complication of their disease. Based on this risk, many physicians choose to start prophylactic anticonvulsants at the time of diagnosis. However, this practice must be weighed against the potential adverse effects of anticonvulsants, which include:

- Allergic reaction, including Steven–Johnson syndrome;
- Hepatic dysfunction;
- Cognitive impairment and imbalance;
- Myelosuppression;
- Alteration of cytochrome P-450 enzyme system.

The latter is an important consideration in patients receiving chemotherapeutic agents that are metabolized by the liver such as taxanes or vinca alkaloids. The American Academy of Neurology has published a practice parameter finding no evidence to support the use of prophylactic anticonvulsant medication in patients with brain tumors who have not experienced a seizure (4).

Definitive Therapy

Treatment of brain metastases is aimed at improving neurologic function, enhancing quality of life, and extending survival. Multiple treatment modalities are now available that may lengthen survival, including surgery, various forms of radiation therapy, and chemotherapy. Treatment strategies often involve a combination of two or more modalities. The following three factors should be considered when designing a treatment regimen:

- Patient (age, functional status, comorbidities);
- Primary tumor (histology, degree of local control, presence of extracranial metastases);
- Metastatic brain disease (location, size, number).

SURGERY   *Solitary lesion*   The goal of surgery is to relieve neurologic symptoms, establish a pathologic diagnosis, and achieve local control. Patients with a single metastatic brain deposit and stable extracranial disease achieve longer survival, improved functional status, and better local control when treated with surgery plus whole brain radiation therapy (WBRT) as compared with WBRT alone (3, 5). Younger patients (age <60) and those with stable extracranial disease realize the most benefit from surgery. The majority of patients show symptomatic improvement after resection, often apparent in the immediate postoperative period.

Multiple lesions   When evaluated by contrast-enhanced MRI, the majority (70%) of patients with metastatic brain disease have multiple lesions. The role of surgery in these patients is less clear, but may be considered in the following circumstances:

- Dominant lesion causing significant symptoms or impending herniation;
- Two lesions accessible by a single craniotomy;
- Need for pathologic diagnosis;
- Young age, good functional status, and stable extracranial disease.

RADIOTHERAPY   Radiation therapy has been the cornerstone of treatment for brain metastases since the 1950s. Although surgery is a viable option for selected patients, many patients are not candidates for this intervention or do not wish to undergo an operation. Radiation therapy can be administered safely to most patients with the goal of palliation of neurological symptoms.

Whole brain radiation therapy   Whole brain fractionated external beam radiotherapy is delivered to the entire brain down to the bottom of the C2 vertebral body. A variety of schedules are employed; a widely used dosing regimen consists of 30 Gy delivered in 10 daily fractions over 2 weeks. WBRT is widely available and results in symptom palliation in many patients when used in combination with corticosteroids. Short-term side effects of WBRT include fatigue, nausea, anorexia, skin irritation, and hair loss. In long-term survivors, delayed toxicity may result in memory loss, dementia, gait ataxia, incontinence, and/or neuroendocrine dysfunction (e.g., hypothyroidism). The incidence of late neurotoxicity may be reduced by avoiding daily fractions greater than 3 Gy. When administered postoperatively in conjunction with surgical resection of a solitary lesion, WBRT decreases the likelihood of both local recurrence (10% with postoperative WBRT versus 46% with surgery alone) and distant recurrence (14% vs. 37%) (6).

Stereotactic radiosurgery   Stereotactic radiosurgery (SRS) is a form of external beam radiation that uses multiple convergent beams to deliver a single high dose of radiation to a discreet target volume. The technique is generally used for lesions up to 3 cm in diameter. Several approaches exist, each of which employs a different source of radiation:

- LINAC, using high-energy X-ray radiation from a linear accelerator;
- Gamma knife, using gamma radiation from a fixed array of cobalt 60 sources;
- Cyclotron, using protons generated from a large accelerator.

For most techniques, precise localization is accomplished using a stereotactic head frame that is anchored to the patient's skull by bone screws (placed under local anesthesia). The treatment itself lasts only minutes, and the frame is removed immediately afterwards. Tumors can be safely and effectively treated using a single dose of radiation ranging from 15 to 24 Gy according to lesion size. It is important to note that SRS produces excellent local control for metastases but does not treat "micrometastases" that are not evident on imaging. The addition of SRS to WBRT has been shown to increase survival in patients with single brain metastasis and achieve effective palliation in patients with one to three brain metastases (7). Complications of stereotactic radiation include seizures, headache, exacerbation of neurologic deficits, nausea, hemorrhage, and radiation necrosis.

Radiosurgery versus surgery   For single brain metastases, both surgery and radiosurgery are effective options, and thus debate remains regarding which modality should be considered first-line therapy. Randomized trials comparing surgery and radiosurgery have not yet been performed to address this question.

For large metastatic tumors with extensive edema and mass effect, surgery is probably superior to radiation for quick and reliable relief of symptoms, provided the lesion can be safely resected. Because even minor swelling in the posterior fossa after radiosurgery can cause hydrocephalus, surgery is often recommended for cerebellar metastases. Radiosurgery has the advantage of being non-invasive and therefore associated with less morbidity and mortality than surgery. Moreover, radiosurgery can be used to treat metastases in surgically inaccessible areas of the brain, such as the brainstem or basal ganglia. Multiple, minimally symptomatic metastases are more simply treated with radiation (WBRT with or without radiosurgery) than surgery.

CHEMOTHERAPY   The role of chemotherapy in the treatment of metastatic brain tumors has historically been confined to patients who have failed surgery, WBRT, and radiosurgery. Temozolomide, an oral alkylating agent that is widely used in the treatment of malignant primary brain tumors, has excellent bioavailability and relatively high central nervous system penetration (20% of plasma levels). Multiple studies have now examined the effects of concurrent temodozolomide and WBRT in patients with newly diagnosed brain metastases, and the results show that the combination is well tolerated and may have more clinical activity than WBRT alone (8). However, larger well-controlled trials will be necessary to confirm these results. Other agents have shown activity in small trials, but a complete discussion is beyond the scope of this review.

Recent data suggest that patients with HER2-positive breast cancer treated with trastuzumab (Herceptin) are at increased risk for isolated CNS progression (9). This may reflect improved peripheral disease control and patient survival with trastuzumab-based therapy; poor CNS penetration of trastuzumab; and/or a predilection for CNS localization by HER2-positive cancers.

PROGNOSIS

Patients with untreated brain metastases have a median survival of 1 month. Corticosteroids improve median survival to 2 months. The addition of WBRT extends median survival to 4–6 months (10). Patients with solitary brain lesions and limited extracranial disease who are treated with surgery or SRS plus WBRT have a median survival of 10–15 months. Favorable prognostic factors include:

- Absence of systemic disease;
- Young age (less than 60 years);
- Good performance status (Karnofsky performance status of 70 or greater);
- Long interval from systemic cancer diagnosis to development of brain metastasis;
- Surgical resection;
- Fewer than three brain lesions;
- Certain primary cancer types (breast, lymphoma).

REFERENCES

1. Barnholtz-Sloan JS, Sloan AE, Davis FG, Vigneau FD, Lai P, Sawaya RE. Incidence proportions of brain metastases in patients diagnosed (1973 to 2001) in the metropolitan detroit cancer surveillance system. J Clin Oncol. 2004; 22: 2865–2872.
2. Posner JB. In "Neurologic Complications of Cancer," FA Davis Company, Philadelphia, 1995.
3. Patchell RA, Tibbs PA, Walsh JW, et al. A randomized trial of surgery in the treatment of single metastases to the brain. N Engl J Med. 1990; 322: 494–500.

4. Glantz MJ, Cole BF, Forsyth PA, et al. Practice parameter: anticonvulsant prophylaxis in patients with newly diagnosed brain tumors. Report of the quality standards subcommittee of the American Academy of Neurology. Neurology. 2000; 54: 1886–1893.
5. Vecht CJ, Haaxma-Reiche H, Noordijk EM, et al. Treatment of single brain metastasis: radiotherapy alone or combined with neurosurgery? Ann Neurol. 1993; 33: 583–590.
6. Patchell RA, Tibbs PA, Regine WF, et al. Postoperative radiotherapy in the treatment of single metastases to the brain: a randomized trial. JAMA. 1998; 280: 1485–1489.
7. Andrews DW, Scott CB, Sperduto PW, et al. Whole brain radiation therapy with or without stereotactic radiosurgery boost for patients with one to three brain metastases: phase III results of the RTOG 9508 randomised trial. Lancet. 2004; 363: 1665–1672.
8. Verger E, Gil M, Yaya R, et al. Temozolomide and concomitant whole brain radiotherapy in patients with brain metastases: a phase II randomized trial. Int J Radiat Oncol Biol Phys. 2005; 61: 185–191.
9. Burnstein H, Lieberman G, Slamon D, et al. Isolated central nervous system metastases in patients with HER2-overexpressing advanced breast cancer treated with first-line trastuzumab-based therapy. Ann Oncol. 2005; 16: 1772–1777.
10. Gaspar L, Scott C, Rotman M, et al. Recursive partitioning analysis (RPA) of prognostic factors in three radiation therapy oncology group (RTOG) brain metastases trials. Int J Radiat Oncol Biol Phys. 1997; 37: 745–751.

PARANEOPLASTIC NEUROLOGIC SYNDROMES

INTRODUCTION

Paraneoplastic neurologic syndromes (Table 65-1) occur prior to or in the setting of cancer and are not related to tumor invasion, infection, ischemia, or treatment toxicities. These syndromes occur in fewer than 1% of cancer patients, but higher risk is associated with certain cancers, such as small cell lung cancer (SCLC), neuroblastoma, and thymoma.

Many paraneoplastic syndromes are related to production of antibodies that target antigens shared by a tumor and by tissues of the nervous system. The consequence is a humoral and cell-mediated immune response against this antigen. The antigens can be cytoplasmic (for example anterior horn cells and Purkinje

Table 65-1

Classical Presentation of Paraneoplastic Syndromes

Syndrome	Symptoms
PCD	Abrupt onset (over hours to weeks) truncal and appendicular ataxia, dizziness, nausea, diplopia, dysphagia, UMN signs, LMN signs, nystagmus
PEM	Subacute mental status change; short-term memory defects, emotional lability, seizures
POM	Opsoclonus = large-amplitude ocular saccades and other eye symptoms, often associated with ataxia and not myoclonus in breast cancer
	Myoclonus = muscle twitches, hypotonia, irritability; occurs in the setting of opsoclonus, often accompanied by ataxia and encephalopathy, can progress to coma
CAR	Photosensitivity and visual loss, may start unilaterally and then progress to bilateral blindness over 6–18 months
MAR	Sudden visual shimmering, flickering, night blindness, and mild peripheral field visual loss, not progressing to full blindness
SPS	Axial stiffness, spine deformities, board-like abdomen; painful muscle spasms are triggered by sudden movement, noise, or emotional upset
Dorsal root ganglionitis	Abnormal sensations (pain, temperature, touch, and proprioception)
Sensorimotor polyneuropathy	Motor and/or sensory weakness, sometimes with tremor and/or gait disorder
Autonomic neuropathy	Orthostatic hypotension, impotence, intestinal pseudo-obstruction
Neuromyotonia	Fasciculations, delayed muscle relaxation, weakness
LEMS	Proximal weakness, with some patients improving with repetitive action
Myopathy	Proximal muscle weakness

cells of cerebellum) or on the cell surface (for example voltage gated potassium channels) or at synaptic junctions. Therefore, for most conditions the antibodies themselves are not directly damaging cells, and it is more likely that a concurrent cell-mediated immune response or antibody reaction with a peptide on the cell surface is actually causing the neurologic symptoms (1).

The immune reaction is characterized by elevations of CSF white count, and in situ synthesis of IgG. Imaging MRI flair or gadolinium studies may suggest an inflammatory reaction, as seen on the rare biopsy or on autopsy examination. The causative antibodies can sometimes be isolated in serum and/or CSF, but their detection may require a research investigation that identifies a novel antibody. A recent evaluation of 60,000 patients tested for paraneoplastic syndromes at the Mayo Clinic over 4 years showed that only 553 (0.9%) possessed known autoantibodies. Some patients had multiple autoantibodies concurrently (2). It is likely that 40% of patients with definite paraneoplastic syndrome do not have a detectable characterizing autoantibody (3).

The diagnosis of paraneoplastic syndromes is primarily clinical, and is usually made in the following circumstances: (1) Development of a classical paraneoplastic neurologic syndrome in a patient known to have had cancer within the past 5 years; (2) Non-classical neurologic syndrome with an onconeural antibody identified (not necessarily a well-characterized one) in the context of a cancer diagnosis within 5 years; (3) A novel neurologic syndrome that improves after cancer treatment without immuno-suppressive therapy; and (4) A neurologic syndrome (classical or not) with a well-characterized onconeural antibody found in anticipation of cancer diagnosis (4). Tables 65-2 and 65-3 describe the well-characterized antibodies often associated with paraneoplastic neurologic syndromes.

Because paraneoplastic syndromes often herald cancer, the patient may be diagnosed and treated early in the natural course of the disease. This may partly explain the prolonged survivorship of patients with paraneoplastic syndromes. In addition, earlier cancer diagnosis may correlate with a greater chance of cure. Most provocative is the concept that a better prognosis may reflect the immune control of the underlying tumor. The presence of a paraneoplastic neurologic

Table 65-2

Well-Characterized Antibodies Strongly Associated with Neurologic Paraneoplastic Syndromes

Antibody	Antigens	Predominant syndromes	Common cancers
Anti-Yo (PCA1 = cdr2)	34 and 62 kD in Purkinje cytoplasm	PCD, POM	Ovarian, breast
Anti-Hu (ANNA-1)	35–40 kD, concentrated in nuclei	PEM, autonomic, POM	SCLC, neuroblastoma
Anti-Ri (ANNA-2)	55 and 80 kD, concentrated in CNS nuclei	PEM, POM	Breast, gyn, SCLC
Anti-amphiphysin	128 kD	SPS, PEM, PCD, POM	Breast, SCLC
Anti-Ma (Ta)	40 and 42 kD in nuclei	PEM, POM	Testicular, lung
Anti-CRMP5 (CV2)	66 kD in CNS cytoplasms	PCD, PEM peripheral neuropathy	SCLC, thymoma

Table 65-3

Antibodies that are Only Partially Characterized or Often Seen Independent of Malignancy

Antibody	Antigen	Predominant syndromes	Common cancers
Anti-VGCC	64 kD in NMJ and Purkinjes	LEMS, PCD	SCLC, lymphoma
Anti-Zic4	Zinc-finger	PCD	SCLC
Anti-Tr		PCD	Hodgkin's
Anti-mGluR1		PCD	Hodgkin's
ANNA-3	170 kD	PEM	SCLC
Anti-recoverin		CAR	SCLC
Anti-gephyrin	23 kD in photoreceptor	SPS	Breast, SCLC
Anti-VGKC		Neuromyotonia	Thymoma, SCLC, Hodgkin's
Anti-MAG		Peripheral neuropathy	Waldenström's macroglobulinemia

syndrome introduces new considerations into treatment planning for a cancer patient. Cancer therapy strives to achieve a balance between maximizing antitumor effects and minimizing treatment side effects, including further damage to the nervous system. For example, radiation fields, which include the spinal cord, may worsen paraneoplastic myelopathy, as well platinum analogs given to patients with subacute neuronopathies.

Treatments for these syndromes involve both cancer therapy to attenuate the cancer-derived immune response and direct suppression of the immune response with steroids, Rituxan, immunoglobulin, or plasmapheresis. Syndromes of neuronal death (such as cerebellar or spinal cord or retinal degeneration) are most difficult to treat, while inflammatory syndromes (of limbic structures, dorsal root, or root exit zones [Guillain–Barre]) are moderately treatable. Most responsive are syndromes (Myasthenic, stiff person) involving blockade of neuromuscular junction (NMJ) signaling (5). This chapter will review the clinical evaluation, biology, and management of various paraneoplastic syndromes.

SYNDROMES OF THE CENTRAL NERVOUS SYSTEM

Paraneoplastic Cerebellar Degeneration

Paraneoplastic cerebellar degeneration (PCD), often associated with anti-Yo Purkinje-cell antibody-1 (PCA-1), also termed cerebellar degeneration related-2 (cdr2), occurs in women with breast or ovarian cancer. Yo antibodies are directed against two proteins (one 34 kDa and the other 62 kDa) in the cytoplasm of cerebellar Purkinje cells (6). Cell loss is associated with progressive gait and then appendicular ataxia with scanning speech. Essentially irreversible are associated brain stem and cerebellar symptoms such as double vision, dysphagia, and nystagmus in all directions of gaze. Although the cerebellum is not considered a control center for emotion and intelligence, 20% of patients experience emotional lability and memory defects. The syndromes seldom are "pure." An upper motor neuron Babinski's reflex is found in half of patients and lower motor neuron distal sensory loss in a minority.

Symptoms develop over weeks and commonly progress to virtually complete dependence. Only 30% of patients are able to walk unassisted and many are unable to write, feed themselves, or swallow (7).

Brain MRI and CT seldom reveal abnormalities other than loss of cerebellar architecture and prominence of folia of the cerebellum. The CSF contains T-lymphocytes and elevated protein and IgG. Treatment is usually not effective in the setting of cellular loss and thus immediate therapy of both tumor and the paraneoplastic sequelae is mandated (7). For example, Phuphanich and Brock report two cases of ovarian-cancer related anti-Yo PCD that remitted with three cycles of immunoglobulin and four cycles of carboplatin and paclitaxel (8).

Because anti-Yo disease is so frequently linked to breast and ovarian cancer, every woman who develops acute or subacute cerebellar symptoms should have testing for anti-Yo. If this autoantibody is detected, radiologic studies should be performed to exclude ovarian cancer (underlying 46% of anti-Yo associated PCDs) and breast cancer (underlying 24%). These studies may require repetition as neurologic symptoms may signal the presence of very small localized tumors. Two-thirds of patients with anti-Yo PCD do not have a known cancer diagnosis at the time the neurologic symptoms begin and as a general rule PCD occurs in the setting of antibody production without cancer in 10% of cases. Other gynecologic cancers, adenocarcinomas of unknown primary, bronchial carcinomas, Hodgkin's disease, and gastric carcinomas are less frequently the underlying cause of PCD.

PCD also occurs in conjunction with autoantibodies other than anti-Yo. In patients with SCLC, PCD has been linked to the following antibodies: (1) Collapsin-response mediator protein 5 (CRMP5) (in which peripheral neuropathy also occurs); (2) Zic4 (in which PEM also occurs); (3) Voltage-gated calcium channel (VGCC) (from which Lambert–Eaton syndrome also results); and (4) PCA-2. Anti-Zic4 frequently appears in the setting of other autoantibodies, but it is only associated with PCD when it is found alone (9).

In Hodgkin's disease, anti-Tr (found in Purkinje cell cytoplasm) and anti-metabotropic glutamate receptor (anti-mGluR1) antibodies are found in serum and/or CSF in association with PCD. PCD has been seen even in patients in complete remission, as well, but may develop at the time of initial diagnosis or of recurrence. PCD in the setting of Hodgkin's is more likely to remit with anti-tumor treatment than is the same syndrome related to anti-Yo (7).

Paraneoplastic Encephalomyelitis (PEM)

Paraneoplastic encephalomyelitis may affect the mesial temporal lobes, midbrain, pons, or spinal cord. Symptoms depend on the site(s) of T-cell infiltrates. *Limbic encephalitis* produces short-term memory disturbances, depression, and emotional lability Inflammation of the temporal and frontal lobes, may cause seizures. The MRI findings include Flair and gadolinium abnormalities, and resemble herpes simplex virus (HSV) encephalitis. PEM presents over weeks to months, rather than days, as in HSV. Brainstem encephalitis is associated with gaze abnormalities and nystagmus, and afflictions of the midbrain cause movement disorders. As a general rule, PEM is also commonly associated with subacute sensory neuropathy and autonomic changes including cardiac arrhythmias and hypotension.

Limbic encephalitis typically occurs in the setting of SCLC (or NSCLC) with anti-Hu (also called type 1 antineuronal nuclear antigen or ANNA-1) antibodies. The Hu antigens against which these antibodies are targeted are four 35–40 kDa RNA binding proteins. These proteins upregulate mRNAs that encode proteins essential for neuron development (6).

Other antibodies have also been linked to PEM. In breast cancer, anti-Ri antibody (type 2 antineuronal nuclear antigen or ANNA-2) targets the 53–61 kDa and 79–84 kDa RNA-binding proteins termed Ri (also known as Nova1 and

Nova2), which are found predominantly in the nuclei of CNS neurons (6). In thoracic cancers (especially SCLC), antibody to type 3 antineuronal nuclear antigen (ANNA-3) binds to nuclei of cerebellar neurons (10). In SCLC, thymoma, and gynecologic cancers, anti-CV2 and anti-CRMP5 bind 62 and 66 kDa proteins found in cytoplasm of neurons, oligodendrocytes, and retinal cells, optic nerve, and PNS axons. Anti-amphiphysin targets a 125-kDa protein that is associated with synaptic vesicles to produce PEM in SCLC patients. In testicular, breast, colon, and non-small cell lung cancer (NSCLC), anti-Ma (also termed anti-Ta) binds to 40 kDa (Ma1) and 42 kDa (Ma2) proteins found in the nuclei and nucleoli of CNS neurons (6). In testicular cancer patients, anti-Ma2 may be associated with brainstem encephalitis (6).

Opsoclonus-Myoclonus (POM)

Opsoclonus ("Dancing eyes") refers to spontaneous, arrhythmic, large-amplitude ocular movements occurring in all directions. Opsoclonus can occur spontaneously in young women but its appearance should activate a search for malignancy, especially neuroblastoma in children. Myoclonus ("Dancing feet or extremities") refers to muscle twitches in the limbs and trunk, as well as hypotonia and irritability. The POM due to anti-Hu or anti-amphiphysin afflicts adults with SCLC. These patients also develop encephalopathy. Other common clinical associations of POM are with breast or ovarian cancer (in the setting of anti-Ri or anti-Yo), and with testicular cancer (with anti-Ma2). However, many POM patients do not have identifiable autoantibodies (11).

POM occurs in 2% of children with neuroblastoma. Ten percent of children with opsoclonus-myoclonus have an underlying neuroblastoma. The eye movements may be multi-direction or one direction ('flutter'). As a general rule, POM patients have a better prognosis. Half of POM patients experience neurologic difficulties before the tumor is identified (7).

In women with anti-Ri, opsoclonus also occurs as a separate clinical entity, and in this setting, is often associated with brainstem difficulties of balance, ataxia, and movement disorders. Breast cancer and, less commonly, SCLC are by far the most frequent tumors in which anti-Ri syndromes develop. Although three-quarters of patients with anti-Ri ocular syndromes have opsoclonus, others have ocular flutter, nystagmus, abnormal visual tracking, blepharospasm, and abnormal vestibule-ocular reflexes. Symptoms peak between 1 week and 4 months of onset. Thirty percent of patients become wheelchair-bound within 1 month of symptom onset. Unlike in PEM, the brain MRI is usually normal and CSF contains mild lymphocytic pleocytosis and slightly high protein. Steroids may be beneficial, and symptoms may respond to treating the underlying breast cancer, to intravenous immunoglobulin, or to plasmapheresis. On autopsy, widespread inflammatory infiltrates are found (12).

In contrast, opsoclonus that occurs in adults in the absence of anti-Ri is usually associated with myoclonus. In adults, the underlying cause is most often SCLC, although the syndrome may be post-viral associated with/syndromes. Gait and truncal ataxia, nausea, and encephalopathy are also common. Lethargy and confusion progress to coma in a quarter of patients, but in other cases symptoms stabilize or spontaneously remit. CT and MRI of the brain are usually normal, but EEG may show slowing. Autopsy samples have demonstrated normal or slightly decreased number of Purkinje cells, increased microglia and gliosis, and inflammation of the leptomeninges and subarachnoid space. While SCLC is by far the most common underlying malignancy, opsoclonus-myoclonus may also develop in patients with chondrosarcoma, or with carcinoma of the endometrium, fallopian tube, bladder, thyroid, or testicles.

Retinopathy

Cancer-associated retinopathy (CAR) is characterized by photosensitivity and visual loss, which may start as unilateral fast movements ("rodent-like") and then may become bilateral over days to weeks. CAR usually precedes the diagnosis of cancer. Lumbar puncture typically reveals a pleocytosis in the CSF. On exam, a patient has poor acuity vision, retinal artery narrowing, and scotomata; blindness often results in 6–18 months. CAR is associated with antibodies that target a 23 kDa calcium-binding protein, recoverin, located in photoreceptors, but subtypes of the syndrome may manifest over 20 separate antigenic targets. Consequently, cone and rod dysfunction occurs without abnormal visual evoked potentials. Most cases develop in patients with SCLC, but other associated cancers include gynecologic, breast, pancreatic, prostate, bladder, laryngeal, colon, NSCLC, and lymphoma (7).

Melanoma-associated retinopathy (MAR) presents more acutely than does CAR, but is less likely to progress to blindness. Symptoms include sudden shimmering, flickering, night blindness, and mild peripheral field visual loss, and generally occur in the setting of known metastatic melanoma, rather than before diagnosis of cancer. Anti-rod bipolar cell antibodies are thought to be responsible, but the specific antigen is unknown (7).

Stiff Person Syndrome

Stiff Person Syndrome (SPS) is characterized by axial stiffness, spine deformities, and board-like abdomen. Sudden movement, noise, or emotional upset triggers painful muscle spasms. Sensory, motor, and cognitive exams are normal. EMG shows continuous motor unit activity in the affected muscles at rest. Paraneoplastic SPS is associated with anti-amphiphysin or anti-gephyrin antibodies (less common). The underlying tumor is usually breast cancer or SCLC, or less commonly, Hodgkin's or thymoma (13).

SYNDROMES OF THE PERIPHERAL NERVOUS SYSTEM

Dorsal Root Ganglionitis

Dorsal root ganglionitis is nearly pathognomonic for paraneoplastic disease. All sensory modalities are impaired (pain, temperature, touch, and proprioception), but the prominent complaints are patchy numbness and paresthesias involving face, trunk, or proximal extremities. Severe pain in all limbs develops over time, as does loss of reflexes and vibration sense. The initial pain syndrome may resemble the symptoms of Zoster infiltration of dorsal root ganglia, but loss of proprioception eventually supervenes and prevents patients from walking unassisted. PEM is often associated. Sjögren's disease is the only other cause of this classic collection of symptoms resulting from selective damage to dorsal root ganglia. No specific antibody has been identified, but some of the same antibodies that cause PEM (anti-Hu, anti-CRMP5) have been identified in these patients. SCLC is the most commonly associated cancer, but there are case reports of dorsal root ganglionitis in the setting of NSCLC and lymphoma as well (14).

Sensorimotor Polyneuropathies

A wide variety of sensory neuropathies result from antibodies binding to sensory fibers, inducing inflammation, and causing demyelination. Anti-myelin-associated glycoprotein (MAG), anti-Hu, and anti-CV2 have been found in patients with peripheral polyneuropathy, with a complex array of syndromes resulting, each impacting motor and sensory nerve conduction differently. Gait disorder and tremor are sometimes seen, as are Guillain-Barre, brachial plexopathy, and anterior horn cell disease, particularly in patients with Hodgkin's Disease. Chronic peripheral neuropathy also occurs in SCLC, melanoma, lymphoma, and plasma cell dyscrasia (14).

The neuropathy that occurs with the POEMS syndrome (P = polyneuropathy, O = organomegaly, E = endocrinopathy, M = M protein, S = skin changes) usually occurs in the setting of osteosclerotic myeloma, osteolytic myeloma, or MGUS. Unlike other paraneoplastic syndromes, the involved antibody is produced by the malignancy, not against it. Radiation to bony lesions may improve POEMS neuropathy in the setting of myeloma. With MGUS, chemotherapy or Rituxan ameliorates-associated neuropathies (14). Comorbidity may also result from underlying amyloidosis.

Autonomic Neuropathy

When cancer causes the immune system to target neurons of the autonomic nervous system, orthostatic hypotension, impotence, diaphoresis, cardiac arrhythmias, hypoventilation, and intestinal pseudo-obstruction can result. Anti-Hu, often associated with underlying SCLC, is found in many cases, but this type of neuropathy can also be due to bronchial carcinoma, thymoma, and Hodgkin's lymphoma. Often the same patients who have sensorimotor neuropathy or PEM will experience autonomic effects of their antibodies as well (7).

SYNDROMES OF THE NEUROMUSCULAR JUNCTION AND MUSCLE

Neuromyotonia

Antibodies to voltage-gated potassium channels (VGKC) or to nicotinic acetylcholine receptors cause spontaneous firing of motor unit potentials. Cramps, fasciculations, delayed relaxation, muscle twitches, or weakness may result. Half of patients have a high creatine kinase. Other less common symptoms include arrhythmias, salivation, memory loss, hallucinations, constipation, personality chance, and insomnia. Thymoma is the most commonly associated tumor, followed by SCLC and Hodgkin's. Plasma exchange is often helpful (7).

Lambert–Eaton Myasthenic Syndrome

Lambert–Eaton Myasthenia Syndrome (LEMS) is the most common neurologic paraneoplastic syndrome. Antibodies against the *P/Q* voltage-gated calcium channel (VGCC) impair conduction at the NMJ. Symptoms include proximal weakness (usually starting in the legs) with less impact on cranial nerves than in myasthenia gravis. Sixty percent of cases are caused by SCLC (15). In some cases, weakness and sub-par reflexes improve with repetitive motion. The usual EMG finding is a low muscle action potential at rest, with diminished response at low rates of repetitive stimulation and heightened response at high rates. 3, 4-Diaminopyridine, which facilitates presynaptic acetylcholine release, is often an effective treatment (7).

Myopathy

Cancer-associated acute necrotizing myopathy typically starts as painful proximal weakness, rapidly progressing to generalized weakness and sometimes to death due to respiratory muscle involvement. Serum Creatine kinase is elevated and muscle biopsy shows necrosis without inflammation. SCLC, GI, breast, renal, and prostate cancers have been linked to this devastating condition. In contrast, both polymyositis and dermatomyositis will show significant muscle inflammation on biopsy. When a diagnosis of polymyositis is made, the patient has a 9–18% risk of having an underlying malignancy (7). The risk of non-Hodgkin's Lymphoma is increased 3.7-fold, the risk of lung cancer 2.8-fold, and the risk of bladder cancer 2.4-fold (16).

Dermatomyositis differs from polymyositis in that patients have a V-shaped chest rash, a heliotrope upper eyelid rash, and scaling erythema on the extensor surfaces of the extremities ("Grotton's sign"), and skin cracking of the hands. Dermatomyositis is even more strongly linked to malignancy than polymyositis is; 15–42% of dermatomyositis patients have an underlying tumor (7). After dermatomyositis is diagnosed, the risk of ovarian cancer rises 10.5-fold, the risk of lung cancer rises sixfold, and the risks of non-Hodgkin's Lymphoma and GI (pancreatic, gastric, and colorectal) cancers each rise approximately 3.5-fold (16).

CONCLUSION

Paraneoplastic syndromes are important to identify early because they signal the need for an immediate search for an underlying tumor. Treatment of that malignancy is essential in order to slow or reverse neurologic morbidity. Other useful treatments are targeted at the immune system, as it appears to mediate the nervous system damage via humoral and/or cellular responses to onconeural antigens. These treatments include steroids, IVIG, plasmapheresis, Rituxan, and cyclophosphamide. Unfortunately, these rarely produce long-term remission of symptoms effectively, especially when neuron death has already occurred. Therefore, it is crucial that paraneoplastic neurologic syndromes be diagnosed as early as possible so that oncologic care can begin quickly, maximizing the opportunity to cure underlying tumors and prevent further neurologic decline.

REFERENCES

1. Sillevis Smith PA, et al. Treatment of paraneoplastic neurologic syndromes. In JH Noseworthy (ed.), "Neurological Therapeutics Principles and Practice," 2nd edition, Vol. 1. Taylor & Francis, New York, NY, 2006, pp. 3490.
2. Pittock SJ, Kryzer TJ, Lennon VA. Paraneoplastic antibodies coexist and predict cancer, not neurological syndrome. Ann Neurol. 2004; 56(5): 715–719.
3. Dalmau J, Gonzalez RG, Lerwill MF. Case records of the Massachusetts General Hospital. Case 4-2007. A 56-year-old woman with rapidly progressive vertigo and ataxia. N Engl J Med. 2007; 356(6): 612–620.
4. Graus F, et al. Recommended diagnostic criteria for paraneoplastic neurological syndromes. J Neurol Neurosurg Psychiatry. 2004; 75(8): 1135–1140.
5. Darnell RB, Posner JB. Paraneoplastic syndromes involving the nervous system. N Engl J Med. 2003; 349(16): 1543–1554.
6. Sutton I, Winer JB. The immunopathogenesis of paraneoplastic neurological syndromes. Clin Sci (Lond). 2002; 102(5): 475–486.
7. Darnell RB, Posner JB. Paraneoplastic syndromes affecting the nervous system. Semin Oncol. 2006; 33(3): 270–298.
8. Phuphanich S, Brock C. Neurologic improvement after high-dose intravenous immunoglobulin therapy in patients with paraneoplastic cerebellar degeneration associated with anti-Purkinje cell antibody. J Neurooncol. 2007; 81(1): 67–69.
9. Bataller L, et al. Antibodies to Zic4 in paraneoplastic neurologic disorders and small-cell lung cancer. Neurology. 2004; 62(5): 778–782.
10. Chan KH, Vernino S, Lennon VA. ANNA-3 anti-neuronal nuclear antibody: marker of lung cancer-related autoimmunity. Ann Neurol. 2001; 50(3): 301–311.
11. Bataller L, Dalmau J. Neuro-ophthalmology and paraneoplastic syndromes. Curr Opin Neurol. 2004; 17(1): 3–8.
12. Luque FA, et al. Anti-Ri: an antibody associated with paraneoplastic opsoclonus and breast cancer. Ann Neurol. 1991; 29(3): 241–251.

13. Murinson BB. Stiff-person syndrome. Neurologist. 2004; 10(3): 131–137.
14. Rudnicki SA, Dalmau J. Paraneoplastic syndromes of the spinal cord, nerve, and muscle. Muscle Nerve. 2000; 23(12): 1800–1818.
15. Rees JH. Paraneoplastic syndromes: when to suspect, how to confirm, and how to manage. J Neurol Neurosurg Psychiatry. 2004; 75(suppl 2): ii43–ii50.
16. Hill CL, et al. Frequency of specific cancer types in dermatomyositis and polymyositis: a population-based study. Lancet. 2001; 357(9250): 96–100.

| 66 | John R. Clark, Paul M. Busse, Daniel Deschler |

HEAD AND NECK CANCER

INTRODUCTION

Cancers of the head and neck include a spectrum of malignant neoplasms. Most commonly, however, "head and neck cancer" refers to epithelial carcinomas, squamous cell cancers and their variant histologic types that arise from the mucosal surfaces of the upper aerodigestive tract and constitute over 85% of the malignant tumors encountered in this region. Those caring for patients with head and neck neoplastic conditions must be conversant with the natural history and preferred forms of treatment for the many different malignant tumors as well as the occasional locally aggressive but benign lesions that arise in this region.

The head and neck are traditionally divided into nine distinct anatomic regions where epithelial cancers of mucosal surfaces originate (Table 66-1). Within these nine regions and associated areas such as the base of skull, orbit, orbital cavity, and the neck itself, other neoplastic conditions may arise

Table 66-1

Sites of the Head and Neck Region from Which Epithelial Cancers of the Upper Aerodigestive Tract may Arise

Oral cavity:	Mobile tongue anterior to circumvallate papillae, hard palate, floor of mouth, buccal surface of cheeks, alveolar ridges, and underlying mandible
Pharynx: subdivided into three sites	
Nasopharynx:	Pharyngeal walls posterior to the nasal cavity and superior to the level of the soft palate
Oropharynx:	Pharyngeal walls from the level of the soft palate inferiorly to the level of the base of the tongue, tonsillar fossas, soft palate, base of tongue posterior to circumvallate papilla
Hypopharynx:	Pharyngeal walls posterior and lateral to the larynx, and pyriform sinuses
Larynx: subdivided into three sites	
Supraglottis:	All laryngeal structures above the true vocal cords: the epiglottis, arytenoids, aryepiglottic folds, false vocal cords, and laryngeal vestibule.
Glottis:	Restricted to the true vocal cords
Subglottis:	The region 0.5 cm inferior to the true vocal cords to the bottom of the cricoid cartilage.
Nasal cavity:	Nasal vestibule, nasal septum, and cribiform plate region
Paranasal sinuses:	Frontal, sphenoid, ethmoid and maxillary sinuses

including primary tumors of the major or minor salivary glands, the skin, the thyroid or parathyroid glands, or non-epithelial tissues of the neck. Sarcomas and hematologic malignancies may also arise in the head and neck region. Representative classical histopathologies encountered in clinical practice are recorded in Table 66-2.

INCIDENCE AND PREVALENCE

The American Cancer Society estimates that there will be 45,660 new cases of head and neck cancer in the United States in 2007, and 11,210 deaths due to this disease. Overall, this suggests a curative potential of approximately 75% making head and neck cancer one of the most curable of adult invasive malignances. However, the impact of this disease on society is not measured solely by its relatively low absolute mortality, but also by the acute and chronic cosmetic, unctional, and psychological morbidities experienced by all patients. Head and neck cancer thus remains a feared disease associated with significant rates of both morbidity and mortality.

Surveillance Epidemiology and End Results (SEER) data reveal the incidence and prevalence of head and neck cancer to be decreasing in a pattern that approximates declines seen for lung cancer. These parallel changes are likely secondary to a national decline in exposure to a common carcinogen, tobacco. However encouraging these data, several sobering facts must be noted.

Significant gender and race-based differences remain in the incidence of head and neck cancer and its treatment outcomes. SEER data reveal the incidence and mortality of oral and pharyngeal cancer women to be minimally improved from 1975 to 2003 when compared to men, and that the incidence and mortality of this disease in African-American males exceeds that of Caucasian males. Indeed in African-American males, the mortality related to laryngeal cancer in 2003 exceeds that of 1969 (1).

Over the past 10 years, SEER data also indicate a remarkable increase in the incidence of cancers of the tonsil in the younger adults. This increase has been attributed in great part to newly recognized pathogen, Human Papilloma Virus (HPV). Molecular data suggest that HPV contributes to the carcinogenic process in up to 40–50% of patients with oropharyngeal cancer (2). The probability that HPV contributed to a patient's oropharyngeal cancer is greater in the setting of a younger patient with no significant history of alcohol or tobacco abuse.

RISK FACTORS FOR HEAD AND NECK CANCER

Alcohol and tobacco containing products remain the most significant risk factors for this disease. All fermented and distilled alcoholic beverages contain carcinogens that promote the development of head and neck cancer. Tobacco-containing products have carcinogenic effects on the upper aero-digestive tract identical to those reported in the lung. Important to the head and neck region, the local effects of alcohol and tobacco carcinogens are both dose-dependent, and synergistic. Smokeless tobacco abuse results in a local exposure to carcinogens that promotes cancers of the oral cavity and to a lesser extent, the oropharynx.

Other significant risk factors for this disease include prolonged exposure to asbestos (larynx cancer), textile fibers, nickel refining, and wood dust and leather tanning (nasal cavity and paranasal sinus adenocarcinomas). Dietary factors may also contribute. The incidence of head and neck cancer is highest in people with the lowest consumption of fruits and vegetables. Recognizing the latter association, clinical trials of various vitamin and anti-oxidants supplements have been conducted. To date, however, micronutrient supplementation has not led to a reduction in the risk of developing head and neck cancer.

Table 66-2

Neoplasms of the Head and Neck Region

Commonly encountered
- Epithelial lesions:
  - Any mucosal surface of upper aerodigestive tract
    - Hyperplastic to dysplastic to invasive carcinomas associated with EtOH/Tobacco
    - Squamous papillomas
  - Oropharynx, especially tonsil and base of tongue
    - Poorly differentiated or non-keratinzing often basoloid squamous cancer sometimes associated with high-risk HPV sub types identical to those seen in women with cervical cancer
  - Nasopharynx
    - Undifferentiated carcinoma of nasopharyngeal type (UCNT) or non-keratinizing carcinoma, both associated with EBV
    - Keratinizing squamous cell carcinomas
  - Nasal cavity and paranasal sinuses
    - Sinonasal undifferentiated cancer (SNUC)
    - Sinonasal squamous cell cancer
- Thyroid and parathyroid cancers
  - Differentiated papillary, follicular, or mixed cancers
  - Anaplastic thyroid cancers
  - Hurthle Cell cancers
  - Medullary Thyroid Cancer
- Major and minor salivary gland tumors
  - Pleomorphic adenoma
  - Warthin's tumor
  - Basal cell adenoma
  - Mucoepidermoid carcinoma
  - Adenoid cystic carcinoma
  - Acinic cell carcinoma
  - Salivary duct carcinoma
  - Carcinoma ex-pleomorphic adenoma
Infrequently encountered
- Neuroendocrine tumors
  - Poorly differentiated carcinomas of neuroendocrine type (commonly seen in nasal cavity or paranasal sinuses)
  - Small cell carcinoma (commonly seen in larynx)
- Olfactory neuroblastomas (a.k.a. esthesioneuroblastomas), commonly located about the upper nasal septum or cribiform plate
- Paragangliomas arising in neck or base of skull
- Merkel cell tumors of scalp
- Small cell cancers, typically of larynx
- Hematologic malignancies
  - Non-Hodgkin's lymphoma involving neck, or oropharynx originaing in Waldier's Ring
  - Hodgkin's Disease presenting as cervical adenopathy
  - Plasmacytomas, typically located in nasopharynx or base of skull
- Sarcomas
  - Soft tissue sarcomas of any site and histopathology
  - Rhabdomyosarcomas of maxillary sinus
  - Osteosarcoma of peri-orbital region in survivors of childhood retinoblastoma
- Mucosal melanomas (typically seen in nasal cavity)
- Primary mandible tumors
  - Dentigerous cysts
  - Odontogenic keratocysts
  - Squamous cell carcinoma

Exposure and prolonged local infection by Epstein–Barr virus or the high-risk HPV subtypes (16 and 18, and to a lesser extent 31 and 33) are associated with cancers of the epithelial cancers of the nasopharynx and oropharynx, respectively (2, 3). For both viruses, transient infection without long-term sequelae is common. Persistence of the viral genome and induction of malignant transformation is a rare event. Nasopharyngeal cancer occurs endemically in some countries of the Mediterranean and Far East, where EBV antibody titers can be measured to screen high-risk populations. Nasopharyngeal cancer is also endemic in Native Americans of Alaska, the Inuit. Nasopharyngeal cancer has also been associated with consumption of salted fish. Nasopharyngeal cancer and HPV-associated oropharyngeal cancer may occur in the absence of significant alcohol or tobacco exposure. There is evidence however, that exposure to alcohol and tobacco increases the risk of HPV-associated oropharyngeal cancer.

Leukoplakia and erythroplakia are pre-malignant mucosal lesions associated with a risk for transformation to in-situ and invasive cancers. Both lesions are commonly found in the oral cavity and oropharynx where chronic exposure to alcohol and tobacco carcinogens is most significant. Leukoplakia is a white, often lacey-appearing hyperkeratotic lesion that may be post-traumatic and non-dysplastic with a low probability of malignant transformation. Persistent leukoplakia should be biopsied and surgically removed if histologically dysplastic. Erythroplasia is a more serious focal reddish lesion associated with mucosal atrophy. Erythroplasia is commonly found to be dysplastic and aneuploid upon biopsy. The probability that an erythroplastic lesion will undergo malignant transformation is high. This lesion should be surgically removed upon discovery.

Perhaps the single greatest risk factor for developing a squamous cancer of the head and neck region is having had one at an earlier time. Similar to the situation with breast, colorectal, bladder, and lung cancer, having one cancer is associated with a significant risk for the development of a second cancer. Indeed, following the curative treatment of a primary head and neck cancer, the annual risk for developing a second unrelated squamous cancer of the upper aero-digestive tract is approximately 2%.

HISTOPATHOLOGY, MOLECULAR BIOLOGY, AND NATURAL HISTORY

Histopathology

Squamous cell cancers of the head and neck are commonly divided into well-, moderated well-, and poorly differentiated types. Patients with poorly differentiated lesions fare less well than those with well-differentiated lesions, but the spectrum of outcomes is not as profound as that associated with well- to poorly differentiated adenocarcinomas. EBV-associated nasopharyngeal cancers are pathologically distinct non-keratinizing or undifferentiated cancers.

Salivary gland cancers can arise from any of the three major (parotid, submandibular, and sublingual) or thousands of minor salivary glands located in the submucosa of the upper aerodigestive tract. The site of the salivary gland tumor predicts its malignant potential as only 10% of parotid tumors are malignant, while 50% of submandibular and sublingual gland tumors, and the majority of minor salivary gland tumors are cancerous at presentation. The spectrum of malignant salivary gland tumor pathology is shown in Table 66-2.

Molecular Biology

Molecular markers are increasingly important in the understanding of head and neck cancer and in its diagnosis and treatment. Chromosomal deletions and other alterations, most frequently involving chromosomes 3p, 9p, 17p, and 13q have been identified in pre-malignant and malignant squamous lesions, as have mutations in tumor suppressor genes such as p53. Amplification of oncogenes is less common, but overexpression of PRAD-1/bcl-1 (cyclin D1), bcl-2, transforming growth factor, and the epidermal growth factor receptor have been described. The latter finding correlates positively with tumor size and poor outcome and is a new target for treatment of advanced cancers. The tumor suppressor p16 when elevated in tumors is a specific measure of HPV-associated cancer. HPV-positivity and an elevated p16 in squamous tumors are correlated with a good prognosis.

Natural History

Squamous cell cancers of the head and neck region are occasionally discovered during routine dental examinations. More commonly, they are discovered after weeks to months of relatively non-specific symptoms arising from the primary site, such as altered speech or swallowing, bleeding, localized pain or referred otalgia. Alternatively, many patients will present with new onset cervical adenopathy of unknown origin. Such patients are often treated empirically for infection, and later discovered to have head and neck cancer after the adenopathy persists or enlarges and the primary physician or a surgical consultant consequently performs a detailed examination of the head and neck region. Distant metastatic disease at presentation is unusual, and symptomatic disease related to such is rarely seen.

The natural history of head and neck cancer is best communicated using the TNM staging system (4). This system has great clinical value, but it is understandably complex given that the many anatomic subdivisions of the head and neck region that have their own unique definitions of T-stage. N-stage and the combined overall TNM-stage are consistent for all mucosal sites except in the unique case of nasopharyngeal cancer. Representative definitions for the T-stages of oropharyngeal cancer, and the common definitions of N-stage and TN-stage groupings are shown in Table 66-3.

A site-specific review of the common presenting symptoms, natural history and treatment of head and neck cancer is beyond the scope of this text. In general, squamous cell cancers of the head and neck region are locally aggressive and carry a moderate risk of spread to regional lymph nodes and a low probability of spread to more distant sites. This common natural history has several site-specific exceptions. For example, certain primary sites are more likely associated with regional disease at presentation (e.g., the nasopharynx, hypopharynx, base of tongue, and supraglottic larynx). In contrast, other sites have a relatively low risk for regional spread (e.g., paranasal sinuses, small lesions of true glottis).

Clinically evident distant spread to lungs, bone, and liver at presentation is uncommon. Such spread is more closely correlated with the extent of regional lymph node metastases (N-stage) than to primary site location or T-stage.

STANDARD EVALUATION AND TREATMENT

Evaluation

The surgeon remains paramount in the definitive evaluation of patients with signs or symptoms relating to possible cancer in head and neck region. Depending on the setting, that surgeon may be general surgeon evaluating an asymptomatic lesion of the neck, an oral surgeon evaluating a lesion of the oral cavity or mandible, or an otolaryngologist or head and neck surgeon consulting for a primary complaint of otalgia, hoarseness, or dysphagia with or without

Table 66-3

TNM Definitions and TN-Stage Grouping for Oropharyngeal Cancer

Primary tumor (T)—Stage definition

T1	Tumor <2 cm in greatest dimension
T2	Tumor >2 cm but not more than 4 cm in greatest dimension
T3	Tumor >4 cm in greatest dimension
T4a	Tumor invades the larynx, deep/intrinsic muscle of tongue, medial pterygoid muscle, hard palate, or mandible
T4b	Tumor invades the lateral pterygoid muscle, pterygoid plates, lateral nasopharynx, or skull base or encases carotid artery

Regional lymph node (N)—Stage definition

NX	Regional nodes cannot be assessed
N0	No regional lymph node metastasis
N1	Metastasis in a single ipsilateral lymph node, ≤3c m in greatest dimension
N2a	Metastasis in a single ipsilateral lymph node, >3 cm but not more than 6 cm in greatest dimension
N2b	Metastasis in multiple ipsilateral lymph nodes, none more than 6 cm in greatest dimension
N3	Metastasis in a lymph node more >6 cm in greatest dimension

Distant metastases (D)—Stage definition

MX	Distant metastasis cannot be assessed
M0	No distant metastasis
M1	Distant metastasis present

Overall stage based on TN-stage groupings

N-stage		T-stage			
		T1	T2	T3	T4
	N0	Stage I	Stage II		
	N1	Stage III			
	N2	Stage IV			
	N3				

regional adenopathy. Regardless of the specialty of the initial surgeon, ultimate evaluation, diagnosis, staging and follow-up must be undertaken be a head and neck surgical specialist with sufficient training and expertise to achieve all the above tasks.

A complete physical examination should include inspection of all visible mucosal surfaces of the head and neck including indirect mirror or fiberoptic laryngoscopy, as well as palpation of the floor of mouth, tongue and tonsil regions, and neck. Obvious tumor masses should be identified along with potential second primary lesions and pre-malignant regions of leukoplakia or erythroplasia. Suspicious lesions should be defined by primary site location, extension into adjacent areas, and overall size. Associated cervical adenopathy should be assessed and if significantly enlarged, the regional extent of disease should be quantified for use in clinical staging. Independent of whether surgical resection will ever be deemed appropriate, the potential for resection of suspected primary site and neck lesions should be determined. As examples, lesions of the lateral tongue are often resectable while those of the nasopharynx or posterior pharyngeal wall are not. Neck lesions fixed to deep tissues are not resectable.

In addition to physical examination, staging procedures include computed tomography (CT) and magnetic resonance imaging (MRI) of the head and neck to identify the extent of the disease. Patients with a large T4 primary lesions or significant (>N1) lymph node involvement should also undergo chest CT and perhaps a bone scan to screen for distant metastases. PET scanning has a limited value in the diagnosis, staging, and management of untreated head and neck cancer, and is generally not recommended. Research studies designed to quantify the value of PET scans in this setting are in progress.

The definitive staging procedure is an examination under anesthesia, which may include laryngoscopy, esophagoscopy, and bronchoscopy (a.k.a. triple endoscopy). During this procedure biopsy samples are obtained to pathologically confirm a primary diagnosis, to define the extent of primary site disease, and to identify additional pre-malignant lesions or second primary cancers. An accurate description of anatomical involvement is critical to determine the potential morbidity of an initial surgical resection, or to define regions that should be included in a salvage surgical procedure if initial non-surgical treatment failed to control disease.

Of special consideration, is the evaluation of a neck mass of unknown origin. Supraclavicular neck disease should raise the question of a primary thoracic or thyroidal cancer, or perhaps an intra-abdominal cancer in the case of a left-sided supraclavicular lesion. Higher neck lesions are more likely to represent spread from a primary lesion in head and neck. Pathological confirmation of a squamous malignancy metastatic to a lymph node can usually be achieved with high accuracy by fine needle aspiration (FNA). The regional lesion can be approached by FNA if a potential primary mucosal abnormality of the upper aero-digestive tract or a salivary gland is not identified after a thorough physical exam that includes a thorough head and neck exam that includes a mirror or fiberoptic examination of the entire pharynx and larynx. Should an FNA prove inconclusive, an excision lymph node biopsy can be considered. In the latter case, consideration should be given to an immediate neck dissection at the time of this biopsy if frozen section analysis indicates a non-lymphomatous malignancy. Such a neck dissection would assist in the control of potential extra-capsular spread of the disease and additional malignant adenopathy. However tempting, an incisional nodal biopsy should be avoided. The latter often compromises subsequent treatment of the neck, and is associated with a lower probability of disease control in the neck. When a regional lymph node of unknown origin is found to contain a non-keratinizing or undifferentiated tumor, the specimen can be evaluated for EBV DNA. A positive test in this setting raises the probability of an occult nasopharyngeal primary cancer, especially if posterior triangle adenopathy is present.

Principles of Treatment

GENERAL PRINCIPLES   Once a patient's primary diagnosis is established and initial staging studies are completed, secondary referrals are made to radiation and medical oncology. The application of modern multidisciplinary treatments requires early input for all potential care providers. A team approach to care is clearly superior, that team commonly including a head and neck cancer nurse specialist, a nutritionist, a social worker, a psychiatrist, and maxillo-facial prosthedontist, among others.

As head and neck cancers differ greatly in local–regional stage and primary site, a detailed review of treatment options is beyond the scope of this chapter. However, a standard approach to treatment can be related. In general, all patients with untreated local–regional head and neck cancer are considered potentially curable if there is no evidence for distant metastatic disease. Treatment decisions begin with an understanding of primary site extent and a decision as to whether the lesion is resectable (removable with a high probability of negative surgical margins). If a lesion is resectable, careful consideration must be given to the specific morbidity that would attend curative surgical resection. With few exceptions, primary lesions that are both resectable and operable (resectable with acceptable morbidity) benefit from primary resection. Lesions that are classically unresectable (e.g., sphenoid sinus, nasopharynx, and posterior pharyngeal wall), or in which primary surgery would have high-associated morbidity (e.g., base of tongue necessitating total glossectomy) are offered primary radiation for cure. Exceptions to this general approach exist. For example, cancers of the hypopharynx and larynx are usually resectable, but primary therapy is often radiation in an effort to preserve native vocal function by avoiding laryngectomy. In this case laryngectomy is reserved for management of persistent or recurrent disease after radiation. The oropharynx is another "resectable" site that is often suitable for organ preservation. Many oropharyngeal cancers are HPV-related and uniquely sensitive to radiation. Even limited, resectable lesions of the oropharynx are generally advised primary treatment with radiation.

Regional nodal disease from head and neck cancer is strategically approached as a separate entity. With rare exception, all patients with defined nodal disease should receive radiation therapy, either before or after surgical resection of the involved nodes. Traditionally, patients underwent surgical resections of the neck when nodal disease was advanced (>N1, or more than a single ipsilateral node of 3 cm) and not fixed to underlying structures. Exceptions include patients with nasopharyngeal cancers that are uniquely sensitive to radiation, and patients with large unresectable primary site lesions who will be treated with definitive radiation to the primary site.

Advances in the multidisciplinary care of patients with chemotherapy have altered the historic paradigms for treating patients with head and neck cancer. For example, concurrent chemotherapy with radiation has replaced traditional surgery and post-operative radiation for advanced lesions of the sites with high-associated surgical morbidity such as the hypopharynx, larynx, and oropharynx.

Management of malignant cervical lesions has also changed with the introduction of multidisciplinary programs involving either induction chemotherapy or concurrent chemotherapy with radiation prior to surgery. In the modern era, the decision to resect regional nodes is often deferred pending re-evaluation after either induction chemotherapy, or current chemotherapy with radiation. Patients whose regional disease has completely regressed (by CT, MR, or PET/CT) after such programs of chemotherapy appear to have excellent outcomes with minimal to no added benefit from additional neck surgery. Multidisciplinary treatment strategies that allow "primary site" preservation without surgical intervention are now firmly established. Similar strategies for the preservation of "regional" nodal tissue are commonly practiced, but admittedly less well established at this time.

Having related general principles for the treatment of head and neck cancer therapy, it is of value to review treatment options according to standard disease groupings.

MANAGEMENT OF LIMITED HEAD AND NECK CANCER   About one-third of patients present with limited, T1, or T2 cancers without associated lymph node involvement or distant disease (Stage I–II disease). In general, these patients can be treated by single modality therapy, with either surgery or radiation therapy alone with a projected 5-year survival of 60–90%. Radiation therapy is administered to maximally tolerated doses (e.g., 72 Gy). Comprehensive radiation treatment to the primary site and regional lymphatics carries a high risk of chronic morbidities such as xerostomia, accelerated dental decay, and mild dysphagia; and a low risk for more severe complications such as osteonecrosis of the mandible or condronecrosis of larynx, or accelerated atherosclerosis of the carotid artery.

Definitive surgical resection of limited cancers is preferred in several settings. For example, limited oral cavity lesions can often be resected with minimal impact on speech and swallowing. In this setting, patients often undergo primary site resection with a limited staging neck dissection for identification of possible occult spread to regional nodes. Indications for post-operative radiation therapy include the risk factors for local–regional relapse such as: close or positive primary site margins, perineural spread of disease, lymphovascular spread of disease, or evidence for spread to regional nodes on the staging neck dissection.

MANAGEMENT OF LOCALLY OR REGIONALLY ADVANCED CANCER

About 50% of patients with head and neck cancer present with locally or regionally advanced disease (stage III or IV disease with either a T3 or T4 primary lesion or regional lymph node metastases). Such patients can still be treated with curative intent in the absence of distant metastatic disease. However, the curative potential of such patients at 3 years is more limited, perhaps 10–50% by traditional therapies, or 40–60% in the modern era with multidisciplinary approaches that include chemotherapy (Table 66-4). In the following sections, we outline options for combined modality regimens for locally advanced or regionally advanced disease.

Surgery Followed by Post-Operative Radiation ± chemotherapy   For many patients with Stage III/IV disease, primary surgery is advised provided that all sites of known disease are resectable and operable, including all regional neck disease. In this setting, recent evidence from two randomized trials provides insight into the optimal post-operative treatment (5–7). Both trials compared standard post-operative radiation to the identical regimen of radiation plus 3 courses of concurrent full-dose cisplatin in patients at high-risk for recurrence (i.e., pathologic evidence for positive margins at the primary site, perineural or lymphovacular spread of disease, multiple involved regional lymph nodes, or extra-capsular extension of disease in the neck). While the toxicity of concurrent chemotherapy with radiation was significant, such therapy was associated with significantly

Table 66-4

Opportunities for Medical Intervention in Head and Neck Cancer

Opportunity	Initial treatment	Outcome	Salvage
Palliative	Surgery/radiation	→ Cure → Relapse	→ Observation → Chemotherapy
Adjuvant	Surgery ⟋ RT → chemotherapy ⟍ chemotherapy/RT	⟋ Cure ⟍ Relapse	→ Observation → ? Chemotherapy
Induction	Chemotherapy → surgery/RT	⟋ Cure Relapse	→ Observation → ? Chemotherapy
Concurrent	Chemotherapy/radiation	→ Cure → Relapse	→ Observation → ? Surgery
Combined	Chemotherapy → chemo/RT	⟋ Cure Relapse	→ Observation → ? Surgery
Prevention	Prevention therapy	→ Relapse	→ ? Surgery/RT

improved local–regional control of disease in both studies, improved overall survival in one trial, and a trend toward improved survival in the second.

At this time, post-operative radiation is standard for all patients with resected stage III or IV head and neck cancer. Selected patients felt at high risk for local–regional relapse despite surgery should be considered for post-operative radiation with concurrent chemotherapy. Ongoing clinical trials seek to identify radiation sensitizers (chemotherapy, anti-cancer antibodies, or small molecule inhibitors) that will enhance the effects of radiation to degrees greater than cisplatin but with less toxicity.

Definitive Radiation with Concurrent Chemotherapy or Cetuximab For the patient with operable and resectable head and neck cancer, an alternative treatment approach to primary site surgery is that of definitive radiation with concurrent chemotherapy. In this setting, primary site preservation is the therapeutic endpoint with surgery reserved for either a planned post-radiation neck dissection, or for urgent salvage of recurrent or persistent disease despite radiation. Multiple randomized trials have proven the validity of this approach (8–14) (Table 66-5). Definitive radiation with concurrent high-dose cisplatin every 21 days (?3) is the currently accepted standard therapy. However, four additional regimens are commonly used by oncologists during the 6- to 7-week course of definitive radiation: moderate-dose cisplatin administered weekly, full-dose cisplatin with a 96 h infusion of 5-flurouracil (5FU), full-dose carboplatin with 5FU, and a carboplatin and paclitaxel combination delivered weekly (15).

Another option for drug sensitization of radiation recently received FDA approval. Cetuximab is an IgG1 chimeric monoclonal antibody that targets the EDGF receptor that is present on essentially all squamous cancers. In a phase III study, weekly cetuximab with radiation improved local–regional control and survival when compared to treatment with definitive radiation alone (16). Equally significant in this study was the observation that the mucosal toxicity of combined cetuximab and radiation was similar to that with radiation alone. The mucosal toxicity of cetuximab with radiation may therefore be less than that associated with the known heightened toxicity of concurrent chemotherapy and radiation. Of additional importance, the magnitude of improved survival with cetuximab and radiation compared to radiation therapy alone was similar to that seen in trials of concurrent chemotherapy and radiation versus radiation alone.

Induction Chemotherapy Followed by Surgery or Radiation Therapy Historically, 40–60% of patients with local-regionally advanced head and neck cancer can be cured by existing regimens of concurrent chemotherapy with radiation. Of those not cured, 75% of patients recur at local–regional sites while 25% relapse only at a distant site. The relative efficacy of recent regimens of concurrent chemotherapy with radiation is supported by evidence that the natural history of advanced head and neck cancer has been altered. In recent trials of concurrent chemotherapy with radiation up to 70% of patients and cured, and in some studies, local–regional failures are less common than distant relapses (17).

The latter observation has rekindled interest in the use of chemotherapy as "induction" therapy, prior to radiation with concurrent chemotherapy, in order to address maximally the potential presence of micrometastatic disease as well as to minimize local–regional disease prior to definitive treatment. From earlier trials of induction chemotherapy, given prior to radiation alone, it was clear that induction therapy reduced relapse at distant sites. However, it was also clear that local–regional control, the primary problem in head and neck cancer, is inferior when induction chemotherapy precedes radiation therapy alone (18).

The most recent trials of induction chemotherapy have included concurrent chemotherapy with radiation. Results from this approach are very promising

Table 66-5

Selected Randomized Trials of Radiation Therapy Versus Concurrent Chemotherapy and Radiation

Study (reference)	Stage/site	N	Treatment	Overall survival (%)	Local–regional control (%)
Merlano et al. (8)	Stages III–IV Unresectable OC,OP,HP,Lx	77	RT	5 yr: 10	5 yr: 32
		80	RT + cisplatin/5FU	5 yr: 24*	5 yr: 64*
Jeremic et al. (9)	Stages III–IV Unresectable All sites	53	RT	5 yr: 15	5 yr: 27
		53	RT + cisplatin	5 yr: 32*	5 yr: 51*
		53	RT + carboplatin	5 yr: 29*	5 yr: 48*
Brizel et al. (10)	Stages II–IV Resectable	60	RT bid	3 yr: 34	3 yr: 41
	Unresectable All sites	56	RT bid + cisplatin/5FU	3 yr: 55	3 yr: 61*
Wendt et al. (11)	Stages III–IV Unresectable OC, OP, HP, Lx	140	RT bid	3 yr: 24	3 yr: 17
		130	RT bid + cisplatin/5FU	3 yr: 49*	3 yr: 36*
Staar et al. (12)	Stages III–IV Unresectable OC, HP	127	RT	2 yr: 39	2 yr: 45
		113	RT + carboplatin/5FU	2 yr: 48	2 yr: 51

(Continued)

Table 66-5 (*Continued*)

Selected Randomized Trials of Radiation Therapy Versus Concurrent Chemotherapy and Radiation

Study (reference)	Stage/site	N	Treatment	Overall survival (%)	Local–regional control (%)
Adelstein et al. (13)	Stages III–IV Resectable	95	RT	3 yr: 23	NA
	Unresectable	87	RT + cisplatin	3 yr: 35*	NA
	OC, OP, HP, Lx	89	RT + cisplatin/5FU	3 yr: 27	NA
Denis et al. (14)	Stages III–IV Resectable	113	RT	5 yr: 16	5 yr: 25
	Unresectable OP	109	RT + carboplatin/5FU	5 yr: 22*	5 yr: 48*
Bonner et al. (15) Stages III–IV Resectable	Unresectable	213	RT	3 yr: 45	3 yr: 34
	OP, HP, Lx	211	RT+cetuximab	3 yr: 55*	3 yr: 47*

OC = oral cavity; OP = oropharynx; HP = hypopharynx; Lx = larynx; PSN = paranasal sinuses; RT = radiation therapy; 5FU = 5-fluorouracil; NA = not available.

*p <0.05 versus RT control.

with phase II studies reporting ~70% survival in patients with stages III and IV disease, and an equal proportion of local–regional and distant relapses (19). This approach is currently being validated in ongoing phase III trials that directly compare outcomes after concurrent chemotherapy and radiation, with or without initial induction therapy.

Management of Recurrent or Metastatic Disease   Management of local–regional disease after an earlier attempt at cure with surgery or radiation begins with exclusion of distant metastatic disease and consideration of salvage options for cure. Patients with resectable local–regional relapses, and no distant metastases should be considered for salvage surgical procedures. Previously unacceptable attendant surgery associated morbidity, such as aphonia after laryngectomy or severe dysphagia after resections of the tongue, may become acceptable in the context of surgery as the only remaining curative option.

Similar patients with unresectable relapses can be treated with definitive radiation if not previously administered, or repeated radiation in selected cases. Patients with favorable prognostics factors such as good performance status, small volume recurrences, previous radiation >6 months earlier, no previous chemotherapy, or radiation sensitive disease (e.g., the nasopharynx) can realized cure rates approaching 10–20% (20). Salvage radiation in this setting is nearly always administered with concurrent chemotherapy.

Candidates for palliation include all those with local–regional relapse but no potentially curative options of salvage surgery or radiation, as well as those with distant metastatic disease. Palliative care begins with control of common problems related to chronic pain, dysphagia with malnutrition, progressive cancer-related wounds, and psychosocial dysfunction. Once these problems are addressed, consideration can be given toward direct medical intervention against cancer.

Chemotherapy has been used with moderate success in the treatment of patients with recurrent or metastatic disease. While there is little evidence that chemotherapy in this setting meaningfully prolongs survival, quality of life can be transiently improved or maintained in those who respond to treatment. In general, single agents are used, and high-dose cisplatin every 3–4 weeks is the historic standard. In common practice however, many patients have been previously treated with cisplatin and the expected toxicity of this treatment is generally considered too toxic for this setting. Commonly used single-agent alternatives are carboplatin, paclitaxel, or docetaxel. Additional agents less commonly used are capecitabine and methotrexate. In general, these agents have a 10–20% chance of producing a meaningful response of several months duration. Factors predicting a response include: a good performance status, an EBV- or HPV-associated cancer, distant metastatic lesions versus local–regional relapse, and disease sites not previously treated with radiation or chemotherapy.

Combination chemotherapy (e.g., cisplatin or carboplatin with either infusional 5-fluorouracil (5FU) or capecitabine, or the combination of carboplatin with paclitaxel) leads to higher initial rates of response and longer progression free survival. However, in direct comparison to single-agent therapy, such combinations are more toxic and are not associated with improvements in overall survival. Therefore, treatment with combination therapy is generally reserved for patients with good performance status and immediately threatening disease that "needs" the rapid early response occasionally seen with combination chemotherapy.

Biologic or targeted therapies are newly available for the palliation of patients with refractory squamous cancers of the head and neck. Cetuximab is approved for use in this setting after previous failure of cisplatin or carboplatin. Clinical trials are evaluating the activity of other targeted therapies such as: a humanized IgG2 monoclonal anti-EGFR antibody (panitumumab), numerous small molecule tyrosine kinase inhibitors, and anti-angiogenic agents.

Clinical trials of chemotherapy and targeted therapies are in progress as components of palliative therapy, induction therapy, and as concurrent therapy with radiation.

Cancer Prevention Therapy   Considerable research has been devoted to the development of medications that might prevent or delay the formation of head and neck cancer. This effort attempts to address the prevalence of this disease in patients who abuse alcohol and tobacco containing products, as well as the 2% annual risk of second primary epithelial cancers in the head and neck, and lung, in patients that are cured of their original lesion.

To date, several trials of *beta*-carotene and *cis*-retinoic have been performed which clearly demonstrate transient regression of an established pre-malignant lesions, leukoplakia. However, there is no evidence that such therapy reduces second primary cancers in high-risk patients. Trials of other medical agents that might delay head and neck cancer formation are in progress.

It is generally accepted that cessation of tobacco and alcohol abuse will reduce the risk of primary head and neck cancer, but the impact of such cessation on second primary cancer formation is speculative.

The incidence of HPV-associated head and neck cancer is increasing. This increase may reverse in years ahead given the recent introduction of effective vaccines against HPV-16 and HPV-18.

Salivary Gland Tumors   Malignant salivary gland cancers are primarily treated with surgery. Post-operative radiation is often advised to reduce the risk of local–regional relapse with indications being: close surgical margins (a common occurrence with facial nerve preservation), an intermediate- to high-grade cancer, or nodal disease at presentation. Surgical resection without post-operative radiation is generally reserved for patients with benign salivary gland tumors, or low-grade invasive carcinomas that are resected with adequate margins.

Adenoid cystic cancer of salivary gland origin is an unusual cancer with a distinct natural history characterized by a high incidence of peri-neural spread retrograde along nerve tracts, more distant than regional relapses, and late recurrences up to 10–20 years after initial diagnosis. Post-operative treatment of this lesion often requires radiation targeted not only to the primary site, but also along nerve tracts between the primary tumor and the base of the skull whenever peri-neural invasion is demonstrated.

Patients with unresectable salivary gland tumors are treated by definitive radiation, often with poor results. Selected patients in this setting may benefit by the use of concurrent chemotherapy with radiation.

For metastatic lesions or refractory local–regional disease, therapy is given with palliative intent, usually chemotherapy with such agents as doxorubicin, cisplatin or carboplatin, and the taxanes.

ADVANCES IN SURGERY AND RADIATION THERAPY

Advances in head and neck surgery parallel those in other surgical oncology disciplines. In general, enhanced pre-operative staging via CT and MRI scans has allowed identification of patients who should, or more importantly, should not undergo major ablative procedures. The trend to avoid unnecessary surgery has been supported by the increased effectiveness of radiation therapy when administered with concurrent medical radiation sensitizers (chemotherapy or cetuximab). Primary site preservation is now a well-established goal in multi-disciplinary treatment programs designed to avoid relatively morbid procedures such as orbital exenterations, and laryngectomies. When surgery is necessary, procedures that preserve function are often possible (e.g., modified vs. radical neck dissections, partial vs. total laryngectomy). An experience with transoral laser and robotic surgery of pharyngeal and laryngeal carcinomas is evolving with decreased functional morbidity. When surgery is ablative of significant function or cosmesis, modern reconstructive techniques can be restorative. The use of microvascular free tissue transfer has allowed significant strides in functional reconstruction with acceptable cosmetic appearance. These techniques have allowed for highly successful reconstruction of mandible and pharyngoesophageal defects, as well as the management of wounds previous felt to be irreparable.

Advances in radiation therapy fall into two broad categories: improvements in targeting of the radiation fields and enhancements in radiation delivery. In the former category, improvements in anatomic staging of cancer by CT/MR scans and fused images allow precise definition of target tissues and delineation of adjacent normal structures. This has led to a more complete coverage of gross disease by radiation and a tighter correlation between dose and the extent of disease. In theory, the benefit from this is enhanced local–regional control of disease, and reduced injury to normal tissues. Advances in radiation treatment delivery systems such as intensity modulated radiation therapy (IMRT) and tomotherapy take advantage of the advances in pre-treatment target definition and deliver radiation therapy in a highly conformal way that further limits radiation exposure to adjacent normal tissue.

While most radiation treatments involve photons, neutron, and proton beam therapy are alternative forms of treatment for selected patients. Fast neutron beam therapy derives its benefit from a more effective biologic dose that overcomes radio-resistant elements of a tumor such as hypoxia. Clinical trials suggest that neutrons may be advantageous for treatment of unresectable salivary gland tumors. Normal tissues also experience the greater biologic effect of neutrons. The potential benefit in tumor control with neutrons must be weighed against an increase in normal tissue injury. Proton beam therapy takes advantage of the unique properties of protons that allow treatment to be exquisitely targeted. As a result, even higher doses of radiation can be delivered than with techniques such as IMRT. Proton beam therapy is a preferred radiation treatment for an increasing number of head and neck sites including periorbital and base of skull tumors where adjacent normal tissue toxicity might result in blindness, or brain or spinal cord injury.

ACUTE AND CHRONIC TOXICITIES OF TREATMENT

The complications of surgery are principally in the categories of pain, function (speech and swallowing), and cosmesis. In general, pain is transient and well managed. Dramatic improvements in post-treatment speech, swallowing, and cosmesis have been achieved by two means: the avoidance or limiting of surgical intervention in selected patients through the use of concurrent chemotherapy and radiation, and the use of novel reconstructive techniques. For example, up to 75% of patients who undergo total laryngectomy will regain intelligible speech, many via the surgical construction of a minute one-way tracheoesophageal fistula. This fistula allows diversion of exhaled air back into the pharynx with resultant oral speech. Palatal prosthetics and dental implantation into revascularized bone grafts after mandibular reconstruction can similar augment functional oral rehabilitation.

Complications of radiation therapy are divided into acute and chronic (late) toxicities. Acute toxicities principally relate to radiation dermatitis and mucositis with consequent issues of wound care, dysphagia, excess oral secretions, and aspiration. These risks are not trivial as recent trials of concurrent chemotherapy and radiation report a near 100% use of prophalactic gastric feeding tubes during radiation and 1–2% acute treatment-related mortality. Chronic or late radiation toxicities can vary from mildly disabling (abnormal taste, xerostomia, and accelerated dental disease), to severely disabling (soft tissue fibrosis with neck stiffness or tongue restriction, second primary cancers, accelerated carotid artery atherosclerosis, and permanent gastric tube dependence in up to 5% of patients).

Complications of chemotherapy vary depending on the specific agents used and the setting. Full dose chemotherapy brings expected risks of myelosuppression, mucositis, diarrhea, nausea and vomiting, alopecia, and nephrotoxicity (with cisplatin). When chemotherapy is used with radiation, chemotherapy-specific toxicities are often minimal as the dose of chemotherapy is often less than maximal. However, all forms of chemotherapy with radiation significantly increase the risk of radiation-induced dermatitis and mucositis. The latter increase has prompted clinical trials evaluating agents that may limit mucositis (e.g., keratinocyte growth factor). The severe mucositis seen with concurrent chemotherapy and radiation has also stimulated interest in cetuximab as an alternative radiation sensitizer. In the one phase III trial of cetuximab and radiation published to date, there was a substantial improvement in local–regional control of disease and survival without an apparent increase in radiation-induced mucositis (16).

REFERENCES

1. Surveillance Epidemiology and End Results (SEER) Fast Stats data from the National Cancer Institute. Available at: http://www.seer.cancer.gov/faststats/ sites.php?stat=Incidence&site=Oral+Cavity+and+Pharynx+Cancer&x=14&y=15 and http://www.seer.cancer.gov/faststats/sites.php?site= Larynx+Cancer& stat= Mortality. Accessed April 11, 2007.
2. Fakry C, Gillison ML. Clinical implications of human papillomavirus in head and neck cancers. J Clin Oncol. 2006; 24: 2606–2611.
3. Lo KW, To KF, Huang DP. Focus on nasopharyngeal cancer. Cancer Cell. 2004; 5: 423–428.
4. National Comprehensive Cancer Network Clinical Practice Guidelines in Oncology: Head and Neck Cancers, V.I.2006. Available at: http://www.nccn.org/professionals/physician_gls/PDF/head-and-neck.pdf. Accessed April 8, 2007.
5. Bernier J, Domenge C, Ozsahin M, et al. Postoperative irradiation with or without concomitant chemotherapy for locally advanced head and neck cancer. N Engl J Med. 2004; 350: 1945–1952.
6. Cooper JC, Pajak TF, Forastierre AA, et al. Postoperative concurrent radiotherapy and chemotherapy for high-risk squamous-cell carcinoma of the head and neck. N Engl J Med. 2004; 350: 1937–1944.
7. Bernier J, Cooper JS, Pajak TF, et al. Defining risk levels in locally advanced head and neck cancers: a comparative analysis of concurrent postoperative radiation plus chemotherapy trials of the EORTC (#22931) and RTOG (# 9501). Head Neck. 2005; 27: 843–850.
8. Merlano M, Bennasso M, Corvo R, et al. Five-year update of a randomized trial of alternating radiotherapy and chemotherapy compared with radiotherapy alone in treatment of unresectable squamous cell carcinoma of the head and neck. J Nat Cancer Inst. 1996; 88: 583–589.
9. Jeremic B, Shibamoto Y, Stanisavljevic B, et al. Radiation therapy alone or with concurrent low-dose daily either cisplatin or carboplatin in locally advanced unresectable squamous cell carcinoma of the head and neck: a randomized trial. Radiother Oncol. 1997; 43: 29–37.

10. Brizel DM, Albers ME, Fisher SR, et al. Hyperfractionated irradiation with or without concurrent chemotherapy for locally advanced head and neck cancer. N Engl J Med. 1998; 338: 1798–1804.

11. Wendt TG, Grabenbauer GG, Rodel CM, et al. Simultaneous radiochemotherapy versus radiotherapy alone in advanced head and neck cancer: a randomized multicenter study. J Clin Oncol. 1998; 16: 1318–1324.

12. Staar S, Rudat V, Stuetzer H, et al. Intensified hyperfractionated accelerated radiotherapy limits the additional benefit of simultaneous chemotherapy— results of a multicentric randomized German trial in advanced head and neck cancer. Int J Radiat Oncol Biol Phys. 2001; 50: 1161–1171.

13. Adelstein DJ, Li Y, Adams GL, et al. An intergroup phase III comparison of standard radiation therapy and two schedules of concurrent chemoradiotherapy in patients with unresectable squamous cell head and neck cancer. J Clin Oncol. 2003; 21: 92–98.

14. Denis F, Garaud P, Bardet E, et al. Final results of the 94-01 French Head and neck Oncology and Radiotherapy Group randomized trial comparing radiotherapy alone with concomitant radiochemotherapy on advanced-stage oropharynx carcinoma. J Clin Oncol. 2004; 22: 69–76.

15. Wong SJ, Agha Z, Milligan S. Concurrent chemotherapy practice patterns for head and neck cancer: what is standard of care? J Clin Oncol. ASCO Annual Meeting Proceedings. 2006; abstract 5542.

16. Bonner JA, Harari PM, Giralt J, et al. Radiotherapy plus Cetuximab for Squamous-Cell Carcinoma of the Head and Neck. New Engl J Med. 2006; 354: 567–578.

17. Adelstein DJ, Saxton JP, Lavertu P, et al. Maximizing local control and organ preservation in stage IV squamous cell head and neck cancer With hyperfractionated radiation and concurrent chemotherapy. J Clin Oncol. 2002; 20: 1405–1410.

18. Forastierre AA, Goepfert H, Moar M, et al. Concurrent chemotherapy and radiotherapy for organ preservation in advanced laryngeal cancer. New Engl J Med. 2003; 349: 2091–2098.

19. Vokes EE, Stenson K, Rosen FR, et al. Weekly carboplatin and paclitaxel followed by concomitant paclitaxel, fluorouracil, and hydroxyurea chemoradiotherapy: curative and organ-preserving therapy for advanced head and neck cancer. J Clin Oncol. 2003; 21: 320–326.

20. Kramer NM, Horwitz EM, Cheng J, et al. Toxicity and outcome analysis of patients with recurrent head and neck cancer treated with hyperfractionated split-course reirradiation and concurrent cisplatin and paclitaxel chemotherapy from two prospective phase I and II studies. Head Neck. 2005: 27:406–414.

INDEX